Hospital-Acquired Infection in the Pediatric Patient

Hospital-Acquired Infection in the Pediatric Patient

Edited by

Leigh G. Donowitz, M.D.

Associate Professor of Pediatrics
Division of Infectious Diseases
University of Virginia
School of Medicine
Charlottesville, Virginia

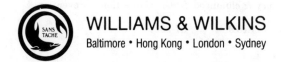

WILLIAMS & WILKINS
Baltimore • Hong Kong • London • Sydney

Editor: Carol-Lynn Brown
Associate Editor: Victoria M. Vaughn
Copy Editor: Judith F. Minkove
Design: Norman Och
Illustration Planning: Lorraine Wrzosek
Production: Raymond E. Reter

Accurate indications, adverse reactions, and dosage schedules for drugs are
provided in this book, but it is possible that they may change. The reader is
urged to review the package information data of the manufacturers of the
medications mentioned.

Printed in the United States of America

Library of Congress Cataloging in Publication Data

Hospital acquired infection in the pediatric patient.

  Includes bibliographies and index.
  1. Nosocomial infections in children. I. Donowitz, Leigh G. [DNLM:
1. Cross Infection—in infancy & childhood. 2. Cross Infection—prevention &
control. WX 167 H8277]
RJ406.N68H67 1988   616.9   87-25244
ISBN 0-683-02612-7

88 89 90 91 92
1 2 3 4 5 6 7 8 9 10

In memory of my mother and father,
Sylvea and Morton C. Grossman,
*my closest friends and
finest role models.*

Preface

Hospitalized pediatric patients are at significant risk of developing hospital-acquired infection. The neonate in the newborn intensive care unit has a 15–25% risk, the child admitted to an intensive care unit has a 14% risk, and the ward patients have a 5% risk of developing hospital-acquired infection. In the pediatric patient, hospital-acquired infection carries the risk of significant additional morbidity, long-term physical, neurologic and developmental sequelae, and death.

Multiple texts review the infectious diseases of the newborn and child; other references describe nosocomial infections primarily as they occur in the adult surgical and medical patient. The goal of this book is to provide an informative, authoritative reference on the management of hospital-acquired infection in the pediatric patient.

The specific infections that are unique as infection control issues in the pediatric patient are divided into two sections: nosocomial infections by site (e.g., bacteremia, pneumonia, and diarrhea) and nosocomial infection by pathogen (e.g., varicella, tuberculosis, and cytomegalovirus).

A special section of the text has been devoted to the management of patients who have unique and high risks of hospital-acquired infections. This section includes a chapter on the neonate, the immunocompromised patient, and the critical care patient.

The Infection Control Personnel and Policy section of this text will become an important reference for medical personnel caring for infants and children. This section contains recommendations and guidelines on isolation; nursing policies; staff education; visitation policies for families, siblings and pets; toys as potential vectors for infectious pathogens; employee health; microbiologic infection control; and antibiotic restriction. The isolation guidelines are a unique highlighted section of this book, providing a ready reference for how to isolate an infant or child with a potentially transmissible infection.

Employee health issues are of particular importance as they pertain to pediatric patients. The immunity of staff members to rubella, chickenpox, mumps, and herpes simplex virus, and the prevalence of viral gastrointestinal and upper respiratory illness and staphylococcal dermatitis may be of lesser importance for personnel involved in adult care. When they occur in the pediatric inpatient setting, these infections can cause major epidemic disease in this nonimmune population and can result in significant morbidity, mortality, and expense in isolation, cohorting, passive immunization, personnel, and ancillary costs.

This book is written for physicians, nurses, medical laboratory personnel, and the many other people who care for hospitalized children. The book is designed to answer specific management questions on the prevention, isolation, and therapies of hospital-acquired infectious disease in the pediatric patient. The goals of the authors in the writing of this informative and current reference text are the prevention of nosocomial infections and optimal management and containment of those infections that are not preventable.

I wish to thank Dick Wenzel, who as a colleague, teacher, and friend initiated my career in nosocomial infections, and John Nelson and Jerry Mandell, who personally encouraged and supported me in this project. I also would like to thank my secretary, Linda Bryant, who maintained a level of organization, editorial and secretarial skills, coupled with a sense of humor, which contributed to making this a far better book.

In conclusion, I wish to acknowledge the authors of this text who not only provided their expertise, time, and scholarship in writing this comprehensive and authoritative text, but who are the scientific investigators who have created the factual information upon which this book is based.

L.D.

Contributors

James W. Bass, M.D., M.P.H.
Clinical Professor of Pediatrics, Uniformed
    Services University of the Health
    Sciences, Bethesda, Maryland
Clinical Professor of Pediatrics, University of
    Hawaii School of Medicine
Chairman, Department of Pediatrics, Tripler Army
    Medical Center, Honolulu, Hawaii

Robert W. Bradsher, M.D.
Chairman, Infection Control Committee of
    University Hospital
Associate Professor of Medicine
University of Arkansas for Medical Sciences
Little Rock, Arkansas

Robert Lee Brawley, M.D., M.P.H.
Commander, Medical Corps
United States Navy
Hospital Epidemiologist
Naval Hospital
Oakland, California

Leigh G. Donowitz, M.D.
Associate Professor of Pediatrics
Division of Infectious Diseases
University of Virginia
    School of Medicine
Charlottesville, Virginia

George B. Fisher, Jr., M.D.
Assistant Professor of Dermatology
University of Virginia Medical Center
Charlottesville, Virginia

Anne A. Gershon, M.D.
Professor, Department of Pediatrics
Columbia University College of Physicians and
    Surgeons
New York, New York

Donald A. Goldmann, M.D.
Hospital Epidemiologist
Director, Bacteriology Laboratory
Associate Professor of Pediatrics
The Children's Hospital
Boston, Massachusetts

Gregory F. Hayden, M.D.
Associate Professor of Pediatrics
University of Virginia Medical Center
Charlottesville, Virginia

J. Owen Hendley, M.D.
Professor, Department of Pediatrics
University of Virginia School of Medicine
Charlottesville, Virginia

Richard F. Jacobs, M.D.
Associate Professor of Pediatrics
Division of Infectious Disease and Immunology
Department of Pediatrics
University of Arkansas for Medical Sciences
Arkansas Children's Hospital
Little Rock, Arkansas

William R. Jarvis, M.D.
Acting Chief, Epidemiology Branch
Hospital Infections Program
Center for Infectious Diseases
Centers for Disease Control
Atlanta, Georgia

Sandra M. Landry, R.N., M.S., C.I.C.
Epidemiology Administrative Coordinator
Division of Hospital Epidemiology
Department of Internal Medicine
University of Virginia School of Medicine
Charlottesville, Virginia

Philip S. LaRussa, M.D.
Assistant Professor, Department of Pediatrics
Columbia University College of Physicians and
    Surgeons
New York, New York

Jacob A. Lohr, M.D.
McLemore Birdsong Professor and Vice Chairman
Department of Pediatrics
Division of Infectious Diseases
University of Virginia
    School of Medicine
Charlottesville, Virginia

Naomi L.C. Luban, M.D.
Director, Hematology/Blood Bank
Department of Laboratory Medicine
Children's Hospital National Medical Center
Professor, Child Health and Development
The George Washington University School of
    Medicine and Health Sciences
Washington, D.C.

William J. Martone, M.D., M.Sc.
Assistant to the Acting Director
Center for Infectious Diseases
Centers for Disease Control
Atlanta, Georgia

M. Dianne Murphy, M.D.
Associate Professor of Pediatrics
Chief, Pediatric Infectious Diseases
The University of Tennessee Medical Center at
    Knoxville
Knoxville, Tennessee

Trudy V. Murphy, M.D.
Assistant Professor of Pediatrics
Southwestern Medical School
University of Texas Health Science Center
Dallas, Texas

John D. Nelson, M.D.
Professor of Pediatrics
University of Texas Health Sciences Center
Southwestern Medical School
Dallas, Texas

Carla M. Odio, M.D.
Assistant Professor of Pediatrics
Infectious Diseases, Hematology-Oncology Section
Hospital Nacional de Niños
San Jose, Costa Rica

Walter A. Orenstein, M.D.
Chief, Surveillance, Investigations and Research
    Branch
Immunization Division
Center for Preventive Services
Centers for Disease Control
Atlanta, Georgia

Robert F. Pass, M.D.
Professor of Pediatrics and Microbiology
University of Alabama at Birmingham
Birmingham, Alabama

Elliott R. Pearl, M.D.
Clinical Associate Professor of Pediatrics
Clinical Assistant Professor of Internal Medicine
University of Virginia School of Medicine
Charlottesville, Virginia

Michael A. Pfaller, M.D.
Associate Professor of Pathology
Co-Director, Clinical Microbiology Laboratory
Director, Special Microbiology Laboratory
University of Iowa Hospitals and Clinics
Director, Clinical Microbiology and Immunology
Veterans Administration Medical Center
Iowa City, Iowa

Larry K. Pickering, M.D.
Professor of Pediatrics
Program in Infectious Diseases and Clinical
    Microbiology
Director, Pediatric Infectious Diseases
University of Texas Medical School
Houston, Texas

Philip A. Pizzo, M.D.
Chief, Pediatric Branch
Head, Infectious Disease Section
National Cancer Institute
National Institutes of Health
Bethesda, Maryland

Randall R. Reves, M.D., M.Sc.
Assistant Professor of Medicine and Epidemiology
Program in Infectious Diseases and Clinical
    Microbiology
Department of Medicine
University of Texas Medical School and
    University of Texas School of Public Health
Houston, Texas

Eugene D. Shapiro, M.D.
Assistant Professor of Pediatrics and Epidemiology
Yale University School of Medicine
New Haven, Connecticut

Jane D. Siegel, M.D.
Associate Professor of Pediatrics
Department of Pediatrics
University of Texas Health Science Center
Dallas, Texas

Jane Skelton, M.D.
Assistant Professor of Internal Medicine
Medical Oncology
McGill University
Montreal, Quebec
Canada

Sergio Stagno, M.D.
Professor of Pediatrics and Microbiology
University of Alabama at Birmingham
Birmingham, Alabama

Russell W. Steele, M.D.
Professor of Pediatrics
Division Head, Pediatric Infectious Diseases/
    Immunology/Allergy
Director, Pediatric Transplantation Center
University of Arkansas for Medical Sciences
Arkansas Children's Hospital
Little Rock, Arkansas

Margaret A. Tipple, M.D.
Hospital Infections Program
Center for Infectious Diseases
Centers for Disease Control
Atlanta, Georgia

Timothy R. Townsend, M.D.
Associate Professor of Pediatrics
The Johns Hopkins University School of Medicine
Hospital Epidemiologist
The Johns Hopkins Hospital
Baltimore, Maryland

Ronald B. Turner, M.D.
Associate Professor, Pediatrics and Laboratory
  Medicine
Medical University of South Carolina
Charleston, South Carolina

Richard P. Wenzel, M.D., M.Sc.
Professor of Medicine and Preventive Medicine
Director, Division of Clinical Epidemiology
Department of Medicine

Director, Hospital Epidemiology Program
University of Iowa Hospitals and Clinics
Iowa City, Iowa

Richard J. Whitley, M.D.
Professor of Pediatrics and Microbiology
Department of Pediatrics and Microbiology
University of Alabama at Birmingham
Birmingham, Alabama

Terry Yamauchi, M.D.
Professor and Chief
Pediatric Infectious Diseases
University of Arkansas for Medical Sciences
Arkansas Children's Hospital
Little Rock, Arkansas

Contents

Section 3. High-Risk Patients

Section 4. Personnel and Policies

1
SITES

1

Bacteremia and Fungemia

**Margaret A. Tipple, M.D., William R. Jarvis, M.D.,
and William J. Martone, M.D., M.Sc.**

INTRODUCTION

Bloodstream infections among pediatric patients have long been recognized as an important problem. Pediatric training programs emphasize recognition of early signs and symptoms of sepsis. Blood cultures are drawn on febrile infants and children as part of "sepsis workups," and antibiotic combinations are chosen carefully for treatment of likely pathogens while culture results are pending.

Extensive literature exists on the problem of community-acquired bloodstream infections in otherwise healthy infants and children, and there is a reasonable understanding of neonatal sepsis (1–3). However, there is little information on the problem of nosocomial, or hospital-acquired bloodstream infections in pediatric patients. Any available information originates mainly from the National Nosocomial Infections Surveillance system (NNIS) and the medical literature. NNIS is a nationwide surveillance system organized by the Centers for Disease Control (CDC) in 1970, and is the only source of current national data on the incidence of nosocomial infections (4). NNIS hospitals are a geographically representative, nonrandom sample of U.S. hospitals; they comprise small hospitals, public hospitals, private hospitals, and teaching hospitals throughout the U.S. Prior to 1986, children's hospitals were underrepresented, and no data were available for pediatric or neonatal intensive care units. Most reports in the medical literature are analyses of nosocomial bloodstream infections among pediatric patients in single institutions.

DEFINITIONS

For this review we have adopted the NNIS system standard definitions (5).

Nosocomial Infection

A nosocomial infection is defined as a localized or systemic condition resulting from the adverse reaction to the presence of an infectious agent(s) or its toxin(s) with no evidence that the infection was present or incubating at the time of hospital admission. Reviews of bacteremia in the literature may use slightly different criteria for designation of nosocomial bacteremia. Usually, infection must have occurred 48 or 72 hours after admission for it to be considered as hospital-acquired. Organisms regarded as likely to have been of community origin (as *Hemophilus influenzae* or *Streptococcus pneumoniae*) may be excluded even if the time requirement has been met. Organisms which commonly occur as contaminants in blood cultures (as coagulase-negative staphylococci, alphahemolytic streptococci or *Bacillus* spp.) may be considered as causing infection only when multiple cultures are positive or only when associated with a vascular catheter. These differences in definitions, plus the possibility that different institutions will have patient populations with different underlying diseases and severity of illness, make it difficult to compare bloodstream infections between hospitals.

Neonatal Nosocomial Infection

When neonates are considered, it is often difficult to determine whether exposure to organisms causing infection occurred at the time of delivery or later. NNIS classifies all neonatal infections as nosocomial unless there is clear evidence of intrauterine infection (as might occur with cytomegalovirus or toxoplasmosis). Neonatal nosocomial infections are divided into two categories: maternal origin, if symptoms are recorded within 48 hours of admission, and hospital-acquired, if the infant becomes symptomatic after 48 hours of age.

Primary versus Secondary Bloodstream Infection

Primary bacteremia is defined as a bloodstream infection occurring in a patient with no evidence of localized infection. However, bacteremia associated with a peripheral intravenous line, a central venous catheter, or an arterial line is regarded as primary even if there is evidence of local site infection. Secondary bacteremia is defined as bloodstream infection with clinical or microbiologic evidence of infection at another site, which is the source of the bloodstream infection. Fungemia refers to the presence of fungi in the bloodstream and generally does not distinguish between primary and secondary infection.

Endogenous versus Exogenous Infection

Endogenous infections result from invasion of the bloodstream by the patient's own flora, while exogenous infections result from invasion of the bloodstream by organisms from the hospital environment. The likely source of organisms may assist in determining if problems with environmental contamination or patient colonization need to be addressed. This may be difficult, however, in the patient with long or frequent hospitalization who may become colonized with hospital organisms and who later develops an endogenous infection with these organisms (6).

Endemic versus Epidemic Infection

Endemic infection refers to the occurrence of disease at a given baseline frequency over a prolonged period of time (7). One purpose of hospital infection control surveillance programs is to establish baseline rates of bacteremia and to determine whether significant changes in these rates have occurred.

Epidemic nosocomial infections, also referred to as outbreaks, are defined as unexpected increases in infection rates (7,8). For determining whether an outbreak exists, rates of infections for different time periods must be compared, making good surveillance data critical.

INCIDENCE OF NOSOCOMIAL BACTEREMIA

Nosocomial infections are estimated to have occurred in 3.4% of all patients hospitalized in the United States during 1984 (9). Data from NNIS suggest that, overall, pediatric patients are less likely to acquire infections than adults, possibly because of shorter average hospital stay. Overall nosocomial infection rates in 1984 were 14.4 per 1000 discharges (1.4%) for newborns and 13.3 per 1000 discharges (1.3%) for general pediatrics patients (Tables 1.1 and 1.2).

NNIS nosocomial infection and bacteremia rates for newborn and general pediatric services are consistent with those reported by various institutions in the United States and Western Europe (Tables 1.1 and 1.2).

Both overall nosocomial infection rates and bacteremia rates are lowest in well newborns. This may be related to their short hospital stay and lack of invasive interventions.

Rates are higher on pediatric services (Table 1.2) with wider variation, especially in overall infection rates, than those seen on newborn services. This wide variation may be explained by the type of surveillance employed (active or passive), inclusion of viral infections, proportion of surgical and medical patients, as well as age, type and severity of underlying disease, number of invasive procedures, length of hospitalization, and possibly other factors. Younger children have been shown to have higher nosocomial infection rates, especially when viral infections are included (14). Centers with a high proportion of oncology patients are also likely to have higher infection rates (15).

Not surprisingly, published studies from individual institutions have shown higher infection rates for pediatric intensive care (PICU) (Table 1.3) and neonatal intensive care (NICU) (Table 1.4) patients than for general pediatric and newborn patients. Nosocomial infection rates in the PICU have been reported to be approximately 4–20 times those for general pediatric patients (Table 1.3). From 5% to over 32% of these nosocomial infections are accounted for by nosocomial bacteremias. The reasons for this wide variability among institutions is unclear, but probably results from differences in study definitions, differences in ages, type and severity of illness, length of stay in the ICU, type and duration of IV therapy, and need for multiple invasive procedures.

As with PICUs, nosocomial infection rates in NICUs have been reported to be, on the average, 4–19 times higher than those in general newborn services (Table 1.4). A larger percentage (averaging about 20%) of nosocomial infections

Table 1.1
Nosocomial Infections in Newborns

Location	Year of Study	Ref. No.	Nosocomial Infection Rate[a]	Nosocomial Bacteremia Rate[b]	Bacteremia as Percent of all Nosocomial Inf.
University of Gottingen	1962–74	10		0.9	
West Germany	1975–82			2.0	
Yale University	1966–78	11		1.0–3.9[c]	
				0.9–2.5[d]	
Karolinska Institute	1969–73	12		1.4	
Sweden	1974–78			3.1	
University of Iowa	1976–77	13	6.0	0.2	3.3
University of South Carolina	1977–81	2		1.2	
Buffalo Children's Hospital	1980–81	14	17.0		
National Nosocomial	1984	9			
Infections Surveillance (NNIS) Study[b]					
Small Hospitals			8.6	0.6	7.0
Small Teaching Hospitals			14.7	2.0	13.6
Large Teaching Hospitals			17.3	3.6	20.7
Total (NNIS)			14.4		

[a]Number of infections per 1000 discharges.
[b]All newborn services—neonatal intensive care units and well-baby nurseries.
[c]Onset at or before 48 hours of age.
[d]Onset after 48 hours of age.

were attributed to bacteremias in NICUs than in any of the other pediatric care services. Risk factors for bacteremias have been shown to include birthweight, presence of infection elsewhere, type and duration of invasive procedures, duration of intravenous therapy, and use of total parenteral nutrition (TPN) (13,19,26,27). An additional risk factor is that neonates admitted to NICUs may not develop "normal" gastrointestinal flora, but instead are colonized with NICU environmental organisms, some of which may become invasive pathogens (28).

Table 1.2
Nosocomial Infection and Bacteremia in Pediatric Patients

Location	Year of Study	Ref. No.	Service	Nosocomial Infection Rate[a]	Nosocomial Bacteremia Rate	Bacteremia as Percent of all Nosocomial Inf.
Boston Children's Hospital	1970	15	AP[b]	46	6.2	14
University of South Carolina	1977–81	2	AP[b]		5.1	
Buffalo Children's Hospital	1980–81	14	AP[b]	32		
University of Virginia	1982–83	16	AP[b]	48	4	8
National Nosocomial Infection Surveillance Study	1984	17	All Pediatric Services			
			Small Hospitals	1.2	<.1	
			Small Teaching Hospitals	14.6	2.4	16.4
			Large Teaching Hospitals	16.6	2.1	12.7
			Total	13.3		

[a]Number of infections per 1000 discharges.
[b]AP—All pediatric medical and surgical patients.

Table 1.3
Nosocomial Infection and Bacteremia in Pediatric Intensive Care Patients

Location	Year of Study	Ref. No.	Service	Nosocomial Infection Rate[a]	Nosocomial Bacteremia Rate[a]	Bacteremia as Percent of all Nosocomial Inf.
Buffalo Children's Hospital	1980–81	14	PICU	110		
Tufts University	1981–83	17	PICU	62		
University of Virginia	1982–83	16	PICU	137	11	8
NNIS	1983–84	Jarvis	PICU	103	33.3	32
Georgia Hosp. A.	1981–82	18	PICU	216	12.2	7
Hosp. B.	1981–82	18	PICU	241	37.6	16

[a]Number of infections per 1000 discharges.

ETIOLOGY AND TRENDS OF NOSOCOMIAL BLOODSTREAM INFECTIONS

This decade has seen significant changes in the causes of nosocomial bloodstream infections. While Gram-positive cocci have continued to predominate as the most common category of pathogen, trends in the etiology of nosocomial bloodstream infection in the past 5–10 years reveal that coagulase-negative staphylococci have emerged as significant and frequently isolated pathogens. In 1984, analyses of the etiology of bloodstream infections on the pediatric and newborn services of NNIS hospitals revealed coagulase-negative staphylococci to be the most commonly isolated organisms. For newborn services, group B streptococcus, enterococci, *E. coli*, and *Klebsiella* spp. were the next most frequently isolated pathogens, while for the pediatric services they were *S. aureus*, *E. coli*, *Klebsiella* spp., and *Candida* sp. (Table 1.5).

Several studies suggest that the reasons for the recent emergence of coagulase-negative staphylococci have included the more frequent and prolonged use of indwelling intravenous catheters, improved survival resulting in prolonged hospitalization, increased use of parenteral nutrition, and the increased use of 2nd and 3rd generation cephalosporins which may select for increasingly antibiotic resistant strains of coagulase-negative staphylococci (27,29–34). In an investigation of increasing incidence of septicemia due to coagulase-negative staphylococci among infants in an institution in the Netherlands, Fleer and associates noted a 10-fold increase in infection among infants who had received contaminated total parenteral nutrition (TPN) solutions (32). Like others, their studies are confounded by an increased proportion of births being of low birthweight, an increased frequency of the use of intravenous cannulae, and frequent courses of antimicrobial agents.

Table 1.4
Nosocomial Bacteremia in Neonatal Intensive Care Patients

Location	Year of Study	Ref. No.	Nosocomial Infection Rate[a]	Nosocomial Bacteremia Rate[a]	Bacteremia as Percent of all Nosocomial Inf.
University of Utah	1970–74	19	246	34	14
University of Virginia	1973–77	20		40[b]	
University of Iowa	1976–77	13	169	27	16
Utrecht, Netherlands	1977–78	21	300	83	27
Buffalo Children's Hospital	1980–81	14	222[c]		
Virginia State Nosocomial Infection Registry	1980–82	22	80	15	19
Tufts University	1981–83	17	59	12	20
University of Liverpool	1981–82	23		51	
University of Pennsylvania	1982–84	24	72	22	31
Freiburg, W. Germany	1982–83	25	239	34	14

[a]Number of infections per 1000 discharges.
[b]Primary and secondary.
[c]Includes nosocomial viral infections.

Table 1.5
Secular Trends in Pathogens: Nosocomial Bacteremia on Newborn and Pediatric Services, NNIS 1980–1984

Newborn Services

Species	Percent of Isolates	
	1980–82	1984
Group B Streptococcus	24.8	15.3
S. aureus	14.5	<8.4
E. coli	11.0	9.4
Coagulase-negative Staphylococci	10.3	20.8
Enterococci	9.9	9.9
Klebsiella spp.	<9.9	8.4
Others	29.5	36.2

Pediatric Services

Species	1980–82	1984
Coagulase-negative Staphylococci	17.6	29.0
S. aureus	14.6	14.0
Klebsiella spp.	9.3	6.5
E. coli	8.9	10.8
Candida spp.	6.6	6.5
Others	43.2	33.2

Their experience, however, may not be generalizable to other institutions. In some centers, the emergence of multiply resistant coagulase-negative staphylococci as a significant bloodstream pathogen has led to changes in recommendations for initial antibiotic therapy for suspected sepsis (33).

During the last 10 years, methicillin-resistant *Staphylococcus aureus* (MRSA) has also emerged as a significant pathogen. Initially noted in tertiary care centers, usually in burn or other special care units, it is now evident that the organism is present in institutions of all types and is a problem on some pediatric and newborn units (23–25,35–37).

Of the Gram-negative organisms causing nosocomial bacteremias on the pediatric and newborn services, *E. coli* and *Klebsiella* spp. continue to be important but with no major changes in incidence rates. However, while rates appear to remain unchanged, outbreaks with antibiotic-resistant organisms have occurred (38,39). NNIS data are inconclusive with regard to nationwide trends in antibiotic resistance within this group of organisms (9).

NNIS data show that fungi are emerging as important pathogens causing disseminated disease among pediatric patients. Among the fungi, *Candida* spp. account for the majority of blood-stream infections. Between 1980–1984, *Candida* spp. were responsible for 79% of fungal bloodstream infections, accounting for 76% of the fungal bloodstream infections among the newborn population, and 81% among the pediatric service population (40). *Candida* spp. sepsis has become a particular problem among low and very low birthweight infants in NICUs. Such infants can be colonized at birth or acquire the organism from the environment and develop sepsis when the organism becomes invasive. Early diagnosis can be difficult; institution of therapy is often late in the course of disease, and fatality rates are high (41,42). The value of more rapid diagnostic tests, such as the use of the lysis centrifugation system and a Mannan enzyme-linked immunoassay are currently being evaluated in this population (43). Several studies have reported outbreaks of invasive Candida infection and suggest that the incidence of endemic infection may be increasing as well, especially among NICU patients and immuno-compromised patients (44–46). Previous or concurrent use of antibiotics, long duration of intravenous therapy, and use of total parenteral nutrition have been associated with outbreaks.

Recently, *Malassezia furfur*, a lipophilic yeast, has been the cause of endemic and epidemic bloodstream infections among neonates receiving intravenous fat emulsions (47,48, unpublished observation).

Organisms most commonly causing primary bacteremia were not necessarily those most often responsible for nosocomial infections in general (Table 1.6). For example, in 1984, *S. aureus* was the most commonly reported cause of all nosocomial infections on both newborn and pediatric services of NNIS hospitals, but was the second most common cause of bacteremia among all pediatric service patients and was not even among the top four organisms causing bacteremia in newborns.

THE COSTS OF NOSOCOMIAL INFECTIONS AND BACTEREMIA

It is estimated that, in 1984, 1% of all hospital-acquired infections caused the patients' deaths and that 3% of infections contributed to death (9). Between 1975 and 1983, 5.9% of nosocomially infected pediatric service patients died. The risk of the death being caused by the infection was 6-fold higher among patients with secondary bacteremia as compared with those without sec-

Table 1.6
Comparison of Pathogens Causing All Nosocomial Infections and Nosocomial Bacteremias on Newborn and Pediatric Services, NNIS, 1984

Newborn Services

Species	Percent of All Nosocomial Infections	Percent of Nosocomial Bacteremias
S. aureus	24.8	<8.4
Coagulase-negative Staphylococci	15.3	20.8
Group B Streptococci	6.2	15.3
E. coli	9.3	9.4
P. aeruginosa	6.7	<8.4
Klebsiella spp.	6.7	8.4
Enterococci	5.7	9.9
Candida spp.	3.8	<8.4

Pediatric Services

Species	Percent of All Nosocomial Infections	Percent of Nosocomial Bacteremias
S. aureus	16.6	14.0
Coagulase-negative Staphylococci	13.2	29.0
E. coli	11.4	10.8
P. aeruginosa	9.6	<6.5
Klebsiella spp.	6.6	6.5
Enterococci	5.3	<6.5
Candida spp.	7.6	6.5

ondary bacteremia. An analysis of NNIS data from 1975–1981 revealed that among patients with nosocomial infection who died, 5.8% of the deaths on pediatric services and 30% of the deaths on the newborn services were attributed to primary bacteremias (Jarvis, unpublished).

Attempts have been made to assess contributions of nosocomial infection to prolongation of hospital stay, and therefore to increased costs of care. Few studies have been done in pediatric patients, and care must be taken in generalizing these to larger numbers and other institutions. A survey done in general hospitals in 1975–76 showed a mean of 4 added hospital days for pediatric patients with nosocomial infection (49). The same study estimated that hospital-acquired bacteremia (adult and pediatric) resulted in 7.4 extra hospital days per episode.

NOSOCOMIAL BLOODSTREAM INFECTIONS

The healthy, immunocompetent individual survives in a world full of microorganisms. As long as a balance is maintained and host defenses remain intact, illness is rare. However, virtually any illness, trauma, or surgical procedure for which a patient is admitted to a hospital involves some breach in host defenses; either mechanical or immunological. Factors important for the acquisition of hospital-acquired bloodstream infection include: a reservoir of pathogenic bacteria, a means of transmission from reservoir to patient, access to the bloodstream, and a susceptible host.

Reservoirs of Pathogenic Bacteria and Fungi

Reservoirs of nosocomial bloodstream pathogens can include the hospital inanimate environment, patients who are colonized, and, rarely, personnel carrier-disseminators. These reservoirs, either directly or indirectly, probably account for the majority of endemic as well as epidemic nosocomial bloodstream infections (Table 1.7).

Table 1.7 is a selected list of outbreaks of nosocomial infection in newborns and children. It is intended to illustrate the variety of implicated organisms, the types of reservoirs, and some of the more common modes of transmission. Some of these outbreaks involved large numbers of colonized patients with few infections; others had a high ratio of infection to colonization. Virtually all involved excess morbidity and, in some cases, increased mortality.

In the past, the role of the hospital inanimate environment as an important reservoir for nosocomial pathogens was overemphasized (63). It is now recognized that environmental contamination with potential pathogens is unavoidable, but with control measures, including disinfection or sterilization of patient care equipment, adequate handwashing, and maintenance of closed IV infusion systems, risk of transmission of infectious agents is small. However, several areas remain problematic and have resulted in a number of outbreaks. These include in-hospital contamination of parenteral solutions during admixture, the use of multiple-dose medication vials, and the reuse of blood pressure transducers (64–68). Undoubtedly, these factors contribute to the endemic occurrence of patient colonization and/or bloodstream infection. A large proportion of outbreaks related to these products have involved *Enterobacteriaceae*, *Pseudomonas* spp., other glucose nonfermenting Gram-negative aerobes, and occasionally, fungi. These organisms are the most readily able

Table 1.7
Nosocomial Outbreaks in Infants and Children Involving the Bloodstream or Disseminated Infection

Organism (Ref.)	Year of Study	Patient Population	Infection Site	Reservoir				Comments
				Hospital Environment	I.V. Fluids Medication	Patients	Personnel	
Gram-negative rods								
Enterobacteriaceae			5 meningitis/ brain abscess					
Citrobacter diversus (50)	1977–78	Nursery	1 bacteremia 140 colonized			X	X	Colonized infants and nurses
Citrobacter diversus (51)	1978	NICU	2 meningitis with sepsis 9 umbilical stump colonization			X	X	Nurse with dermatitis of hands
Enterobacter aerogenes (52)	1976	Gen. ped.	7 bacteremias		X E			i.v. fluid with added KCl
Enterobacter spp. (53)	1984	Gen. ped.	63 bacteremias		X I			i.v. fluid contaminated at time of manufacture
Escherichia coli (39)	1982	NICU	1 bacteremia, 1 sputum isolate, 1 urinary tract infection, 13 colonized			X		Colonized infants
Klebsiella spp. (54)	1978–79	NICU	5 bacteremias	X				Banked breast milk; Contaminated breast pump
Serratia marcescens (55)	1973–74	Nursery	31 colonized 9 abscesses at I.V. site 6 bacteremias			X		Colonized infants Multiple antibiotic-resistant
Multiple Gram-negative rods [a]	1976–77	NICU	13 bacteremias		X E			Lipid emulsion
Multiple Gram-negative rods [a]	1981	NICU	5 bacteremias		X E			Lipid emulsion
Nonfermenters								
Pseudomonas aeruginosa (56)	1971	NICU	9 bacteremias	X				Resuscitation equipment
Pseudomonas aeruginosa [a]	1982	NICU	24 colonized 8 bacteremias			X	X	Colonized infants and nurse with dermatitis
Pseudomonas cepacia (57)	1976	Nursery	2 bacteremias 2 conjunctivitis 1 urinary tract inf. 2 colonized	X				Distilled water used in respiratory therapy equipment
Pseudomonas maltophilia (58)	1980	Open heart surgery	8 bacteremias	X	X E			Reused transducers in arterial pressure monitoring system
Gram-positive cocci								
Coagulase-negative *Staphylococcus* (32)	1980–81	NICU	≥11 bacteremias		X E			Total parenteral nutrition fluid

**Table 1.7
(Cont.)**

Organism (Ref.)	Year of Study	Patient Population	Infection Site	Reservoir Hospital Environment	I.V. Fluids Medication	Patients	Personnel	Comments
Staphylococcus aureus (59)	1981–82	Nursery	1 bacteremia 20 bullous impetigo			X	X	Nurse, nasal carrier-disseminator
Group A *Streptococcus* (60)	1966–67	Nursery	2 bacteremias 48 colonized in 2 outbreaks			X		Colonized infants
Gram-positive rods								
Listeria monocytogenes (61)	1985	Delivery room	1 bacteremia 1 meningitis	X				Resuscitation equipment
Fungi								
Aspergillus spp. (62)	1982–84	Ped. oncology	5 pts. with multiple organ infection	X				Hospital construction
Candida parapsilosis (44)	1982–83	NICU	8 fungemias	X	X E			Reused transducers TPN fluid in line

I = Intrinsic contamination.
E = Extrinsic contamination
ªCDC unpublished data

to proliferate in glucose containing parenteral solutions.

Probably the single most important reservoir for nosocomial bloodstream pathogens are colonized/infected patients. Colonized patients may develop overt illness or may remain as reservoirs for transmission of organisms to other patients, usually via shared equipment, on the hands of caregivers, or both. Infants may remain colonized long after hospital discharge, and they may introduce pathogenic organisms to other areas of the hospital if they require readmission (28). Oncology patients requiring frequent hospitalization may likewise serve as reservoirs. Antibiotic-resistant *Enterobacteriaceae, Pseudomonas* spp., methicillin-resistant *S. aureus*, and multiply resistant coagulase-negative staphylococci have all been identified as being able to persistently colonize the respiratory and gastrointestinal tracts or the injured skin and mucous membranes (69,70).

Personnel may also function as reservoirs by shedding organisms with which they are persistently colonized (personnel carrier-disseminators). Such shedders have been implicated in outbreaks of *S. aureus* and group A streptococcus, and less commonly with outbreaks related to Gram-negative organisms (50,51,59).

Transmission of Pathogens from Reservoir to Patients

A more common problem, however, is transient hand carriage of hospital pathogens, which personnel acquire in the course of their daily caregiving routines. Inadequate and improper handwashing routines may result in patient-to-patient transmission. In this situation, these health care workers are more appropriately described as vectors than as reservoirs.

Situations that make transmission of pathogenic bacteria to a susceptible host more likely include overcrowding and understaffing, inadequate isolation precautions, and lack of accessible facilities for handwashing (26,71). Patients are increasingly likely to be colonized with potential pathogens as the length of their hospital stay increases (28).

Pathophysiology of Primary Bacteremia

Most primary bacteremias are actually secondary in that they are related to intravenous catheters or other intravascular devices. An estimated ⅔ of primary bacteremias occur in association with intravascular devices (72). Bacteria can gain access to the bloodstream directly, as occurs when contaminated fluids are infused, or from the skin along the path of needle or cannula through skin and subcutaneous tissue. Bloodstream infections resulting from migration of organisms through skin and subcutaneous tissue around the needle or cannula are thought to be many times more common than those resulting from infusion of contaminated fluids. It is thus not surprising that skin flora such as coagulase-negative staphylococci and *S. aureus* have been the organisms commonly implicated in cannula-related infections, whereas the *Enterobacteriaceae* and the nonglucose fermenting Gram-negative rods have been the organisms most commonly associated with intrinsic and extrinsic contamination of intravenous products (72,73).

RISK FACTORS FOR NOSOCOMIAL BLOODSTREAM INFECTIONS

Since most nosocomial bacteremias are related to intravenous catheter-related colonization, assessment of risk factors for development of nosocomial bacteremia frequently becomes an exercise in determining risk factors for colonization of the catheter. Currently recognized risk factors include type of cannula (steel needle versus plastic cannula), peripheral versus central placement, duration of use, and number of line manipulations. Presence of a pressure monitoring device and use of TPN are also risk factors.

Host factors are much more difficult to evaluate, particularly because premature and ill newborns and older children with severe illness are likely to both be immunocompromised and to require aggressive intravenous therapy and intravascular monitoring (74–79).

DIAGNOSIS OF NOSOCOMIAL BACTEREMIA

Primary bacteremia and/or fungemia may present as fever without any obvious source. The patient may have chills and/or be hypotensive and appear critically ill. In contrast, the neonate may show only poor feeding or increased number of apnea episodes. Any patient with a documented infection at another site may develop signs and symptoms of secondary bacteremia. Conversely, in any patient with suspected bacteremia, a remote site of infection should be sought and, if found, appropriately treated.

If the bacteremia is catheter or intravascular device-related, there may be erythema, tenderness, or palpable cord at the intravenous (i.v.)

insertion site. Septic thrombophlebitis may occur, but appears to be rare in pediatric patients. The neutropenic patient with catheter-related sepsis may have little inflammatory reaction at an infected i.v. site (72). The patient with bloodstream infection related to a central catheter may have no evidence of exit site infection.

The following observations should make one consider the possibility of i.v. infusion related sepsis:

1. Patient receiving i.v. infusion at the onset of septicemia;
2. Inflammation at the cannula insertion site—especially if there is pus present;
3. Primary septicemia—i.e., no evidence for local infection;
4. Patient has no other risk factors for sepsis;
5. Precipitous onset of symptoms of sepsis;
6. Sepsis refractory to appropriate antimicrobial therapy until the contaminated infusion is discontinued (72).

The definitive test for bloodstream infection is blood culture, and it should be done in any patient where reasonable suspicion of bacteremia exists. Optimum timing, volume of blood, and optimum number of cultures are also important considerations. Bacteremia may precede its visible result of fever and chills by minutes to an hour or more, and may make timing of blood cultures difficult. In the patient who continues to have chills or fever while receiving antibiotics, blood cultures should be done just before the next dose of antibiotic, when antibiotic levels are likely to be low. The laboratory should be notified so that appropriate techniques to adsorb or inactivate the antibiotic can be used (80).

Ideally, several cultures should be obtained over a period of hours before starting antimicrobial therapy. However, this is often difficult to accomplish, particularly in critically ill patients, so a reasonable compromise may be 2 sets of cultures 30 minutes apart, (plus cultures of line and i.v. fluid, etc., if they are suspect) before starting treatment. The largest possible volume of blood should be obtained.

The i.v. site should be examined for signs of inflammation and cultured if indicated. If there is concern that the line is the source of infection, it may be appropriate to culture peripheral blood and blood drawn through the line simultaneously. Methods for semiquantitating blood cultures have been described and may be useful in determining whether the line is colonized and in determining whether true bacteremia is present (81–83). If a line is removed as part of a sepsis workup, an effort should be made to culture the catheter. Although several methods have been described, those that quantitatively or semiquantitatively assess the number of bacteria colonizing the catheter appear to correlate better with risk of sepsis than those that are merely qualitative. In addition, the quantitative count of bacteria present in the blood may be useful to differentiate colonization from infection (83). The hospital infectious diseases consultant and microbiology laboratory should be consulted to obtain instructions and materials required for quantitative cultures.

Rapid methods for detection of bloodstream infections have so far been of limited value, but may be useful in certain clinical situations. These include: Gram stain of blood buffy coat, lysis centrifugation, and antigen tests for body fluids, such as CSF and urine (84–86). Other methods for rapid diagnosis are being evaluated. The microbiology laboratory and infectious disease service should be involved in the evaluation of all suspected nosocomial bacteremia, so new diagnostic procedures can be applied where appropriate.

TREATMENT OF NOSOCOMIAL BACTEREMIA

To determine the appropriate therapy for a nosocomial bacteremia, an important issue is whether the bacteremia is primary or secondary.

If the bacteremic episode is explained by the presence of a remote infection, then treatment is aimed at the remote infection, with treatment of pneumonia, drainage of abscesses, debridement of wounds, etc. Antimicrobial therapy should be initially targeted to the most likely organisms, often guided by Gram stain of purulent material. Therapy can be reviewed and changed, if necessary, when culture results are obtained.

If a bacteremia is presumed to be primary and related to an intravascular device, the following should be included as part of treatment:

1. The entire i.v. system including fluid, tubing, and filters should be changed;

2. If a pressure monitoring device is in use, all components, including transducers and stopcocks, should be changed; and
3. All intravascular cannulas and insertion sites should be evaluated, and changed if necessary. If intrinsic or extrinsic product contamination is suspected, the product should be cultured and saved until contamination has been excluded.

Recent studies indicate that some bacteremias may be successfully treated with the i.v. cannula in place (86–89). However, it has been shown that following successful treatment with the catheter in place, the risk of a second catheter-related bacteremia is greater than the risk associated with an initial or new catheter (86). The possibility of recurrent infection must be balanced against the potential problems of removing and reinserting the catheter.

Treatment with antibiotics should usually begin before culture results are available. Initial therapy of suspected sepsis will depend on the most likely organisms for the patient in question and the setting involved. In an NICU, where Group B streptococci and *Enterobacteriaceae* are frequently encountered, empiric therapy with ampicillin and an aminoglycoside are often prescribed. Centers that have high rates of documented infections with methicillin-resistant coagulase-negative or coagulase-positive staphylococci may need to consider using vancomycin.

Patients in pediatric intensive care units and those who are immunosuppressed will need combination therapy tailored to cover likely organisms. Centers experiencing problems with methicillin-resistant *S. aureus*, coagulase-negative staphylococci, or multiply antibiotic resistant Gram-negative organisms will need to select antimicrobial agents accordingly.

Depending on the severity of illness, antibiotic choice should be broad enough to cover all likely pathogens. Antibiotic regimens should be reevaluated and changed, if appropriate, when final blood culture reports are available. Antibiotic levels should be monitored when indicated and possible.

As the patient is treated, patient care procedures and products should be evaluated and modified, if needed, to prevent recurrence. The case should be discussed with the infection control staff, and if other cases are found, further epidemic investigation should be initiated.

PREVENTION OF NOSOCOMIAL BLOODSTREAM INFECTIONS

Comparison of nosocomial infection rates in an individual institution with those of other hospitals or with NNIS rates must be done with care, since the characteristics of patients in different hospitals may vary significantly. Knowledge of infection rates in one's own institution is more important, to establish baseline rates, which will allow early recognition of problems and assessment of control measures.

If a problem is identified, different control measures may be needed, depending on whether a problem appears to be endemic or epidemic. Low levels of endemic infection are likely to be kept low by attention to aseptic technique, isolation precautions where appropriate, and good handwashing. It is estimated that 25–33% of nosocomial infections in adults are preventable by these measures (90). No information is available for pediatric or newborn services.

Epidemics

It has been estimated that up to 10% of all nosocomial infections, and 8% of all nosocomial bacteremias are related to known outbreaks (8,69,90). The actual percentages may be much higher as an unknown number of outbreaks are unrecognized.

Outbreaks of nosocomial bacteremia require detailed investigation to find the causative factor and may implicate a product or require a systematic change in routine patient care. Coordination of the infection control team, nursing service, pharmacy service, hospital administration, plus outside agencies including state and local health departments, Food and Drug Administration, and Centers for Disease Control may be necessary to effect rapid and effective control of an outbreak.

Intravascular Devices

Because of the importance of intravascular devices in current medical management of hospital patients, and the potential for serious complications, the Centers for Disease Control has developed guidelines for the prevention of intravascular infections. These guidelines should be available to all personnel involved in the placement and maintenance of intravenous lines and intravascular monitoring devices (91). Key recommendations are:

1. Intravenous therapy should be used only when absolutely necessary.
2. Personnel should wash hands before inserting an i.v. cannula and before manipulating any part of the system.
3. The cannula should be secured to prevent movement at the insertion site, and the insertion site should be covered by a sterile dressing.
4. The insertion site should be observed as frequently as necessary for evidence of infiltration or inflammation, and the cannula removed promptly if either complication occurs.
5. Recommendations for adult patients are that steel rather than plastic needles be used where possible, that cannulas be changed every 48–72 hours, and that upper extremity sites be chosen where possible. No studies are available for pediatric patients.
6. Fluids and medications for parenteral use should be handled aseptically, and admixing should be done in the pharmacy, if possible. Pharmacy guidelines for storage and expiration dates should be followed.

Areas requiring further study include the use of topical antibiotics, time intervals for changing i.v. system tubing, and the use of in-line filters.

Central cannulas that are intended to be left in place for prolonged periods require additional care, and individual hospitals must develop guidelines for their insertion and care (92). Important considerations are:

1. Routines for dressing changes and exit site care.
2. Guidelines for administration of blood products and withdrawal of blood for laboratory studies.
3. Standardization of techniques for flushing lines, changing tubing, and other procedures that open the lines to possible bacterial contamination.

Intravascular Pressure Monitoring Devices

Intravascular pressure monitoring devices are increasingly important in the management of the critically ill patient. Since they may need to be used for several days, strict attention must be paid to aseptic technique. Each hospital should develop formal policies regarding use of this equipment, using published guidelines. Recommendations for insertion and maintenance are generally the same as for intravenous cannulas (91).

Some additional suggestions include:

1. Disposable components should be used where possible.
2. Reusable equipment should be cleaned and sterilized according to manufacturer's instructions.
3. A closed flush system (rather than an open syringe and stopcock arrangement) should be used to keep the cannula patent; flush solutions should not contain glucose, and the flush solution should be changed every 24 hours.

REFERENCES

1. McCarthy PL, Grundy GW, Spiesel SZ, Dolan TF: Bacteremia in children: an outpatient clinical review. *Pediatrics* 57:861–868, 1976.
2. Bryan CS, Reynolds KL, Derrick CW, Jr.: Patterns of bacteremia in pediatrics practice: factors affecting mortality rates. *Pediatr Infect Dis* 3:312–316, 1984.
3. Klein JO, Marcy SM: Bacterial sepsis and meningitis. In Remington JS, Klein JO (eds): *Infectious Diseases of the Fetus and Newborn Infant.* Philadelphia, WB Saunders, 1983, pp 679–735.
4. Hughes JM, Culver DH, White JW, Jarvis WR, Morgan WM, Munn VP, Mosser JL, Emori TG: Nosocomial infection surveillance 1980–82. *MMWR.* CDC Surveillance Summaries 32 (Spec. Suppl. 4):1SS–16SS, 1983.
5. US Dept. Health and Human Services, PHS, CDC, Atlanta. National Nosocomial Infections Surveillance System, Procedure Manual, p XIII 1–59, 1988.
6. Brachman PS: Epidemiology of nosocomial infections. In Bennett JV, Brachman PS (eds): *Hospital Infections.* Boston, Little, Brown & Co, 1986, pp 3–16.
7. Dixon, RE: Investigation of endemic and epidemic nosocomial infections. In Bennett JV, Brachman PS (eds): *Hospital Infections.* Boston, Little, Brown & Co, 1986, pp 73–93.
8. Wenzel RP: Epidemics—identification and management. In Wenzel RP (ed): *Prevention and Control of Nosocomial Infections.* Baltimore, Williams & Wilkins, 1987, pp 94–108.
9. Horan TC, White JW, Jarvis WM, Emori TG, Culver DW, Munn VP, Thornsberry C, Olson DR, Hughes JM: Nosocomial infection surveillance 1984. *MMWR:* CDC Surveillance Summaries 35 Suppl 1, p 17SS–29SS, 1986.
10. Speer CP, Hauptmann D, Stubbe P, Gahr M: Neonatal septicemia and meningitis in Gottingen, West Germany. *Pediatr Infect Dis* 4:36–41, 1985.
11. Freedman RM, Ingram DL, Gross I, Ehrenkranz RA, Warshaw JB, Baltimore RS: A half century of neonatal sepsis at Yale: 1928–1978. *Am J Dis Child* 135:140–144, 1981.
12. Bennet R, Eriksson M, Zetterstrom R: Increasing incidence of neonatal septicemia: Causative organisms and predisposing risk factors. *Acta Pediatr Scand* 70:207–210, 1981.
13. Maguire GC, Nordin J, Myers MG, Koontz FP, Hierholzer W, Nassif E: Infections acquired by young infants. *Am J Dis Child* 135:693–698, 1981.
14. Welliver RC, McLaughlin S: Unique epidemiology of nosocomial infection in a children's hospital. *Am J Dis Child* 138:131–135, 1984.
15. Gardner P, Carles DG: Infections acquired in a pediatric hospital. *J Pediatr* 81:1205–1210, 1972.
16. Donowitz LG: High risk of nosocomial infection in the pediatric critical care patient. *Crit Care Med* 14:26–28, 1986.
17. Brown RB, Hosmer D, Chen HC, Teres D, Sands M, Bradley S, Opitz E, Szwedzinski D, Opalenik D: A comparison of infections in different ICUs within the same hospital. *Crit Care Med* 13:472–476, 1985.
18. Jarvis WR: Epidemiology of nosocomial infections in pediatric patients. *Pediatr Infect Dis* 6:344–350, 1987.
19. Hemming VG, Overall JC, Britt MR: Nosocomial infections in a newborn intensive-care unit: Results of forty-one months of surveillance. *N Engl J Med* 294:1310–1316, 1976.
20. Townsend TR, Wenzel RP: Nosocomial bloodstream infections in a newborn intensive care unit: A case-matched control study of morbidity, mortality and risk. *Am J Epidemiol* 114:73–80, 1981.
21. Hoogkamp-Korstanje JAA: Analysis of bacterial infections in a neonatal intensive care unit. *J Hosp Inf* 3:275–284, 1982.
22. Wenzel RP, Thompson RL, Landry SM, Russell BS, Miller PJ, Ponce de Leon S, Miller GB: Hospital-acquired infections in intensive care unit patients: An overview with emphasis on epidemics. *Infect Control* 4:371–375, 1983.
23. Hensey OJ, Hart CA, Cooke RWI: Serious infection in a neonatal intensive care unit: A two-year study. *J Hyg Camb* 95:289–297, 1985.
24. Kumar SP, Delivoria-Papadopoulos M: Infections in newborn infants in a special care unit: a changing pattern of infection. *Ann Clin Lab Sci* 15:351–356, 1985.
25. Dascher F: Letter to the editor: Analysis of bacteria; infections in a neonatal intensive care unit. *J Hosp Inf* 4:90–91, 1983.
26. Goldmann DA, Durbin WA, Jr., Freeman J: Nosocomial infections in a neonatal intensive care unit. *J Infect Dis* 144:449–459, 1981.
27. Anday EK, Talbot GH: Coagulase-negative staphylococcus bacteremia—a rising threat in the newborn infant. *Ann Clin Lab Sci* 15:246–251, 1985.
28. Goldmann DA: Bacterial colonization and infection in the neonate. *Am J Med* 70:417–422, 1981.
29. Brown AE: Management of the febrile, neutropenic patient with cancer: therapeutic considerations. *J Pediatr* 106:1035–1042, 1985.
30. Wade JC, Schimpff SC, Newman KA, Wiernik PH: *Staphylococcus epidermidis:* an increasing cause of infection in patients with granulocytopenia. *Ann Int Med* 97:503–508, 1982.
31. Baumgart S, Hall SE, Campos JM, Polin RA: Sepsis with coagulase-negative staphylococci in critically ill newborns. *Am J Dis Child* 137:461–463, 1983.
32. Fleer A, Senders RC, Visser MR, Bijlmer RP, Gerards LJ, Kraaijeveld CA, Verhoef J: Septicemia due to coagulase-negative staphylococci in a neonatal intensive care unit: clinical and bacteriological features and contaminated parenteral fluids as a source of sepsis. *Pediatr Infect Dis* 2:426–431, 1983.
33. Stillman RI, Wenzel RP, Donowitz LG: Emergence of coagulase-negative staphylococci as major nosocomial bloodstream pathogens. *Infect Control* 8:108–112, 1987.
34. Munson DP, Thompson TR, Johnson DE, Rhame FS, Van Drumen N, Ferrieri P: Coagulase-negative staphylococcal septicemia: Experience in a newborn intensive care unit. *J Pediatr* 101:602–665, 1982.
35. Jarvis WR, Thornsberry C, Boyce J, Hughes JM: Methicillin-resistant *Staphylococcus aureus* at children's hospitals in the United States. *Pediatr Infect Dis* 4:651–655, 1985.
36. Storch GA, Rajagopalan L: Methicillin-resistant *Staphylococcus aureus* bacteremia in children. *Pediatr Infect Dis* 5:59–67, 1986.
37. McNeil MM, Solomon SL: The epidemiology of methicillin-resistant *Staphylococcus aureus. The Antimicrobic Newsletter* 2:49–56, 1985.
38. Anderson EL, Hieber JP: An outbreak of gentamycin-resistant *Enterobacter cloacae* infections in a pediatric intensive care unit. *Infect Control* 4:148–152, 1983.
39. Gaynes RP, Simpson D, Reeves SA, Noble RC, Thornsberry C, Culver D, Allen JR, Martone WJ: A nursery outbreak of multiple-aminoglycoside-resistant *Escherichia coli. Infect Control* 5:519–524, 1984.
40. Jarvis WR: Secular trends in nosocomial fungal infection rates in the United States, 1980–1984 (unpublished).

41. Baley JE, Kliegman RM, Fanaroff AA: Disseminated fungal infections in very low-birth-weight infants: Clinical manifestations and epidemiology. *Pediatrics* 73:144–152, 1984.

42. Johnson DE, Thompson TR, Green TP, Ferrier P: Systemic Candidiasis in very low-birth-weight infants (<1,500 grams). *Pediatrics* 73:138–143, 1984.

43. de Repentigny L, Reiss E: Current trends in immunodiagnosis of Candidiasis and Aspergillosis. *Rev Infect Dis* 6:301–312, 1984.

44. Solomon SL, Alexander H, Eley JW, Anderson RL, Goodpasture HC, Smart S, Furman RM, Martone W: Nosocomial fungemia in neonates associated with intravascular pressure-monitoring devices. *Pediatr Infect Dis* 5:680–685, 1986.

45. Meunier-Carpentier F, Kiehn TE, Armstrong D: Fungemia in the immunocompromised host. *Amer J Med* 71:363–370, 1981.

46. Weese-Mayer DE, Fondriest DW, Brouillette RT, Shulman ST: Risk factors associated with candidemia in the neonatal intensive care unit: a case-control study. *Pediatr Infect Dis* 6:190–196, 1987.

47. Long JG, Keyserling HL: Catheter-related infection in infants due to an unusual lipophilic yeast—*Malassezia furfur*. *Pediatrics* 76:896–990, 1985.

48. Powell DA, Aungst J, Snedden S, Hansen N, Brady M: Broviac catheter-related *Malassezia furfur* sepsis in five infants receiving intravenous fat emulsions. *J Pediatr* 105:987–990, 1984.

49. Haley RW, Schabert DR, Crossley KB, Von Allmen SD, McGowan JE, Jr.: Extra charges and prolongation of stay attributable to nosocomial infections: A prospective interhospital comparison. *Am J Med* 70:51–58, 1981.

50. Graham DR, Anderson RL, Ariel FE, Ehrenkranz NJ, Rowe B, Boer HR, Dixon RE: Epidemic nosocomial meningitis due to *Citrobacter diversus* in neonates. *J Infect Dis* 144:203–209, 1981.

51. Parry MF, Hutchinson JH, Brown NA, Wu CH, Estreller L: Gram-negative sepsis in neonates: A nursery outbreak due to hand carriage of *Citrobacter diversus*. *Pediatrics* 65:1105–1109, 1980.

52. Edwards KE, Allen JR, Miller MJ, Yogev R, Hoffman PC, Klotz R, Marubio S, Burkholder E, Williams T, Davis AT: *Enterobacter aerogenes* primary bacteremia in pediatric patients. *Pediatrics* 62:304–306, 1978.

53. Matsaniotis NS, Syriopoulou VP, Theodoridou MC, Tzanetou KG, Mostrou GI: Enterobacter sepsis in infants and children due to contaminated intravenous fluids. *Infect Control* 5:471–477, 1984.

54. Donowitz LG, Marsik FJ, Fisher KA, Wenzel RP: Contaminated breast milk: A source of Klebsiella bacteremia in a newborn intensive care unit. *Rev Inf Dis* 3:716–720, 1981.

55. Stamm WE, Kolff CA, Dones EM, Javariz R, Anderson RL, Farmer JJ, de Quinones HR: A nursery outbreak caused by *Serratia marcescens*—scalp-vein needles as a portal of entry. *J Pediatr* 89:96–99, 1976.

56. Bobo RA, Newton EJ, Jones LF, Farmer LH, Farmer JJ: Nursery outbreak of *Pseudomonas aeruginosa*: Epidemiological conclusions from five different typing methods. *Appl Microbiol* 25:414–420, 1973.

57. Rapkin RH: *Pseudomonas cepacia* in an intensive care nursery. *Pediatrics* 57:239–243, 1976.

58. Fisher MC, Long SS, Roberts EM, Dunn JM, Balsara RK: *Pseudomonas maltophilia* bacteremia in children undergoing open heart surgery. *JAMA* 246:1571–1574, 1981.

59. Nakashima AK, Allen JR, Martone WJ, Plikaytis BD, Storer B, Cook LM, Wright SP: Epidemic bullous impetigo in a nursery due to a nasal carrier of *Staphylococcus aureus*: Role of epidemiology and control measures. *Infect Control* 5:326–331, 1984.

60. Geil CC, Castle WK, Mortimer EA: Group A streptococcal infections in newborn nurseries. *Pediatrics* 6:849–854, 1970.

61. Nelson KE, Warren D, Tomasi AM, Raju TN, Vidyasagar D: Transmission of neonatal listeriosis in a delivery room. *Am J Dis Child* 139:903–905, 1985.

62. Weems JJ, Davis BJ, Tablan OC, Kaufman L, Martone WJ: Construction activity: An independent risk factor for invasive aspergillosis and zygomycosis in patients with hematologic malignancy. *Infect Control* 8:71–75, 1987.

63. Rhame FS: The inanimate environment. In Bennett JV, Brachman PS (eds): *Hospital Infections*. Boston, Little, Brown & Co. 1986, pp 223–250.

64. Solomon SL, Khabbaz RF, Parker RH, Anderson RL, Geraghty MA, Furman RM, Martone WJ: An outbreak of *Candida parapsilosis* bloodstream infections in patients receiving parenteral nutrition. *J Infect Dis* 149:98–102, 1984.

65. Stamm WE, Colella JJ, Anderson RL, Dixon RE: Indwelling arterial catheters as a source of nosocomial bacteremia: An outbreak caused by *Flavobacterium* species. *N Engl J Med* 292:1099–1102, 1975.

66. Williams WW: Infection control during parenteral nutrition therapy. *J Parenteral and Enteral Nutrition* 9:735–746, 1985.

67. Maki DG, Hassemer CA: Endemic rate of fluid contamination and related septicemia in arterial pressure monitoring. *Am J Med* 70:207–212, 1981.

68. Wenzel RP, Osterman CA, Donowitz LG, Hoyt JW, Sande MA, Martone WJ, Peacock JE, Levine JI, Miller GB: Identification of procedure-related nosocomial infections in high-risk patients. *Rev Infect Dis* 3:701–707, 1981.

69. Haley RW: Incidence and nature of endemic and epidemic nosocomial infections. In Bennett JV, Brachman PS (eds): *Hospital Infections*. Boston, Little, Brown & Co 1986, pp 359–374.

70. Cooperstock MS: Indigenous flora. In Feigin RD, Cherry JD (eds): *Textbook of Pediatric Infectious Diseases*. Philadelphia, WB Saunders, 1987, pp 106–133.

71. Haley RW, Bregman DA: The role of understaffing and overcrowding in recurrent outbreaks of Staphylococcal infection in a neonatal special-care unit. *J Infect Dis* 145:875–885, 1982.

72. Maki DG: Infections due to infusion therapy. In Bennett JV, Brachman PS (eds): *Hospital Infections*. Boston, Little, Brown & Co, 1986, pp 561–580.

73. Hamory BH: Nosocomial bloodstream and intravascular device-related infections. In Wenzel RP (ed): *Prevention and Control of Nosocomial Infections*. Baltimore, Williams & Wilkins, 1987, pp 283–319.

74. Wilson CB: Immunologic basis for increased susceptibility of the neonate to infection. *J Pediatr* 108:1–12, 1986.

75. Miller ME, Stiehm ER: Immunology and resistance to infection. In Remington JS, Klein JO (eds): *Infectious Diseases of the Fetus and Newborn Infant*. Philadelphia, WB Saunders, 1983, pp 27–68.

76. Pizzo PA: Infectious complications in the child with cancer. II. Management of specific infectious organisms. *J Pediatr* 98:513–523, 1981.

77. Pizzo PA: Infectious complications in the child with cancer. I. Pathophysiology of the compromised host and the initial evaluation and management of the febrile cancer patient. *J Pediatr* 98:341–354, 1981.

78. Feigin RD, Matson DO: Opportunistic infections in the compromised host. In Feigin RD, Cherry JD (eds): *Textbook of Pediatric Infectious Diseases*. Philadelphia, WB Saunders, 1981, pp 1008–1043.

79. Klein JO, Remington JS, Marcy SM: Current concepts of infections in the fetus and newborn infant. In Remington JS, Klein JO (eds): *Infectious Diseases of the Fetus and Newborn Infant*. Philadelphia, WB Saunders, 1983, pp 1–26.

80. Tilton RC: The laboratory approach to the detection of bacteremia. *Ann Rev Microbiol* 36:467–493, 1982.

81. Raucher HS, Hyatt AC, Barzilai A, Harris MB, Weiner MA, LeLeiko NS, Hodes DS: Quantitative blood cultures in the evaluation of septicemia in children with Broviac catheters. *J Pediatr* 104:29–33, 1984.

82. Maki DG, Werse CE, Sarafin HW: A semi-quantitative culture method for identifying intravenous-catheter-related infection. *N Engl J Med* 296:1305–1309, 1977.

83. Whimbey E, Kiehn TE, Brannon P, Benezra D, Armstrong D: Clinical significance of colony counts in immunocompromised patients with *Staphylococcus aureus* bacteremia. *J Infect Dis* 155:1328–1330, 1987.

84. Fong JC, Tilton RC: Detection of bacterial antigens by counterimmunoelectrophoresis, coagglutination, and latex agglutination. In Lennett EH, Balows A, Hausler WJ, Shadomy HJ (eds): *Manual of Clinical Microbiology*. Washington, DC, American Society for Microbiology, pp 883–890, 1985.

85. Graham BS: Detection of bacteremia and fungemia: Microscopic examination of peripheral blood smears. *Infect Control* 5:448–452, 1984.

86. Johnson PR, Decker MD, Edwards KM, Schaffner W, Wright PF: Frequency of Broviac catheter infections in pediatric oncology patients. *J Infect Dis* 154:570–578, 1986.

87. Pizzo PA, Commers J, Cotton D, Gress J, Hathorn J, Heimenz J, Longo D, Marshall D, Robichaud KJ: Approaching the controversies in antibacterial management of cancer patients. *Am J Med* 76:436–449, 1984.

88. Wang EEL, Prober CG, Ford-Jones L, Gold R: The management of central intravenous catheter infections. *Pediatr Infect Dis* 3:110–113, 1984.

89. Shapiro ED, Wald ER, Nelson KA, Spiegelman N: Broviac catheter-related bacteremia in oncology patients. *Am J Dis Child* 136:679–681, 1982.

90. Maki DG: Nosocomial bacteremia: An epidemiologic overview. *Am J Med* 70:183–196, 1981.

91. Simmons BP, Hooten TM, Wong ES, Allen JR: *Guidelines for Prevention of Intravascular Infections*. Atlanta, Centers for Disease Control, 1981.

92. Ford R: History and organization of the Seattle-area Hickman catheter committee. *NITA* 8:123–135, 1985.

2

Pneumonia

Richard F. Jacobs, M.D.

BACKGROUND

Nosocomial pneumonia constitutes a common and potentially life-threatening complication of hospitalization (1,2). Along with the recognition that nosocomial pneumonia is an important cause of morbidity and mortality, came the understanding that aerobic Gram-negative bacilli predominate as the major bacterial agents in these infections in adults (3). The emergence of Gram-negative bacilli as the predominate cause of nosocomial pneumonia is felt to be related to the increased use of broad spectrum antibiotics, the use of prolonged ventilatory assistance for critically ill patients, and newly developed respiratory equipment using mainstream reservoir nebulizers. These circumstances have been described in retrospective analyses which suggested a 4-fold increase in the incidence of nosocomial Gram-negative pneumonia occurring among hospitalized patients between the late 1950s and early 1960s (4–6). As the importance of nosocomial pneumonia is more widely acknowledged, so, too, is the role of respiratory viruses in nosocomial pneumonia in children (7). The respiratory viruses are considered to be the leading cause of nosocomial pneumonia in children, accounting for 24% of all nosocomial infections (8). Previously, respiratory viruses were underestimated as a cause of nosocomial pneumonia in children.

Incidence

Nosocomial pneumonia in all ages is currently the third most common site of hospital-acquired infection, accounting for approximately 15% of all nosocomial infections. The lung ranks third in frequency behind the urinary tract and skin as a cause of hospital-acquired infection (7). However, the mortality for these two organ systems range from 1–4%, while the estimated mortality rate associated with nosocomial pneumonia ranges from 20–50%. It has been estimated that as many as 15% of all deaths occurring in hospitalized patients of all ages are directly related to nosocomial pneumonia (2,8,9). Therefore, the significance of nosocomial pneumonia is emphasized as the most common fatal nosocomial infection for all ages in this country.

Over the past two decades, more published reports on the epidemiology and pathogenesis of this disease process have appeared. However, the controversy still exists concerning the proper samples or tests for diagnosis, and the treatment regimens for management in these patients (10,11). This controversy is more notable in the pediatric age group due to high-risk patient populations, the increased risk of viral nosocomial pneumonia, the absence of safe invasive diagnostic testing, the increasing number of new antibacterial and antiviral drugs, and the advent of new vaccines. This greater risk of nosocomial pneumonia with a poor outcome has been accentuated over the past decade because of the rise of modern intensive care facilities with the ability to maintain critically ill patients for prolonged periods of time with the use of invasive life support techniques. In the pediatric population, this has also been evident by the ability of modern pediatricians to maintain life in very low birthweight, premature newborns, and immunocompromised patients (12). These categories have enhanced the risk of nosocomial pneumonia with its subsequent complications, morbidity and mortality.

The incidence of nosocomial pneumonia is highly dependent upon the patient group, patient environment, and the immunologic and nutritional status of the individual patient. The National Nosocomial Infections' Studies (NNIS) for the year 1983 recorded an annual incidence of nosocomial lower respiratory tract infection of approximately 0.55% (5.5 cases per 1000 discharges) for all ages (7). Interestingly, the incidence was much lower in nonteaching hospitals (0.41%) and in small teaching hospitals (0.46%) compared with larger teaching hospitals (0.75%). These figures, however, did not take into account that the larger teaching hospitals were the centers for neonatal intensive care units and pediatric intensive care units. These numbers may reflect a patient population with an increasing disease severity and, therefore, an increased risk for nosocomial pneumonia. This increased risk among teaching hospitals was also found in a separate study evaluating the incidence of bacteremic nosocomial pneumonia in which a 10-fold greater incidence occurred in teaching versus nonteaching hospitals (9,13). In the NNIS report, the highest incidence of nosocomial pneumonia occurred in adult medical-surgical services with a 0.5–1% incidence of nosocomial pneumonia. Pediatric services registered one of the lowest risks at 0.03–0.3% incidence (7). However, as the incidence of nosocomial pneumonia was evaluated in certain patient settings, the increased patient risk groups were evident. Respiratory intensive care units accounted for 20% of all nosocomial pneumonias (11) compared with a 17.5% occurrence rate in postoperative patients (14). Note that neonatal intensive care units accounted for 7% of nosocomial pneumonias under similar circumstances (12). However, these incidence figures for nosocomial pneumonia in pediatric patients do not include a uniform attempt in accounting for viral etiologies. Some pediatric studies have evaluated hospitalized children diligently for a viral etiology of their nosocomial pneumonia and have suggested infection rates much higher than previously reported (7,8).

The postoperative patient has an increased risk to develop nosocomial pneumonia with rates that may approach 15 per 100 operations (14). Within this group, persons undergoing thoracic, thoracoabdominal, and upper abdominal surgical procedures are at greatest risk. Reasons for this presumably high risk include postoperative pain that can result in an inability to clear secretions adequately, sedation and analgesia, as well as the use of chest tubes, which may provide a direct conduit for bacterial entrance into the lower respiratory tract.

Pathophysiology

In hospitalized patients, the pathophysiology of nosocomial pneumonia is felt to occur secondary to altered or circumvented pulmonary antimicrobial defenses in the upper and lower respiratory tract (1,15). The pathogenesis of most cases of nosocomial pneumonia is felt to reflect subclinical aspiration of oropharyngeal secretions that have become colonized by the resident hospital flora. This flora includes aerobic Gram-positive and Gram-negative organisms found to be the common causes of hospital-acquired infections of all body sites at that institution (16,17). In the pediatric hospital, it would also include viral etiologies for patients hospitalized with contagious and seasonal respiratory viral illnesses (18–21). In a study of susceptible hospitalized children, 17% developed a respiratory illness with a viral etiology confirmed in two-thirds. The frequency of nosocomial viral pneumonia in children has been shown to be highest in the youngest patients, those under 2 years of age, in whom the rate of nosocomial infection in winter may reach or exceed 45% (18–21).

The normal flora of most patients upon admission to the hospital consists of both Gram-positive and Gram-negative organisms with species of *Neisseria* and staphylococci predominating. In colder months, many healthy individuals are routinely colonized with *Haemophilus influenzae* and *Streptococcus pneumoniae* (16,17). Children in particular may also be asymptomatically colonized with *Streptococcus pyogenes*. This normal flora routinely protects against colonization with aerobic Gram-negative bacilli and other Gram-positive organisms. The risk of colonization has been verified by studies that have demonstrated that only 3% of healthy individuals are colonized with Gram-negative bacilli upon admission to the hospital (22). Studies in healthy adult volunteers have shown that radioactively labeled concentrations of 10^8 colony forming units per milliliter of *Escherichia coli*, *Klebsiella pneumoniae*, and *Proteus mirabilis* have regularly failed to result in colonization that could be demonstrated for more than a few hours (16). Colonization, which is defined as the presence of these Gram-positive and Gram-negative organisms not considered to be part of normal flora, occurs regularly in hospitalized patients (23,24). This bacterial colonization has been shown to increase with the severity of the patients illness and will be seen in up to 45% of patients hospitalized in an adult medical-surgical intensive care unit after 96 hours. Up to 25% of these patients have been shown to become colonized in the first 24 hours (22). The risk factors for colonization have been identified and include acidosis, endotracheal intubation, hypotension, and broad spectrum antibiotic therapy (25).

Turbulence in the nasal passageways normally results in the impaction of large particles, preventing deposition in the lower respiratory tract. Nasotracheal, orotracheal, or tracheostomy tubes bypass this initial host defense mechanism for preventing colonization of the upper respiratory tract. The importance of this colonization has been demonstrated by the fact that 23% of colonized patients develop nosocomial pneumonia while only 3% of noncolonized hospitalized patients develop nosocomial pneumonia (16).

Fibronectin, an adhesive glycoprotein found in serum and on a variety of cell surfaces, appears important in the resistance of colonization. Under normal conditions, buccal cells coated with fibronectin selectively allow for adherence of Gram-positive bacteria. This prevents the adherence of Gram-negative bacilli on buccal or tracheal cells (26,27). The important factor in this fibronectin selective adherence is the recent documentation that increased levels of salivary proteases occur in seriously ill hospitalized patients. This increased protease content of saliva has been shown to be associated with the loss of fibronectin from buccal cell surfaces and an increased adherence and colonization of airway surfaces with Gram-negative bacilli (28). This disruption of the normal biochemical milieu of the upper respiratory tract would allow environmental Gram-negative bacilli or other nosocomial pathogens to gain a foothold in the upper respiratory tract. Although the implications of these preceding biochemical observations are uncertain, they might form the basis of new strategies in prevention of airway bacterial colonization in high-risk patient groups.

Numerous observations have suggested that respiratory epithelium of hospitalized patients has increased affinity for attachment of Gram-negative bacilli (29–31). In studies of in vitro bacterial adherence using buccal cells from various patient groups, there appears to be a predictive pattern for the risk of subsequent bacteria colonization of the upper and lower respiratory tract (30). Bacterial lectins, such as pili on cell membranes of *Pseudomonas aeruginosa*, have been indentified as important factors in adherence to airway mucosa. Receptors on respiratory epithelial cells may also be important in mediating attachment of Gram-negative bacilli (32). A sialic acid moiety on cell surfaces or tracheal mucin has been implicated as a receptor for *Pseudomonas aeruginosa* (33).

The source of colonizing flora in these patient populations would be important in schemes for prevention of upper airway colonization. A fecal to oral route for bacterial contamination of respiratory airways has historically been suspected for bedridden patients. This route has not been able to readily explain the frequency of colonization by organisms such as *Pseudomonas aeruginosa* and *Acinetobacter species*, which are not usual inhabitants of the human gastrointestinal tract. In studies addressing this circumstance, patients having daily cultures monitored from rectal, hypopharyngeal, and tracheal sites following prolonged intubation commonly have enterobacteriaceae in the hypopharynx and rectum prior to their appearance in tracheal cultures. In contrast, nonenterobacteriaceae, such as *Pseudomonas aeruginosa* and *Acinetobacter species*, were rarely found in these sites prior to their appearance in the trachea. These studies suggest that environmental sources exist primarily for nonenterobacteriaceae and that colonizing enterobacteriaceae originate primarily from the patient's endogenous flora (34,35). From these works, investigators have suggested that the most important factors for transmission of this environmental flora are the hands of health care personnel and respiratory therapy equipment (36). Other factors in the modern intensive care unit that can enhance bacterial colonization of critically ill patients include the increasingly popular nebulized or aerosolized respiratory therapy medications and gastric alkalization to prevent stress gastritis, ulcers, and bleeding. These procedures have been shown to produce larger numbers of patients with extensive bacterial overgrowth in the upper gastrointestinal and respiratory tract. This in turn appears to lead to airway colonization secondary to aspiration of gastric microflora (37–42).

In critically ill patients with prolonged hospitalization, the role of malnutrition on upper respiratory tract colonization has recently been described. The potential for colonization of the buccal mucosa with nonenterobacteriaceae was directly and significantly correlated with the level of malnutrition. In these studies, a nutritional index that measured serum albumin and total lymphocyte counts as an indicator of malnutrition correlated with an increased colonization by these organisms (31).

Nosocomial pneumonia is felt to result when these colonizing organisms evade the mucociliary and cellular defenses of the lower respiratory tract. This may be due to a direct effect on the mucociliary apparatus and cellular host defenses in the lower respiratory tract, as seen with infections such as influenza, or due to a primary or secondary immunodeficiency state, as seen in neutropenic cancer chemotherapy patients (43–45). The most important factor predisposing to nosocomial pneumonia is endotracheal intubation. Both short-term intubation for surgery or airway maintenance as well as longer intubation for respiratory failure are associated with the highest recorded frequencies of nosocomial pneumonia in the range of 15–20%. Recent studies have shown the incidence of nosocomial pneumonia for intubated patients to be 4-fold higher than that of the nonintubated patients; tracheostomy tube placement seems to have an even higher risk of nosocomial pneumonia (17). The fact that these are critically ill patients requiring prolonged hospitalization in intensive care units is an obvious reason for this increased risk. However, the endotracheal tube also eliminates the most effective natural host defense mechanism of the upper airway. The filtration system of the upper airway and the mucociliary clearance system of the larger airways are bypassed during intubation. Accentuating this loss of mucociliary transport is the mechanical irritation and damage of the respiratory epithelium, which can predispose to local colonization with potential bacterial and viral pathogens (11,14).

Finally, the current liberal use of broad spectrum antibiotic therapy in the hospital setting has also been associated with an increased risk of nosocomial pneumonia. The incidence of nosocomial pneumonia in antibiotic-treated hospitalized patients has been reported at several times that reported in general hospital patients not receiving antibiotics. Therefore, the indiscriminate use of broad spectrum antibiotic chemotherapy is felt to be a potential cause of increased colonization with multiple resistant Gram-positive and Gram-negative bacteria (46,47).

Nosocomial pneumonia may also occur as a result of metastatic infections secondary to bacteremia or primary infection at a distant site. Recent investigations have implied that distant infections, such as peritonitis, may also contribute to the establishment of nosocomial pneumonia. The infrequent association of nosocomial pneumonia with bacteremia suggests that primary respiratory infection is the most common route. Distant infection may selectively sequester polymorphonuclear leukocytes away from the lung. This could explain the increased mortality from Gram-negative pneumonia in these cases (43).

Cellular elements of pulmonary host defense in the lung include the resident mononuclear phagocyte, the alveolar macrophage, which forms a vital component of defense against Gram-positive bacterial organisms and viruses. The presence of polymorphonuclear leukocytes (PMNs) has been shown to be more important in effective host defense against Gram-negative bacillary pulmonary infections (48). It has recently been demonstrated that cellular host defense activity by alveolar macrophages may be ineffective in bacterial clearance during sepsis, septic shock, and/or the adult respiratory distress syndrome (49,50). Ineffective cellular host defense capabilities in these situations would increase the risk for morbidity and mortality from nosocomial pneumonia.

Therefore, the factors predisposing to nosocomial pneumonia include age, (premature and low birthweight newborns), poor nutritional status, underlying pulmonary immune status, length of time in the hospital, general anesthesia, endotracheal intubation, tracheostomy, inhalation therapy, antibiotic therapy, and respiratory tract colonization with Gram-negative bacilli.

POPULATION

Understanding the importance of nosocomial pneumonia requires that the major risk factors for acquisition of this disease be compared with the high-risk groups for worst outcome. Any patient hospitalized today would be considered to have an added risk for nosocomial pneumonia. However, the patient groups that manifest stress, including acidosis, hypotension, hypoperfusion, an altered state of conscious-ness, and any patient requiring nasotracheal, or-otracheal or nasogastric intubation have an increased risk for a poor outcome (1,5,11,25). A special category in the pediatric setting are the groups at risk for symptomatic or asymp-tomatic aspiration. These include children with tracheoesophageal fistulae, swallowing dys-coordination, gastroesophageal reflux, and sur-gery patients with unprotected airways. These patients are at increased risk for aspiration of resident flora in the hypopharynx. The circum-stances in which these children have been hos-pitalized for diagnostic workup or treatment of these underlying diseases increases the risk for nosocomial pneumonia with hospital-acquired pathogens. Also included in this group would be patients with primary and secondary myopa-thies with altered swallowing mechanisms, and children with facial burns and smoke inhalation requiring prolonged hospitalization. Children with underlying pulmonary disease, cardiac disease (especially shunt lesions with pulmonary hy-pertension), and primary immunodeficiencies (severe combined immune deficiency) have a marked risk for fatal outcome with nosocomial pneumonia (1,51–53).

Malnutrition is also a risk factor that increases the incidence of nosocomial pneumonia in pe-diatrics. Included in this group of high-risk pa-tients would be immunosuppressed children. The risk for bacterial and viral pneumonia with a fatal outcome in children with primary immu-nodeficiencies has been well-documented. Sec-ondary immunodeficiencies, such as cancer chemotherapy and organ transplant recipients, make up a large group of individuals who are at high risk for nosocomial pneumonia. Included in this group of high-risk children is the pre-mature newborn. A premature newborn requires prolonged hospitalization frequently with ex-tended endotracheal intubation as major risk fac-tors for nosocomial pneumonia. These predisposing factors, coupled with an underly-ing immune system that is not the equivalent of older children and adults, plus the continued problem of nutrition makes the premature new-born one of the highest risk patient groups for nosocomial pneumonia currently in pediatrics (1,7,12,17,51,53). Therefore, these high-risk patients groups in conjunction with predisposing factors for upper respiratory tract colonization, altered local and/or systemic host defense pa-rameters, underlying disease states, and age are at increased risk for nosocomial pneumonia and excessive mortality.

Etiologic Agents

The relationship between etiologic agents and mortality from nosocomial pneumonia has been of great clinical interest and importance. The etiology of nosocomial pneumonia has been shown to be relatively predictable with the ma-jority of cases due to Gram-negative bacillary organisms, while Gram-positive organisms make up the second largest group. In several studies, the mortality associated with Gram-negative ba-cillary pneumonias is frequently estimated to be about 50%. This is compared with a mortality rate from Gram-positive pneumonias which has been reported to be between 5–24%. Among Gram-negative bacillary deaths, those infections associated with *Pseudomonas aeruginosa* have demonstrated the highest mortality rate between 70–80% (1,2,7,9,14). Viral nosocomial pneu-monias, which have been described as being nonfatal in most circumstances, have been par-ticularly prominent in children with secondary immunodeficiency states, such as cancer che-motherapy and organ transplantation (54–56). Nosocomial pneumonia due to respiratory syn-cytial virus in patients with congenital heart dis-ease—in particular, shunt lesions with pulmonary hypertension—have an excessive mortality rate ranging from 40–80% (51,53).

Specific etiologic organisms for nosocomial pneumonia have been variable from institution to institution. Clinicians must therefore be aware of the organisms and the antibiotic susceptibility data of these organisms at their own institutions. The bacteriology of nosocomial pneumonia demonstrates the important role of aerobic Gram-negative bacilli. The Gram-negative bacilli: *Escherichia coli*, *Klebsiella pneumoniae*, and *Pseudomonas aeruginosa* are the most common etiologies and comprise up to 73% of all isolates described in nosocomial pneumonia studies. *Staphylococcus aureus* and *Staphylococcus ep-idermidis* are seen in up to 20% of cases. Other Gram-negative bacilli, including *Acinetobacter species* and *Proteus species*, make up most of the remainder (7,17). In most cases, single path-ogens have been identified. However, in 10–25% of cases, polymicrobial Gram-negative pneumonias have been reported (16). The NNIS data of 1983 indicates that the two most common bacterial etiologic agents causing nosocomial pneumonia in children were Gram-negative rods (Table 2.1). The predominance of Gram-negative bacillary pathogens as etiological agents for nosocomial pneumonia has been noted in community hospitals as well as teaching centers (7). Among the Gram-positive bacteria, *Staphylococcus aureus* is by far the most common. *Streptococcus pneumoniae*, the most frequent bacteria in community-acquired pneumonias for patients over 6 years of age, accounts for less than 3% of all bacterial nosocomial pneumonias (7,17). *Legionella pneumophila* and *Legionella micdadei* have also been implicated in outbreaks of nosocomial pneumonia. The true incidence of nosocomial pneumonia for the *Legionella species* is not known in children and probably varies among hospitals (57–59). In pediatric hospitals, the consideration for nonpneumococcal streptococci and *Haemophilus influenza* type B exist (7,17). Although these organisms are much more common as etiologic agents in community-acquired pneumonias, nosocomial acquisition of these bacterial pathogens secondary to a distant infection with bacteremia or direct respiratory tract spread should be considered (60).

In the neonatal intensive care unit, the consideration of *Staphylococcus epidermidis* as a potential cause of nosocomial infections, including pneumonia, has been recently suggested as an important cause of infection (Table 2.1). Therefore, in the neonatal intensive care unit, Gram-negative bacilli and Gram-positive aerobic infections, including *Staphylococcus epidermidis*, must be considered as potential etiologies in nosocomial pneumonia (12,61).

Nosocomial pneumonia secondary to fungi have been an increasing part of the clinician's dilemma in treating nosocomial pneumonia in the past two decades (62). Fungal infections have become special problems in immunosuppressed children. The lung remains one of the most commonly identifiable sites of infection among immunosuppressed patients. Neutropenic patients are at particular risk for acquiring aerobic Gram-negative bacillary pneumonias, even in the absence of endotracheal intubation. With the use of broad spectrum antibiotic therapy in immunosuppressed patients for suspect bacterial infections, fungal etiologies in pulmonary infections have become increasingly important (Table 2.1) (63). *Aspergillus species* pneumonia has been associated with neutropenia as well as corticosteroid usage. Construction near hospital sites as well as contaminated fireproofing materials and air conditioning equipment have also been associated with nosocomial pulmonary aspergillosis (64,65). *Candida species*, including *Candida albicans, Candida tropicalis, Candida paraspilosis* and *Torulopsis glabrata*, have become an increasing cause of nosocomial infection, including pneumonia in neutropenic cancer chemotherapy patients. The potential importance of fungal infections in these patient groups is recognized by the current use of empiric antifungal therapy in febrile neutropenic patients who are unresponsive to empiric antibacterial chemotherapy (63).

Although viruses have been felt to be a less frequent cause of nosocomial pneumonia in the past, several viral respiratory pathogens are more common than generally acknowledged (Table 2.1). This potential for the underreporting of viral nosocomial pneumonias is primarily due to difficulties with the diagnostic techniques necessary for identifying these etiologic agents. With the advent of improved rapid diagnostic testing and culture capabilities in modern virology laboratories, the true incidence of viral

Table 2.1
Etiologic Agents Causing Nosocomial Pneumonia in Children

Bacteria	Fungi	Viruses
K. pneumoniae	Candida	Respiratory syncytial virus
P. aeruginosa	Aspergillus	Influenzae A/B
S. aureus		Parainfluenza virus
S. epidermidis		Adenovirus
Enterococci		Cytomegalovirus
Other Gram-negative		Varicella-zoster virus
bacilli		Herpes simplex virus
S. pneumoniae		Measles
H. influenzae		

nosocomial pneumonias in pediatric patients is beginning to be elucidated. In a recent survey, it was reported that viral agents accounted for 20% of all nosocomial lower respiratory tract infections during a 17-month surveillance period in a general hospital setting. The majority of these nosocomial viral pneumonia cases in this study occurred on pediatric wards (20). Other recent reports have observed that viral etiologies are in fact the most common cause of nosocomial pneumonia in the pediatric patient population (19,21).

Particular attention has recently been focused on two viral pathogens, respiratory syncytial virus (RSV) and influenza A, as important etiologic agents for nosocomial respiratory infection (66–69). In one study, over 40% of hospitalized infant contacts developed RSV infection during hospitalization (18). In a second report, seven hospitalized adults with debilitating disease developed nosocomial influenza A pneumonia after exposure to a single index case (67). Furthermore, although RSV and influenza appear to be the most common viral agents causing nosocomial pneumonias, occasional outbreaks have been reported with other viral agents, including parainfluenza, adenovirus, measles, and varicella-zoster viruses (19,20). Recently, more clinicans have recognized that rotavirus, the most common cause of nosocomial viral gastroenteritis, has respiratory symptoms as a presenting sign/symptom; pneumonia, however, is not common (70). The importance of viral nosocomial infections has to be considered with the seasonal occurrence of the specific viruses, including RSV and the influenza viruses. The recent availability of the new antiviral drug, ribavirin (Virazole), for the treatment of RSV bronchiolitis–pneumonia in high-risk patient groups has made the rapid diagnosis of RSV disease an important cause of nosocomial pneumonia (71). RSV has been shown to be a common cause of nosocomial viral pneumonia in high-risk patient groups. These include children with primary immunodeficiencies, congenital heart disease (cyanotic lesions, pulmonary hypertension), children with underlying lung disease, which includes bronchopulmonary dysplasia and immunosuppressed children on cancer chemotherapeutic regimens (53). Recently, cancer chemotherapy patients have been shown to have an increased risk for lower respiratory tract infection with a fatal outcome. Keep in mind that the majority of these patients acquired RSV as a nosocomial process. It is also important to note that children with RSV generally have more severe disease with decreasing age, usually under two years of age. However, in the cancer chemotherapy patient group, children over two years of age who acquired nosocomial RSV also developed lower respiratory tract infection with a significant increased risk for intensive care monitoring and a fatal outcome (53).

DIAGNOSIS

The optimal method for diagnosis of nosocomial pneumonia remains undefined and controversial. Diagnosis has historically been made on clinical grounds with an appropriate chest roentgenogram, Gram stain, and culture of respiratory tract secretions. Unfortunately, this definition has probably overestimated the true incidence of nosocomial pneumonia as many other entities can be easily confused in the critically ill patient (72–77). This necessity for proper identification of an infectious process is more important in the adult populations in which pulmonary emboli, myocardial infarction with congestive heart failure, and chronic lung disease can mimic nosocomial pneumonia. The recognition that chest roentgenographic changes seen in the adult respiratory distress syndrome are not necessarily associated with an infectious process have also made the diagnosis of nosocomial pneumonia difficult in some adult patients. This has caused internists to rely on invasive monitoring of pulmonary capillary wedge pressures, central venous, and mean arterial blood pressures in an attempt to delineate cardiac causes for chest roentgenogram alterations. In the pediatric patient, these underlying diseases are not as commonly encountered. However, high-risk patient groups, including children with congenital heart disease, bronchopulmonary dysplasia, and cancer chemotherapy patients receiving irradiation and antimetabolite chemotherapy, have caused similar confusing radiographic circumstances for pediatricians. These situations have been further confused with the finding that fever is associated with pulmonary infiltrates caused by several of these entities (77).

Bacteria

Recent data suggest a poor correlation between culture results obtained from endotracheal suction specimens and those from otherwise sterile sites, such as lung, blood, and pleural cultures (75–77). As many as 75% of upper airway cultures represent colonization rather than invasive infections (22), but up to 30% of the time, infection is mistaken for colonization (75). The difficulty in interpreting upper airway bacterial cultures is accentuated by the fact that patients in the intensive care environment generally have abnormal chest roentgenograms whether or not lung infection is present. Similarly, fever and leukocytosis are common in these patients irrespective of pneumonia. Cough and sputum production have little relevance in the intubated patient and are infrequent diagnostic indicators in children. Even when the tracheobronchial secretions are purulent, the differentiation between tracheobronchitis and pneumonia may be difficult. Therefore, the clinical suspicion is the first and foremost characteristic in the proper diagnosis of nosocomial pneumonia.

Considerations in the diagnosis of nosocomial pneumonia should include a change in the clinical status of the patient that is unexplained by other events. These changes may include a drop in oxygenation, an increased requirement in supplemental oxygen therapy, the presence of metabolic acidosis, or increasing ventilator pressure requirements. A change in the fever pattern with a concomitant increase in the quantity and purulence of respiratory secretions should be clues to the potential presence of an infectious process. These factors, in combination with a sudden increase in a previously diagnosed lung infiltrate or a new infiltrate, should make the clinician suspicious of a potential nosocomial pneumonia. While such criteria may lack both sensitivity and specificity, they may be the only available parameters for the clinician (1). Also included in this consideration is the etiology of the nosocomial pneumonia. This should take into account the epidemiology of the intensive care and patient environment. Close contact with adjacent patients sharing nursing or respiratory therapy personnel should be considered as a potential for the etiology of these changes. Recent patient exposure to respiratory syncytial virus or influenza virus should be considerations as to the etiology of these changes (78,79). Recent transfusions in newborns or organ transplantation recipients would raise cytomegalovirus as a possibility (80,81). Also, the bacteriological flora of the intensive care or patient care facility should be considered at this time.

Once it has been determined that a potential nosocomial pneumonia exists, the clinician must begin to identify the specific etiologic organism. In patients with prolonged intubation and respiratory therapy, serial respiratory tract secretion Gram stains may assist the clinician in determining if an inflammatory and potentially infectious process exists. Microscopic examination of upper respiratory tract secretions by Gram stain will reveal an increased influx of PMNs and the presence or absence of a predominate bacterial organism (2). Unfortunately, these specimens are often contaminated with upper airway flora. Similarly, cultures of such specimens may or may not reflect the microbiology of infected lung tissue. Isolation of a single organism, bacterial or fungal, from blood cultures can help to differentiate between contaminating and infecting bacterial isolates in the respiratory secretions of these patients. However, recent data suggest that only 2–5% of blood cultures are positive for bacterial organisms from patients with nosocomial pneumonia (7). Blood cultures in a patient with suspected nosocomial pneumonia are therefore justified, but a high percentage yield should not be expected. The presence of pleural fluid should always be investigated as a potential microbiologic diagnostic sample. Since microbiologic evaluation of contaminated respiratory specimens can be misleading, a number of invasive methods have been developed to obtain noncontaminated specimens for diagnostic evaluation. The use of quantitative sputum cultures, washed sputum cultures, and microscopic screening of sputa for the presence of upper airway cells suggesting contamination have all been evaluated but have been met with significant controversy regarding their actual usefulness (74–77). Unfortunately, these are the only major specimens available to clinicians treating critically ill intubated children for nosocomial pneumonia.

Transtracheal aspiration in nonintubated patients, percutaneous thin needle lung aspiration, and protected shielded-tip bronchoscopic sampling of lower airway secretions have all been suggested as methods that avoid upper airway contamination of respiratory specimens (82–92). All these methods may in fact increase diagnostic specificity in patients, but they many not be well-tolerated by certain critically ill patients with suspected pneumonia (93,94). The percutaneous thin needle lung aspiration has been considered to be contraindicated in patients on positive pressure breathing modes (91). Quantitative cultures of shielded-tip bronchoscopic sampling have recently been considered to have a rather high rate of false-positive results (90). The recent description of protected transbronchial needle aspiration (pigtail catheter) in adult patients with suspect nosocomial pneumonia has been suggested to be superior to protected specimen brush culture (95). For patients with histologic evidence of pneumonia, excellent microbiologic correlation between lung tissues and bronchoscopic specimens have been noted. However, for patients without pneumonia, a high incidence of false-positive results among the bronchoscopic specimens have been reported.

In a recent study, bronchoalveolar lavage in immunocompromised patients proved to be similar to open-lung biopsy for the diagnosis of cytomegalovirus, *Pneumocystis carinii*, and atypical mycobacteria (96). The ability to do flexible bronchoscopy to obtain these specimens from intubated patients with nosocomial pneumonia and the adult respiratory distress syndrome is a fairly new approach which is being investigated. Results to allow sensitivity and specificity analysis regarding patients with these entities compared with patients without pneumonia are currently being evaluated. These procedures are of less importance in the pediatric age population because of the current lack of a small flexible bronchoscope with access for suctioning or brush passage into the lower respiratory tract for sampling. Therefore, in smaller children who are unable to safely receive an adult flexible bronchoscope, these procedures are unavailable.

Urine bacterial antigen detection systems have recently been shown to be efficacious in identifying common community-acquired etiologic agents for pneumonia in children (97). Bacterial antigen detection systems for *Haemophilus influenzae* type B, *Streptococcus pneumoniae*, and group B streptococci (newborn), have added to the diagnostic capabilities of blood culture isolation in children with community-acquired pneumonia. Since these organisms are not common causes of nosocomial pneumonia in children, its current utility is minimized. Identification of certain bacterial organisms by direct fluorescent antibody microscopy has added to the diagnostic capabilities for nosocomial acquisition

of *Legionella pneumophila* and *Bordetella pertussis* (98). These specimens taken from the nasopharynx and/or endotracheal tube are examined by direct fluorescent antibody microscopy using fluorescenated monoclonal antibody stained specimens. Therefore, for the diagnosis of bacterial nosocomial pneumonia in the pediatric population, the reliance upon blood cultures with a 2–5% yield, direct fluorescent antibody microscopy, bacterial antigen detection systems, and the occasional patient who will tolerate a thin needle direct lung aspiration are the mainstays for the diagnosis for bacterial nosocomial pneumonia. Although an influx of PMNs with a predominant organism in the endotracheal tube culture suggests a nosocomial infectious process, these procedures have not been proven to be diagnostic. The potential use of a double-lumen plugged catheter by blind passage has been proposed in critically ill children, but awaits further study before its usefulness and safety are determined (99).

Fungi

In immunocompromised children with nosocomial pneumonias unresponsive to broad-spectrum antibiotic therapy regimens, the alternative of open-lung biopsy with special histologic stains and cultures has been used in a number of situations. The diagnosis of nosocomial pneumonia due to *Aspergillus* and *Candida species* may be suspected by examination of wet preps of endotracheal tube secretions. Confirmation may be proven by histological examination and culture of tracheobronchial or open-lung biopsy material.

Viruses

The diagnosis of viral nosocomial pneumonia has been enhanced significantly over the past decade by the advent of better virologic tissue culture capabilities and by rapid diagnostic testing (98). Compared with the problems of bacterial colonization of the upper respiratory tract, the presence of a viral pathogen in the upper respiratory tract in patients with a compatible chest roentgenogram and clinical presentation has been felt to be diagnostic. We currently have the ability to culture influenza viruses, respiratory syncytial virus, adenovirus, and varicella-zoster virus; cytomegalovirus and herpes simplex virus are now proven causes of pneumonia in immunocompromised and organ transplant patients. Rapid diagnostic tests for cell-associated antigens have improved our capability for the identification of these etiologies for nosocomial pneumonia. Fluorescent microscopic analysis (FA) and enzyme-linked immunosorbent assay (ELISA) antigen detection systems have increased the ability to make the rapid diagnosis of respiratory syncytial virus and influenzae virus from upper respiratory tract secretions and cellular debris in these patients (98). The cultures of these specimens and the rapid diagnostic testing capabilities are highly dependent upon proper specimen collection. The necessity for acquiring upper respiratory tract cellular debris is paramount for reliable diagnoses. Fluorescent antibody and ELISA techniques require cellular debris for the detection of cellular antigens from these viruses. For viral culture, similar types of specimens are important for increasing the yield from a nasal wash or lavage. It is up to the clinician to inform the virology laboratory of the major viruses considered in the diagnostic workup. This will allow the virology laboratory to select the appropriate tissue culture cell lines to increase the yield for a positive culture.

The sensitivity and specificity of the rapid diagnostic tests for viral etiologies from properly collected specimens have varied between 85–95%. Therefore, for select viral groups, rapid diagnostic capabilities have the possibility for accurate diagnosis of the nosocomial pneumonia (98). Improved antiviral chemotherapy over the past decade provides an added incentive for the clinician to confirm cultures for viral nosocomial pneumonias which are not currently accessible by rapid diagnostic tools.

The future of rapid diagnostic capabilities in nosocomial pneumonia has recently been enhanced by the advent of DNA probes. These DNA/DNA, RNA/DNA probes with their high degree of specificity from properly collected specimens should provide an increased sensitivity for the diagnosis of an etiologic cause of nosocomial pneumonia for organisms that have in the past been difficult to identify. They should also broaden and increase the number of organisms that would be identifiable from the respiratory tract and tissue samples (100).

Although rapid diagnostic tests have recently improved our capabilities for diagnosing viral and bacterial nosocomial pneumonias, culture confirmation remains important. Culture of bacterial isolates is significant because of its availability for antibiotic susceptibility testing. In an era of widespread use and abuse of antibiotics, susceptibility data are important in allowing the clinician to select the appropriate antibiotic(s) to be used in empiric and specific therapy regimens.

TREATMENT

Treatment of nosocomial pneumonia may be empiric or specific. Empiric treatment is employed for cases of clinically suspected pneumonia in which an identified etiologic agent is not available to guide specific therapy. When a specific bacterial etiology is identified and antibiotic susceptibility data are available, specific therapy may be chosen. Intravenous antibiotics remain the conventional form of treatment for nosocomial bacterial pneumonia, although recent investigation with inhaled endobronchial antibiotics (101,102) and passive immunization (103) have been reported. Several factors must be considered in the selection of an appropriate empiric antibiotic therapy regimen (1). Patient records must be reviewed to identify recently administered antibiotics which could select resistant organisms as the etiology for this nosocomial infection. The parents must be interviewed for the possibility of underlying disease states, such as cystic fibrosis, which would predispose the patient to *Pseudomonas species* and *Staphylococcus aureus* infections. Special groups, including premature newborns with an increased risk for *Staphylococcus epidermidis* infections, and the potential for empiric antifungal therapy in immunocompromised patients should be taken into account. Recent surveillance cultures of the patient's sputum have consistently identified a particular organism. These findings should be taken into account, and antibiotic therapy should cover the individual organism and its susceptibility pattern. Although this organism may not be the etiologic agent involved in the lower respiratory tract, it is advisable to be sure that the empiric antibiotic regimen includes that organism. It would also be important to review recent patterns of nosocomial pathogens in the specific hospital or intensive care unit. If the environment has a particularly high incidence of pneumonia or other nosocomial infections caused by multiple antibiotic-resistant *Pseudomonas species* or *Acine-*

tobacter antitratus during the past several months, empiric antibiotic therapy should cover those susceptibility antibiograms. Another important consideration is the presence or absence of *Legionella species* in the proven cases of nosocomial pneumonia in that institution. In the pediatric wards, seasonal or recent nosocomial outbreaks of viral or mycoplasmal respiratory infections in the community should likewise be considered.

In general, empiric treatment of nosocomial pneumonias should include coverage of aerobic Gram-negative bacilli. In high-risk patients, this should also include highly resistant organisms, such as *Pseudomonas* and *Acinetobacter*. Empiric therapy should also include Gram-positive organisms, such as *Staphylococcus aureus*. The identification of a high frequency of methicillin-resistant *Staphylococcus aureus* (104) and/or the consideration of *Staphylococcus epidermidis* in the premature newborn would guide the clinician in selecting the specific antistaphylococcal regimen that would include vancomycin. Based upon these considerations, several regimens have been employed for empiric treatment of nosocomial pneumonia (Table 2.2). These regimens provide broad spectrum antibacterial activity for nosocomial pneumonia in pediatrics. In the event

that a specific etiologic agent is identified, specific antibacterial therapeutic regimens of single or multiple drugs may be considered. They should be selected based upon the antibiotic susceptibility data for that pathogen.

Recent controversies include the role of aminoglycosides in treating Gram-negative pneumonia. Select investigations have questioned the usefulness of aminoglycosides in treating pneumonia (105–108). The narrow therapeutic ratios for achievable levels in the serum of aminoglycosides and the difficulty in penetration from blood into the respective respiratory secretions and tissues may result in local drug concentrations insufficient for treating the infecting organisms (107,108). An alternative consideration is the recent suggestion that aminoglycosides are more active than β-lactam antibiotics against certain resistant Gram-negative bacilli, such as *Pseudomonas*. With these considerations and with the advent of the newer third generation cephalosporins, the potential use of alternative drug therapy or direct intratracheal instillation of aminoglycosides has emerged (109,110). In a recent report, patients receiving parenteral antibiotics plus aerosol aminoglycoside therapy in saline suspension instilled into the respiratory tract every 8 hours, versus saline aerosol instillations,

Table 2.2
Empiric Treatment of Nosocomial Pneumonia

	Immunocompetent		
Intubated/instrumented	nafcillin[a] clindamycin	plus	aminoglycoside[b] cephalosporin cefotaxime
Methicillin-resistant organisms prevalent	vancomycin[c]	plus	aminoglycoside cephalosporin cefotaxime
Nonintubated, age less than 6 years[d]	nafcillin clindamycin	plus	cephalosporin cefotaxime
	Immunocompromised		
No prior antibiotics	nafcillin clindamycin	plus	aminoglycoside cephalosporin ceftazidime
Prior antibiotics ± indwelling catheter	vancomycin	plus	aminoglycoside[e] cephalosporin ceftazidime
Unresponsive to antibiotics	erythromycin[f] amphotericin B		

[a]Substitute methicillin in the neonate.
[b]Gentamicin, tobramycin, amikacin dependent on susceptibility data for individual institution.
[c]Vancomycin also indicated in the neonatal intensive care unit if *S. epidermidis* is prevalent.
[d]Includes *H. influenzae* as metastatic site from primary infection.
[e]Change of aminoglycoside, cephalosporin, or addition of a ticarcillin, Timentin, piperacillin, azlocillin, or imipenem to cover resident *Pseudomonas species*.
[f]Added to existing regimen to cover *Legionella species*, if endemic.

revealed an increased treatment success rate with the inhaled aminoglycoside therapy (111). This was in spite of the fact that an equal superinfection rate with resistant flora was found between the two groups. The present usage of aerosolized or directly instilled aminoglycosides should be limited to multiple resistant Gram-negative bacilli with borderline achievable serum concentrations compared with the mean inhibitory concentration (MIC) of the organism.

In addition to antibiotics, immunologic methods of treatment of Gram-negative pneumonia have emerged with the availability of passive immune antisera, J-5 cross-protective antisera, and hyperimmune globulin (103,111). These modes of therapy are currently being evaluated in experimental models of Gram-negative pneumonia, but the clinical efficacy and role for these modes of therapy in nosocomial pneumonia are not available at this time.

The treatment of nosocomial pneumonia still relies upon intravenous antibiotics as the mainstay. The consideration for amphotericin B with or without 5-flucytosine should be considered for certain *Candida species*. There are no prospective studies evaluating the imidazoles (ketoconazole, itraconazole, or miconazole) versus amphotericin B for the treatment of fungal infections frequently involved in nosocomial pneumonia. Although the imidazoles have been shown to be effective in certain dimorphic fungal pulmonary infections such as cryptococcosis, blastomycosis, and histoplasmosis, their usefulness in invasive fungal infections caused by *Aspergillus* and *Candida species* have not been verified.

With the advent of acyclovir for the treatment of herpes simplex and varicella-zoster viral infections, antiviral therapy in immunocompromised patients with visceral involvement secondary to these viruses should be considered. herpes simplex and varicella-zoster virus have been shown to cause pneumonia in patients with community-acquired infections and less frequently as a cause of nosocomial pneumonia. These circumstances dictate that antiviral therapy with acyclovir should be instituted promptly based on the epidemiologic and clinical presentation of the patient. The recent licensing of the antiviral drug, ribavirin (Virazole), has brought widespread debate regarding its role in the treatment of viral respiratory pathogens. Certainly, the accumulated data support its efficacy against

respiratory syncytial virus in high-risk patient groups (71). These data should make ribavirin a prompt and early consideration for aerosol treatment in patients with RSV bronchiolitis-pneumonia who fall into these high-risk patient groups for a fatal outcome. These high-risk patients include congenital heart disease, pulmonary disease, and immunocompromised infants and children. Although not licensed, the use of ribavirin in patients on assisted ventilation via the endotracheal tube should be considered in these high-risk patient groups (53). Ribavirin has in vitro activity against other viral respiratory pathogens, including parainfluenza and influenza viruses. It is currently not approved for these indications, however.

PREVENTION

The prevention of nosocomial pneumonia involves environment, patient, and personnel. The fundamental object in preventing nosocomial pneumonia is to reduce the acquisition of potential pathogens in the upper airways and to thus reduce the potential for aspiration of these organisms into the lower respiratory tract. In the area of environment, compulsive care of the ventilator apparatus is always indicated. Ventilated patients should be suctioned regularly to decrease intrabronchial secretions. Those without support instrumentation should be routinely coughed and deep-breathed with respiratory therapy. Care should be taken to insure that medications and other material used for respiratory support are sterile. Disposable substances should be used when feasible. Patients should be treated on the ventilator for the shortest possible time with extubation remaining a constant consideration to be weighed against the risk of nosocomial pneumonia. For situations in which resistant strains of organisms exist within an intensive care area, appropriate isolation precautions must be maintained. Patients who are either infected or colonized should be selectively grouped or isolated (cohorted). Aerosolized antibiotics for prophylaxis (112,114) against bacterial colonization should not be considered as a routine procedure. However, in outbreaks of pneumonia caused by a single pathogen, such as *Acinetobacter*, the use of this modality for short periods may prove beneficial.

The appropriate design and staffing of critical care areas is an important environmental consideration for the prevention of nosocomial pneumonia. Attention to environmental factors such as hand washing between patient contacts, compliance with hospital infection control policy, adherence to isolation procedures, reporting of communicable diseases with a multidisciplined approach between infection control personnel, infectious disease specialists, and primary care clinicians would assist in preventing or diminishing the importance of nosocomial pneumonia (114).

While most attention has been focused upon prevention of nosocomial Gram-negative pneumonia, effective methods for reducing endemic nosocomial bacterial and viral infections have also been reported. Regarding *Legionella species*, measures that have largely employed hyperchlorination of contaminated potable water within the hospital have been shown to reduce the incidence of nosocomial infection (58). In addition, limited success has been achieved in controlling nosocomial viral respiratory infections. Respiratory syncytial virus is spread primarily by direct inoculation of large droplets or by direct contact. Thus, secretion precautions have been advocated for known cases. In a single study, isolation cohorting of staff to infected infants reduced the spread of RSV among patients, but not among hospital personnel (18). In a recent attempt to minimize nosocomial RSV during an outbreak, a disposable eye-nose goggle was used with promising results (115).

Influenza virus, on the other hand, may also be spread by small-particle aerosol. Thus, influenza may be spread more rapidly and is generally even more difficult to control during outbreaks (68,69). A surveillance system that monitors the emergence of viruses in the community can assist in the diagnosis of nosocomial pneumonia cases. An attempt to limit the number of contacts with other children, personnel, and symptomatic visitors will diminish traffic and exposure to respiratory viruses. Personnel with any respiratory symptoms need to be recognized as a potential hazard to very young or high-risk children. The length of hospitalization should be limited, personnel should not simultaneously care for uninfected and infected patients, and the limitation of elective hospitalization of high-risk patients during peak viral seasons may diminish infection rates (18).

Immunization may be an effective means for diminishing the significance of disease by nosocomial pneumonia for specific pathogens. Seasonal immunization of high-risk groups with influenza vaccines to include hospital workers is currently the most rational approach to controlling nosocomial influenza respiratory infection. An alternative to antibiotic prophylaxis, immunization is then proposed as a rational method for prevention of some bacterial nosocomial pneumonias. This approach has been evaluated in adults for *Pseudomonas aeruginosa* pneumonia using prophylactic immunization with a lipopolysaccharide vaccine (111). Although results from that study suggested that immunization reduced the incidence and mortality of *Pseudomonas* pneumonia, the experiment was limited to only 34 vaccinated patients. The recent development of hyperimmune anti-*Pseudomonas* globulin offers the potential for rapid immunization using passive administration of type-specific antibodies. An alternative and perhaps more rational suggestion would be to confer protection against Gram-negative species which serve as potential pathogens for the human respiratory tract. The use of cross-protective vaccines or antisera, such as the J-5 mutant of *E. coli* OlII might be a candidate immunogen (103). Even with recent clinical studies of J-5 antisera suggesting a protective role against Gram-negative septicemia, the relative degree of pulmonary protection provided by J-5 antisera has not been determined.

It is the opinion of most infection control personnel that many of the causes of nosocomial pneumonia are currently not preventable. The best chance to decrease morbidity and mortality lies in the early diagnosis and treatment with appropriate anti-infectives. Supportive therapy should be aggressive, and attempts to decrease or reverse organ failure should be vigorous.

SUMMARY

Nosocomial pneumonia continues to be a leading cause of fatal nosocomial infection in the United States. Although there are differences in pathogens by age, the importance of nosocomial pneumonia is apparent in the adult population as well as in the pediatric patient groups. The ability to diagnose these infections utilizing clinical suspicion and microbiologic/rapid diagnostic tests will allow the clinician to treat nosocomial pneumonia effectively in the critically ill patient. Unfortunately, these treatment modalities and preventive measures have not kept pace with our understanding of the pathogenesis of this infection. The pediatric patient population presents several unique and specific infection control, diagnostic, and treatment problems for the practicing clinician. The appropriate infection control and isolation policies for specific viral and multiple antibiotic-resistant bacterial isolates remains a cornerstone in the prevention of nosocomial pneumonia. The judicious use of empiric antibacterial chemotherapy remains important in the treatment of patients with nosocomial pneumonia. However, in the pediatric patient population, the recognition that viral and fungal etiologies are important causes of nosocomial pneumonia challenges the clinician to apply the appropriate diagnostic and effective treatment regimens in pediatric nosocomial pneumonias. The epidemiologic data for the clinician's own institution in determining the etiologic causes of nosocomial pneumonia, drug susceptibility patterns, and the seasonal and patient distribution of these infections are critical. Nosocomial pneumonia will continue to remain a significant cause of morbidity, mortality, and hospital cost in the United States in the forthcoming decades. The advent of new rapid diagnostic testing and improved treatment modalities for effective therapy and prevention will be aided by the increased availability of immunologic therapy for these disease states. Although these modalities show great promise, it will be up to the clinician to stay current on the field of nosocomial pneumonia, since it will continue to be a significant problem in the United States.

REFERENCES

1. Pennington JE: Hospital acquired pneumonia. In Wenzel RP (ed): *Prevention and Control of Nosocomial Infections*. Baltimore, Williams & Wilkins, 1987, pp 321–334.
2. Graybill JR, Marshall LW, Charache P, Wallace CK, Melvin VB: Nosocomial pneumonia: A continuing major problem. *Am Rev Respir Dis* 108:1130–1140, 1973.
3. Johanson WG, Pierce AK, Sanford JP: Changing pharyngeal bacterial flora of hospitalized patients: Emergence of Gram-negative bacilli. *N Engl J Med* 281:1137–1170, 1969.
4. Pierce AK, Sanford JP, Thomas GD, Leonard JS: Long-term evaluation of decontamination of inhalation-therapy equipment and the occurrence of necrotizing pneumonia. *N Engl J Med* 282:528–531, 1970.
5. Veazey JM, Jr: Hospital-acquired pneumonia. In Wenzel RP (ed): *CRC Handbook of Hospital Acquired Infections*. Boca Raton, FL, CRC Press, 1981, pp 341–369.
6. Bartlett JG, O'Keefe P, Tally FP, Louie TJ, Gorbach SL: Bacteriology of hospital-acquired pneumonia. *Arch Intern Med* 146:868–871, 1986.
7. Centers for Disease Control: National nosocomial infectious study report, annual summary, 1983. *MMWR* 33, 255:955–2155, 1985.
8. Welliver RC, McLaughlin S: Unique epidemiology of nosocomial infection in a children's hospital. *Am J Dis Child* 138:131–135, 1984.
9. Bryan CS and Reynolds KL: Bacteremic nosocomial pneumonia. *Am Rev Respir Dis* 129:668–671, 1984.
10. Bartlett JG: Invasive diagnostic techniques in respiratory infections. In Pennington JE (ed): *Respiratory Infections: Diagnosis and Management*. New York, Raven Press, 1983, pp 55–77.
11. Stevens RM, Teres D, Skillman JJ, Feingold DS: Pneumonia in an intensive-care unit. *Arch Intern Med* 134:106–111, 1974.
12. Hemming VG, Overall JC Jr, Britt MR: Nosocomial infections in a newborn intensive care unit. *N Engl J Med* 294:1310–1316, 1976.
13. Gross PA, Neu HC, Aswapokee P, VanAntwerpen C, Swapokee A: Deaths from nosocomial infections: Experience in a university hospital and a community hospital. *Am J Med* 68:219–223, 1980.
14. Garibaldi RA, Britt MR, Coleman ML, Reading JC, Pace NL: Risk factors for postoperative pneumonia. *Am J Med* 70:677–680, 1981.
15. Brown RB, Ryczak M, Sands M: Management of nosocomial pneumonia. *Hosp Form* 21:1208–1217, 1986.
16. LaForce FM, Hopkins J, Trow R, Wang WLL: Human oral defenses against Gram-negative rods. *Am Rev Respir Dis* 114:929–935, 1976.
17. Brook I: Bacterial colonization, tracheobronchitis, and pneumonia following tracheostomy and long-term intubation in pediatric patients. *Chest* 76:420–424, 1979.
18. Hall CB, Douglas RG Jr, Geiman JM, Messner MK: Nosocomial respiratory syncytial virus infections. *N Engl J Med* 293:1343–1346, 1975.
19. Wenzel RP, Deal EC, Hendley JO: Hospital-acquired viral respiratory illness on a pediatric ward. *Pediatrics* 60:367–371, 1977.
20. Valenti WM, Hall CB, Douglas RG Jr, Menegus MA, Pincus PH: Nosocomial viral infections. Epidemiology and significance. *Infect Control* 1:33–37, 1979.
21. Hall CB: Nosocomial viral respiratory infections: Perennial weeds on pediatric wards. *Pediatrics* 70:670–676, 1981.
22. Johanson WG, Pierce AK, Sanford JP: Nosocomial respiratory infections with Gram-negative bacilli. *Ann Intern Med* 77:701–706, 1972.
23. Johanson WG Jr, Pierce AK, Sanford JP: Changing pharyngeal bacterial flora of hospitalized patients. Emergence of Gram-negative bacilli. *N Engl J Med* 281:1437–1440, 1969.
24. Rose HD, Babcock JB: Colonization of intensive care unit patients with Gram-negative bacilli. *Am J Epidemiol* 101:495–501, 1975.
25. Craven DE, Kunches LM, Kilinsky V, Lichtenberg DA, Make BJ, McCabe WR: Risk factors for pneumonia and fatality in patients receiving continuous mechanical ventilation. *Am Rev Respir Dis* 133:792–796, 1986.
26. Woods DE, Straus DC, Johanson WG Jr, Bass JA: Role of fibronectin in the prevention of adherence of pseudomonas aeruginosa on buccal cells. *J Infect Dis* 143:784–790, 1981.
27. Abraham SN, Beachey EG, Simpson WA: Adherence of streptococcus pyogenes, Escherichia coli and Pseudomonas aeruginosa to fibronectin-coated and uncoated epithelial cells. *Infect Immun* 41:1261–1268, 1983.
28. Woods DE, Straus DC, Johanson WG Jr, Bass JA: Role of salivary protease activity in adherence of Gram-negative bacilli to mammalian buccal epithelial cells in vivo. *J Clin Invest* 68:1435–1440, 1981.
29. Johanson WG Jr, Higuchi JH, Chaudhuri TR, Woods DE: Bacterial adherence to epithelial cells in bacillary colonization of the respiratory tract. *Am Rev Respir Dis* 121:55–63, 1980.
30. Niederman MS, Rafferty TD, Sasaki CT, Merrill WM, Matthay RA, Reynolds HY: Comparison of bacterial adherence to ciliated and squamous epithelial cells obtained from the human respiratory tract. *Am Rev Respir Dis* 127:85–90, 1983.

31. Niederman MS, Merrill WM, Ferranti RD, Pagano K, Palmer LB, Reynolds HY: Nutritional status and bacterial binding in the lower respiratory tract in patients with chronic tracheostomy. *Ann Intern Med* 100:795–800, 1984.

32. Ramphal R, Sadoff JC, Pyle M, Silipigni JD: Role of pili in the adherence of Pseudomonas aeruginosa to injured tracheal epithelium. *Infect Immun* 44:38–40, 1984.

33. Ramphal R, Pyle M: Evidence of mucins and sialic acid as receptors for Pseudomonas aeruginosa in the lower respiratory tract. *Infect Immun* 41:339–344, 1983.

34. Schwartz SN, Dowling JN, Benkovic C, DeQuittner-Buchanan M, Prostko T, Yee RB: Sources of Gram-negative bacilli colonizing the trachea of intubated patients. *J Infect Dis* 138:227–231, 1978.

35. Sottile FD, Marrie TJ, Prough DS, Hobgood CD, Gower DH, Webb LX, Costerton JW, Gristinia AG: Nosocomial pulmonary infection: Possible etiologic significance of bacterial adhesion to endotracheal tubes. *Crit Care Med* 14:265–270, 1986.

36. Maki DG, Alvarado CJ, Hassemer CA, Zily MA: Relation of the inanimate hospital environment to endemic nosocomial infection. *N Engl J Med* 25:1562–1566, 1982.

37. Severe JL: Possible role of humidifying equipment in spread of infections from the newborn. *Pediatrics* 24:50–53, 1959.

38. Reinarz JA, Pierce AK, Mays BB, Sanford JP: Potential role of inhalation therapy equipment in nosocomial pulmonary infection. *J Clin Invest* 44:831–839, 1965.

39. Cross AS, Roupe B: Role of respiratory assistance devices in endemic nosocomial pneumonia. *Am J Med* 70:681–685, 1981.

40. Hoffman MA, Finberg L: Pseudomonas infections in infants associated with high-humidity environment. *J Pediatr* 46:626–630, 1985.

41. DuMoulin GC, Hedley-Whyte J, Paterson DG, Lisbon A: Aspiration of gastric bacteria in antacid treated patients: A frequent cause of postoperative colonization of the airway. *Lancet* 1:242–245, 1982.

42. Atherton ST, White DJ: Stomach as a source of bacteria colonizing respiratory tract during artificial ventilation. *Lancet* 2:968–969, 1978.

43. White JC, Nelson S, Winkelstein JA, McL. Booth FV, Jakab GJ: Impairment of antibacterial defense mechanisms of the lung by extrapulmonary infection. *J Infect Dis* 153:202–208, 1985.

44. Glezen WP: Viral pneumonia as a cause and result of hospitalization. *J Infect Dis* 147:765–770, 1983.

45. Segreti J, Bone RC: Nosocomial pneumonia and pneumonia in immunocompromised patients. *J Crit Illness* 1:55–65, 1986.

46. Louria DB, Kaminski T: The effects of four antimicrobial drug regimens on sputum superinfection in hospitalized patients. *Am Rev Respir Dis* 85:649–665, 1962.

47. Tillotson JR, Finland M: Bacterial colonization and clinical superinfection of the respiratory tract complicating antibiotic treatment of pneumonia. *J Infec Dis* 119:597–624, 1969.

48. Onofrio JM, Toews GB, Lipscomb MF, Pierce AK: Granulocyte-alveolar macrophage interaction in the pulmonary clearance of *Staphylococcus aureus. Am Rev Respir Dis* 127:335–341, 1983.

49. Jacobs RF, Kiel DP, Balk RA: Alveolar macrophage function in a canine model of endotoxin-induced lung injury. *Am Rev Respir Dis* 134:745–751, 1986.

50. Shennib H, Chiu RCJ, Mulder DS, Richards GK, Prentis J: Pulmonary bacterial clearance and alveolar macrophage function in septic shock lung. *Am Rev Respir Dis* 130:444–449, 1984.

51. MacDonald NE, Hall CB, Suffin SC, Alexson C, Harris PJ, Manning JA: Respiratory syncytial viral infection in infants with congenital heart disease. *N Engl J Med* 307:397–400, 1982.

52. Johanson WG Jr: Pathogenesis and prevention of nosocomial pneumonia in a nonhuman primate model of acute respiratory failure. *Am Rev Respir Dis* 130:502–504, 1984.

53. Hall CB, Powell KR, MacDonald NE, Gala CL, Menegus ME, Suffin SC, Cohen HJ: Respiratory syncytial viral infection in children with compromised immune function. *N Engl J Med* 315:77–81, 1986.

54. Meyers JD, Thomas ED: Nonbacterial pneumonia after allogeneic marrow transplantation: A review of ten years' experience. *Rev Infect Dis* 4:1119–1132, 1982.

55. Ramsey PG, Fife KH, Hackman RC, Meyers JD, Corey L: Herpes simplex virus pneumonia: Clinical virologic and pathologic features in 20 patients. *Ann Intern Med* 97:813–820, 1982.

56. Shields AF, Hackman RC, Fife KH, Corey L, Meyers JD: Adenovirus infections in patients undergoing bone marrow transplantation. *N Engl J Med* 312:529–533, 1985.

57. Dowling JN, Kroboth FJ, Karpf M, Yee RB, Pasculli AW: Pneumonia and multiple lung abscesses caused by dual infection with *Legionella micdadei* and *Legionella pneumophila. Am Rev Respir Dis* 127:121–125, 1983.

58. Helms CM, Massanari RM, Zeitler R, Streed S, Gilchrist MJR, Hall N, Hausler WJ, Sywassink J, Johnson W, Wintermeyer L, Hierholzer WJ: Legionnaires' disease associated with a hospital water system: A cluster of 24 nosocomial cases. *Ann Intern Med* 99:172–178, 1983.

59. Meyer RD: Legionella infections: A review of five years of research. *Rev Infect Dis* 5:258–278, 1983.

60. Mylotte JM, Beam TR Jr: Comparison of community-acquired nosocomial pneumococcal bacteremia. *Am Rev Respir Dis* 123:265–268, 1981.

61. Christensen GD, Bisno AL, Parisi JT, McLaughlin B, Hester MG, Luther RW: Nosocomial septicemia due to multiply antibiotic-resistance *Staphylococcus epidermidis. Ann Intern Med* 96:1–10, 1982.

62. Degregorio MW, Lee WMF, Linker CA, Jacobs RA, Ries CA: Fungal infections in patients with acute leukemia. *Am J Med* 73:543–548, 1982.

63. Pizzo PA, Robichaud KJ, Gill FA, Wistebsky FG: Empiric antibiotic and antifungal therapy for cancer patients with prolonged fever and granulocytopenia. *Am J Med* 72:101–111, 1982.

64. Lentino JR, Rosenkranz MA, Michaels JA, Kurup VP, Rose HD, Rytel MW: Nosocomial aspergillosis. A retrospective review of airborne disease secondary to road construction and contaminated air conditioners. *Am J Epidemiol* 116:430–437, 1982.

65. Andrews CP, Weiner MH: Aspergillus antigen detection in bronchoalveolar lavage fluid from patients with invasive aspergillosis and aspergillomas. *Am J Med* 73:372–380, 1983.

66. Hall CB, Douglas RG Jr: Modes of transmission of respiratory syncytial virus. *J Pediatr* 99:100–103, 1981.

67. Kapila R, Lintz DI, Tecson FT, Ziskin L, Louria DB: A nosocomial outbreak of influenza A. *Chest* 71:576–579, 1977.

68. Hall CB, Douglas RG Jr: Nosocomial influenza infection as a cause of intercurrent fevers in infants. *Pediatrics* 55:673–677, 1975.

69. Meibalane R, Sedmak GV, Sasidharan P, Garg P, Grausz JP: Outbreak of influenza in a neonatal intensive care unit. *J Pediatr* 91:974–976, 1977.

70. Goldwater PN, Chrystie IL, Banatvala JE: Rotaviruses and the respiratory tract. *Br Med J* 15:1551–1552, 1979.

71. Hall CB, McBride JT, Walsh EE, Bell DM, Gala CL, Hildreth S, TenEycr LG, Hall WJ: Aerosolized ribavirin treatment of infants with respiratory syncytial viral infection. *N Engl J Med* 308:1443–1447, 1983.

72. Zavala D: The diagnosis of pulmonary disease by nonthoracotomy techniques. *Chest* 64:100–102, 1973.

73. Lorber B, Swenson RM: Bacteriology of aspiration pneumonia. *Ann Intern Med* 81:329–331, 1974.

74. Murray PR, Washington JA II: Microscopic and bacteriologic analysis of sputum. *Mayo Clin Proc* 50:339–344, 1975.

75. Andrews CP, Coalson JJ, Smith JD, Johanson WG: Diagnosis of nosocomial bacterial pneumonia in acute, diffuse lung injury. *Chest* 80:254–258, 1981.

76. Tobin MJ, Grenvik A: Nosocomial lung infection and its diagnosis. *Crit Care Med* 12:191–199, 1984.

77. Berger R, Arango L: Etiologic diagnosis of bacterial nosocomial pneumonia in seriously ill patients. *Crit Care Med* 13:833–836, 1985.

78. Hoffman PC, Dixon RE: Control of influenza in the hospital. *Ann Intern Med* 87:725–728, 1977.
79. Hall CB, Geiman JM, Douglas RG Jr, Meagher MP: Control of nosocomial respiratory syncytial viral infections. *Pediatrics* 62:728–732, 1978.
80. Brady MT, Milam JD, Anderson DC, Hawkins EP, Speer ME, Seavy D, Bijou H, Yow MD: Use of deglycerolyzed red blood cells to prevent post transfusion infection with cytomegalovirus in neonates. *J Infect Dis* 150:334–339, 1984.
81. Taylor BJ, Jacobs RF, Baker RL, Moses EB, McSwain BE, Shulman G: Frozen deglycerolyzed blood prevents transfusion-acquired cytomegalovirus infections in neonates. *Ped Infect Dis* 5:188–191, 1986.
82. Bartlett JG, Rosenblatt JE, Finegold SM: Percutaneous transtracheal aspiration in the diagnosis of anaerobic pulmonary infection. *Ann Intern Med* 79:535–540, 1973.
83. Bartlett JG: Diagnostic accuracy of transtracheal aspiration bacteriologic study. *Am Rev Respir Dis* 115:777–782, 1977.
84. Fossieck B, Parker R, Cohen M, Kane RC: Fiberoptic bronchoscopy and culture of bacteria from the lower respiratory tract. *Chest* 72:5–9, 1977.
85. Wimberley N, Faling L, Bartlett J: A fiberoptic bronchoscopy technique to obtain lower uncontaminated airway secretions for bacterial culture. *Am Rev Respir Dis* 119:337–343, 1979.
86. Boyd B, Wimberley N, Bass J: A new fiberoptic bronchoscopy technique diagnosis of pulmonary infections: Clinical results in 50 patients. Abstr. *Am Rev Respir Dis* 121:114, 1980.
87. Hayes D, McCarthy L, Friedman M: Evaluation of two bronchofiberscopic methods of culturing the lower respiratory tract. *Am Rev Respir Dis* 122:319–323, 1980.
88. Teague R, Wallace R Jr, Awe R: The use of quantitative sterile brush culture and Gram stain analysis in the diagnosis of lower respiratory tract infection. *Chest* 79:157–161, 1981.
89. Higuchi JH, Coalson JJ, Johanson WG Jr: Bacteriologic diagnosis of nosocomial pneumonia in primates: Usefulness of the protected specimen brush. *Am Rev Respir Dis* 125:53–57, 1982.
90. Chastre J, Viau F, Brun P, Pierre J, Dauge MC, Bouchama A, Akesbi A, Gibert C: Prospective evaluation of the protected specimen brush for the diagnosis of pulmonary infections in ventilated patients. *Am Rev Respir Dis* 130:924–929, 1984.
91. Davidson M, Tempest B, Palmer DL: Bacteriologic diagnosis of acute pneumonia: Comparison of sputum, transtracheal aspirates, and lung aspirates. *JAMA* 235:158–163, 1976.
92. Palmer DL, Davidson M, Lusk R: Needle aspiration of the lung in complex pneumonias. *Chest* 78:16–21, 1980.
93. Spencer C, Beaty H: Complications of transtracheal aspiration. *N Engl J Med* 286:304–306, 1972.
94. Unger K, Moser K: Fatal complication of transtracheal aspirations. *Arch Intern Med* 132:437–439, 1973.
95. Lorch D, John J, Miller KS, Tomlinson J, Strange C, Wooten S, Sahn S: Transbronchial needle aspiration and protected specimen brush in the etiologic diagnosis of pneumonia. *Am Rev Respir Dis* 133:A125, 1986.
96. Coleman DL, Dodek PM, Luce JM, Golden JA, Gold WM, Murray JF: Diagnostic utility of fiberoptic bronchoscopy in patients with pneumocytis carinii penumonia and the acquired immune deficiency syndrome. *Am Rev Respir Dis* 128:795–799, 1983.
97. Ramsey BW, Marcuse EK, Foy HM, Cooney MK, Allan I, Brewer D, Smith AL: Use of bacterial antigen detection in the diagnosis of pediatric lower respiratory tract infections. *Pediatrics* 78:1–9, 1986.
98. Jacobs RF: Rapid diagnosis of infections in pulmonary disease. *Amer Rev Respir Dis* 134:829–831, 1986.
99. Zucker A, Pollack M, Katz R: Blind use of the double-lumen plugged catheter for diagnosis of respiratory tract infections in critically ill children. *Crit Care Med* 12:867–870, 1984.
100. Kohne DE: The application of DNA probes to the diagnosis of infectious disease. *Infect Dis Newsletter* 4:43–45, 1985.
101. Klastersky J, Meunier-Carpentier F, Kahan-Coppens L, Thys JP: Endotracheally administered antibiotics for Gram-negative pneumonia. *Chest* 75:586–591, 1979.
102. Gough PA, Jordan NS: A review of the therapeutic efficacy of aerosolized and endotracheally instilled antibiotics. *Pharmacotherapy* 2:367–377, 1982.
103. Ziegler EJ, McCutchan JA, Fierer J, Glauser MP, Sadoff JC, Douglas H, Braude AI: Treatment of Gram-negative bacteremia and shock with human antiserum to a mutant *Escherichia coli*. *N Engl J Med* 307:1225–1228, 1982.
104. Haley RW, Hightower AW, Khabbaz RF, Thornsberry C, Martone WJ, Allen JR, Hughes JM: The emergence of methicillin-resistant *Staphylococcus aureus* infections in United States hospitals: Possible role of the house staff-patient transfer circuit. *Ann Intern Med* 97:297–308, 1982.
105. Klastersky J, Geuning C, Mouawad E, Daneau D: Endotracheal gentamicin in bronchial infections in patients with tracheostomy. *Chest* 61:117–120, 1972.
106. Pennington JE, Reynolds HY: Tobramycin in bronchial secretions. *Antimicrob Agents Chemother* 4:299–301, 1973.
107. Pennington JE, Reynolds HY: Pharmacokinetics of gentamicin sulfate in bronchial secretions. *J Infect Dis* 131:158–162, 1975.
108. Moore RD, Smith CR, Lietman PS: Association of aminoglycoside plasma levels with therapeutic outcome in Gram-negative pneumonia. *Am J Med* 77:657–662, 1984.
109. Klastersky J, Huysmans E, Weerts D, Henfgens C, Daneau D: Endotracheally administered gentamicin for the prevention of infections of the respiratory tract in patients with tracheostomy: A double-blind study. *Chest* 65:650–655, 1974.
110. Klastersky J, Hensgens C, Noterman J, Mouawad E, Meunier-Carpentier F: Endotracheal antibiotics for the prevention of tracheobronchial infections in tracheostomized unconscious patients. *Chest* 68:302–306, 1975.
111. Collins MS, Roby RE: Protective activity on an intravenous immune globulin (human) enriched in antibody against lipopolysaccharide antigens of *Pseudomonas aeruginosa*. *Am J Med* 76:168–174, 1984.
112. Greenfield S, Teres D, Bushnell LS, Hedley-Whyte J, Feingold DS: Prevention of Gram-negative bacillary pneumonia using aerosol polymyxin as prophylaxis. I. Effects on the colonization pattern of the upper respiratory tract of seriously ill patients. *J Clin Invest* 52:2935–2940, 1973.
113. Feeley TW, DuMoulin GC, Hedley-Whyte J, Bushnell LS, Gilbert JP, Feingold DS: Aerosol polymyxin and pneumonia in seriously ill patients. *N Engl J Med* 293:471–475, 1975.
114. Simmons BP, Wong ES: Guideline for prevention of nosocomial pneumonia. *Infect Control* 3:327–333, 1982.
115. Gala CL, Hall CB, Schnabel KC, Pincus PH, Blossom P, Hildreth SW, Betts RF, Douglas RG: The use of eye-nose goggles to control nosocomial respiratory syncytial virus infection. *JAMA* 256:2706–2708, 1986.

3

Urinary Tract Infection

Jacob A. Lohr, M.D.

BACKGROUND

The urinary tract remains the most frequently involved site of primary infection in patients with hospital-acquired infections. In the 1984 report from the National Nosocomial Infections Surveillance System (NNIS) (1), the urinary tract accounted for 38.5% of the nosocomial infections in nonteaching, small teaching, and large teaching hospitals. This percentage was more than twice the 17.8% distribution for lower respiratory infection, the second most frequently involved site. The overall infection rate for the urinary tract was 12.9 cases per 1,000 discharges.

The infection rates for the pediatric and newborn services for the three hospital categories in the NNIS report are shown in Table 3.1. Urinary tract infections (UTIs) were not represented on pediatric services in the nonteaching hospitals, but had a prominent role on pediatric services in large teaching hospitals where they ranked second to lower respiratory infections. On the newborn services, the UTIs ranked low on the list of leading sites. However, most of the included newborns were in well-baby nurseries where infection rates do not represent the nosocomial milieu of newborn intensive care units.

A recently completed study of a 5-year experience with hospital-acquired UTIs at the University of Virginia Children's Medical Center (UVCMC) included the center's newborn intensive care unit (NICU) patients and non-NICU patients. These latter patients represented the pediatric intensive care unit (PICU), burn unit (BU), preschool-age ward (PAW), and school-age ward (SAW) (2). The overall UTI rate was 14.2 cases per 1,000 admissions (NICU patients, 7.9 cases/1,000 admissions; non-NICU patients, 15.0 cases/1,000 admissions). This overall rate compares with that from most of the 1984 NNIS large teaching hospital adult services (surgery, 19.5 cases/1,000 discharges; medicine, 19.5 cases/1,000 discharges; and gynecology, 14.4 cases/1,000 discharges), and exceeds the rate from the obstetrical services (4.2 cases/1,000 discharges) (1).

The unit-specific rates for the UVCMC study are shown in Table 3.2. There were six non-NICU patients who were chronically hospitalized and differed from those patients with limited hospitalization in that each was hospitalized a total of more than 365 days during the study period. All six patients had greater than 15 infections, and one had at least 50 infections during the study period.

The UVCMC NICU rate of 7.9 cases/1,000 admissions far exceeds that from the NNIS newborn services; but, as noted, the NNIS primarily included well babies. The BU rate of 28.4 cases/1,000 admissions can be compared with the rate of 13 cases/1,000 admissions reported from the National Burn Information Exchange (3). The UVCMC BU rates were based on the infections in only three patients and cannot be conclusive, but imply that pediatric patients in such units are at high risk for nosocomial urinary tract infection. The BU rate in the UVCMC study was higher than the rate for all other units in the study but was not significantly higher than that for the PICU. Excluding the chronically hospitalized patients, the combined rates of infection in intensive care units (NICU, PICU, BU) were significantly higher than the combined rates for the general wards. This is not surprising since nosocomial infection rates in general are higher for intensive care units than for general wards (4,5).

Nosocomial UTIs impact on costs of hospitalization, patient morbidity, and, possibly, pa-

Table 3.1
Site-Specific Infection Rates (Cases/1,000 Discharges), by Service[a]

				Site[b]			
Service[c]	UTI	SWI	LRI	BACT	CUT	Other	All Sites
1. Nonteaching hospitals							
PED	0.0	0.1	0.1	0.0	0.1	0.9	1.2
NEW	0.5	0.2	1.8	0.6	2.6	2.9	8.6
2. Small teaching hospitals							
PED	2.0	0.6	2.0	2.4	2.3	5.2	14.6
NEW	0.6	0.2	1.4	2.0	4.8	5.6	14.7
3. Large teaching hospitals							
PED	2.8	1.6	3.9	2.1	1.2	4.9	16.6
NEW	1.0	0.3	2.9	3.6	3.7	5.6	17.4

[a]Adapted from Nosocomial infection surveillance, 1984 (1).
[b]UTI, urinary tract infection; SWI, surgical wound infection; LRI, lower respiratory infection; BACT, primary bacteremia; CUT, cutaneous infection.
[c]PED, pediatric services; NEW, newborn services.

tient mortality. Several studies have identified that the costs for antibiotic treatment ranged from $150–$300 per nosocomial UTI, and each infection added 2 days to the hospital stay (6–8). The impact of these modest results is magnified by the high frequency of hospital-acquired UTIs. Efforts leading to decreases in the overall rate of these infections constitute a significant cost containment issue.

In addition to prolonged hospitalization, short-term morbidity includes symptomatic UTI and the possibilities of secondary wound infection and secondary bacteremia. Only 35% of adult patients with hospital-acquired bacteriuria are symptomatic (9). The severity of symptoms is related more to the seriousness of the patient's

underlying disease than to the type of infecting organism (10–12). In adult patients, most nosocomial UTIs are benign and are resolved with catheter removal, regardless of the use or nonuse of antibiotics (13). However, one study suggests that bacteriuria may persist for up to 3 months in a majority, even if antibiotics are used (14). In the UVCMC study, 28% of the patients in whom clinical findings at documentation were recorded were asymptomatic (2).

Secondary infections associated with nosocomial UTIs are well-documented. Surgery patients with nosocomial bacteriuria may develop secondary postoperative wound infections with the same organisms isolated from the urine (15). Secondary bacteremia is defined as a blood-

Table 3.2.
Inpatient Unit-Specific Infected Patient Rates and Infection Rates (2)

Group[a]	Unit[a]	Number of Patients	Number of Infections	Number of Admissions	Number of Infected Patients per 1000 Admissions	Number of Infections per 1000 Admissions
NICU Patients	NICU	12	15	1,910	6.3	7.9
	PICU	10	19	1,846	5.4	10.3
Non-NICU Patients Limited Hospitalization	PAW	8	12	6,511	1.2	1.8
	SAW	21	55	6,126	3.4	9.0
	BU	3	4	141	21.3	28.4
Non-NICU Patients Chronic Hospitalization	PICU PAW SAW	6	~130	Included in Above Non-NICU Patient Admissions	~0.4	~9.0
Total	ALL	60	~235	16,534	~3.6	~14.2

[a]NICU, Neonatal intensive care unit; PICU, pediatric intensive care unit; PAW, preschool-age ward; SAW, school-age ward; BU, burn unit.

stream infection with the same organism that is also isolated from another site (1). In the 1984 NNIS report, the urinary tract was the least frequent of the primary sources of secondary bacteremias, regardless of the type of hospital category (Table 3.3) (1). Only 3.3% of hospital-acquired UTIs were complicated by secondary bacteremia. The rate was 5.6% for all sites combined. On the other hand, hospital-acquired UTIs are the primary site of 40% of Gram-negative bacteremias (16–21). In children, the risk of secondary bacteremia may be smaller; secondary bacteremia was not documented in any of the 60 children in the UVCMC study (2).

The long-term morbidity of hospital-acquired UTIs is not well-defined. The risks for developing chronic pyelonephritis, hypertension, or renal failure as a result of these infections is not known.

The mortality attributed to hospital-acquired UTIs is either directly associated with the complication of secondary bacteremia or is associated in an undefined manner with the infection itself. The apparent impact of secondary bacteremia is striking in certain studies that reported a 20–50% mortality rate in adult patients with this complication (16,18,20). An additional study determined an overall mortality rate of 31% in patients with nosocomial UTIs who became bacteremic (22). The mortality that could be attributed specifically to the hospital-acquired UTI was 13%, and all of those patients were at high risk with poor prognosis from their underlying disease.

Other studies have found that bacteremic UTIs contribute little to death rates (23–25). The impact of the UTI itself may be significant. In a recently reported prospective study, the acquisition of UTI during indwelling bladder catheterization was associated with nearly a 3-fold increase in mortality among hospitalized adult patients (26). This increased mortality was not related to the patients' underlying debility or to the development of secondary bacteremia. Thus, the reason for the associated mortality was not clear. A subsequent study in hospitalized patients did not confirm a relationship between bacteriuria and death (27).

In the UVCMC study, no mortality could be directly attributed to the UTIs (2). Only two of the 60 children died. Neither had a secondary bacteremia. Only one had a UTI at death. One patient had never been catheterized, and one was undergoing intermittent catheterization at the time of death. Therefore, these patients cannot be compared with the adult patients experiencing a 3-fold increase in mortality, since all of the adult patients had indwelling urinary catheters (26).

POPULATION AT RISK

The major risk factors that predispose patients to infection of the urinary tract are urethral catheterization and periurethral colonization with potential urinary tract pathogens (9,28–30). The presence of urinary tract catheterization defines a group of adults at risk for nosocomial UTI (9,28–30). In children, urinary tract catheterization appears to have a similar significance. In the UVCMC study, 40 of the 42 infected non-NICU patients with limited hospitalization had undergone catheterization, and 87 of the 90 infections in the 42 patients were associated with catheterization (2). In the NICU population, eight of the 12 infected patients had been catheterized, and 10 of the 15 infections in the 12 patients were associated with catheterization. Overall in these UVCMC study patients, 89% of those infected were catheterized, and 92% of the infections occurred in catheterized patients.

Table 3.3
Percentage of Infection with Secondary Bacteremia, by Site[a] and Hospital Category[b]

Hospital Category	Site[c]					
	UTI	SWI	LRI	CUT	Other[d]	All Sites
Nonteaching	3.1	3.5	3.3	4.1	8.9	3.8
Small Teaching	2.7	4.2	6.1	9.4	9.6	4.9
Large Teaching	3.9	6.0	5.9	9.4	14.3	6.8
All Hospitals	3.3	4.9	5.4	8.6	12.0	5.6

[a]Excluding primary bacteremia.
[b]Adapted from Nosocomial infection surveillance, 1984 (1).
[c]UTI, urinary tract infection; SWI, surgical wound infection; LRI, lower respiratory infection; BACT, primary bacteremia; CUT, cutaneous infection.
[d]Most frequently associated with cardiovascular (70.8%) and intraabdominal infections (10.5%).

Periurethral colonization by potential urinary tract pathogens precedes UTI in both catheterized and noncatheterized patients (31). The virulence of these organisms is probably the result of a combination of the ability of the organisms to adhere to uroepithelial cells and the increased affinity of these cells for bacterial attachment. Organisms that colonize the periurethral area are usually from the patients' own flora (endogenous infection), primarily gastrointestinal (*Escherichia coli, Enterococcus* spp., *Klebsiella* spp., *Enterobacter* spp., and others) (31,32). Although not part of normal flora, hospital-acquired *Pseudomonas* spp. often inhabit the gastrointestinal tract prior to colonizing the periurethral area (32–34). Skin or distal urethral organisms (coagulase-negative staphylococci, *Candida* spp., and others) also play a significant role in endogenous infections (35,36). Less frequently, organisms from the hands of medical personnel may be involved when a breach of proper catheter management technique occurs (exogenous infection) (29,37,38). These organisms may have their origins from many sources, including the nose, mouth, or rectum of the personnel (39), hand lotions (40), and other patients (41,42). Exogenous infection can be responsible for case clusters and epidemics of nosocomial UTIs.

The catheter offers to potential pathogens several routes of entry into the urinary tract. First, organisms may be pushed into the bladder at the time of catheterization (43,44). Infection can occur in this manner with organisms residing in the distal urethra (35,36), or the catheter itself may be contaminated prior to its use and may thus be a source of pathogens (37). Second, organisms may migrate from the periurethral area to the bladder along the outside of the indwelling catheter. This process was first demonstrated by Kass (45) and later confirmed by others (46–49). It is the most important mechanism of infection in catheterized patients (70–80%) (29,37,50). Third, organisms can reach the bladder through reflux or urine inside the catheter tubing. This route accounts for about 20–30% of the infections in adults (29,37,50) and results from a flaw in the care of the patients' catheter systems.

An enormous population of hospitalized patients are placed at risk of infection because of urinary tract catheter utilization. Ten percent of hospitalized adult patients are exposed to temporary indwelling urinary catheters (9,28). One percent of children are catheterized during hospitalization (51). The overall risk of developing bacteriuria while catheterized ranges between 6–23% in adult studies (9,29,37,52) and was 9% in pediatric patients in a single study (51). The risks will vary, depending on a number of factors: overall duration of exposure to catheter use, type of catheterization (indwelling versus intermittent), type of system (open versus closed), sex, associated urologic surgery, and underlying medical condition.

The risk of infection increases as the duration of exposure to a catheter increases. A single in and out catheterization in adult patients is associated with a 0.5–8% risk of subsequent bacteriuria (53–56). It is generally held that the attendant risk resides at the lower end of this range, unless other additional risk factors are involved. The risk of single in and out catheterization in children is not well-defined. Of adults who are not bacteriuric at the time of catheterization and who remain catheterized for at least a day, as many as 10% will become bacteriuric during their period of catheterization (9,29,37,52).

In adult patients, the use of intermittent catheterization has a beneficial effect on the rate of infection in patients with neurogenic bladders using clean self-catheterization (57). A prospective controlled study comparing intermittent versus indwelling catheterization has not been done in adult or pediatric patients. In the UVCMC study, the total number of children exposed to catheterization of any type was not documented; therefore, rates of infection for intermittent versus indwelling catheter use could not be determined (2). However, of 97 UTIs associated with catheter use, 49 followed intermittent catheter exposure only, and 48 followed indwelling catheter use, either alone or in sequence with intermittent or condom catheter use. In addition, in the 42 non-NICU patients with limited hospitalization, the mean duration of catheter use before documentation of infection for patients with only intermittent catheterization (15.7 days) was not significantly different from the mean durations for patients exposed to indwelling catheters, either alone (14.3 days) or in sequence with in and out or condom catheter use (16.8 days). These data imply similar risks; but without denominator data, no conclusions can be drawn.

It is well-documented that a closed drainage system markedly decreases the risks attendant with an open drainage system (58,59). The cumulative risk of infection with a closed system is about 25% at 14 days (58). With open drainage, virtually all patients will be bacteriuric after 4 days of indwelling catheterization (59,60). One study recorded a significant decrease in Gram-negative bacteremia in association with the introduction of the closed system (16).

Adult females have two and a half times as great a risk for acquisition of nosocomial UTIs as do males (29). The reason for this difference is assumed to be the shorter female urethra that provides less of a barrier to organisms moving toward the bladder in the space outside the catheter.

With associated urologic surgery, risk of infection in adult patients is increased (61). An increased risk in children is not documented.

The patient's underlying condition can affect risk of infection acquisition. Risks are increased in certain groups, such as bedridden patients or women with complicated labors and deliveries (55,61,62). In debilitated patients, an increased risk is at least partially related to periurethral colonization with more pathogenic organisms (46,48). No data regarding the degree of risk associated with specific underlying disorders is available for pediatric populations. In the UVCMC study, 52% of the children had a principal neurologic diagnosis, and 18% had an underlying primary renal disorder (2). These diagnoses could reflect increased risk for UTI, but may simply reflect conditions in which patients frequently undergo urinary tract catheterization.

Patients with nosocomial UTIs acquired without urinary tract instrumentation fall into a small, ill-defined group. In the UVCMC study, 33% of the NICU patients were infected without catheterization (2). All were premature. Otherwise, no common characteristics were apparent. Of the two non-NICU patients infected without prior catheterization, both had leukemia and were neutropenic when their infections occurred. These latter two patients may represent a special high-risk category within the group of hospitalized children who have not had urinary tract invasion.

ETIOLOGIC ORGANISMS

Virtually any organism should be considered a pathogen for nosocomial UTIs. In the 1984 NNIS report (1), *Escherichia coli* was the organism most frequently isolated from the urinary tract in all the adult services. *Enterococcus* spp. ranked

second on all services, except surgery, where *Pseudomonas aeruginosa* occurred more frequently. *Escherichia coli* was also the premier pathogen on the pediatric (30.4%) and newborn (35.2%) services. *Pseudomonas aeruginosa* ranked second (13.4%) on the pediatric services, and *Klebsiella* spp. ranked second (15.5%) on the newborn services. Coagulase-negative staphylococci occupied a prominent position on the newborn services (9.9%; ranking third) but did not appear as one of the five most frequently isolated organisms on the pediatric services. *Candida* spp. ranked fifth in both the pediatric (10.7%) and newborn services (8.5%).

The pathogens in the UVCMC study (2) are shown in Table 3.4. *Escherichia coli* was the most frequently isolated organism (22.1%) in the non-NICU patients with limited hospitalization, but ranked third (15.8%), along with *Enterococcus* spp. on the NICU service. Coagulase-negative staphylococci ranked third (12.5%) on the non-NICU services, but was the number one isolate (31.6%) in the NICU. *Candida* spp. were isolated uncommonly (2.9%) in the non-NICU patients and were not isolated from any of the NICU patients.

Certain organisms (*Serratia marcescens, Pseudomonas aeruginosa*, and *Citrobacter freundii*) are more likely to appear with case, clustering, whereas others (*Escherichia coli*) are infrequently spread by cross-contamination or single-source infection (63,64).

In adult patients, polymicrobic bacteriuria is the rule in patients with chronic indwelling catheters (65–67). In the UVCMC study, more than one organism was isolated in 15% of the infections and more than two in 2% of the infections (Table 3.4) (2). This experience included eight infections (8%) in patients without catheters, and 49 (47%) in patients exposed only to intermittent catheterization.

DIAGNOSIS

The clinical presentation of nosocomial UTIs is usually more subtle than that associated with UTIs in otherwise healthy, noncatheterized patients. In nonhospitalized, noncatheterized patients, symptoms of acute UTIs often include fever, dysuria, urinary frequency, incontinence or nocturia, urgency, and abdominal and/or flank pain. In contrast, acute UTIs in catheterized patients must be recognized in the midst of an often complex clinical setting. Dysuria, increased frequency, and urgency may be either absent or

Table 3.4
Microbiology[a] (2)

Group	Newborn Intensive Care Unit Patients	Non-Newborn Intensive Care Unit Patients: Limited Hospitalization
Number of Infections	15	90
Single Organism	11	78
Two Organisms	4	10
Three Organisms	0	2
Total Organisms	19	104
Organisms (%)		
Escherichia coli	3 (15.8)	23 (22.1)
Pseudomonas spp.	1 (5.3)	22 (21.2)
Klebsiella spp.	1 (5.3)	11 (10.6)
Enterobacter spp.	4 (21.1)	4 (3.9)
Proteus spp.	0 (0)	3 (2.9)
Serratia spp.	1 (5.3)	1 (1.0)
Acinetobacter spp.	0 (0)	2 (1.9)
Morganella spp.	0 (0)	2 (1.9)
Citrobacter spp.	0 (0)	1 (1.0)
Coagulase-negative staphylococci	6 (31.6)	13 (12.5)
Staphylococcus aureus	0 (0)	3 (2.9)
Enterococcus spp.	3 (15.8)	10 (9.6)
Nonhemolytic streptococci	0 (0)	5 (4.8)
Candida spp.	0 (0)	3 (2.9)
Other fungi	0 (0)	1 (1.0)
Total	19 (100.0)	104 (100.0)

not apparent. Conversely, fever may be present because of the underlying disease, complications such as pneumonia, postoperative wound infection, postanesthesia atelectasis, thrombophlebitis, drug fever, or other nosocomial infection.

Just as with UTIs in otherwise healthy, noncatheterized patients, many catheterized patients have asymptomatic infections. Sixty-five percent of adult patients with nosocomial bacteriuria are asymptomatic (9). In the UVCMC study, 33% of the infections in NICU patients and 27% of the infections in non-NICU patients with limited hospitalization were asymptomatic (2). Not surprisingly, fever was the only symptom in 67% of the infections in the NICU patients. It was also the only symptom in 47% of the infections in the non-NICU patients. The catheterized patients old enough to report symptoms noted only abdominal or flank pain and did not describe dysuria, urgency, or increased frequency.

Microscopic examination of an uncentrifuged or centrifuged urine specimen has some diagnostic usefulness in nosocomial UTIs. As is true with other UTIs, the presence or absence of pus cells is not accurately predictive of the presence or absence of a UTI (68,69). Pyuria can occur secondary to a number of causes, including ure-

thral or bladder irritation secondary to catheter use (69,70). Conversely, a nosocomial UTI can be present without pyuria. In the UVCMC study, more than five polymorphonuclear leukocytes per high-power field were identified in only 51% of the centrifuged infected urine specimens subjected to urinalysis (2).

A recent review of urine microscopy for bacteriuria outlined criteria for the proper interpretation of findings from uncentrifuged or centrifuged, stained, or unstained specimens (Table 3.5) (71). The most reliable and reproducible method is examination of a stained, centrifuged sediment. The Gram stain is the choice over a methylene blue stain, since the latter stain is too sensitive and frequently reveals organisms at concentrations of 1,000–10,000 per ml (72).

No test can replace bacteriologic culture. For surveillance purposes, the Centers for Disease Control has previously defined nosocomial UTI as a urine culture with a colony count of $>10^5$ colony forming units per ml (CFU/ml) from a symptomatic or asymptomatic patient without previous manifestations of infection or previous positive culture (73). Infection is also diagnosed if the patient develops suggestive symptoms, and if a urinalysis reveals >10 white blood cells per high-power microscopic field. A patient with previously diagnosed bacteriuria who becomes

Table 3.5
Criteria for Interpretation of Urine Microscopy for Maximum Sensitivity and Specificity[a] (71)

Method	Methodology	Criteria for Significance ($>10^5$ CFU[b]/ ml)	Sensitivity %	Specificity %
1. Examination of unstained, uncentrifuged urine	1 drop of urine from Pasteur pipette, cover-glassed slide, $\times 40$ objective, low-intensity light, high technical skill	Any/HPF[b]	61–88	65–94
2. Examination of unstained, centrifuged urine	10 mL of urine, centrifuge at 2,500–3,000 rpm for 5 min, 1 drop of sediment from cover-glassed slide, $\times 40$ objective, trained observers	Any/HPF ≥ 1/HPF >10/HPF	91 93–97 82	84 ≤ 88 >95
3. Examination of stained, uncentrifuged urine	1–2 drops of urine from Pasteur pipette, Gram's stain, observe ≥ 5 fields, $\times 100$ objective, trained observers	Any/OIF[b] ≥ 1/OIF ≥ 2/OIF ≥ 5/OIF	93 87 94 83	79 89 98 99
4. Examination of stained, centrifuged urine	10 mL of urine, centrifuge at 2,500–3,000 rpm for 5 min, 1–2 drops of sediment from Pasteur pipette, Gram's stain, $\times 100$ objective	Any/OIF ≥ 1/OIF ≥ 5/OIF	97 98 87	66 89 96

[a]Copyright 1986, American Medical Association.
[b]CFU, colony-forming units; HPF, high-power field; OIF, oil-immersion field.

colonized with a new pathogen is also considered to have a new nosocomial infection.

The components of the definition require modification when applied to routine hospital practice. The definitions should be different for each method of urine collection (Table 3.6) (74–76). In addition, criteria for midstream collections are different for males and females. Probability of infection is affected by the following: number of species identified, Gram-stain character of the organism, colony counts, presence of symptoms, and presence of pyuria. The guidelines apply only to patients not on antimicrobial agents. In patients without catheters, the criteria are consistent with those for otherwise healthy, nonhospitalized patients with acute UTIs. In patients with indwelling catheters, likely infections require colony counts of only 10^3 CFU/ml, if symptoms are present. Counts less than 10^5 CFU/ml from catheter urine have been shown to progress to counts $>10^5$ CFU/ml in subsequent cultures, if patients are untreated (77). Some investigators consider colony counts as low as 10^2 CFU/ml in urine collected aseptically from catheter tubing to be "significant" bacteriuria (29,30,78,79).

The infections defined above are considered nosocomial if symptoms occur later than 48 hours

after admission or if a previously collected urine has revealed no evidence of incubating infection.

TREATMENT

Treatment of a hospital-acquired urinary tract infection requires detailed knowledge of the individual patient. The therapeutic issues may be relatively simple in an otherwise healthy patient who acquires a catheter-related urinary tract infection in the postoperative period of uncomplicated surgery. On the other hand, the issues can be complex in a catheterized, postoperative, immunosuppressed, intensive care unit patient with a wound infection under therapy, pulmonary infiltrates, chronic bacteriuria, and a new onset of fever and pyuria. Because of the spectrum of patients with hospital-acquired UTIs, it is not possible to recommend a single therapeutic regimen for all such infections. Therefore, the following guidelines should be considered with each infection.

Urinary Catheter Use.   Is the catheter still necessary? If not, it should obviously be removed. In adults, many hospital-acquired UTIs will resolve with catheter removal whether or not antibiotics are used (13).

Table 3.6
Definition of Urinary Tract Infection[a]

Method of Collection	Colony Count	Probability of Infection

Suprapubic Aspiration	One species
	  Gram-negative bacilli:
	    any number
	  Gram-positive cocci:
	    >1,000
		
		>90%
		
		>90%

	Two species (at least 1 Gram-negative)
	  >10^4
	  10^3–10^4
	  <10^3
		
		Infection likely
		Suspicious; repeat
		Infection unlikely

Catheterization	One species
	  >10^5
	  10^4–10^5
	  10^3–10^4
	  <10^3
		
		95%
		Infection likely
		Suspicious; repeat
		Infection unlikely

	Two species
	  >10^4
	  10^3–10^4
	  <10^3
		
		Infection likely
		Suspicious; repeat
		Infection unlikely

Midstream, Clean-voided[b] (Male)	One species
	  >10^4
	  10^3–10^4
	  <10^3
		
		Infection likely
		Suspicious; repeat
		Infection unlikely

	Two species >10^5 <10^5	 Suspicious; repeat Infection unlikely

Midstream, Clean-voided (Female)	One species
	  3 specimens: >10^5
	  2 specimens: >10^5
	  1 specimen:
	    >10^5
	    10^4–10^5
	    <10^4
		
		95%
		90%
		
		80%
		Suspicious; repeat
		Infection unlikely

	Two species
	  1–3 specimens: >10^5
	  1 specimen:
	    >10^5
	    <10^5
		
		Infection likely
		
		Suspicious; repeat
		Infection unlikely

Urine Bag	One-two species
	  Any growth
	  No growth
		
		Unreliable
		Infection unlikely[c]

[a]Modified from Hellerstein (74) and Garibaldi (75).
[b]In males, cleansing of the urethral meatus prior to urine collection may not be necessary (76).
[c]1. All of the guidelines apply only to patients not on antimicrobial therapy.
2. The presence of symptoms and/or the presence of pyuria (>5 polymorphonuclear leukocytes/high-power field) should move a patient from the category of "Infection unlikely" to the category of "Suspicious; repeat" or from the category of "Suspicious; repeat" to the category of "Infection likely."
3. The presence of more than two species most likely represents specimen contamination.

Has a breach of catheter-care technique occurred? The infection may resolve with institution of appropriate technique. In addition, the infection is not likely to respond to antibiotics if a source of contamination continues to be present.

Previous Bacteriuria.   Is this a recurrence? If so, does it represent inadequate treatment of a previous infection, or does it represent continued exposure to the hazard of catheterization?

Does this patient have persistent bacteriuria? Some patients requiring catheterization, such as those with a neurogenic bladder, have continuous colonization of bladder urine with organisms. Treatment will not necessarily sterilize the urine; and if the organisms are eradicated, they may be replaced by more resistent bacteria. Treatment should be limited in this setting to those patients who are symptomatic.

Symptoms.   Is the patient symptomatic? If so, the infection should be treated. It is debatable whether an asymptomatic infection requires therapy. If the catheter is to be removed in the ensuing 5–7 days, antibiotics may be useful in the asymptomatic patient. If the catheter is to remain for an undefined period, antibiotics may complicate the long-term care by selecting out resistant organisms.

Underlying Disease.   Is any underlying disorder going to have an impact on antibiotic selection? Debilitated patients may become infected more frequently and may be infected with more resistant organisms (32,80).

Urinary Tract Abnormalities.   Is an anatomic or functional abnormality of the urinary tract present that would make therapy less effective?

Other Drug Therapies.   Has concomitant therapy, such as immunosuppressive drugs, extended the spectrum of likely pathogens?

Other Infections.   Are other infections already under therapy with antibiotics which may alter microbiologic evaluation of the UTI? Will antibiotics have to be selected for treatment of other infections as well as for treatment of the UTI? Has antibiotic therapy affected bacteria sensitivity patterns?

Reactions to Antibiotics.   Many patients with hospital-acquired UTIs have had multiple drug exposures, and a history of possible drug sensitivity is not unusual.

Altered Drug Metabolism.   Does the patient have renal or liver disease warranting a change in drug choice or dose?

Recent Infection History on Patient's Inpatient Unit.   Have patients in the unit experienced infections with unusually resistant organisms? Many patients with hospital-acquired UTIs are cared for in intensive care units where highly resistant organisms have been selected out (4,5).

Common Hospital-Acquired UTI Pathogens

Gram-negative Coloforms.   Initial therapy should provide coverage for Gram-negative organisms, including *Pseudomonas* spp. (1,2).

Coagulase-Negative Staphylococci.   Therapy for coagulase-negative staphylococci should be included in initial therapy in all NICU patients (2). In non-NICU patients, specific therapy should be included if the Gram stain of a urine specimen reveals Gram-positive cocci.

Enterococcus **Spp.**   Antibiotic therapy selected for the other groups of organisms needs to be effective against *Enterococcus* spp., or an additional antibiotic is required (1,2).

Candida **Spp.**   Therapy for candidal infection should be considered when microscopic examination of an unstained sediment from a centrifuged urine reveals a yeast form, although indications for treatment of candiduria remain inexact (81,82). Specific fungal culture media should be utilized for species identification.

Antibiotic Sensitivity Patterns.   Therapy should be altered to fit the sensitivity patterns of the organisms isolated from the infected urine.

Antibiotic Route.   With few exceptions, initial therapy should be parenteral. After sensitivities are known, therapy in selected cases can be oral.

Duration of Therapy.   Appropriate duration is not well-defined. Single dose or short-course therapy (1–3 days) cannot be recommended at this time. Routine therapy should be for a minimum 7–10 days.

FOLLOW-UP

Urine cultures should be repeated during the initial part of therapy, and the urine should be sterile 48–72 hours after therapy, or an alteration of therapy is indicated.

Cultures should be repeated in the 1st week after therapy is discontinued to identify early recurrences. Subsequent cultures should be performed when the patient is symptomatic in order to identify later recurrences. It is probably not necessary to do routine cultures on asymptomatic patients. It is debatable whether there is any value to routinely culturing the urine when the catheter is removed.

Radiographic evaluation is indicated only for selected patients. It is not required for all patients with hospital-acquired UTIs. It should be considered in patients infected without urinary catheter exposures.

PREVENTION

It is doubtful that all hospital-acquired UTIs can be prevented. However, their occurrence can be minimized if appropriate guidelines are utilized. Many guidelines are simple, inexpensive, and of proven efficacy. Some seem prudent, but are of unproven benefit. Still others appear useful, but their expense makes adoption unlikely in many hospitals.

The following approaches have been considered in the prevention of hospital-acquired UTIs.

Identification of At-Risk Patients

It is clear that the pediatric at-risk population is composed almost exclusively of patients exposed to urinary tract catheterization (2). It is essential that personnel caring for such patients be educated in correct techniques of catheter insertion and care.

Limitation of Catheterization

Beeson, in his classic 1958 editorial entitled "The Case Against the Catheter" admonished physicians concerning unnecessary catheter use (83). The caveat remains true today. Many catheters are inserted without justification, and others remain longer than necessary.

Selection of Type of Catheterization

Alternatives to indwelling catheterization have been sought in order to avoid the complications of the indwelling method. Intermittent catheterization, suprapubic catheterization, and condom drainage are proposed alternatives. Intermittent clean self-catheterization, with or without urinary antisepsis, has been shown to be effective in small numbers of adult patients with neurogenic bladders (57). However, the advantage of intermittent catheterization over indwelling catheterization in comparable pediatric or adult patient populations has not been proven in a prospective, randomized, controlled clinical trial. In addition, in the UVCMC study, the number of patients with catheter-associated bacteriuria was composed of almost equal representation from patients exposed to indwelling catheterization and patients exposed only to intermittent catheterization (2). This suggests no advantage of one approach over the other. Suprapubic catheterization, likewise, has no proven efficacy over indwelling catheterization. Lastly, condom drainage has not been compared with indwelling catheterization under study conditions; but complications such as local irritation, urine obstruction, and high rates of bacteriuria make the condom catheter a less attractive choice (84,85).

Selection of Indwelling Catheter System (Open Versus Closed Catheter System)

Closed drainage systems have significantly lower infection rates than do open drainage systems (43,58,59,86,87). Rates of catheterization-associated bacteriuria approach 100% after 2–4 days of catheterization with an open system (29,37). The rates with closed systems have been reduced to approximately 20% (29,58). Any indwelling urinary catheter should be connected to a closed system.

Care of the Closed System

The following indwelling catheter care procedures, if followed, should be carried out by specifically trained individuals (29,88) or, if economically practical, by a specific team with responsibility for catheter insertion and maintenance (88,89).

Aseptic Insertion of Catheters

Prevention of contamination at the time of any catheter insertion has obvious benefits. Use of an iodophor preparation at the time of insertion provides an appropriate antibacterial spectrum and has limited adverse side effects, such as local skin reactions (90). Benzalkonium chloride has been advocated, but is less effective and can serve as a culture medium (91).

Securing of the Catheter

This procedure prevents movement and urethral traction (92). The practice seems prudent but is unproven in preventing the ascent of periurethral organisms through the space around the catheter. Little expense and inconvenience are involved in the procedure so it is recommended.

Maintenance of the "Closed" System

Disconnection of junctions or improper care of drainage bags occurred in approximately 30% of patients in one study predisposing patients to bacteriuria (29). Use of plastic junction seals may be appropriate (37). All urine samples should be obtained aseptically and without opening junctions for procurement of the sample.

Prophylactic Antibiotics

Since 80% of infections involve periurethral organisms (29,37,50), these bacteria have been the target of varying prophylactic maneuvers.

Systemic Antibiotics.   The use of systemic antibiotics might affect periurethral organisms indirectly by altering intestinal flora or directly, by inhibiting or decreasing periurethral colonization. Systemic antibiotic prophylaxis is effective in decreasing rates of catheter-associated bacteriuria (29,37), but the effect is limited to 4 days (29). Patients receiving prophylactic antibiotics are more likely to develop bacteriuria with resistant organisms (34,80,93). Prophylactic systemic antibiotics are not recommended.

Meatal Antibiotics.   Studies in adults have not demonstrated effectiveness of daily meatal washing with soap and water or application of polyantibiotic ointment or povidone-iodine in decreasing rates of bacteriuria (52,94); in some patients, their use was associated with an increased rate of bacteriuria. A more recent study demonstrated effectiveness of a water-soluble polyantimicrobic cream applied to the catheter-meatal junction (95). Until their effectiveness is confirmed, the use of meatal antibiotics is not recommended.

Prevention of Bladder Contamination

Antimicrobial Agents on or Impregnated in Catheters.   Antibacterial lubricants or antibacterial substances impregnated in catheters offer no benefit (96,97), and their use is not recommended.

Bladder Irrigation.   Irrigation with antibiotics is effective in preventing bacteriuria with open systems but not with closed systems because their instillation requires frequent opening of the system (38). In addition, infection with resistant organisms is increased with their use. Their routine use is contraindicated.

Unobstructed Urine Flow.   Maintenance of free urine flow should decrease the likelihood of bladder urine infection.

Surveillance Cultures.   Most patients have a brief lag time between colonization of bladder urine and the appearance of symptoms, making treatment prior to true infection impossible (9). Routine surveillance is not recommended.

Prevention of Bag Contamination

Instillation of povidone-iodine (98), hydrogen peroxide (99,100), or chlorhexidine solution (101) appeared useful in uncontrolled studies, but prospective clinical trials have not supported their utilization (50,102). Their use is not recommended.

Prevention of Reflux of Infected Bag Urine into Bladder

No antireflux device is 100% effective. One study did not demonstrate a difference in rates of bacteriuria associated with systems with or without devices (97). They are not recommended for routine use at this time. It is recommended that the bag be kept in a dependent position at all times in order to avoid reflux (87).

Cohorting of Patients with Nosocomial UTI

The greater the number of catheterized patients, the more difficult it would be to spatially isolate patients with catheters. However, it is recommended that patients with hospital-acquired UTIs be spatially isolated if practical. In addition, patients with catheters should be spatially isolated from patients colonized at any site or infected at any site with highly resistant pathogens. In every circumstance, careful handwashing cannot be overemphasized.

Replacement of Catheter

Replacement may be useful if the sterility of the closed system has been violated, but replacement at arbitrarily fixed intervals is not recommended.

Epidemic Surveillance

Epidemics of nosocomial UTIs can develop insidiously. Early recognition depends on routine monitoring for increased rates, clustered cases, appearance of unusual organisms in more than one case, or unusual resistance patterns in urine isolates. Certain measures are appropriate if case clustering or epidemic spread is recognized. These include a reemphasis on careful handwashing, gloving, and spatial isolation of infected patients. Instillation of urinary antiseptics into drainage bags may be of benefit in this setting (101,103). Use of urinary suppressants or blad-

Table 3.7
Guidelines for Prevention of Catheter-Associated Urinary Tract Infections

DO:

1. Educate personnel in correct techniques of catheter insertion and care.
2. Catheterize patients only when necessary and remove the catheter as soon as possible.
3. Use closed systems for indwelling catheterizations and maintain the integrity of the closed system.
4. Aseptically insert the catheter.
5. Secure the catheter properly.
6. Maintain unobstructed urine flow and keep the collection bag in a dependent position.
7. Obtain urine samples aseptically.
8. Emphasize careful handwashing.
9. Spatially isolate patients with urinary tract infections, if practical.
10. Spatially isolate catheterized patients from patients known to be colonized or infected with highly resistant organisms.
11. Monitor for features of epidemics.

DO NOT:

1. Use systemic prophylactic antibiotics.
2. Use daily meatal care with povidone-iodine or polymicrobic ointment.
3. Perform continuous irrigation of the bladder through the catheter, unless obstruction to urine flow necessitates.
4. Change the catheter at arbitrarily fixed intervals.
5. Perform routine bacteriologic monitoring.

der irrigation in colonized patients has been suggested (63).

Guidelines for the prevention of catheter-associated UTIs are outlined in Table 3.7.

REFERENCES

1. Horan TC, White JW, Jarvis WR, Emori TG, Culver DH, Munn VP, Thornsberry C, Olson DR, Hughes JM: Nosocomial infection surveillance, 1984. *Morbidity and Mortality* 35:17ss–29ss, 1984.
2. Lohr JA, Donowitz LG, Sadler JA: Hospital-acquired urinary tract infections in children. Presented at the Interscience Conference on Antimicrobial Agents and Chemotherapy. New York, October, 1987.
3. Feller I: The National Burn Information Exchange, University of Michigan, Ann Arbor, 1978.
4. Donowitz LG, Wenzel RP, Hoyt JW: High risk of hospital-acquired infection in the ICU patient. *Crit Care Med* 10:355–357, 1982.
5. Donowitz LG: High risk of nosocomial infection in the pediatric critical care patient. *Crit Care Med* 14:26–28, 1986.
6. Krieger JN, Kaiser DL, Wenzel RP: Nosocomial urinary tract infections: secular trends, treatment and economics in a university hospital. *J Urol* 130:102–106, 1983.
7. Haley RW, Schaberg DR, Crossley KB, Von Allmen SD, McGowan JE Jr: Exra charges and prolongation of stay attributable to nosocomial infections: A prospective interhospital comparison. *Am J Med* 70:51–58, 1981.
8. Givens CD, Wenzel RP: Catheter-associated urinary tract infections in surgical patients: A controlled study on the excess morbidity and costs. *J Urol* 124:646–648, 1980.
9. Garibaldi RA, Mooney BR, Epstein BJ, Britt MR: An evaluation of daily bacteriologic monitoring to identify preventable episodes of catheter-associated urinary tract infection. *Infect Control* 3:466–470, 1982.
10. Edebo L, Laurell G: Hospital infection of the urinary tract with proteus. *Acta Pathol Microbiol Scand* 43:93–105, 1958.

11. Edwards LD, Cross A, Levin S, Landau W: Outbreak of a nosocomial infection with a strain of *Proteus rettgeri* resistant to many antimicrobials. *Am J Clin Pathol* 61:41–46, 1974.
12. Lancaster LJ: Role of *Serratia* species in urinary tract infections. *Arch Intern Med* 109:82–85, 1962.
13. Cox CE, Hinman F Jr: Incidence of bacteriuria with indwelling catheter in normal bladders. *JAMA* 178:919–921, 1961.
14. Paterson ML, Barr W, MacDonald S: Urinary infection after colporrhaphy: Its incidence, causation, and prevention. *J Obstet Gynaecol Br Commonw* 67:394–401, 1960.
15. Krieger JN, Kaiser DL, Wenzel RP: Nosocomial urinary tract infections cause wound infections postoperatively in surgical patients. *Surg Gynecol Obstet* 156:313–318, 1983.
16. Martin CM, Bookrajian EN: Bacteriuria prevention after indwelling urinary catheterization. *Arch Intern Med* 110:703–711, 1962.
17. McCabe WR, Jackson GG: Gram-negative bacteremia. I. Etiology and ecology. *Arch Intern Med* 110:847–855, 1962.
18. McCabe WR, Jackson GG: Gram-negative bacteremia. II. Clinical, laboratory and therapeutic observations. *Arch Intern Med* 110:856–864, 1962.
19. Freid MA, Vosti KL: The importance of underlying disease in patients with Gram-negative bacteremia. *Arch Intern Med* 121:418–423, 1968.
20. DuPont HL, Spink WW: Infections due to Gram-negative organisms: An analysis of 860 patients with bacteremia at the University of Minnesota Medical Center. *Medicine* 48:307–332, 1969.
21. McGowan JE Jr, Parrott PL, Duty VP: Nosocomial bacteremia: Potential for prevention of procedure-related cases. *JAMA* 237:2727–2729, 1977.
22. Bryan CS, Reynolds KL: Hospital-acquired bacteremic urinary tract infection: Epidemiology and outcome. *J Urol* 132:494–498, 1984.
23. Daschner F, Nadjem H, Langmaack H, Sandritter W: Surveillance, prevention and control of hospital-acquired infections. *Infection* 6:261–265, 1978.
24. Quintiliani R, Klimek J, Cunha BA, Maderazo EG: Bacteremia after manipulation of the urinary tract. The importance of pre-existing urinary tract disease and compromised host defenses. *Postgrad Med J* 54:668–671, 1978.
25. Gross PA, Neu HC, Aswapokee P, Van Antwerpen C, Aswapokee N: Deaths from nosocomial infections: Experience

in a university hospital and a community hospital. *Am J Med* 68:219–223, 1980.

26. Platt R, Polk BF, Murdock B, Rosner B: Mortality associated with nosocomial urinary-tract infection. *N Engl J Med* 307:637–642, 1982.

27. Gross PA, Van Antwerpen C: Nosocomial infections and hospital deaths. *Am J Med* 75:658–662, 1983.

28. Haley RW, Hooton TM, Culver DH, Stanley RC, Emori TG, Handison CD, Quade D, Shadtman RH, Schaberg DR, Shah BV, Schaty GD: Nosocomial infections in US hospitals, 1975–1976. Estimated frequency by selected characteristics of patients. *Am J Med* 70:947–959, 1981.

29. Garibaldi RA, Burke JP, Dickman ML, Smith CB: Factors predisposing to bacteriuria during indwelling urethral catheterization. *N Engl J Med* 291:215–219, 1974.

30. Burke JP: Status of methods to prevent urinary catheter-associated infections. Presented to a symposium at Harvard Medical School in honor of Dr. Maxwell Finland, Boston, March 13, 1982.

31. Sobel JD, Kaye D: Host factors in the pathogenesis of urinary tract infections. *Am J Med* 76:122–130, 1984.

32. Rose HD, Schreier J: The effect of hospitalization and antibiotic therapy on the Gram-negative fecal flora. *Am J Med Sci* 255:228–236, 1968.

33. Shooter RA, Cooke EM, Gaya H, Jumar P, Patel N, Parker MT, Thom BT, France DR: Food and medicaments as possible sources of hospital strains of *Pseudomonas aeruginosa. Lancet* 1:1227–1229, 1969.

34. Montgomerie JZ, Morrow JW: *Pseudomonas* colonization in patients with spinal cord injury. *Am J Epidemiol* 108:328–336, 1978.

35. Cox CE: The urethra and its relationship to urinary tract infection: The flora of the normal female urethra. *South Med J* 59:621–626, 1966.

36. Helmholz HF Sr: Determination of the bacterial content of the urethra: A new method, with results of a study of 82 men. *J Urol* 64:158–166, 1950.

37. Platt R, Polk BF, Murdock B, Rosner B: Reduction of mortality associated with nosocomial urinary tract infection. *Lancet* 1:893–897, 1983.

38. Warren JW, Platt R, Thomas RJ, Rosner B, Kass EH: Antibiotic irrigation and catheter-associated urinary-tract infections. *N Engl J Med* 299:570–573, 1978.

39. Burke JP, Ingall D, Klein JO, Gezon HM, Finland M: *Proteus mirabilis* infections in a hospital nursery traced to a human carrier. *N Engl J Med* 284:115–121, 1971.

40. Morse LJ, Schonbeck LE: Hand lotions—a potential nosocomial hazard. *N Engl J Med* 278:376–378, 1968.

41. Sinclair WJ: *Semmelweis—His Life and His Doctrine*, London, Sherratt & Hughes, 1909, p. 49.

42. Williams REO, Blowers R, Garrod LP, Shooter RA: *Hospital Infection: Causes and Prevention*, London, Lloyd-Luke, 1960.

43. Gillespie WA, Linton KB, Miller A, Slade N: The diagnosis, epidemiology and control of urinary infection in urology and gynaecology. *J Clin Pathol* 13:187–194, 1960.

44. Emmett JL: Preoperative and postoperative care in transurethral prostatectomy. *Surg Clin North Am* 20:1061–1075, 1940.

45. Kass EH, Schneiderman LJ: Entry of bacteria into the urinary tracts of patients with inlying catheters. *N Engl J Med* 256:556–557, 1957.

46. Garibaldi RA, Burke JP, Britt MR, Miller WA, Smith CB: Meatal colonization and catheter-associated bacteriuria. *N Engl J Med* 303:316–318, 1980.

47. Shackman R, Messent D: The effect of an indwelling catheter on the bacteriology of the male urethra and bladder. *Br Med J* 2:1009–1012, 1954.

48. Bultitude MI, Eykyn S: The relationship between the urethral flora and urinary infection in the catheterized male. *Br J Urol* 45:678–683, 1973.

49. Brehmer B, Madsen PO: Route and prophylaxis of ascending bladder infection in male patients with indwelling catheters. *J Urol* 108:719–721, 1972.

50. Thompson RL, Haley CE, Searcy MA, Guenthner SM, Kaiser DL, Gröschel DHM, Gillenwater JY, Wenzel RP: Catheter-associated bacteriuria. Failure to reduce attack rates using periodic instillation of a disinfectant into urinary drainage systems. *JAMA* 251:747–751, 1984.

51. Wenzel RP, Osterman CA, Hunting KJ: Hospital-acquired infections. II. Infection rates by site, service and common procedures in a university hospital. *Am J Epidemiol* 104:645–651, 1976.

52. Burke JP, Jacobson JA, Garibaldi RA, Conti MI, Alling DW: Evaluation of daily meatal care with poly-antibiotic ointment in prevention of urinary catheter-associated bacteriuria. *J Urol* 129:331–334, 1983.

53. Guze LB, Beeson PB: Observations on the reliability and safety of bladder catheterization for bacteriologic study of the urine. *N Engl J Med* 255:474–475, 1956.

54. Kass EH: Bacteriuria and diagnosis of infections of the urinary tract with observations on the use of Methionine as a urinary antiseptic. *Arch Intern Med* 100:709–714, 1957.

55. Turck M, Goffe B, Petersdorf RG: The urethral catheter and urinary tract infection. *J Urol* 88:834–837, 1962.

56. Turck M, Petersdorf RG: The role of antibiotics in the prevention of urinary tract infections. *J Chronic Dis* 15:683–689, 1962.

57. Lapides J, Diokno AC, Lowe BS, Kalish MD: Followup on unsterile, intermittent self-catheterization. *J Urol* 111:184–186, 1974.

58. Kunin CM, McCormack RC: Prevention of catheter-induced urinary-tract infections by sterile closed drainage. *N Engl J Med* 274:1155–1161, 1966.

59. Kass EH: Asymptomatic infections of the urinary tract. *Trans Assoc Am Phy* 69:56–64, 1956.

60. Roberts JBM, Linton KB, Pollard BR, Mitchell JP, Gillespie WA: Long-term catheter drainage in males. *Brit J Urol* 37:63–72, 1965.

61. Lytton B: Urinary infection in cystoscopy. *Br Med J* 2:547–549, 1961.

62. Brumfitt W, Davies BI, Rosser EI: Urethral catheter as a cause of urinary-tract infection in pregnancy and puerperium. *Lancet* 2:1059–1062, 1961.

63. Schaberg DR, Haley RW, Highsmith AK, Anderson RL, McGowan JE Jr: Nosocomial bacteriuria: A prospective study of case clustering and antimicrobial resistance. *Ann Intern Med* 93:420–424, 1980.

64. Winterbauer RH, Turck M, Petersdorf RG: Studies on the epidemiology of *Escherichia coli* infections. V. Factors influencing acquisition of specific serologic groups. *J Clin Invest* 46:21–29, 1967.

65. Garibaldi RA, Brodine S, Matsumiya S: Infections among patients in nursing homes. Policies, prevalence and problems. *N Engl J Med* 305:731–735, 1981.

66. Warren JW, Tenney JH, Hoopes JM, Muncie HL, Anthony WC: A prospective microbiologic study of bacteriuria in patients with chronic indwelling urethral catheters. *J Infect Dis* 146:719–723, 1982.

67. Eddeland A, Hedelin H: Bacterial colonization of the lower urinary tract in women with long-term indwelling urethral catheter. *Scand J Infect Dis* 15:361–365, 1983.

68. Pryles CV, Eliot CR: Pyuria and bacteriuria in infants and children. *Am J Dis Child* 110:628–635, 1965.

69. McGuckin M, Cohen L, MacGregor RR: Significance of pyuria in urinary sediment. *J Urol* 120:452–454, 1978.

70. Stansfeld JM: The measurement and meaning of pyuria. *Arch Dis Child* 37:257–262, 1962.

71. Jenkins RD, Fenn JP, Matsen JM: Review of urine microscopy for bacteriuria. *JAMA* 255:3397–3403, 1986.

72. Sanford JP, Favour CB, Mao FH, Harrison JH: Evaluation of "positive" urine culture: Approach to differentiation of significant bacteria from contaminants. *Am J Med* 20:88–93, 1956.

73. Garner JS, Bennett JV, Scheckler WE, Maki DG, Brackman PS: Surveillance of nosocomial infections. *Proc Inter Conf*

Nocosomial Infections, Centers for Disease Control, Atlanta, August 3–6, 1970, 277.

74. Hellerstein S: Recurrent urinary tract infections in children. *Ped Infect Dis* 1:271–281, 1982.

75. Garibaldi RA: Hospital acquired urinary tract infections. In Wenzel RP (ed): *CRC Handbook of Hospital-Acquired Infections*. Boca Raton, CRC Press, 1981, pp. 513–537.

76. Lohr JA, Donowitz LG, Dudley SM: Bacterial contamination rates for non-clean-catch and clean-catch midstream urine collections in boys. *J Pediatr* 109:659–660, 1986.

77. Stark RP, Maki DG: Bacteriuria in the catheterized patient. What quantitative level of bacteriuria is relevant? *N Engl J Med* 311:560–564, 1984.

78. Daifuku R, Stamm WE: Association of rectal and urethral colonization with urinary tract infection in patients with indwelling catheters. *JAMA* 252:2028–2030, 1984.

79. Kevorkian CG, Merritt JL, Ilstrup DM: Methenamine mandelate with acidification: An effective urinary antiseptic in patients with neurogenic bladder. *Mayo Clin Proc* 59:523–529, 1984.

80. Gaynes RP, Weinstein RA, Smith J, Carman M, Kabins SA: Control of aminoglycoside resistance by barrier precautions. *J Infect Control* 4:221–224, 1983.

81. Kohn DB, Uehling DT, Peters ME, Fellows KW, Chesney PJ: Short-course amphotericin B therapy for isolated candiduria in children. *J Pediatr* 110:310–313, 1987.

82. Turner RB, Donowitz LG, Hendley JO: Consequences of Candidemia for Pediatric patients. *Am J Dis Child* 139:178–180, 1985.

83. Beeson PB: Editorial: The case against the catheter. *Am J Med* 24:1, 1958.

84. Johnson ET: The condom catheter: Urinary tract infection and other complications. *South J Med* 76:579–582, 1983.

85. Hirsch DD, Fainstein V, Musher DM: Do condom-catheter collecting systems cause urinary tract infections? *JAMA* 242:340–341, 1979.

86. Ansell J: Some observations on catheter care. *J Chronic Dis* 15:675–682, 1962.

87. Kunin CM: *Detection, Prevention and Management of Urinary Tract Infections*, ed 2. Philadelphia, Lea & Febiger, 1974.

88. Lindan R: The prevention of ascending, catheter-induced infections of the urinary tract. *J Chronic Dis* 22:321–332, 1969.

89. Keresteci AG, Leers WD: Indwelling catheter infection. *Can Med Assoc J* 109:711–713, 1973.

90. Lawrence CA, Block SS: *Disinfection, Sterilization and Preservation*. Philadelphia, Lea and Febiger, 1968.

91. Sanford JP: Disinfectants that don't. *Ann Intern Med* 72:282–283, 1970.

92. Viant AC, Linton KB, Gillespie WA, Midwinter A: Improved method for preventing movement of indwelling catheters in female patients. *Lancet* 1:736–737, 1971.

93. Selden R, Lee S, Wang WLL, Bennett JV, Eickhoff TC: Nosocomial *Klebsiella* infections: Intestinal colonization as a reservoir. *Ann Intern Med* 74:657–664, 1971.

94. Burke JP, Garibaldi RA, Britt MR, Jacobson JA, Conti M, Alling DW: Prevention of catheter-associated urinary tract infections. Efficacy of daily meatal care regimens. *Am J Med* 70:655–658, 1981.

95. Larsen RA, Burke JP: Determinants of the efficacy of meatal care in preventing catheter-associated urinary infections. *Clin Res* 33:100A, 1985.

96. Butler HK, Kunin CM: Evaluation of Polymyxin catheter lubricant and impregnated catheters. *J Urol* 100:560–566, 1968.

97. Kunin CB, Finkelberg Z: Evaluation of an intraurethral lubricating catheter in prevention of catheter-induced urinary tract infections. *J Urol* 106:928–930, 1971.

98. Evans AT, Cicmenec JF: The role of Betadine microbicides in urine bag sterilization. In *Proceedings of the Second World Congress on Antiseptics 1980*. New York, HP Publishing, 1980, pp. 85–86.

99. Maizels M, Schaeffer AJ: Decreased incidence of bacteriuria associated with periodic instillation of hydrogen peroxide into the urethral catheter drainage bag. *J Urol* 123:841–845, 1980.

100. Desautels RE, Chibaro EA, Lang RJ: Maintenance of sterility of urinary drainage bags. *Surg Gynecol Obstet* 154:838–840, 1982.

101. Southampton Infection Control Team: Evaluation of aseptic techniques and chlorhexidine on the rate of catheter-associated urinary tract infections. *Lancet* 1:89–91, 1982.

102. Gillespie WA, Jones JE, Teasdale C, Simpson RA, Nashef L, Speller DCE: Does the addition of disinfectant to urine drainage bags prevent infection in catheterized patients? *Lancet* 1:1037–1039, 1983.

103. Noy MF, Smith CA, Watterson LL: The use of chlorhexidine in catheter bags. *J Hosp Infect* 3:365–367, 1982.

4

Surgical Wound Infection

Robert Lee Brawley, M.D., M.P.H.

BACKGROUND

The nationwide nosocomial infection rate in the Study on the Efficacy of Nosocomial Infection Control (SENIC) in acute care hospitals was 5.7 infections per 100 admissions. Surgical wound infections were second among the most common sites for nosocomial infections, with over 500,000 infections per year (1). More importantly, surgical wound infections constituted 24% of all nosocomial infections but accounted for 55% of additional hospital days and 42% of extra costs attributable to nosocomial infections (2).

Etiology

Almost all surgical wound infections are acquired at the time of operation (3). Risk for developing surgical wound infection is largely determined by complex interaction of three factors: the amount and type of wound contamination; wound condition at the end of surgery (related to surgical technique); and host resistance to infection (4). Wounds contamination can come from extraneous sources (exogenous contamination), such as the surgeon's hands, other surgery team members, or the operating room environment. Contamination more likely comes from the patient's own bacteria (endogenous contamination) from some area of the body next to or sometimes remote from the surgical site (3,5,6).

Incidence

Pediatric and newborn services and children's hospitals were specifically excluded from the SENIC study, and no incidence rates for surgical wound infections in children were calculated. However, these pediatric nationwide surveillance data were collected by the National Nosocomial Infections Surveys (NNIS), which categorized hospitals as nonteaching, small

teaching (≤ 500 beds), and large teaching (> 500 beds). From 1980–1982, pediatric surgical wound infection rates per 1000 discharges for these hospital categories were 0.6, 0.8, and 1.6, respectively. Newborn surgical wound infection rates per 1000 discharges were 0.2, 0.4, and 0.7, respectively. These data compare with overall surgical wound infection rates per 1000 discharges from NNIS hospitals for all surgical services of 4.6, 6.4, and 8.2, respectively (7).

Prospective studies of surgical wound infections in children have been infrequent (6,8–17). Surgical wound infections have comprised from 0.9%–30% of all nosocomial infections in newborns and children. Surgical wound infection rates in children have varied widely from 0.4–150 infections per 1000 admissions (Table 4.1). Surgical wound infections per 1000 admissions have been determined for various surgical services (Table 4.2), with highest rates occurring in neurosurgery and cardiovascular surgery.

The incidence of pediatric surgical wound infections in clean wounds has varied by location from 2.1% in Toronto (8), to 3.1% in Milwaukee (16), and 7.9% in London (13). Cruse and Foord (18) studied 62,939 wounds over ten years and reported that a clean wound infection rate of <1% was ideal, a rate of 1%–2% was acceptable, and >2% was a rate for concern and investigation.

Organisms Causing Surgical Wound Infections

Surgical wound infections in children principally have been bacterial infections with viral and fungal infections being rare in normal children. NNIS surveys in the early 1970s reported that *Staplylococcus aureus*, *Escherichia coli*, and *Pseudomonas aeruginosa* were the pathogens most frequently isolated from pediatric and

Table 4.1
Studies of Pediatric Surgical Wound Infections in the Literature

Site	Ref.	Year Reported	Total No. of Adm.	No. Surg. Wound Infect.	Surg. Wound Infect. Rate[a]	Percent of Nosocomial Infect.
Sick Children's, Toronto	8	62	17,836	157	8.8	13.5
University of Kentucky	9	67	376	6	16.0	30.0
Childrens Hosp., Boston	10	72	12,209	145	11.9	26.0
University of Virginia	11	75	5050 Peds	2	0.4	0.9
			344 NICU	1	2.9	1.2
Adelaide Child., Australia	12	76	37,674	181	4.8	17.0
Rush-Presbyterian-St. Lukes, Chicago	6	76	5968		26.4 specialty surg. 40.7 general surg.	
Sick Children's, London	13	76	459	69	150.3	21.0
University of Iowa	14	81	7339	38	5.2	9.8
Childrens Hosp., Buffalo	15	84	17,221	59	3.4	8.4
Milwaukee Childrens	16	84	1045 cases	44	4.2	
University of Virginia	17	86	3084	17	5.5	9.1

[a]Infections per 1000 admissions.

Table 4.2
Surgical Wound Infection Rates for Pediatric Surgical Services

Surgical Service	Chicago (6)	Boston Children's (10)	U. Virginia (17)
Cardiovascular	108.0		
General surgery	40.7	16.8	
Neurosurgery	90.9	41.8	
Orthopaedics	23.1	20.8	
Pediatric surgery			19.6
Plastic surgery	22.5		37.7
Thoracic surgery	38.5		

[a]Infections per 1000 admissions.

newborn surgical wound infections (19). During the early 1980s, *S. aureus* continued as the most common bacterial pathogen; *E. coli*, and *P. aeruginosa* were among the top five pathogens likely to cause surgical wound infections (Table 4.3). Newborn surgical wound infections in the early 1980s had an increase in predominance of *P. aeruginosa* and coagulase-negative *Staphylococci* (20,21).

These data have been similar in other reports of pediatric surgical wound infections. *S. aureus*, either alone or combined with *E. coli*, was cultured from 30% of infected wounds reported by Doig and Wilkinson (13). *S. aureus*, *E. coli*, and *Pseudomonas* spp. were the three most common pathogens recovered from surgical wound infections by Welliver and McLaughlin (15), with *S. aureus* and Gram-negative bacilli caus-

Table 4.3
Most Common Bacterial Pathogens in Pediatric and Newborn Surgical Wound Infections

Pathogen	Percentage of Surgical Wound Infections					
	NNIS 80–82 (7)		NNIS 83 (20)		NNIS 84 (21)	
	P[a]	N	P	N	P	N
S. aureus	27.1	35.1	28.8	30.4	34.8	23.1
E. coli	15.8	13.1	8.2		10.6	
Coagulase-neg. *Staph* spp.		11.3	16.4	26.1	10.6	23.1
P. aeruginosa	6.2		6.8	8.7	10.6	15.4
Enterococci	8.9		6.8	13.0	7.6	7.7
Klebsiella spp.		9.5	6.8	13.0		7.7
Bacteroides spp.	6.5					
Enterobacter spp.		6.6				

[a]P–pediatric; N–newborn

ing almost an equal number of cases. Gardner and Carles (10), had *S. aureus* isolated from 48% of wound infections, *E. coli* from 20%, and *Klebsiella*-Enterobacter from 17%. *S. aureus* was the most frequent pathogen isolated from surgical wound infections in a surgical special care nursery (14) and at a children's hospital in Australia (12). Roy and coworkers (8) studied admissions to a pediatric hospital in 1959; *S. aureus* caused 89% of surgical wound infections in clean wounds, and 57% of those in wounds not classified as clean, mostly related to operations on the intestinal tract.

Since surgical wound infections have been defined clinically by the presence of pus in the incision site, a positive culture is not required; and cultures may never be performed. However, cultures were obtained from 69% of infected wounds in the 1959 study of Roy and coworkers (8) and from 83% of wounds studied by Welliver and McLaughlin (15) in 1980–1981.

POPULATION

The population at risk for surgical wound infections in newborns and children has not been specifically defined from prospective studies. High-risk surgical patients could be predicted with a multivariable index developed by logistic regression from the SENIC study data (22). Four risk factors predicted a subgroup of patients developing 90% of surgical wound infections. These risk factors were abdominal operation, operation longer than two hours, contaminated or dirty wound class, and having three or more underlying diagnoses. This multivariate index has not been validated for pediatric patients; targeted surveillance for surgical wound infections in high-risk children would be the advantage of this index.

Culbertson and coworkers (23) stated that surgical wound infection risk varied inversely with host resistance. Pediatric patients with abnormalities in host resistance by virtue of age, underlying conditions or diseases, and/or medications should then be more susceptible to surgical wound infections.

Age

Davis and coworkers (16) reported no significant differences in mean age between infected and uninfected pediatric surgical patients having clean surgical procedures. Doig and Wilkinson's study (13), however, showed significantly

increased rates for younger patients, with 38.4% of neonatal wounds becoming infected compared with 12.4% of wounds in children 5 years and older. Mead and coworkers (24) noted that children <1 year old had higher clean wound infection rates (2.7%) than children 1–14 years old (0.3%). Donowitz (25) has reviewed the immunologic deficiencies of the newborn which increase their risk for nosocomial infections. Particularly important for surgical wound infections was the poor development of the stratum corneum in premature infants less than 32 weeks gestation.

Underlying Conditions

Intensive Care.   Maguire and coworkers (14) demonstrated increased risk for surgical wound infections among patients in a surgical special care nursery. Donowitz (17) reported that pediatric intensive care patients had significantly more surgical wound infections than pediatric ward admissions (1.5 infections per 100 admissions vs. 0.5 infections per 100 admissions; $P = 0.03$).

Trauma.   Caplan and coworkers (26) reported the increased risk for nosocomial infections in trauma patients. No comparable series has been reported in pediatric trauma patients.

The surgical wound classification system has been modified to estimate the relative probability of surgical wound infections after trauma based on bacterial contamination and time from injury to operative treatment (27). A similar classification for pediatric trauma patients would more accurately estimate their risk of surgical wound infections.

Tertiary Care.   Pediatric tertiary care centers have not been specifically studied as a variable affecting surgical wound infections. The rise in popularity of ambulatory surgery with removal of relatively simple surgical cases from these hospitals would tend to increase the surgical wound infection rates. Longer preoperative stays and longer surgery in more complex surgical cases would be risk factors for higher surgical wound infection rates in tertiary care hospitals (16).

DIAGNOSIS

Surgical wound infection has been defined as the presence of pus at the incision site. For burn wounds, infection was defined as either $\geq 10^6$

organisms per gram of biopsied tissue, or new inflammation or new pus not present on admission (28).

Diagnosis of surgical wound infection is usually empirically determined with prediction of bacterial etiology based on clinical presentation. Clinicians should be encouraged to obtain purulent material for Gram stain and culture prior to instituting antimicrobial therapy.

Early Detection of Surgical Wound Infections

Clinical characteristics of surgical wound infections which depend upon the bacterial etiology have been described (5,29,30). Group A Streptococcal infection, rarely a modern cause of surgical wound infections, causes rapidly spreading erythema with systemic toxicity within 24–48 hours after surgery. Wound infections with systemic toxicity caused by *Clostridium* spp. may also appear one or two days postoperatively.

Surgical wound infections caused by other bacterial pathogens generally present from 4–14 days postoperatively. *S. aureus* and *Staphylococcus* spp. infections appear from 3–7 days postoperatively. Induration, erythema, wound tenderness, thick purulent drainage, or abscess formation are prominent features of *S. aureus* infections; systemic toxicity may predict dissemination from the wound to other organs. Mixed infections with Gram-negative enteric bacilli and anaerobes generally cause infections 4–6 days postoperatively. Infections caused by enteric Gram-negative bacilli, alone, usually present 7–14 days after surgery; induration is prominent with little erythema. Systemic toxicity is common with enteric Gram-negative bacilli infections, especially with dissemination to other body sites.

Most gastrointestinal tract surgical wound infections are polymicrobial, caused by Gram-negative enteric bacilli, *Pseudomonas* spp., enterococci, and anaerobic bacteria. Bacterial species can be predicted by the gastrointestinal site that was the source of contamination. In general, the small bowel contains predominantly aerobic Gram-negative bacilli, but the distal ileum and colon has a predominance of anaerobes mixed with enterococci and aerobic Gram-negative bacilli (31). Peritonitis in the child is almost invariably the result of intestinal contamination from a ruptured appendicitis or perforated bowel. *E. coli*, enterococci, and *Bacteroides fragilis* have been common causes of peritonitis (29).

Surveillance for Surgical Wound Infections

Surgical wound infections may be detected by prospective surveillance using either wound classification-specific or procedure-specific surveillance techniques (32–35).

The amount and type of microbial contamination of the wound is one risk factor for developing surgical wound infections (4,29). A surgical wound classification system based on clinical estimation of contamination and subsequent risk of infection (32,33) has been widely used to define four categories of surgical procedures: clean wounds, clean-contaminated wounds, contaminated wounds, and dirty (i.e., definitely infected) wounds. Several studies have found increasing surgical wound infection rates proportional to the degree of contamination (13,16,23,36). The Centers for Disease Control (CDC) has recommended that all operations be classified by this method (4).

Procedure-specific surgical wound infection surveillance has been used at the University of Virginia since 1972 (34) and in statewide surveillance of surgical wound infections in Virginia hospitals (35). This surveillance method for pediatric surgical patients has not been reported at other hospitals. Surveillance and tabulation of procedure-specific surgical wound infection rates have also been recommended by the CDC (4).

Surgical wound infection rates may vary considerably for procedures within even clean wound categories. A major advantage of procedure-specific wound surveillance is to focus surveillance and control efforts on surgical procedures at high risk for developing surgical wound infections (37).

TREATMENT

Many treatment principles of surgical wound infections are similar to those applied for antibiotic prophylaxis prior to surgery (29,37). For effective treatment, the bacterial pathogens must be determined empirically at clinical presentation of the surgical wound infection. Antibiotics must then be selected for their known activity against these predicted pathogens, with consideration of toxicity, side effects, pharmacologic half-life, and cost.

Clinicians should be encouraged to obtain Gram stains of purulent material and culture prior to treatment. Definitive antimicrobial therapy should replace the empiric regimen based on these laboratory results and clinical progress. A table of susceptibility of certain bacteria to available antibiotics has been compiled by Young (38). Blumer and coworkers (39) reviewed the treament of pediatric skin and soft tissue infections and recommended guidelines for therapy with oral antibiotics.

Antibiotic Recommendations

Gram-positive Infections

Infections that can be caused by either *Staphylococcus aureus* or the Group A *Streptococcus* can be treated with nafcillin, oxacillin, or early generation cephalosporins, such as cefazolin. Nafcillin is primarily metabolized by the liver and should be avoided in the jaundiced neonate and in patients with liver diseases (40). Oral antistaphyloccal agents, such as dicloxacillin or cloxacillin, should be used to treat only mild or moderately severe infections (38,39).

When methicillin resistant *S. aureus* is a potential pathogen in a hospital, vancomycin should be the empiric therapy, pending culture and sensitivity results. Vancomycin is also the empiric treatment of choice for coagulase-negative *Staphylococci*, which are often resistant to multiple antibiotics. Vancomycin, alone or combined with rifampin, would be the empiric treatment of choice for central nervous system (CNS) shunt infections caused by Gram-positive cocci, since coagulase-negative *Staphylococci* cause 60%–75% of shunt infections (41). Definitive therapy for coagulase-negative *Staphylococci* should be guided by culture and sensitivity results.

Penicillin G, ampicillin, vancomycin, or mezlocillin usually are given for uncomplicated enterococcal infections. More serious enterococcal infections can be treated with synergistic combinations of penicillin G or ampicillin plus gentamicin. In penicillin allergic patients, vancomycin plus gentamicin would be recommended with caution because of potential nephrotoxicity (42).

Gram-negative Infections

Peritonitis and infections from gastrointestinal surgery may be empirically treated with cefoxitin (29,43,44); or ampicillin, gentamicin, and clindamycin (29,45); or ampicillin, amikacin, and often, clindamycin or metronidazole (46). Early limitation of the antibiotic spectrum, based on aerobic and anaerobic bacteriologic data, is highly recommended.

Since appendicitis is the most common reason for intraabdominal surgery in childhood, antibiotic treatment of appendicitis continues to be studied. David and coworkers (45) reviewed 300 cases of gangrenous and perforated appendicitis. Children treated with ampicillin, gentamicin, and clindamycin had shorter hospital stays with fewer wound infections than children treated with ampicillin and/or gentamicin. The Danish study of perforated appendicitis (44) had a 3% incidence of intraabdominal abscesses with 5 days of cefoxitin compared with an 11.3% incidence with ampicillin and metronidazole ($P < 0.05$). Lau and coworkers (47) treated patients with gangrenous, perforated, or abscessed appendicitis with 5 days of antibiotics; moxalactam significantly decreased ($P < 0.05$) septic complications compared with either cefotaxime or cefoperazone.

Surgical Management

Operative management and antibiotics are usually necessary for satisfactory resolution of surgical wound infections involving either closed anatomical spaces or abscess formation (29). Most wound infections require suture removal, and opening of the incision with appropriate drainage and wound debridement. Antibiotics should be given before surgical drainage to ensure that drug concentrations in the blood and tissues are adequate to inhibit the growth of any bacteria disseminated by the procedure (5,38). For intraabdominal infections, drainage of the infection focus is mandatory in combination with antibiotic therapy (30).

PREVENTION

Modifying Risk Factors for Surgical Wound Infections

Many recommendations in the literature for preventing surgical wound infections were derived from studies of general surgical patients. A superb summary of this literature was completed by Mayhall (3) who concluded that only seven recommendations were supported by proper epidemiologic studies. These recommended prevention techniques were: 1. minimizing preoperative hospitalization; 2. weight reduction for obesity; 3. eradication of remote infections; 4. hair removal by clipping or shaving with a razor just prior to surgery; 5. minimizing the duration of surgery; 6. prophylactic antibiotics; and 7. prospective surveillance with feedback of surgical wound infection rates to individual surgeons. These recommendations could be applied to the prevention of pediatric surgical wound infections as follows:

Preoperative Hospitalization.   Cruse (5) conducted a prospective 10-year study of surgical wound infections. The clean wound infection rate with a 1-day preoperative stay was 1.2%; it was 2.1% with a 1-week stay, and 3.4% with a preoperative stay of more than 2 weeks. These increasing rates inferred that colonization of the patient's skin by nosocomial organisms increased during the period of preoperative hospitalization. A Swedish study (48) reported that surgical wound infection rates increased from 4.5% with a 1-day preoperative hospital stay to 12.5% with longer preoperative stays; however, this study was confounded by three or more other variables associated with high surgical wound infection rates in 85% of the patients with longer preoperative stays.

Only Davis and coworkers (16) have demonstrated significant differences (P < 0.04) in the mean duration of preoperative hospitalization between infected (6.5 days) and uninfected (5.0 days) patients in a children's hospital.

Future studies of this factor in pediatric surgical wound infections will have to control for changing patterns of surgical practice, since ambulatory surgery has become more common. One study of ambulatory surgery has demonstrated an overall surgical wound infection rate of less than 1% (49).

Obesity.   Obesity has not been confirmed as a risk factor in pediatric surgical wound infections. The National Research Council (NRC) (32) prospective study reported a surgical wound infection rate for obese patients of 16.5%. Cruse and Foord (50) reported an overall clean wound infection rate of 1.8%, which increased to 13.5% in obese patients. Weight control, prior to surgery, for obese, older pediatric patients with elective surgical procedures, thus, seems prudent pending definitive study of this possible risk factor.

Remote Infections.   Active infections remote from the surgery site have been shown to increase the risk for surgical wound infections. In the NRC study (32), remote infections increased the surgical wound infection rate from 6.7% to 18.4%; genitourinary and respiratory infections were the most frequent remote infections. Birkenstock (51) in South Africa had the surgical wound infection rate increased from 6.0% to 31.6% by remote infections. Edwards (6) reported that 61.3% of surgical wound infections were associated with remote infections. These remote infections were mostly in the urinary tract or lower respiratory tract and were associated with medical devices in these sites, intravascular devices, or prostheses.

Children with known remote sites of infection should not have elective surgery until the infection is eradicated or under appropriate control with definitive treatment. Special attention should also be given to the proper use and control of medical devices, especially intravascular devices, which may predispose the surgical patient to occult remote infections (6).

Hair Removal.   Techniques of hair removal for surgery have been studied in adults. Seropian and Reynolds (52) had significantly higher surgical wound infection rates after hair removal by razor (5.6%) than with no preoperative hair removal (0.6%). Cruse (5) reported a 0.9% clean surgical infection rate in patients with no hair removal; it was 1.4% in patients shaved with an electric razor, and 2.3% in patients shaved with a standard razor. Alexander and coworkers (53) reported that hair removal by clippers instead of razors had significantly lower surgical wound infection rates both at hospital discharge and 30 days after surgery.

Hair removal in pediatric patients requiring surgery should be done with electric clippers or electric razors. The occasional patient who requires hair removal with a standard razor should have the procedure performed by the surgeon in the operating room.

Duration of Surgery.   Risk of surgical wound infection was strongy associated with the duration of surgery. Operation longer than two hours was a variable in the simplified index for predicting surgical wound infections developed from the SENIC study (22). Doig and Wilkinson (13) showed a doubling of surgical wound infection rates with each hour of surgery. Davis and coworkers (16) reported significantly longer (P < 0.02) mean duration of surgery in pediatric patients with wound infections (333 minutes) compared with children who did not develop wound infections (222 minutes).

Duration of surgery should be a variable reported in the surveillance of pediatric surgical wound infections. Stratification of surgical wound infection rates by both procedure and duration of surgery would enhance feedback of surgical wound infection rates to individual surgeons.

Prophylactic Antibiotics. Antibiotic prophylaxis was defined as the use of antimicrobial agents in the absence of suspected or documented infection (54). Antibiotic prophylaxis should be given only when the risk of infection outweighs the risks of therapy. Rational antibiotic prophylaxis may be prospectively based on the surgical wound classification (29).

Antibiotic prophylaxis is indicated when there is a high risk of infection following surgery (i.e., alimentary tract surgery); when the risk of infection is low but has disastrous consequences when it occurs, such as cardiovascular or orthopaedic prosthetic implant surgery; and for invasive surgical procedures in patients with immunosuppression (i.e., leukemia, high-dose steroids) (3,30,54). Several important principles were recommended for antibiotic prophylaxis. First, the antibiotic(s) used must be active against the majority of anticipated pathogens. In addition, antibiotic inhibitory levels must be continuously present when contaminating organisms have access to exposed tissue until final wound closure. Finally, antibiotic prophylaxis should not be continued beyond 48 hours (3,30,55).

Kaiser (37) has reviewed the recent features of antimicrobial prophylaxis in surgery and has tabulated recommended antibiotic prophylaxis for most commonly performed surgical procedures. Prophylactic antibiotics in pediatric surgical procedures can be recommended for many alimentary tract and biliary tract procedures, urinary tract surgery, or instrumentation in children with bacteriuria or obstructive uropathy (13), cardiac surgery for structural defects, surgery with prosthetic materials, and surgery in the immunocompromised host (29,30).

Prospective Wound Surveillance Program. The SENIC nationwide controlled study of surgical wound infections (2,22) reported that hospitals with organized infection control programs with intensive surveillance and reporting of surgical wound infection rates to surgeons reduced surgical wound infection rates by 20% compared to hospitals without those programs. Moreover, hospitals with these active infection control programs, plus a physician with a special interest in infection control, were able to reduce surgical wound infection rates by 38% compared to hospitals without similar programs.

Reduction in surgical wound infection rates with prospective surveillance and feedback of rates to individual surgeons has been found in other studies (2,18,24,56,57). Haley (2) cited the 1915 paper by Brewer where clean wound infection rates dropped from 39% in 1895 to 1.2% by 1913–1914. Cruse and Foord (18) had clean wound infection rates over their 10-year study decline from 2.5% to 0.6%; Mead and coworkers (24) reported a 42% reduction in clean wound infection rates from 1.9% to 1.1%. A 5-year study by Olson and coworkers (56) reported a significant decline (P < 0.05) in overall surgical wound infection rates from 4.2% to 1.9%. Condon and coworkers (57) reported that the clean wound infection rate significantly decreased (P < 0.01) from 3.5% to < 1%.

Prospective surveillance for surgical wound infections using SENIC (2,22) and CDC guidelines (4) should be part of every hospital's infection control program.

Infection Control Guidelines-Surgical Wound Infections. Guidelines for the prevention of surgical wound infections have been published by the CDC (4). Some guidelines needed special emphasis. First, handwashing was the single most important infection control measure for preventing the transmission of infectious diseases in hospitalized patients (58). Handwashing should be especially emphasized in intensive care units where compliance has been low (59). Health care personnel should be required to wash their hands before and after surgical wound care. Also, contact isolation was recommended for major surgical wound infections. Patients with significant *S. aureus* wound infections, especially, should not share a room with other preoperative or postoperative patients (60). Outbreaks of wound infections caused by the same organism, such as methicillin-resistant *S. aureus* may require cohort isolation techniques (61). Drainage/secretion precautions were designed to prevent the spread of infection by direct or indirect contact with purulent material and may be used for minor surgical wounds (60).

REFERENCES

1. Haley RW, Culver DH, White JW, Morgan WM, Emori TG: The nationwide nosocomial infection rate: A new need for vital statistics. *Am J Epidemiol* 121:159–167, 1985.

2. Haley RW: Surveillance by objective: A new priority-directed approach to the control of nosocomial infections. *Am J Infect Control* 13:78–89, 1985.

3. Mayhall CG: Surgical infections including burns. In Wenzel RP (ed): *Prevention and Control of Nosocomial Infections.* Baltimore, Williams & Wilkins, 1987, pp 344–384.

4. Garner JS: CDC guidelines for prevention of surgical wound infection, 1985. *Infect Control* 7:193–200, 1986.

5. Cruse P: Surgical infection: Incisional wounds. In Bennett JV, Brachman PS (eds): *Hospital Infections,* ed 2. Boston, Little, Brown, & Company, 1986, pp 423–436.

6. Edwards LD: The epidemiology of 2056 remote site infections and 1966 surgical wound infections occurring in 1865 patients: A four year study of 40,923 operations at Rush-Presbyterian-St. Luke's Hospital, Chicago. *Ann Surg* 184:758–766, 1976.

7. Centers for Disease Control. Nosocomial infection surveillance, 1980–1982. In *CDC Surveillance Summaries.* 32:1SS–16SS, 1983.

8. Roy TE, McDonald S, Patrick ML, Keddy JA: A survey of hospital infection in a pediatric hospital. Part II. The distribution of hospital infections in different areas of the hospital, postoperative wound infections and the consequences of infection. *Can Med Assoc J* 87:592–599, 1962.

9. McNamara MJ, Hill MC, Balows A, Tucker EB: A study of the bacteriologic patterns of hospital infections. *Ann Intern Med* 66:480–488, 1967.

10. Gardner P, Carles DG: Infections acquired in a pediatric hospital. *J Pediatr* 81:1205–1210, 1972.

11. Wenzel RP, Osterman CA, Hunting KJ: Hospital acquired infections. II. Infection rates by site, service, and common procedures in a university hospital. *Am J Epidemiol* 104:645–651, 1976.

12. Cooper RG, Sumner C: Hospital infection data from a children's hospital. *Med J Austr* 2:1110–1113, 1970.

13. Doig CM, Wilkinson AW: Wound infection in a children's hospital. *Br J Surg* 63:647–650, 1976.

14. Maguire GC, Nordin J, Myers MG, Koontz FP, Hierholzer W, Nassif E: Infections acquired by young infants. *Am J Dis Child* 135:693–698, 1981.

15. Welliver RC, McLaughlin S: Unique epidemiology of nosocomial infection in a children's hospital. *Am J Dis Child* 138:131–135, 1984.

16. Davis SD, Sobocinski K, Hoffmann RG, Mohr B, Nelson DB: Postoperative wound infections in a children's hospital. *Pediatr Infect Dis* 3:114–116, 1984.

17. Donowitz LG: High risk of nosocomial infection in the pediatric critical care patient. *Crit Care Med* 14:26–28, 1986.

18. Cruse PJE, Foord R: The epidemiology of wound infection. A 10-year prospective study of 62,939 wounds. *Surg Clin North Am* 60:27–40, 1980.

19. Cruse PJE: Wound infections: Epidemiology and clinical characteristics. In Simmons RL, Howard RJ (eds): *Surgical Infectious Diseases,* New York, Appleton-Century Crofts, 1982, pp 429–441.

20. Centers for Disease Control. Nosocomial infection surveillance, 1983. In *CDC Surveillance Summaries* 33:9SS–21SS, 1984.

21. Centers for Disease Control. Nosocomial infection surveillance, 1984. In *CDC Surveillance Summaries* 34:17SS–29SS, 1986.

22. Haley RW, Culver DH, Morgan WM, White JW, Emori TG, Hooten TM: Identifying patients at high risk of surgical wound infection. A simple multivariate index of patient susceptibility and wound contamination. *Am J Epidemiol* 121:206–215, 1985.

23. Culbertson WR, Altemeier WA, Gonzalez LL, Hill EO: Studies on the epidemiology of postoperative infection of clean operative wounds. *Ann Surg* 154:599–603, 1961.

24. Mead PB, Pories SE, Hall P, Vacek PM, Davis JH, Gamelli RL: Decreasing the incidence of surgical wound infections. Validation of a surveillance notification program. *Arch Surg* 121:458–461, 1986.

25. Donowitz LG: Infection in the newborn. In Wenzel RP (ed): *Prevention and Control of Nosocomial Infections.* Baltimore, Williams & Wilkins, 1987, pp 481–493.

26. Caplan ES, Hoyt N, Cowley RA: Changing patterns of nosocomial infections in severely traumatized patients. *Amer Surgeon* 45:204–210, 1979.

27. Weigelt JA: Risk of wound infections in trauma patients. *Am J Surg* 150:782–784, 1985.

28. Wenzel RP, Osterman CA, Hunting KJ, Gwaltney JM: Hospital-acquired infections. I. Surveillance in a university hospital. *Am J Epidemiol* 103:251–260, 1976.

29. Mollitt DL: Pediatric surgical infection and antibiotic usage. *Pediatr Infect Dis* 4:326–329, 1985.

30. Stone HH: Infection in postoperative patients. *Am J Med* 81 (Suppl 1A):39–44, 1986.

31. Stone HH, Kolb LD, Geheber CE: Incidence and significance of intraperitoneal anaerobic bacteria. *Ann Surg* 181:705–710, 1975.

32. National Academy of Sciences—National Research Council. Division of Medical Sciences Ad Hoc Committee of the Committee on Trauma: Postoperative wound infections: The influence of ultraviolet irradiation of the operating room and of various other factors. *Ann Surg* 160 (Suppl 2):2–192, 1964.

33. Definitions and classifications of surgical infections. In Committee on Control of Surgical Infections of the Committee on Pre- and Postoperative Care. American College of Surgeons. Altemeier WA, Burke JF, Pruit BA, Sandusky WR (eds): *Manual on Control of Infections in Surgical Patients,* ed 2. Philadelphia, JB Lippincott, 1982, pp 27–29.

34. Wenzel RP, Hunting KJ, Osterman CA: Postoperative wound infection rates. *Surg Gynecol Obstet* 144:749–752, 1977.

35. Farber BF, Wenzel RP: Postoperative wound infection rates: Results of prospective statewide surveillance. *Am J Surg* 140:343–346, 1980.

36. Lennard ES, Hargiss CO, Schoenknecht FD: Postoperative wound infection surveillance by use of bacterial contamination categories. *Am J Infect Control* 13:147–153, 1985.

37. Kaiser AB: Antimicrobial prophylaxis in surgery. *N Engl J Med* 315:1129–1138, 1986.

38. Young LS: Antimicrobial therapy. In Wyngaarden JB, Smith LH (eds): *Cecil Textbook of Medicine,* ed 17. Philadelphia, WB Saunders, 1985, pp 96–108.

39. Blumer JL, Lemon E, O'Horo J, Snodgrass DJ: Changing therapy for skin and soft tissue infections in children: Have we come full circle? *Pediatr Infect Dis* 6:117–122, 1987.

40. Nelson JD: *1987–1988 Pocketbook of Pediatric Antimicrobial Therapy,* ed 7. Baltimore, Williams & Wilkins, 1987, p 6.

41. Yogev R: Cerebrospinal fluid shunt infections: A personal view. *Pediatr Infect Dis* 4:113–118, 1985.

42. Gullberg RM: The enterococcus. *Infect Control* 7:600–606, 1986.

43. Kager L, Nord CE: Use of beta-lactam antibiotics in intra-abdominal surgery. *Scand J Infect Dis* Suppl 42:143–150, 1984.

44. The Danish Multicenter Study Group: A Danish multicenter study: Cefoxitin versus ampicillin and metronidazole in perforated appendicitis. *Br J Surg* 71:144–146, 1984.

45. David IB, Buck JR, Filler RM: Rational use of antibiotics for perforated appendicitis in childhood. *J Pediatr Surg* 17:494–500, 1982.

46. Chadwick EG, Yogev R, Shulman ST: Combination antibiotic therapy in pediatrics. *Am J Med* 80 (Suppl 6B):166–171, 1986.

47. Lau W, Fan S, Chu K, Suen H, Yiu T, Wong K: Randomized, prospective, and double-blind trial of new β-lactams in the treatment of appendicitis. *Antimicrob Agents Chemother* 28:639–642, 1985.

48. Hasselgren P, Aaljo A, Fornander J, Lundstam S, Seeman T: Postoperative wound infections in patients with long preoperative hospital stay. *Acta Chir Scand* 148:473–477, 1982.

49. Craig CP: Infection surveillance for ambulatory surgery patients: An overview. *QRB* 9:107–111, 1983.

50. Cruse PJE, Foord R: A five-year prospective study of 23,649 surgical wounds. *Arch Surg* 107:206–210, 1973.

51. Birkenstock WE: Surgical sepsis. *S Afr Med J* 47:436–440, 1973.

52. Seropian R, Reynolds BM: Wound infections after preoperative depilatory versus razor preparation. *Am J Surg* 121:251–254, 1971.

53. Alexander JW, Fischer JE, Boyajian M, Palmquist J, Morris MJ: The influence of hair-removal methods on wound infections. *Arch Surg* 118:347–352, 1983.

54. Committee on Infectious Diseases, Committee on Drugs, and Section on Surgery. Antimicrobial prophylaxis in pediatric surgical patients. *Pediatrics* 74:437–439, 1984.

55. Platt R: Antibiotic prophylaxis in surgery. *Rev Infect Dis* 6 (Suppl 4):S880–S886, 1984.

56. Olson M, O'Connor M, Schwartz ML: Surgical wound infections. A 5-year prospective study of 20,193 wounds at the Minneapolis VA Medical Center. *Ann Surg* 199:253–259, 1984.

57. Condon RE, Schulte WJ, Malangoni MA, Anderson-Teschendorf MJ: Effectiveness of a surgical wound surveillance program. *Arch Surg* 118:303–307, 1983.

58. Wenzel RP: Prevention and treatment of hospital-acquired infections. In Wyngaarden JB, Smith LH (eds): *Cecil Textbook of Medicine*, ed 17. Philadelphia, WB Saunders, 1985, pp 1485–1492.

59. Albert RF, Condie F: Hand-washing patterns in medical intensive-care units. *N Engl J Med* 304:1465–1466, 1981.

60. Garner JS, Simmons BP: Isolation precautions. In Bennett JV, Brachman PS (eds): *Hospital Infections*, ed 2. Boston, Little, Brown, & Co, 1986, pp 143–150.

61. Ford-Jones EL: The special problems of nosocomial infection in the pediatric patient. In Wenzel RP (ed): *Prevention and Control of Nosocomial Infections*. Baltimore, Williams & Wilkins, 1987, pp 494–540.

5

Diarrhea

Larry K. Pickering, M.D. and Randall R. Reves, M.D., M.Sc.

BACKGROUND

Introduction and Incidence

Diarrhea is a major cause of morbidity and mortality in infants and children worldwide (1). Hospitalized children can develop diarrhea as a result of acquisition of the organism prior to admission or during their course of hospitalization. In either instance, the risk of spreading it to other children is significant if appropriate infection control measures are not instituted. For an episode of diarrhea to be considered nosocomial in nature, the onset of disease must occur during hospitalization or shortly after discharge, and the infection should not be present or incubating at the time of the patient's admission.

Available data on the true frequency, morbidity and mortality associated with nosocomial gastrointestinal tract infections are limited. Data gathered by the Centers for Disease Control as part of the National Nosocomial Infections Study (NNIS), which included 79 hospitals in 31 states in 1977, showed that the rate of recognized nosocomial gastrointestinal tract infections on all services was 1.6 infections per 10,000 patient discharges. The rate varied from a low of 0 per 10,000 discharges on the obstetrics service to 6.1 per 10,000 discharges on the pediatric service, and 7.6 per 10,000 discharges on the newborn service (2). The overall nosocomial gastrointestinal tract rate was considerably lower than rates for nosocomial urinary tract, surgical wound, lower respiratory tract, primary bacteremia and cutaneous infections (2).

Data from the CDC summarizing nosocomial infections from 1984 showed that the most common types of nosocomial infections were urinary tract, surgical wound, respiratory tract, and bacteremia; gastrointestinal tract infections were not mentioned (3).

In January 1974, the CDC initiated the SENIC Project (Study on the Efficacy of Nosocomial Infection Control) which was designed to evaluate various techniques of infection control in preventing nosocomial infections at four sites: surgical wound, urinary tract, lower respiratory tract, and blood. The frequency of nosocomial gastroenteritis was not mentioned in reports of this study (4,5). Both the NNIS and SENIC studies were not designed to specifically evaluate pediatric patients, in whom the majority of nosocomial gastrointestinal tract infections occur (6,7).

Many reports have appeared in the literature describing outbreaks of nosocomial gastrointestinal tract infections due to specific enteropathogens. Most of these outbreaks have occurred in children. Although these reports are useful in highlighting the problem of nosocomial gastroenteritis in pediatric patients, the true medical and economic significance of this problem remains unknown.

Etiology

Many bacterial, viral, and parasitic organisms produce diarrhea in humans (Table 5.1), but the relative importance of each organism as a cause of nosocomial diarrhea is not known. Nosocomial outbreaks of gastroenteritis can be classified into one of two epidemiologic patterns: common source and person-to-person transmission. Those organisms which have a low inoculum dose are more important in person-to-person transmission of disease than those with a higher inoculum dose. Common source outbreaks are generally food- or waterborne and may involve many patients and staff in a hospital, or may be confined to a small number of patients exposed to a specific food item or contaminated water (8,9). Common source outbreaks may also be

Table 5.1
Enteropathogens which Cause Gastroenteritis

BACTERIA
Aeromonas species
Campylobacter jejuni
Clostridium difficile
Escherichia coli
   enterotoxigenic
   enteropathogenic
   invasive
   enterohemorrhagic (0157:H7)
Salmonella species
Shigella species
Vibrio cholerae
Vibrio parahemolyticus
Yersinia enterocolitica

PARASITES
Cryptosporidium
Entamoeba histolytica
Giardia lamblia

VIRUSES
Enteric adenovirus
Norwalk-like viruses
Rotavirus

caused by contaminated instruments or medications. Outbreaks of gastroenteritis that occur due to person-to-person transmission generally occur on pediatric units, including neonatal nurseries. Table 5.2 summarizes the factors that are important in the introduction of nosocomial infectious gastroenteritis. Enteropathogens are most commonly introduced into a pediatric hospital unit by an infant or child and less frequently by hospital personnel. Specific enteropathogens which have been associated with nosocomial outbreaks will be discussed below.

Aeromonas

Species of Aeromonas including *A. caviae*, *A. hydrophila* and *A. sobria* have been shown in some studies to be causes of acute gastroenteritis; other studies do not support this observation (10). The illness associated with Aeromonas appears to be seasonal with a mid-

Table 5.2
Factors Important in the Introduction of Nosocomial Infectious Gastroenteritis

- Short-term carriers of enteropathogens.
- Patient-to-patient transmission via hands of hospital personnel, generally after contact with a child with diarrhea.
- Contaminated medications, food, or medical instruments.

summer peak. Gastroenteritis is more common in children under two years of age, and often presents with relatively nonspecific clinical symptoms. Watery diarrhea with mild fever or brief duration is most common, but both prolonged diarrhea and dysentery-like illness have been reported. The true frequency of Aeromonas in stool cultures is probably underestimated because the organism may resemble normal enteric flora. Aeromonas has not been reported to cause nosocomial diarrhea.

Campylobacter

C. fetus subspecies *jejuni* is an enteric pathogen that has been shown by DNA homology studies to be two organisms, *C. jejuni* and *C. coli*. These organisms are generally not distinguished in clinical microbiology laboratories and are reported as *C. jejuni*. In North America, Campylobacter is increasingly being recognized as a common cause of bacterial diarrhea (11) and has been shown to produce outbreaks of diarrhea in day care centers (12). Selective techniques are required to culture Campylobacter in the laboratory.

A thermophilic strain of Campylobacter, referred to as *C. lardis* has been distinguished from *C. jejuni*. This organism has been shown to produce diarrhea in humans and birds. *C. pylori* has been isolated from the gastric antrum of patients with histologically confirmed gastritis. Although nosocomial spread of Campylobacter is uncommon, many outbreaks due to *C. jejuni* have been reported due to contaminated raw milk, water, food, or through a person-to-person transmission or contact with infected animals (13).

Escherichia Coli

Several recognized categories of *E. coli* produce diarrhea: enterotoxigenic *E. coli* (ETEC), enteropathogenic *E. coli* (EPEC), enteroinvasive *E. coli* (EIEC), and enterohemorrhagic *E. coli* (14–16). *E. coli* is one of the most common bacterial causes of diarrhea in humans worldwide. The best understood mechanisms for *E. coli* disease are those due to heat-stable (ST) and heat-liable (LT) enterotoxins. ETEC belong to many different subgroups and cause disease in patients of all ages, especially infants and children in developing countries and persons who travel from developed to developing countries.

Foodborne outbreaks due to ETEC have been documented, but relatively few nosocomial outbreaks have been documented in association with enterotoxigenic *E. coli*. In 1976 in special care nurseries of a large pediatric hospital, the association of an heat-stable enterotoxin producing *E. coli* 078:k80:H12 and diarrhea was made (17). Fifty-five of 205 infants admitted to the nurseries over a 7-month period developed a diarrheal illness characterized by nine or more loose stools a day. The epidemic organism was isolated from several environmental sources, including the walls of isolettes and washbasins, as well as the formula being fed to one infant. A widespread colonization among hospital personnel was not documented. The epidemic disappeared coincident with cohorting of culture-positive infants in a separate nursery which was staffed by separate personnel. An outbreak associated with ST producing *E. coli* 0159 occurred over 3 months among 25 infants in the Glasgow Royal Maternity Hospital (18). An outbreak of infantile diarrhea in a newborn intensive care unit was associated with enterotoxigenic organisms that represented multiple serotypes of different organisms (*E. coli*, Klebsiella, and Citrobacter) (19).

Enteropathogenic *E. coli* (EPEC) have been incriminated as causing both sporadic and epidemic diarrhea in infants (20,21). Originally, EPEC was a term used to describe all *E. coli* associated with diarrheal syndromes, but the term EPEC is now defined more narrowly (22). When toxin production and invasiveness were recognized as mechanisms of *E. coli* disease, there was doubt for several years that EPEC organisms were pathogens since they are not invasive and do not make ST or LT. The EPEC are those *E. coli* epidemiologically incriminated in outbreaks of infantile diarrhea, which can be defined by serogroup and can be demonstrated to lack known virulence traits (enterotoxin production and invasiveness). Volunteer studies (23) and studies comparing isolation rates from sick and well children have demonstrated that EPEC organisms are pathogens; however, the specific mechanism(s) of disease production is not known.

The serotypes of EPEC that have been associated classically with infantile diarrhea include: 026, 055, 086, 0111, 0119, 0125, 0126, 0127, 0128ab and 0142 as the most important; and 018, 044, 0112 and 0114 as less important. They are infrequently found among healthy infants or adults not exposed to cases, and are different from *E. coli* found in nonenteric *E. coli*

infections. Outbreaks of infantile enteritis associated with *E. coli* 0142 were described in 54 infants in Dublin (24). In another nursery outbreak of gastroenteritis, *E. coli* 0142 occurred among 56 infants admitted to contiguous high-risk nurseries at a county general hospital in Arizona (25). Four diarrhea-associated deaths occurred, and 17 other infants had intractable diarrhea. The incriminated *E. coli* 0142 was isolated from the hands of five personnel, suggesting hand transmission of the pathogen. A more insidious nosocomial illness was described over 7 months in association with *E. coli* 0114 (26). Other serotypes have been recognized in association with epidemic diarrhea in newborn nurseries (27). Recognition of a nosocomial infantile enteritis outbreak may require monitoring of illnesses that occur after discharge from a brief hospitalization following birth.

Invasive *E. coli* (EIEC) are closely related antigenically, and biochemically to Shigella and cause a dysentery-like illness. They possess a large (140 Mdalton) plasmid, which encodes for invasiveness (28), just as has been found in Shigella. Infections generally occur in adults; foodborne outbreaks have been reported (14). Invasive *E. coli* have not been described in nosocomial outbreaks to date.

Enterohemorrhagic *E. coli* produces bloody diarrhea without fever. This hemorrhagic colitis syndrome has been recognized to be caused primarily by a single serotype of *E. coli* 0157:H7, which produces large amounts of cytotoxin (29), similar to the cytotoxin produced by *S. dysenteriae* serotype 1. Enterohemorrhagic *E. coli* lack the 140 Mdalton plasmid that is associated with the invasiveness characteristic of EIEC, but it does possess a 70 Mdalton plasmid (30). *E. coli* that produce high levels of cytotoxin are clinically important because like Shigella, they have been incriminated as etiologic agents of hemolytic uremic syndrome (31). The role of this organism is nosocomial diarrhea needs further clarification.

Salmonella. Currently, three species of Salmonella are differentiated on the basis of biochemical characteristics: *S. cholera-suis*, *S. typhi* and *S. enteritidis*. Nearly all of the 1700 serotypes of Salmonella are now grouped under the single species name *S. enteritidis*. Determining serotypes remains a useful epidemiologic tool for outbreak situations in both the hospital and community setting. Many outbreaks of Salmonella gastroenteritis in hospitalized patients have been published. In one food-borne outbreak, five patients developed salmonellosis caused by three different serotypes of Salmonella over a 3-month period (32). This outbreak could have gone unrecognized because of the multiple serotypes responsible. The outbreak was controlled following cessation of use of contaminated brewer's yeast.

Food-borne salmonellosis outbreaks may simultaneously affect patients in multiple hospitals. In 1962 and 1963, a large interstate outbreak of nosocomial gastroenteritis affecting patients, medical staff, and employees of 53 hospitals in 13 states was caused by *S. derby* (33). Contaminated eggs, which were eaten either raw or undercooked, were responsible for this multistate outbreak. In 1973, eggnog containing raw eggs caused nosocomial gastroenteritis in 18 patients (34). Person-to-person spread to hospital staff as well as hospitalized patients was documented.

Common source Salmonella outbreaks have also been traced to contaminated diagnostic reagents, medications, and medical instruments. These types of outbreaks generally do not present as typical common source outbreaks, and therefore may be difficult to recognize. An interstate outbreak of *S. cubana* infection occurred in 1966 (35–37), due to contaminated carmine dye used as a marker of gastrointestinal transit. Nosocomial outbreaks of salmonellosis have also been traced to bile salts, gelatin, pancreatin, pepsin, vitamins, and extracts of various endocrine glands (38,39). In these outbreaks, cases of salmonellosis frequently appeared to be sporadic, requiring a high index of suspicion to document their association with a common vehicle. Outbreaks of Salmonella gastroenteritis have been associated with upper gastrointestinal endoscopy (40), rubber tubing attached to a suction apparatus, (41) and plastic tubing of an intermittent suction machine (42).

An epidemic caused by *S. kottbus* was traced to contaminated pooled breast milk. Donor mothers, appeared to asymptomatically excrete the organisms in breast milk (43,44). Contaminated breast milk has also caused neonatal outbreaks of Klebsiella bacteremia (45) and *E. coli* gastroenteritis (46).

Outbreaks of Salmonella infections have been reported in nurseries. The organism is generally introduced into the nursery by an infant recently born to a mother with clinical or asymptomatic salmonellosis (47,48), or into pediatric wards by a child who has acquired salmonellosis in the community (49,50). Both infants and adults may be involved in an outbreak (51). In these outbreaks, organisms appear to be spread from person-to-person by hospital staff, and an outbreak may persist for months (49,52,53). On occasion, Salmonella have been isolated from many sources, including hands of hospital staff members, dust, water in infant bottle warmers, delivery room resuscitators, bedside tables and cribs, thermometers and towels (47,52,54–57). The significance of environmental isolates of Salmonella is uncertain. Considerable morbidity may be associated with salmonellosis outbreaks both in newborns and in patients on medical and surgical wards (49,58). In a total of 46 Salmonella cross infection outbreaks reported to CDC from both hospitals and custodial institutions, the case fatality ratio was 5% (38).

Shigella

There are 4 serogroups of Shigella containing 40 serotypes. *S. sonnei* is the most common cause of bacillary dysentery in the United States and Europe, while *S. flexneri* serotypes account for a majority of the remaining cases. Nosocomial transmission of Shigella is not often documented, even though the infectious dose is in the range of 10–100 organisms (59). In one reported outbreak, one of twins born to a mother with a history of diarrhea during the 4 weeks prior to delivery developed *S. sonnei* diarrhea on day 5 of life (60). A stool culture obtained from the mother also yielded *S. sonnei*. In addition, a nurse caring for the infected infant subsequently developed diarrhea and had a stool culture positive for *S. sonnei*. All three isolates had the same pattern of multiple antibiotic resistance. In a review of eight previously reported cases of neonatal shigellosis, Shigella was isolated from stool specimens from six mothers, three of whom had diarrhea at the time of delivery (61). Four additional nosocomial cases occurred in infants who acquired the organisms from their mothers at the time of delivery.

The role of hospital staff in the transmission of nosocomial shigellosis is illustrated in an outbreak of nine cases of shigellosis in an infirmary of a custodial institution (62). Since patients were bedridden, direct person-to-person spread from one patient to another seemed unlikely.

The epidemic strain in this outbreak also had a multiple antibiotic-resistance pattern.

Vibrio Cholerae

Strains of *V. cholerae* are classified according to somatic or 0 groups. *V. cholerae* strains are further separated into two main serotypes (Ogawa and Inaba), and two biotypes (classical and El Tor). *V. cholerae* 0 group 1 (01 strains) are those responsible for epidemic cholera, and all other strains are referred to as ''non01 *V. cholerae*.'' In countries with endemic cholera, all ages are affected, although children over 1 year of age are disproportionately involved. *V. cholerae* 01 is primarily a problem in Asia and Africa, although a focus is present in the Gulf Coast of the United States where it has been associated with undercooked shellfish consumption (63). All clinical isolates of *V. cholerae* 01 from the U.S. have been hemolytic, biotype El Tor, serotype Inaba and have had the same unique phage type and toxin-gene sequence (64). Nosocomial transmission of cholera has been described in developing countries, but not in the United States.

Vibrio Parahemolyticus

V. parahemolyticus is a common marine isolate that has been found in water, shellfish, fish, and plankton. Although widely disseminated in coastal waters, *V. parahemolyticus* is an uncommon cause of diarrhea except in Japan, where consumption of raw seafood is common. Although outbreaks of diarrhea due to *V. parahemolyticus* have been reported (65), nosocomial outbreaks in the United States due to Vibrio species are rare.

Yersinia Enterocolitica

Gastroenteritis due to *Y. enterocolitica* currently is uncommon in the United States, although it is a frequent cause of gastroenteritis among children in Canada and Europe. Illness occurs more commonly in children during the first 4 years of life than in older children or adults and may resemble shigellosis or acute appendicitis, although endemic infection usually results in diarrhea, vomiting, abdominal pain, and fever (66).

In 1982, a multistate outbreak of infections due to *Y. enterocolitica* transmitted by pasteurized milk was reported (67). A fatal episode of *Y. enterocolitica* sepsis occurred in a man following receipt of blood contaminated with this organism (68). In both instances, the cold temperature at which the milk and blood were stored may have facilitated growth of *Y. enterocolitica*. A nosocomial outbreak of *Y. enterocolitica* enteritis was reported from Finland (69). The index case was a girl admitted to a pediatric surgical ward with fever, abdominal pain, diarrhea, and suspected appendicitis. She did not undergo surgery, and after her clinical status improved, she was transferred to a pediatric ward. Within two weeks, six cases of *Y. enterocolitica* infection occurred among hospital staff on the two wards in which she was housed. Each infection was caused by *Y. enterocolitica* sereotype 9. All but one of the six staff members infected had been working on one of the two wards while the index case was hospitalized on that ward. The organism appeared to have spread by person-to-person transmission from patient to staff and possibly among staff members. The possibility of a common vehicle among the hospital staff members was not excluded.

Viral Enteropathogens

Rotarvirus, Norwalk-like virus, and enteric adenovirus are recognized causes of acute infectious gastroenteritis. Other viruses that may cause infectious gastroenteritis include astroviruses, calicivirus, coronavirus, and minirotavirus (70,71). These viruses exhibit different epidemiologic and clinical features, although most episodes are self-limited and are characterized by various combinations of diarrhea, nausea, vomiting, abdominal cramps, headache, myalgia, and low-grade fever. Rotavirus is the only one of these agents for which commercial kits are available for diagnosis and is the major one responsible for nosocomial gastroenteritis.

Rotavirus. Rotavirus is one of the most important enteric pathogens throughout the world, particularly in infants. It is found in nearly 50% of stools from children admitted to the hospital with gastroenteritis (72–75). The majority of patients with rotavirus infection are between 6 and 24 months. Illness is prevalent in temperate climates in winter months. When infection occurs, virus excretion is greatest during the 2nd and 3rd days of illness and is rarely detected after the 8th day. Because there are multiple serotypes, reinfection can occur.

Nosocomial transmission of rotavirus has been well-documented on pediatric wards. Seven–59% of children admitted to the hospital with other diagnoses acquire rotavirus in the hospital (76–82). Twelve–25% of immunocompromised patients acquire rotavirus in the hospital, have an extended period of virus excretion, and may be a source of virus for transmission to others (83–87). Adults are likely to have either mild or asymptomatic infection (88,89) and may transmit the disease, although nosocomial outbreaks involving adult patients in the hospital have been reported (90,91).

Nosocomial rotavirus infection may cause both outbreaks and endemic diarrheal disease in newborn nurseries; however, in most cases, infection is asymptomatic (92–100). Asymptomatic rotavirus infections also occur in older children (101,102), with evidence of asymptomatic rotavirus infection being 24–50% in infants less than 2 years of age during rotavirus season. The role of asymptomatic excretors in nosocomial rotavirus infection is not known.

In these nursery settings, the modes of introduction and transmission were not well-characterized. Since asymptomatic infection in adult household contacts of pediatric cases and hospital personnel has been documented, it is possible that infants become infected during or shortly after birth from either a maternal or a hospital staff source. Infection may then spread within the nursery either by person-to-person transmission or, alternatively, may be frequently reintroduced, particularly during the winter months.

Enteric Adenoviruses. At least two distinct subgroups of enteric adenovirus, F (type 40) and G (type 41), have been described. These agents primarily affect children under 2 years of age (103). Diagnosis can be made by electron microscopy or by ELISA, but commercial assays are not available. These agents cause a gastrointestinal tract illness with fever and may be associated with respiratory tract findings. Treatment is nonspecific, and fluid replacement is dictated by the patient's condition. Enteric adenovirus can be an important cause of acute gastroenteritis in hospitalized infants and young children (104). Infections with these viruses have been shown to be a major cause of morbidity in hospitalized children who have undergone ileostomy or colostomy procedures for necrotizing enterocolitis (105).

Norwalk Virus. Norwalk-like virus agents are much smaller than rotavirus (27 nm vs. 70 nm); therefore, diagnosis is made by immune electron microscopy (IEM) of stools or by serology. Commercial assays are not available. The illness is characterized by an incubation period of 18–48 hours, followed by diarrhea, and low-grade fever lasting 1–2 days (106). The only natural host of virus appears to be humans. Serologic studies indicate that between 50–70% of residents in the United States have developed antibodies to Norwalk agent by 30 years of age (107). These serum antibodies do not necessarily confer immunity.

Epidemics of Norwalk-like viruses have been reported in nursing homes, schools, recreational areas, and hospitals (106,108,109). Waterborne, foodborne and person-to-person transmission have all been implicated in epidemics (110), and the results of volunteer studies suggest fecal-oral transmission. Outbreaks of gastroenteritis due to Norwalk-like virus have been reported in hospitals (108,109). In one outbreak, 55% of elderly patients and 61% of the nursing employees on one floor became ill (108). Infection was most likely spread from patient-to-patient by nursing employees. Another outbreak affected 57 patients and 69 staff members over a 26-day period. The index case was a patient admitted with acute abdominal pain and diarrhea 2 days prior to the outbreak (109). The epidemic curve indicated person-to-person transmission. Calicivirus, astroviruses, and minirotaviruses may also cause nosocomial diarrhea in infants, but their detection is currently possible only in research laboratories (71,111).

Parasitic Enteropathogens

The parasites that are the most frequent causes of parasitic diarrhea in persons in the United States are *Giardia lamblia*, *Entamoeba histolytica*, and *Cryptosporidium*.

Giardia Lamblia. *G. lamblia* is a flagellated protozoan that exists in trophozoite and cyst forms. Disease caused by this organism is common in certain high-risk populations and in persons who travel to hyperendemic areas (112,113). Chronic diarrhea with malabsorption and significant weight loss over many months may also occur. Studies in day care centers have shown that Giardia cysts, and even trophozoites are common in children manifesting no symptoms (114). Giardia cysts can remain viable and infectious in water for more than 3 months. Although nosocomial hospital-based outbreaks are uncommon, transmission of Giardia among children in day care centers is common (113).

Entamoeba Histolytica. Amebiasis is a major health problem in Asia, Latin America, and Africa. The influx of refugees into the United States during the last 10 years has increased the likelihood that physicians will see children with amebiasis (115,116). Childhood intestinal amebiasis generally presents with diarrhea containing blood and mucus and no fever. Diarrhea without blood, fulminating colitis, appendicitis, and ameboma occur infrequently in children. The cyst form is resistant to environmental stresses and is the infective stage. Nosocomial infection is rare, although a colonic irrigation machine was implicted in an outbreak of amebiasis (117).

Cryptosporidium. In 1976, the first human infection due to Cryptosporidium was reported. With the onset of the acquired immunodeficiency syndrome (AIDS) epidemic, many patients with chronic malabsorption syndrome and severe protracted, watery diarrhea were recognized as having cryptosporidiosis (118,119). Other reports have demonstrated that Cryptosporidium is a common intestinal parasite of immunocompetent humans, particularly of children in the first 4 years of life. Potential sources of infection with Cryptosporidium include pet cats or dogs, farm animals, laboratory animals, contaminated water, attendance at day care centers, following international travel, and exposure to infected persons. Cryptosporidium may be transmitted from person-to-person in the hospital environment (120,121). Serologic evidence of infection has been shown to be common among hospital personnel (121).

Other Organisms

Any infectious agent transmitted by food or water, or spread from one infected person to another and causing gastroenteritis, may be associated with outbreaks of nosocomial gastrointestinal illness. Recently recognized causes of acute gastrointestinal tract infections may be anticipated to cause outbreaks of nosocomial gastroenteritis, which may be documented by the use of recently developed laboratory techniques (122).

POPULATIONS

On the basis of epidemiologic and etiologic considerations, nosocomial infectious diarrhea in

children can be divided into a number of major categories which include antimicrobial agent associated colitis, foodborne or waterborne diarrhea, diarrhea in immunosuppressed hosts, necrotizing enterocolitis and diarrhea acquired by children who do not fall into the above categories.

Antimicrobial Agent-Associated Colitis

An important consideration among patients with diarrhea who are taking or have recently taken an antibiotic is pseudomembranous or antimicrobial-associated colitis (AAC). This condition refers to the presence of a pseudomembrane or of multiple plaque-like lesions in the colon induced by an antimicrobial agent. The specific cause is a toxin produced by *Clostridium difficile* (123). The most commonly implicated antimicrobial agents are ampicillin, the cephalosporins, and clindamycin (124). Patients with AAC present with diarrhea that is watery and often contains blood and mucus. Diarrhea is either the only manifestation of disease or occurs in association with nausea, vomiting, abdominal pain or cramps, fever, and leukocytosis. The most important aspect of therapy in patients with AAC is discontinuation of the antimicrobial agent. If this is done, symptoms usually resolve within 1–2 weeks. If symptoms persist or worsen, specific therapeutic agents such as vancomycin or metronidazole should be considered (125). It should be stressed that many children who receive antibiotics develop diarrhea, and that AAC is rare.

C. difficile can be recovered from 83% of patients with AAC, but from only 11% of patients with diarrhea-associated with antimicrobial therapy in which AAC is not present (126). In addition, *C. difficile* can be recovered from stools of healthy children in an age-related relationship (45% less than 1 year of age and 18% over 1 year of age) (127). These findings indicate that although *C. difficile* can be associated with AAC, its role in gastroenteritis not associated with AAC in children is not known. Nosocomial outbreaks of diarrhea due to *C. difficile* have been reported (128,129), as has isolation of the organism from the environment and contacts in both the hospital (129) and day care setting (130).

Foodborne or Waterborne Disease

An outbreak of foodborne or waterborne disease has been defined as an incident in which two or more persons experience gastrointestinal tract disease after ingesting a common food or water which has been epidemiologically implicated as the source of illness (8,9). Determination of the incubation period and the presence or absence of selected clinical findings (especially vomiting and fever) often lead the physician toward the correct diagnosis in outbreaks of foodborne diarrhea. Table 5.3 outlines characteristics of foodborne and waterborne disease. As a general rule, when outbreaks are divided by incubation period of the illness, those less than 1 hour are due to chemical poisoning; those of 1–7 hours, either *Staphylococcus aureus* or *Bacillus cereus* preformed enterotoxins; those of 8–14 hours, *C. perfringens* toxin; and those over 14 hours, other infectious or toxic agents. Salmonella organisms can contaminate many types of food, with poultry and eggs being the most common sources. *Vibrio parahemolyticus* is a marine organism that commonly contaminates shellfish, as does *V. cholerae*. Unpasteurized milk can be contaminated with Salmonella, Campylobacter, or *Yersinia enterocolitica* (131). Nonbacterial pathogens that cause waterborne or foodborne illness include Norwalk virus, *G. lamblia*,

Table 5.3
Characteristics of Foodborne or Waterborne Outbreaks of Diarrhea

Incubation Period	Presumptive Causative Agent
5 mins–18 hours (usually <3 hours)	Chemical
1–6 hours	*Staphylococcus aureus* enterotoxin *Bacillus cereus* enterotoxin
6–16 hours	*Clostridium perfringens* enterotoxin *B. cereus* enterotoxin
16–36 hours	Shigella Salmonella *Vibrio parahemolyticus* Invasive *Escherichia coli* *Yersinia enterocolitica*
16–72 hours	*E. coli* enterotoxin *V. parahemolyticus* enterotoxin *V. cholerae* enterotoxin
72–120 hours	*Escherichia coli* 0157:H7
1–3 days	Norwalk virus
1–7 days	*Campylobacter jejuni*

E. histolytica, and rarely, rotavirus. Noninfectious causes, such as fish and shellfish poisoning syndromes or mushroom poisoning, have been implicated in foodborne outbreaks (132). An outbreak of gastroenteritis due to food poisoning should be considered when hospitalized patients and/or hospital staff members develop acute gastroenteritis characterized by vomiting and fever. The laboratory approach used to confirm the cause of an outbreak will depend somewhat upon the etiologic agent.

Immunocompromised Patients

A diverse group of enteropathogens should be considered among patients with compromised immune defenses, including bone marrow transplant recipients and those with AIDS (83–87,133–136). Diseases caused by a wide range of pathogenic and opportunistic microorganisms significantly increase the morbidity and mortality of the preexisting condition (134). In addition to conventional enteropathogens, other organisms should be considered, including Cryptosporidium, *Isospora belli*, Herpes viruses (H. simplex and cytomegalovirus), *Candida albicans*, *C. difficile*, *Mycobacterium avium-intracellulare* complex, and Salmonella. Intestinal disease occurs in 50% of patients with AIDS in the United States and in over 90% of patients with AIDS in Africa and Haiti. The potential for nosocomial spread varies by organism.

Necrotizing Enterocolitis (NEC)

The most common nosocomial setting in which necrotizing enterocolitis occurs is in the newborn infant less than 1 week of age. Risk factors include prematurity, maternal infections during delivery, and manipulation, such as umbilical vessel exchange transfusion (137). A newborn infant may develop abdominal distension, vomiting, or apneic spells. The illness rapidly progresses to bloody diarrhea, intestinal perforation, shock, septicemia, and pneumatosis intestinalis, with a mortality that may exeed 70%. The pathogenesis of NEC appears to involve some type of ischemic mucosal injury which may result from hypoxemia or hypertension. Several organisms have been implicated, such as *Pseudomonas*, *Klebsiella*, *E. coli* and Clostridia species, including *C. butyricum*, *C. perfringens*, *C. difficile* and rotavirus (137,138). Management of necrotizing enterocolitis must include early suspicion and recognition, discontinuation of oral feeding, parenteral fluid and nutritional therapy, administration of antimicrobial therapy, and aggressive surgical excision of necrotic bowel if evidenced by pneumatosis intestinalis, peritonitis, or obstruction. Necrotizing enterocolitis appears to be rare in breastfed infants. Outbreaks have been reported from many nurseries, making an infectious agent suspect in the pathogenesis of this condition (138,139).

Others

Many cases of diarrhea occur in patients who do not fall into one of the aforementioned categories (140,141). The episodes are often caused by highly contagious organisms (Shigella, *G. lamblia*, or rotavirus). If children are hospitalized with infectious diarrhea or develop diarrhea during hospitalization, a potential for nosocomial spread exists, especially in areas of the hospital where close contact is facilitated, such as intensive care units, neonatal nurseries, and crowded wards.

DIAGNOSIS

Surveillance and Outbreak Evaluation

Surveillance for diarrheal diseases, as for other nosocomial infections, includes routine surveillance and the more intensive surveillance required when an outbreak is suspected. Routine surveillance can be conducted by review of laboratory isolates from stool cultures and, in some cases, blood cultures; from reports from nursing or medical staff who are generally aware of diarrhea in pediatric patients; from contacts with patients who may have been discharged during the incubation period; from reports from physicians of severe cases, such as necrotizing enterocolitis; and from employee health if transmission within the hospital staff occurs. If an outbreak is suspected and more intensive surveillance is deemed necessay, case finding can be improved by daily contact with nursing personnel and medical staff. The decision to initiate a more thorough investigation should be made if a point source is suspected or if contamination of a commercial item is possible as an etiologic factor.

The microbiology laboratory can be utilized for surveillance for nosocomial diarrhea, although the ability of the laboratory to detect most pathogens will be limited. Depending upon the availability of more specialized techniques in the hospital and upon the frequency with which stool specimens are tested for various pathogens, the value of the microbiology laboratory to function as a sensitive indicator of an increase in the prevalence of enteropathogens in the hospital will vary. Many hospitals will process stools only for Salmonella, Shigella, Campylobacter, and rotavirus, while others, particularly tertiary care hospitals, may have testing available upon request for Yersinia, Vibrio species, *C. difficile*, and its toxin, Cryptosporidium, Isospora, and even electron microscopy for Norwalk agent and enteric adenovirus. One can readily see that even small clusters of food- or medication-borne salmonellosis, if due to an unusual serotype, may be detected by the laboratory. The more protracted person-to-person spread of rotavirus with generally mild or subclinical cases may go undetected if virologic studies are unavailable or are not ordered by the physician. One would expect that the published surveillance data for nosocomial diarrhea represents an underestimate of the true incidence, particularly in pediatrics, where viral agents are exceedingly common. Acute diarrhea in the pediatric patient, whether community- or hospital-acquired, should be considered infectious until an alternative diagnosis is made.

To establish an alternate diagnosis to a nosocomial gastrointestinal tract infection, a careful review of the patient's medical history, including current medications, should be undertaken. There are many noninfectious causes of diarrhea that can be mistakenly labeled as nosocomial infections if appropriate evaluation is not undertaken (142).

Clinical Manifestations and Diagnosis

The approach to hospitalized patients with acute infectious diarrhea begins with a carefully obtained medical history, including epidemiologic considerations and a physical examination. Information that is gathered can then be used to guide selection of laboratory tests and to provide optimal therapy.

Acute diarrhea can be caused by one of a number of organisms (Table 5.1). Clinical manifestations occurring in patients with diarrhea are a reflection of either localized involvement of the gastrointestinal tract (nausea; vomiting; abdominal discomfort; or number, volume, and character of stools; or ileus) or generalized symptoms or signs (fever, dehydration, skin lesions, pneumonia). The latter symptoms are indicative of a more extensive involvement produced by some enteropathogens. The presence of a specific clinical manifestation is not pathognomonic of any causative agent; however, some clinical features occur more frequently as a result of infection by certain microorganisms. Virulence properties of enteropathogens that produce disease are enterotoxin production, cytotoxin production, invasion of intestinal mucosa, or adherence to intestinal mucosa. Bacterial organisms that invade intestinal mucosa often cause fever, and if the colon is primarily involved, also cause abdominal cramps, tenesmus, fecal urgency, and passage of stools containing blood and mucus. Patients with secretory diarrhea have abdominal cramps and pass a low to moderate number of large volume stools which when passed, may be associated with temporary relief. Patients with acute giardiasis or cryptosporidiosis often have watery, foul-smelling stools associated with nausea and flatulence or chronic diarrhea with malabsorption and abdominal distension. Diarrhea due to rotavirus and enteric adenovirus generally occurs in infants who present with low-grade fever, vomiting, and watery diarrhea, which is due to damage to the microvilli.

The patient should be carefully assessed to determine what diagnostic evaluation and therapy might be necessary. In patients with mild diarrhea who are otherwise healthy, laboratory evaluation is probably not indicated except to establish a diagnosis for isolation purposes or as part of an outbreak evaluation. Patients with blood or mucus in their stools should have cultures performed to detect one of the invasive bacteria, which often respond to antimicrobial therapy. Patients with bloody diarrhea who have stool cultures testing negative for bacteria as well as *E. histolytica* should be evaluated for invasive and hemorrhagic *E. coli* infection as well as inflammatory bowel disease and other noninfectious causes of bloody stools. Attention should be given to vital signs, moistness of mucous membranes, skin tugor, urine output, weight loss, presence of emesis, and amount of diarrhea. These factors are all important in determining the state of dehydration (143).

Laboratory Diagnosis

Many laboratory tests are available to assist in the evaluation of the cause of gastroenteritis. Identifying the cause of an episode of acute diarrhea facilitates appropriate therapy (Table 5.4),

Table 5.4
Laboratory Tests Used to Diagnose the Cause of Gastroenteritis

Laboratory Test	Organisms Suggested or Identified
Microscopic observation of stool	
fecal leukocytes	Invasive or cytotoxin producing bacteria
trophozoites, cysts, or oocysts	*Giardia lamblia*, *Entamoeba histolytica*, *Cryptosporidium*
spiral or S-shaped Gram-negative bacilli	*Campylobacter jejuni*
Stool culture standard special	Shigella, Salmonella *Campylobacter jejuni*, *Yersinia enterocolitica*, *Vibrio cholerae*, *V. parahemolytica*, *Clostridium difficile*
Enzyme immunoassay or latex agglutination	Rotavirus, *C. difficile* toxin
Serotyping	*E. coli* 0157:H7, EPEC, epidemic of diarrhea due to *E. coli*
Intestinal biopsy duodenum or small bowel	*G. lamblia*, strongyloides, adherent *E. coli*
colon	*E. histolytica*
Tests performed in research laboratories	Detection of labile toxin, stable toxin, or cytotoxin produced by bacteria, enteric adenovirus, Norwalk-like viruses, invasive *E. coli*

but probably won't alter isolation procedures, since enteric precautions generally do not vary by specific enteropathogen.

Observation of stool with regard to color, form, and the presence of blood or mucus may help to categorize the cause. Small quantities of stool containing blood and mucus more commonly indicate infection with Shigella, Salmonella, or Campylobacter, but may occur with any of the other enteropathogens that involve the colon, including invasive *E. coli*, *C. difficile*, *Y. enterocolitica*, and *V. parahemolyticus*. Grossly bloody stools with little or no mucus may be indicative of infection due to *E. histolytica* or enterohemorrhagic *E. coli* 0157:H7. Frothy, greasy, foul-smelling stools suggest malabsorption and can be an indication of infection with Giardia. Stool containing large amounts of water and sodium occur as a result of toxin-producing organisms such as *V. cholerae* or enterotoxigenic *E. coli*.

Stools can be observed under the microscope to detect leukocytes, red blood cells, or parasites. Electron microscopy or immune electron microscopy can be used to visualize rotavirus, Norwalk virus, or enteric adenovirus. Examination of diarrheal stool specimens for fecal leukocytes provides information concerning the anatomic location and extent of mucosal inflammation. Fecal leukocytes are produced in response to bacteria that diffusely invade the colonic mucosa and indicate that the patient has colitis (144). The most common causes of a marked fecal exudate are Shigella, Campylobacter, and Salmonella, although ulcerative colitis, Crohn's disease, AAC, invasive *E. coli*, *Y. enterocolitica*, and, occasionally, *V. parahemolytica* are associated with large numbers of fecal leukocytes. Fecal leukocytes are generally not present in stools from patients with diarrhea secondary to enterotoxigenic bacteria, viruses, or parasites.

Patients with amebiasis may have a low number of leukocytes found on examination of stool, but a striking exudate will be lacking unless a bacterial infection of the colonic ulcers produced by amebiasis has occurred (145). Patients with diarrhea should have their stools examined for ova and parasites if there is a history of exposure to people with giardiasis or recent travel to high-risk areas; stool cultures are repeatedly negative for other enteropathogens; the patient is immunocompromised; diarrhea persists for longer than 1 or 2 weeks; or amebiasis is suspected. Giardiasis should be considered in the diagnosis of any patient with diarrhea lasting 1 week or longer (112).

Cryptosporidium oocysts may be detected from fecal material by preliminary determination using the iodine wet mount technique; definitive identification requires use of the modified Kinyoun acid-fast staining technique. If both tests are negative, a more effective and time-consuming method of concentrating oocysts using Sheather's sugar coverslip flotation method can be employed (119). A diagnosis of *E. histolytica* can be made by examination of fresh stool specimens or bowel wall scrapings for cysts or trophozoites. Trophozoites are generally found in liquid stools, whereas cysts are detected in formed stools. Confusion in differentiating amebic cysts from fecal leukocytes may occur (115). A number of serologic tests are available for amebiasis and are almost always positive in acute amebic dysentery and hepatic amebiasis (79). A liver scan may indicate the presence of a liver abscess. Gram stain of Campylobacter colonies reveals small spiral or S-shaped Gram-negative bacilli. Direct phase microscopy of feces has been reported to be a rapid method for tentative identification of this organism, although insufficient data now exist to mandate routine use of this test.

Stool Cultures

Salmonella, Shigella, and Campylobacter are enteropathogens which should be detected in most microbiology laboratories. *Y. enterocolitica* can be identified by most hospital laboratories if personnel are alerted to look for this organism. Recovering the organism from blood, joint fluid, or other normally sterile fluid can be accomplished without difficulty; however, isolating the organism from feces is difficult due to overgrowth by normal flora. To maximize recovery of *V. parahemolyticus* or *V. cholerae*, stool specimens should be streaked directly onto thiosulfate-citrate-bile salts-sucrose (TCBS) or tellurite-taurocholate-gelatin agars (TTGA). These organisms may grow on some more selective laboratory media (MacConkey), but are inhibited by most selective media, such as those used to isolate Salmonella and Shigella. The TCBS and TTGA media are generally not used in routine processing of stool specimens, but are available commecially.

Aeromonas hydrophilia can easily be overlooked on standard stool cultures. A specialized blood agar has been suggested for isolation. Oxidase testing of organisms that resemble *E. coli* can select organisms as possible aeromonas. If oxidase-positive colonies are found, they can be evaluated further biochemically to determine species. *C. difficile* can be isolated by anaerobic stool culture on agar containing cycloserine, cefoxitin, and fructose (CCFA). For definitive diagnosis, it is necessary to demonstrate the presence of toxin in stool specimens and its neutralization with antitoxin.

Special Diagnostic Tests

Rotavirus can be detected by examination of stool specimens for typical particles by electron microscopy or by use of commercially available qualitative enzyme immunoassay kits (146). The technique of immune electron microscopy (IEM) has proved useful in the study of volunteers with experimentally induced Norwalk virus gastroenteritis. Enteric adenoviruses can be identified by immune electron microscopy of stool specimens; however, these tests are not commercially available.

Enterohemorrhagic E. coli should be suspected if the isolates ferment sorbitol. These strains can be definitively identified by serotyping them as 0157:H7 (147,148). Most enterotoxigenic E. coli, EPEC, and invasive E. coli may be of relatively few serotypes, indicating the need to determine the relationship between these strains and the serotypes of E. coli. Although microbiology laboratories can isolate E. coli, specialized laboratory facilities are necessary to identify enterotoxigenicity and invasiveness. Commercial assays also are available for detection of the toxins produced by C. difficile (149).

Intestinal Biopsy

The value of proctosigmoidoscopy and colonic biopsy in patients with acute infectious diarrhea is limited; however, there are conditions in which this procedure can be of diagnostic value, including patients with AAC, E. histolytica infection, and diarrhea caused by other chronic disorders, such as ulcerative colitis or adults with obstructive carcinoma or villous adenoma. In addition, patients with immune deficiency can benefit from this procedure. Since the organisms that involve the colon are varied and difficult to diagnose in patients with various immune deficiencies, including AIDS, biopsy may be helpful in establishing the diagnosis and guiding therapy. Biopsy of the duodenum or upper small bowel may help to establish the diagnosis of disease due to Giardia, Strongyloides, Cryptosporidium, or adherent E. coli.

Evaluation of Outbreaks

Greater applications in genetic engineering have helped to unravel many problems in microbiology. Use of DNA probes and monoclonal antibodies allow the area of molecular epidemiology to be applied to the evaluation of nosocomial outbreaks (150). Genetic probes have been used to study several enteropathogens (151–153).

TREATMENT

Enteric infections are generally self-limited conditions, but the occurrence of diarrhea in a hospitalized child with an underlying disease or at a young age can be devasting to the child and hazardous to contacts. Therapy of infants and children with diarrhea should be considered under two headings: fluid and electrolyte therapy and dietary manipulation; and specific therapy with antimicrobial agents.

Fluid and Electrolyte

Loss of fluid and electrolytes via the gastrointestinal tract is a significant complication in patients with diarrhea. If vomiting occurs, this loss is compounded. Continued loss of fluid and/or electrolytes leads to dehydration, which is the most severe sequela of diarrheal disease. Children, especially infants, are more susceptible to dehydration. Maintaining optimal hydration and electrolyte balance is critical in such patients (143,154). Oral therapy generally consists of rehydration and maintenance for a 6–12 hour period with a glucose electrolyte solution followed by initiation of a modified diet (155). Commercial preparations of ready-to-feed glucose electrolyte solutions are available and should be utilized (143). In some patients, oral fluid will not be adequate, and intravenous fluids must be administered.

Antimicrobial Therapy

In selected patients with diarrhea, antimicrobial agents will decrease symptoms and/or reduce fecal shedding of the organism. Decreasing fecal shedding is especially important in hospitalized patients to lessen the chance for nosocomial spread. Treatment is not indicated for patients with mild self-limited illness due to Aeromonas, although for those with an illness that persists for weeks or presents in a dysentery-like fashion, trimethoprim/sulfamethoxazole (TMP/SMX) is recommended. The treatment of choice for shigellosis where susceptibility is unknown is trimethoprim plus sulfamethoxazole (Table 5.5). In children with ampicillin-susceptible strains of Shigella, ampicillin will eradicate clinical symptoms and fecal shedding (156,157). Amoxicillin is not as effective as ampicillin in the treatment of shigellosis and should not be used (158). Approximately half of the S. sonnei strains are resistant to ampicillin, whereas

Table 5.5
Antimicrobial Therapy for Patients with Diarrhea Due to Bacterial Enteropathogens

Enteropathogens	Antimicrobial Agent	Dosage for Children	Maximum Dose
Aeromonas hydrophila	None for most patients; TMP/SMX for severe or prolonged illness	TMP 10 mg/kg/day plus SMX 50 mg/kg/day orally, in 2 divided doses for 5 days	TMP 160 mg plus SMX 800 mg every 12 h
Antimicrobial-associated (Clostridium difficile)	Vancomycin	20 mg/kg/day orally in 4 divided doses for 7 days	500 mg/day
Campylobacter jejuni	Erythromycin	40 mg/kg/day orally, divided 4 times daily for 5–7 days	1 gm/day
E. coli			
Enterotoxigenic	None or TMP/SMX	See above	
Enteropathogenic	None or TMP/SMX	See above	
Enteroinvasive	TMP/SMX	See above	
Enterohemorrhagic	TMP/SMX	See above	
Shigella species	TMP/SMX	See above	
	or		
	Ampicillin	50–75 mg/kg/day orally, divided 4 times daily for 5 days	6 gm/day
Salmonella			
Carrier state	None	None	
Acute gastroenteritis	None	None	
Bacteremia and/or enteric fever	Ampicillin	200 mg/kg/day IV, divided every 4 hours for 2 weeks	6 gm/day
	or		
	Chloramphenicol	75 mg/kg/day orally or IV divided every 6 hours for 2 weeks	3 gm/day
	or		
	TMP/SMX	TMP 10 mg/kg/day plus SMX 50 mg/kg/day in two divided doses for 2 weeks	TMP 160 mg plus SMX 800 mg every 12 h
V. cholerae	TMP/SMX	Dose as above; treat for 2 days	
Vibrio parahemolyticus	None (?)	None	
Y. enterocolitica	None (?)	None	

S. flexneri strains have generally remained relatively susceptible to ampicillin.

The type of syndrome produced by Salmonella influences the selection and duration of antimicrobial therapy. Antibiotics are not indicated in the treatment of persons who are nontyphoid Salmonella carriers. In most patients with Salmonella gastroenteritis, antimicrobial therapy is not given unless the patient is less than 6 months of age, has an underlying disease, including hemoglobinopathy (i.e., sickle cell anemia), malignancy, liver disease, or appears toxic with a high temperature. Therapy is given to these patients to prevent dissemination. Antimicrobial therapy is also administered to patients with typhoid fever, bacteremia caused by nontyphoidal strains, and dissemination with localized suppuration (Table 5.5). Chloramphenicol, ampicillin, and trimethoprim/sulfamethoxazole are the current drugs of choice (159). Third-generation cephalosporins and the new quinolones may be useful in treatment of patients with resistant organisms (160).

AAC is treated by removing the offending antibiotic and by treating the patient according to the degree of symptomatology. Mild cases

Table 5.6
Antimicrobial Therapy of Parasites That Cause Gastroenteritis

Enteropathogens	Therapy	Dosage for Children	Maximum Dose
Giardia lamblia	Quinacrine	6 mg/kg/day orally divided 3 times daily for 7 days	300 mg/day
	or		
	Metronidazole	15 mg/kg/day orally divided 3 times daily for 7 days	750 mg/day
	or		
	Furazolidone	9 mg/kg/day orally divided 3 times daily for 10 days	400 mg/day
Entamoeba histolytica asymptomatic cyst excretor	Iodoquinol	30 mg/kg/day divided 3 times daily for 20 days	2 gm/day
	or		
	Paromomycin	25–30 mg/kg/day divided 3 times daily for 7 days	Same
	or		
	Diloxanide furoate[a]	20 mg/kg/day divided 3 times daily for 10 days	1500 mg/day
Intestinal amebiasis	Metronidazole	30–50 mg/kg/day divided 3 times daily for 10 days	2250 mg/day
	plus		
	Iodoquinol	See above	
	or		
	Dehydroemetine[a]	1 to 1.5 mg/kg/day IM in 2 doses for up to 5 days	90 mg/day
	plus		
	Iodoquinol	See above	
Cryptosporidium	None		

[a]Available from the CDC Drug Service Centers for Disease Control in Atlanta, Georgia, (404) 329-3670 or (404) 329-3311.

generally require no additional treatment. Moderate to severe illness is best treated with vancomycin (125). An alternate form of therapy that can be given is metronidazole. Recurrence of colitis after discontinuation of vancomycin or metronidazole has been documented in 10–20% of patients (161). Relapses are treated with a second course of either vancomycin or metronidazole. In patients with Campylobacter enteritis, erythromycin is the agent of choice. Therapy reduces fecal excretion in all patients, and will alter clinical symptoms only if administered early in the course of disease. Antimicrobial agents improve diarrhea associated with cholera by reducing fluid loss, decreasing required fluid replacement, and by eradicating organisms from the gastrointestinal tract.

Antimicrobial agents may be given orally or intravenously. No data exist to support the use of antimicrobial agents in diarrheal disease due to *V. parahemolyticus* or *Y. enterocolitica*.

Quinacrine hydrochloride, metronidazole, and furazolidone are effective in treating patients with infection due to *Giardia lamblia* (Table 5.6) (162,163). The cure rate with these three preparations ranges from 84%–93% (163). Furazolidone is the only preparation available in a liquid form. In treating patients with amebiasis, iodoquinol is the best lumenal amebicide presently available commercially in the United States (162). This drug is effective against both cysts and trophozolites in the lumen of the gut, but is ineffective against tissue forms of disease. Invasive amebiasis of the intestine, liver, or other organs necessitates the additional use of a tissue amebicide, such as metronidazole. Optimal therapy of patients with cryptosporidiosis is not known.

PREVENTION

Recommendations for prevention of transmission of nosocomial diarrhea in pediatric patients should include routine handwashing and care in handling of fecal material in all children, since asymptomatic excretion of many enteropathogens is well-documented. In addition, children hospitalized because of acute diarrhea should be placed in "Enteric Precautions" according to guidelines developed at the Centers for Disease Control (Table 5.7) (164). These children should not be a source of hospital cross-infection. Occasionally, children are hospitalized during the incubation period of a diarrheal disease. Exposed hospital contacts are then at risk. Patients in the same room as the index patient should be managed with enteric precautions. The exposed roommates may be incubating the contagious diarrheal agent, and they should not be transferred into a room with unexposed children. These exposed patients should be isolated as a cohort.

In handling children with diarrhea, gowns are recommended if soiling is likely; hospital personnel should wear gloves when handling fecal material or the patient. Wearing of masks is not helpful and is not recommended. Children documented to have infection with the same agent can be isolated in the same room. Table 5.7 shows the recommended specifications for enteric precautions. In outbreaks that are prolonged and caused by person-to-person

Table 5.7
Recommended Enteric Precautions

Enteric Precautions
Visitors—Report to Nurses' Station
Before Entering Room[a]

1. Masks are not indicated.
2. Gowns are indicated if soiling is likely.
3. Gloves are indicated for touching infective material.
4. Hands must be washed after touching the patient or potentially contaminated articles and before taking care of another patient.
5. Articles contaminated with infective material should be discarded or bagged and labeled before being sent for decontamination and reprocessing.

[a]Adapted from reference 164.

Table 5.8
Diseases Requiring Enteric Precautions[a]

Amebic dysentery
Cholera
Coxsackievirus disease
Diarrhea, acute illness with suspected infectious etiology
Echovirus disease
Encephalitis (unless known not to be caused by enteroviruses)
Enterocolitis caused by *Clostridium difficile*
Enteroviral infection
Gastroenteritis caused by:
  Campylobacter species
  Cryptosporidium
  Dientamoeba fragilis
  Escherichia coli (enterotoxic, enteropathogenic, enteroinvasive, or enterohemorrhagic)
  Giardia lamblia
  Isospora
  Salmonella species
  Shigella species
  Vibrio cholerae
  Vibrio parahemolyticus
  Viruses, including Norwalk agent, rotavirus, and enteric adenovirus
  Yersinia enterocolitica
  Unknown etiology but presumed to be an infectious agent
Hand, food, and mouth disease
Hepatitis, viral, type A
Herpangina
Meningitis, viral (unless known not to be caused by enteroviruses)
Necrotizing enterocolitis
Pleurodynia
Poliomyelitis
Typhoid fever (*Salmonella typhi*)
Viral pericarditis, myocarditis, or meningitis (unless known not to be caused by enteroviruses)

[a]Adapted from reference 164.

transmission, more radical measures, such as cohorting infected patients with the same hospital staff, have appeared to be effective measures in several outbreaks. Table 5.8 shows diseases that require a patient to be placed into Enteric Precautions.

REFERENCES

1. DuPont HL, Pickering LK (eds) *Infections of the Gastrointestinal Tract. Microbiology, Pathophysiology, and Clinical Features*. New York, Plenum, 1980.
2. Centers for Disease Control, National Nosocomial Infections Study Report (NNIS), Annual Summary 1977, U.S. Dept. of Health, Education and Welfare, 1979.
3. Horan TC, White JW, Jarvis WR, Emori TG, Culver DH, Munn VP, Thornsberry C, Olson DR, Hughes JM: Nosocomial infection surveillance, 1984. *Morbid Mortal Weekly Rep* 35(1SS):17–29, 1986.

4. Haley RW, Culver DH, White JW, Morgan WM, Emori TG, Munn VP, Hooton TM: The efficacy of infection surveillance and control programs in preventing nosocomial infections in US hospitals. *Am J Epidem* 121:182–205, 1985.

5. Haley RW, Culver DH, White JW, Morgan WM, Emori TG: The nationwide nosocomial infection rate: a new need for viral statistics. *Am J Epidem* 121:159–167, 1985.

6. Moffet H: Pediatric nosocomial infections in the community hospital. *Pediatr Infect Dis* 1:430–442, 1982.

7. Welliver RC, McLaughlin S: Unique epidemiology of nosocomial infection in a children's hospital. *Am J Dis Child* 138:131–135, 1984.

8. Foodborne Disease Surveillance. Centers for Disease Control. Annual Summary 1981. US Dept Health and Human Services, Public Health Service. HHS Publication No. 1983;(CDC) 83–8185.

9. Harris JR, Cohen ML, Lippy EC: Water-related disease outbreaks in the United States, 1981. *J Infect Dis* 148:759–762, 1983.

10. Kindschuh M, Pickering LK, Cleary TG, Ruiz-Palacios G: Clinical and biochemical significance of toxin production by *Aeromonas hydrophila. J Clin Microbiol* 25:916–921, 1987.

11. Blaser MJ, Wells JG, Feldman RA, Pollard RA, Allen JR, and the Collaborative Diarrhea Disease Study Group: Campylobacter enteritis in the United States. *Ann Intern Med* 98:360–365, 1983.

12. Pickering LK, Bartlett AV, Woodward WE: Acute infectious diarrhea in day care children: epidemiology and control. *Rev Infect Dis* 8:539–547, 1986.

13. Blaser MJ, Penner JL, Wells JG: Diversity of serotypes in outbreaks of enteritis due to *Campylobacter jejuni. J Infect Dis* 146:826, 1982.

14. Levine MM: *Escherichia coli* that cause diarrhea: Enterotoxigenic, enteropathogenic, enteroinvasive, enterohemorrhagic and enteroadherent. *J Infect Dis* 155:377–389, 1987.

15. DuPont HL, Formal SB, Hornick RB, Merrill JS, Libonati JP, Sheahan DG, LaBrec EH, Kalas JP: Pathogenesis of *Escherichia coli* diarrhea. *N Engl J Med* 285:1–9, 1971.

16. Edelman R, Levine MM: Summary of a workshop on enteropathogenic *Escherichia coli. J Infect Dis* 147:1108–1118, 1983.

17. Ryder RW, Wachsmuth IK, Buxton AE, Evans DG, DuPont HL, Mason E, Barrett FF: Infantile diarrhea produced by heat-stable enterotoxigenic *Escherichia coli. N Engl J Med* 295:849–853, 1976.

18. Gross RJ, Rowe B, Henderson A, Byatt ME, MacLaurin JC: A new *Escherichia coli* 0-group 0159, associated with outbreaks of enteritis in infants. *Scand J Infect Dis* 8:195–198, 1976.

19. Guerrant RL, Dickens MD, Wenzel RP, Kapikian AZ: Toxigenic bacterial diarrhea: nursery outbreak involving multiple bacterial strains. *J Pediatr* 89:885–891, 1976.

20. Levine MM, Edelman R: Enteropathogenic *Escherichia coli* of classic serotypes associated with infant diarrhea: Epidemiology and pathogenesis. *Epidemiol Rev* 6:31–51, 1984.

21. Toledo MRF, Alvariza MCB, Murahovschi J, Ramos SRTS, Trabulsi LR: Enteropathogenic *Escherichia coli* serotypes and endemic diarrhea in infants. *Infect Immun* 39:586–589, 1983.

22. Gangarosa EJ, Merson MH: Epidemiologic assessment of the relevance of the so-called enteropathogenic serogroups of *Escherichia coli* in diarrhea. *N Engl J Med* 296:1210–1213, 1977.

23. Levine MM, Bergquist EJ, Nalin DR, Waterman DH, Hornick RB, Young CR: *Escherichia coli* strains that cause diarrhea but do not produce heat-labile or heat-stable enterotoxins and are noninvasive. *Lancet* 1:1119–1122, 1978.

24. Hone R, Fitzpatrick S, Keane C, Gross RJ, Rowe B: Infantile enteritis in Dublin caused by *Escherichia coli* 0142. *J Med Microbiol* 6:505–510, 1973.

25. Boyer KM, Petersen NJ, Farzaneh I, Pattison CP, Hart MC, Maynard JE: An outbreak of gastroenteritis due to *E. coli* 0142 in a neonatal nursery. *J Pediatr* 86:919–927, 1975.

26. Jacobs SI, Holzel A, Wolman B, Keen JH, Miller V, Taylor J, Gross RJ: Outbreak of infantile gastroenteritis caused by

Escherichia coli 0114. *Arch Dis Child* 45:656–663, 1970.

27. Rowe B, Gross J, Lindop R, Baird RB: A new *E. coli* 0 Group 0158 associated with an outbreak of infantile enteritis. *J Clin Pathol* 27:832–833, 1974.

28. Harris JR, Wachsmuth IK, Davis BR, Cohen ML: High molecular weight plasmid correlates with *Escherichia coli* enteroinvasiveness. *Infect Immun* 37:1295–1298, 1982.

29. O'Brien AD, Lively TA, Chen ME, Rothman SW, Formal SB: Purification of *Shigella dysenteriae* 1 (Shiga)-like toxin from *Escherichia coli* 0157:H7 strain associated with haemorrhagic colitis. *Lancet* 2:573, 1983.

30. Riley LW, Remis RS, Helgerson SD, McGee HB, Wells JG, Davis BR, Herbert RJ, Olcott ES, Johnson LM, Hargrett NT, Blake PA, Cohen ML: Hemorrhagic colitis associated with a rare *Escherichia coli* serotype. *N Engl J Med* 308:681–685, 1983.

31. Karmali MA, Petric M, Lim C: The association between idiopathic hemolytic uremic syndrome and infection by verotoxin producing *Escherichia coli. J Infect Dis* 151:775–782, 1985.

32. Kunz LJ, Ouchterlony OTB: Salmonellosis originating in a hospital: a newly recognized source of infection. *N Engl J Med* 253:761–763, 1955.

33. Sanders E, Sweeney FJ Jr, Friedman EA, Boring JR, Randall EL, Polk LD: An outbreak of hospital-associated infections due to *Salmonella derby. JAMA* 186:984–986, 1963.

34. Steere AC, Hall WJ III, Wells JG, Craven PJ, Leotsakis N, Farmer JJ, Gangarosa EJ: Person-to-person spread of *Salmonella typhimurium* after a hospital common-source outbreak. *Lancet* 1:319–322, 1975.

35. Lang DJ, Kunz LJ, Martin AR, Schroeder SA, Thomson LA: Carmine as a source of nosocomial salmonellosis. *N Engl J Med* 276:829–832, 1967.

36. Komarmy LE, Oxley ME, Brecher G: Hospital-acquired salmonellosis traced to carmine dye capsules. *N Engl J Med* 276:850–852, 1967.

37. Eickhoff TC: Nosocomial salmonellosis due to carmine. *Ann Intern Med* 66:813–814, 1967.

38. Baine WB, Gangarosa EJ, Bennett JV, Barker WA Jr: Institutional salmonellosis. *J Infect Dis* 128:357–360, 1973.

39. Glencross EJG: Pancreatin as a source of hospital-acquired salmonellosis. *Br Med J* 2:376–378, 1972.

40. Chmel H, Armstrong D: *Salmonella oslo*: a focal outbreak in a hospital. *Am J Med* 60:203–208, 1976.

41. Ip HMH, Sin WK, Chau PY, Tse D, Teoh-Chan CH: Neonatal infection due to *Salmonella worthington* transmitted by a delivery room suction apparatus. *J Hyg* 77:307–314, 1976.

42. Aber RC, Banks WV: An outbreak of nosocomial *Salmonella typhimurium* infection linked to environmental reservoir. *Infect Control* 1:386–390, 1980.

43. Centers for Disease Control, *Salmonella kottbus* meningitis-associated with contaminated breast milk. *Morbid Mortal Weekly Rep* 20:154, 1971.

44. Ryder RW, Crosby-Ritchie A, McDonough B, Hall WJ: Human milk contaminated with *Salmonella kottbus*: a cause of nosocomial illness in infants. *JAMA* 238:1533–1534, 1977.

45. Donowitz LG, Marsik FJ, Frisler KA, Friesen P, White FMM: Contaminated breast milk: A source of *Klebsiella bacteremia* in a newborn intensive care unit. *Rev Infect Dis* 3:716–720, 1981.

46. Stiver HG, Albritten WL, Clark J, Friesen P, White FMM: Nosocomial colonization and infection due to *E. coli* 125:k70 epidemiologically linked to expressed breast milk feedings. *Can J Public Health* 68:479–482, 1977.

47. Epstein HC, Hochwald A, Ashe R: Salmonella infections of the newborn infant. *J Pediatr* 38:723–731, 1951.

48. Abramsom H: Infection with *Salmonella typhimurium* in the newborn. *Am J Dis Child* 74:576–586, 1947.

49. Rice PA, Craven PC, Wells JG: *Salmonella heidelberg* enteritis and bacteremia: an epidemic on two pediatric wards. *Am J Med* 60:509–516, 1976.

50. Lamb VA, Mayhall CG, Spadora AC, Markowitz SM, Farmer JJ, Dalton HP: Outbreak of *Salmonella typhimurium* gastroenteritis due to an imported strain resistant to ampicillin, chlor-

amphenicol and trimethoprim/sulfamethoxazole in a nursery. *J Clin Microbiol* 20:1076–1079, 1984.

51. Datta N, Pridie RB: An outbreak of infection with *Salmonella typhimurium* in a general hospital. *J Hyg* 58:229–241, 1960.

52. Mushin R: An outbreak of gastroenteritis due to *Salmonella derby*. *J Hyg* 46:151–157, 1948.

53. Hirsch W, Sapiro-Hirsch R, Berger A, Winter ST, Mayer G, Mertzbach D: *Salmonella edinburg* infection in children: a protracted hospital epidemic due to a multiple-drug-resistant strain. *Lancet* 2:828–830, 1965.

54. Watt J, Wegman ME, Brown OW, Schliessmann DJ, Maupin E, Hemphill EC: Salmonellosis in a premature nursery unaccompanied by diarrheal disease. *Pediatrics* 22:689–705, 1958.

55. Bate JG, James U: *Salmonella typhimurium* infection dust-borne in a children's ward. *Lancet* 2:713–715, 1958.

56. Rubenstein AD, Fowler RN: Salmonellosis of the newborn with transmission by delivery room resuscitators. *Am J Public Health* 45:1109–1114, 1955.

57. Edgar WM, Lacey BW: Infection with *Salmonella heidelberg*. *Lancet* 1:161–163, 1963.

58. Abrams IF, Cochran WD, Holmes LB, Marsh EB, Moore JW: A *Salmonella newport* outbreak in a nursery with a one-year follow-up: effect of ampicillin following bacteriologic failure of response to kanamycin. *Pediatrics* 37:616–623, 1966.

59. DuPont HL, Hornick RB: Clinical approach to infectious diarrheas. *Medicine* (Baltimore) 52:265–270, 1973.

60. Salzman TC, Scher CD, Moss R: Shigellae with transferable drug resistance: outbreak in a nursery for premature infants. *J Pediatr* 71:21–26, 1967.

61. Haltalin KC: Neonatal shigellosis: report of 16 cases and review of the literature. *Am J Dis Child* 114:603–611, 1967.

62. Weissman JB, Hutcheson RH, Jr: Shigellosis transmitted by nurses. *South Med J* 69:1341–1346, 1976.

63. Morris JG, Black RE: Cholera and other vibrioses in the United States. *N Engl J Med* 312:343–350, 1985.

64. Kaper JB, Bradford HB, Roberts NC, Falkow S: Molecular epidemiology of *Vibrio cholerae* in the U.S. Gulf Coast. *J Clin Microbiol* 16:129–134, 1982.

65. Barker WH Jr: *Vibrio parahaemloyticus* outbreaks in the United States. *Lancet* 1:551–554, 1974.

66. Kohl S, Jacobson JA, Nahmias A: *Yersinia enterocolitica* infections in children. *J Pediatr* 89:77–79, 1976.

67. Tackett CO, Narain JP, Sattin R, Lofgren JP, Konigsberg C, Rendtorff RC, Rausa A, Davis BR, Cohen ML: A multistate outbreak of infections caused by *Yersinia enterocolitica* transmitted by pasteurized milk. *JAMA* 251:483–486, 1984.

68. Wright CD, Selss IF, Vinton KJ, Pierce RN: Fatal *Yersinia enterocolitica* sepsis after blood transfusion. *Arch Pathol Lab Med* 109:1040–1042, 1985.

69. Toivanen P, Toivanen A, Olkkonen L, Aantaa S: Hospital outbreak of *Yersinia enterocolitica* infection. *Lancet* 1:801–803, 1973.

70. Cukor G, Blacklow NR: Human viral gastroenteritis. *Microbiol Rev* 48:157–179, 1984.

71. Dolin R, Treanor JJ, Madore HP: Novel agents of viral enteritis in humans. *J Infect Dis* 155:365–376, 1987.

72. Kapikian AZ, Kim HW, Wyatt RG, Cline WL, Arrobio JO, Brandt CD, Rodriguez WJ, Sack DA, Chanock RM, Parrott RH: Human reovirus-like agent as the major pathogen associated with 'winter' gastroenteritis in hospitalized infants and young children. *N Engl J Med* 294:965–972, 1976.

73. Rodriguez WJ, Kim HW, Arrobio JO, Brandt CD, Chanock RM, Kapikian AZ, Wyatt RG, Parrott RH: Clinical features of acute gastroenteritis associated with reovirus-like agent in infants and young children. *J Pediatr* 91:188–193, 1977.

74. Middleton PJ, Szymanski MT, Petric M: Viruses associated with acute gastroenteritis in young children. *Am J Dis Child* 131:733, 1977.

75. Vesikari T, Maki M, Sarkkinen HK, Arstilla PP, Haloneu PE: Rotavirus, adenovirus and non-viral enteropathogens in diarrhoea. *Arch Dis Child* 56:264–270, 1981.

76. Flewett TH, Bryden AS, Davies H: Epidemic viral enteritis in a long stay children's ward. *Lancet* 1:4–5, 1975.

77. Ryder RW, McGowan JE, Jr, Hatch MH, Palmer EL: Reo-

78. Dennehy PH, Peter G: Risk factors associated with nosocomial rotavirus infection. *Am J Dis Child* 139:935–939, 1985.

79. Chapin M, Yatabe J, Cherry JD: An outbreak of rotavirus gastroenteritis on a pediatric unit. *Am J Infect Control* 11:88–91, 1983.

80. Noone C, Banatvala JE: Hospital acquired rotaviral gastroenteritis in a general pediatric unit. *J Hosp Infect* 4:297–299, 1983.

81. Builtenwerf J, Muilwijkevan AM, Schaap GJP: Characterization of rotaviral RNA isolated from children with gastroenteritis in two hospitals in Rotterdam. *J Med Virol* 12:71–78, 1983.

82. Berger R, Hadziselimovic F, Just M, Reigel P: Effect of feeding human milk on nosocomial rotavirus infections in an infant ward. *Dev Biol Stand* 53:219–228, 1983.

83. Jarvis WR, Middleton PJ, Gelfand EW: Significance of viral infections in severe combined immunodeficiency disease. *Pediatr Infect Dis* 2:187–192, 1982.

84. Booth IW, Chrystie IL, Levinsky RJ, Marshall WC, Pincott J, Harries JT: Protracted diarrhoea, immunodeficiency and viruses. *Eur J Pediatr* 138:271–272, 1982.

85. Chrystie IL, Booth IW, Kidd AH, Marshall WC, Banatvala JE: Multiple faecal virus excretion in immunodeficiency. *Lancet* 1:282, 1982.

86. Yolken RH, Bishop CA, Townsend TR, Bolyard EA, Bartlett J, Santos GW, Saral R: Infectious gastroenteritis in bone-marrow-transplant recipients. *N Engl J Med* 306:1009–1012, 1982.

87. Saulsbury FT, Winkelstein JA, Yolken RH: Chronic rotavirus infection in immunodeficiency. *J Pediatr* 97:61–65, 1980.

88. Vollet JJ, Ericsson CD, Gibson D, Pickering LK, DuPont HL, Kohl S, Conklin RH: Human rotavirus in an adult population with travelers' diarrhea and its relationship to the location of food consumption. *J Med Virol* 4:81–87, 1979.

89. Kim HW, Brandt CD, Kapikian AZ, Wyatt RG, Arrobio JO, Rodriguez WJ, Chanock RM, Parrott RH: Human reovirus-like agent infection: occurrence in adult contacts of pediatric patients with gastroenteritis. *JAMA* 238:404–407, 1977.

90. Cubitt WD, Holzel H: Hospital acquired rotavirus infection in adults. Who is at risk? *J Hosp Infect* 1:327–331, 1980.

91. Holzel H, Cubitt DW, McSwiggan DA, Sanderson PJ, Church J: An outbreak of rotavirus infection among adults in a cardiology ward. *J Infect* 2:33–37, 1980.

92. Bishop RF, Hewstone AS, Davidson GP, Townley RRW, Holmes IH, Ruck BJ: An epidemic of diarrhea in human neonates involving a reovirus-like agent and 'enteropathogenic' serotypes of *Escherichia coli*. *J Clin Pathol* 29:46–49, 1976.

93. Murphy AM, Albrey MB, Crewe EB: Rotavirus infections of neonates. *Lancet* 2:1149–1150, 1977.

94. Cameron DJS, Bishop RF, Veenstra AA, Barnes GL: Non-cultivatable viruses and neonatal diarrhea: fifteen-month survey in a newborn special care nursery. *J Clin Microbiol* 8:93–98, 1978.

95. Crewe E, Murphy AM: Further studies on neonatal rotavirus infections. *Med J Aust* 1:61–63, 1980.

96. Van Renterghem L, Borre P, Tilleman J: Rotavirus and other viruses in the stool of premature babies. *J Med Virol* 5:137–142, 1980.

97. Rocchi G, Vella S, Resta S, Cochi S, Donnelli G, Tangncci F, Menichella D, Varveir A, Inglese R: Outbreak of rotavirus gastroenteritis among premature infants. *Br Med J* 283:886, 1981.

98. Dearlove J, Latham P, Dearlove B, Pearl K, Thomson A, Lewis IG: Clinical range of neonatal rotavirus gastroenteritis. *Br Med J* 286:1473–1475, 1983.

99. Rotbart HA, Levin MJ, Yolken RH, Manchester DK, Jantzen J: An outbreak of rotavirus-associated neonatal necrotizing enterocolitis. *J Pediatr* 103:454–459, 1983.

100. Rudd PT, Carrington D: A prospective study of chlamydial, mycoplasmal and viral infections in a neonatal intensive care unit. *Arch Dis Child* 59:120–125, 1984.

101. Champsaur H, Questiaux E, Prevot M, Henry-Amar M,

Goldszmidt D, Bourjonane M, Bach C: Rotavirus carriage, asymptomatic infection, and disease in the first two years of life. I. Virus shedding. *J Infect Dis* 149:667–674, 1984.

102. Keswick BH, Pickering LK, DuPont HL, Woodward WE: Prevalence of rotavirus in children in day care centers. *J Pediatr* 103:85–86, 1983.

103. Brandt CD, Kim HW, Rodriguez WJ, Arrobio JO, Jeffries BC, Stallings EP, Lewis C, Miles AJ, Gardner MK, Parrott RH: Adenoviruses and pediatric gastroenteritis. *J Infect Dis* 151:437–443, 1985.

104. Yolken RH, Lawrence F, Leister F, Takiff HE, Strauss SE: Gastroenteritis associated with enteric type adenovirus in hospitalized infants. *J Pediatr* 101:21–26, 1982.

105. Yolken RH, Franklin CC: Gastrointestinal adenovirus: an important cause of morbidity in patients with necrotizing enterocolitis and gastrointestinal surgery. *Pediatr Infect Dis* 4:42–47, 1985.

106. Kaplan JE, Gary W, Baron RC, Singh N, Schonberger LB, Feldman R, Greenberg HB: Epidemiology of Norwalk gastroenteritis and the role of Norwalk virus in outbreaks of acute nonbacterial gastroenteritis. *Ann Intern Med* 96:756–761, 1982.

107. Blacklow NR, Cukor G, Bedigian MK, Echeverria P, Greenberg HB, Schreiber DS, Trier JS: Immune response and prevalence of antibody to Norwalk virus as determined by radioimmunoassay. *J Clin Microbiol* 10:903–909, 1979.

108. Gustafson TL, Kobylik B, Hutcheson RH, Schaffner W: Protective effect of anticholinergic drugs and psyllium in a nosocomial outbreak of Norwalk gastroenteritis. *J Hosp Infect* 4:367–374, 1983.

109. Leers W-D, Kasupski G, Fralick R, Wartman S, Garcia J, Gary W: Norwalk-like gastroenteritis epidemic in a Toronto hospital. *Am J Public Health* 77:291–295, 1987.

110. Morse DL, Guzewich JJ, Nanrahan JP, Stricoff R, Shayegain M, Deibel R, Grabau G, Nowak N, Hervman JE, Cukor G, Blacklow NR: Widespread outbreaks of clam- and oyster-associated gastroenteritis. Role of Norwalk virus. *N Engl J Med* 314:678–681, 1986.

111. Spratt HC, Marks MI, Gomersall M, Gill P, Pai CH: Nosocomial infantile gastroenteritis associated with minirotavirus and calcivirus. *J Pediatr* 93:922–926, 1978.

112. Craft JC: Giardia and giardiasis in childhood. *Pediatr Infect Dis* 1:196–211, 1982.

113. Pickering LK, Evans DG, DuPont HL, Vollet JJ, Evans DJ: Diarrhea caused by Shigella, Rotavirus and Giardia in day care centers: prospective study. *J Pediatr* 99:51–56, 1981.

114. Pickering LK, Woodward WE, DuPont HL, Sullivan PS: Occurrence of *Giardia lamblia* in children in day care centers. *J Pediatr* 104:522–526, 1984.

115. Krogstad DJ, Spencer HC Jr, Healy GR, Gleason NN, Sexton DJ, Herron CA: Amebiasis: epidemiologic studies in the United States, 1971–1974. *Ann Intern Med* 88:89–97, 1978.

116. Fuchs G, Pickering LK: Amebiasis in the pediatric population. In Ravdin JI (ed): *Amebiasis: Human Infection by Entamoeba histolytica.* New York, John Wiley & Sons (in press).

117. Istre GR, Kreiss K, Hopkins RS, Healy GR, Benziger M, Caufield TM, Dickinson P, Englert TR, Comptom RC, Mathews HM, Simmons RA: An outbreak of amebiasis spread by colonic irrigation at a chiropractic clinic. *N Engl J Med* 307:339–342, 1982.

118. Fayer R, Unger BLP: Cryptosporidium spp and cryptosporidiosis. *Microbiol Rev* 50:458–483, 1986.

119. Tzipori S: Cryptosporidiosis in animals and humans. *Microbiol Rev* 47:84–96, 1983.

120. Baxby D, Hart CA, Taylor C: Human cryptosporidiosis: a possible cause of hospital cross infection. *Br Med J* 287:1760–1761, 1983.

121. Koch KL, Phillips DJ, Aber RC, Current WL: Cryptosporidiosis in hospital personnel. Evidence for person-to-person transmission. *Ann Intern Med* 102:593–596, 1985.

122. Cleary TG, Pickering LK: Update on infectious diarrhea. In Aronoff SC, Hughes WT Jr, Kohl S, Speck WT, Walt ER (eds): *Advances in Pediatric Infectious Diseases.* Chicago: Year Book 1:117–143, 1986.

123. Bartlett JG: Antibiotic-associated pseudomembranous colitis. *Rev Infect Dis* 1:530–539, 1979.

124. Bartlett JG: Antimicrobial agents implicated in *Clostridium difficile* toxin-associated diarrhea or colitis. *Johns Hopkins Med J* 149:6–9, 1981.

125. Teasley DG, Gerding DN, Olson MM, Peterson LR, Gebhard RL, Schwarts MJ, Lee JT: Prospective randomized trial of metronidazole versus vancomycin for *Clostridium difficile* associated diarrhea and colitis. *Lancet* 2:1043–1046, 1983.

126. George WL, Rolfe RD, Finegold SM: *Clostridium difficile* and its cytotoxin in feces of patients with antimicrobial agent-associated diarrhea and miscellaneous conditions. *J Clin Microbiol* 15:1049–1053, 1982.

127. Elstner CL, Lindsay AN, Book LS, Matsen J: Lack of relation of *Clostridium difficile* to antibiotic-associated diarrhea in pediatric patients. *Pediatr Infect Dis* 2:364–366, 1983.

128. Bender BS, Bennett R, Laughon BE, Gaydos C, Forman MS, Bennett R, Greenough WB, III, Sears SD, Bartlett JG: Is *Clostridium difficile* endemic in chronic-care facilities? *Lancet* 2:11–13, 1986.

129. Kim KH, Fekety R, Batts DH, Brown D, Cudmore M, Silva J, Waters D: Isolation of *Clostridium difficile* from the environment and contacts of patients with antibiotic-associated colitis. *J Infect Dis* 143:42–50, 1981.

130. Kim KH, DuPont HL, Pickering LK: Outbreaks of diarrhea associated with *Clostridium difficile* and its toxin in day care centers: evidence of person-to-person spread. *J Pediatr* 120:376–382, 1983.

131. Potter ME, Kaufmann AF, Blake PA, Feldman RA: Unpasteurized milk. The hazards of a health fetish. *JAMA* 252:2048–2054, 1984.

132. Hanrahan JP, Gordon MA: Mushroom poisoning. Case reports and a reivew of therapy. *JAMA* 251:1057–1061, 1984.

133. Whiteside ME, Barkin JS, May RG, Weiss SD, Fischl MA, MacLeod CL: Enteric coccidiosis among patients with the acquired immunodeficiency syndrome. *Amer J Trop Med Hyg* 33:1065–1072, 1984.

134. Bodey GP, Fainstein V, Guerrant R: Infections of the gastrointestinal tract in the immunocompromised patient. *Ann Rev Med* 37:271–281, 1986.

135. Jacobs JL, Gold JWM, Murray HM, Roberts RB, Armstrong D: Salmonella infections in patients with the acquired immunodeficiency syndrome. *Ann Intern Med* 102:186–188, 1986.

136. Malebranche R, Arnoux E, Guerin JM, Pierre GD, Laroche AC, Pean-Guichard C, Flie R, Morisset PH, Spira T, Mandeville R, Drotman P, Seemayer T: Acquired immunodeficiency syndrome with severe gastrointestinal manifestations in Haiti. *Lancet* 2:873–877, 1983.

137. Kliegman RM, Fanaroff AA: Necrotizing enterocolitis. *N Engl J Med* 310:1093–1103, 1984.

138. Rotbart HA, Levin MJ: How contagious is necrotizing enterocolitis? *Pediatr Infect Dis* 2:406–413, 1983.

139. Book LS, Overall JL, Herbst JJ, Britt MR, Epstein B, Jung AL: Clustering of necrotizing enterocolitis: interruption by infection-control measures. *N Engl J Med* 297:984–986, 1977.

140. Pickering LK, Evans DJ, Munoz O, DuPont HL, Coello-Ramirez P, Vollet JJ, Conklin RH, Olarte J, Kohl S: Prospective evaluation of enteropathogens in children with diarrhea in Houston and Mexico. *J Pediatr* 93:383–388, 1978.

141. Gurwich MJ, Williams TW: Gastroenteritis in children: A two-year review in Manitoba. I. Etiology. *J Infect Dis* 136:239–247, 1977.

142. Gleason W, Pickering LK: Chronic diarrhea in children. In Gillis SS, Kagan BM, (eds): *Current Pediatric Therapy* 12:231–241, 1986. Philadelphia: WB Saunders.

143. Bartlett AV, Pickering LK: Pediatric diarrhea. In Callaham M (ed): *Current Therapy in Emergency Medicine.* Toronto: BC Decker, 1026–1032, 1987.

144. Pickering LK, DuPont HL, Orlate J, Conklin R, Ericsson C: Fecal leukocytes in enteric infections. *J Clin Pathol* 68:562–565, 1977.

145. Mahmound AAF, Warren KS: Amebiasis. *J Infect Dis* 134:639–643, 1976.

146. Knisley CV, Bednarz-Prashad AJ, Pickering LK: Detection of

rotavirus in stool specimens using monoclonal and polyclonal antibody based assay systems. *J Clin Microbiol* 23:897–900, 1986.

147. Riley LW, Remis RS, Helgerson SD, McGee HB, Wells JG, Davis BR, Herbert RJ, Olcott ES, Johnson LM, Hargrett NT, Blake PA, Cohen ML: Hemorrhagic colitis with a rare *Escherichia coli* serotype. *N Engl J Med* 308:681–685, 1983.

148. Wells JG, David BR, Wachsmuth K, Riley LW, Remis RS, Sokolow R, Morris GK: Laboratory investigation of hemorrhagic colitis outbreaks associated with a rare *Escherichia coli* serotype. *J Clin Microbiol* 18:512–520, 1983.

149. Laughon BE, Viscidi RP, Gdovin SL, Yolken RH, Bartlett JG: Enzyme immunoassay for detection of *Clostridium difficile* toxins A and B in fecal specimens. *J Infec Dis* 149:781–788, 1984.

150. Eisenstein BI, Engleberg NC: Applied molecular genetics: new tools for microbiologists and clinicians. *J Infect Dis* 153:416–430, 1986.

151. Jiwa SF: Probing for enterotoxigenicity among the salmonellae: an evaluation of biological assay. *J Clin Micro* 14:463–472, 1981.

152. Kaper JV, Moseley SL, Falkow S: Molecular characterization of environmental and non-toxigenic strains of *Vibrio cholerae*. *Infect Immun* 32:661–667, 1981.

153. Georges MC, Wachsmuth IK, Birkness KA, Moseley SL, Georges AJ: Genetic probes for enterotoxigenic *Escherichia coli* isolated from childhood diarrhea in the Central African Republic. *J Clin Microbiol* 18:199–202, 1983.

154. Sack RB, Pierce NF, Hirschhorn N: The current status of oral therapy in the treatment of acute diarrheal disease. *Am J Clin Nutrit* 31:2252–2257, 1978.

155. Brown KH, McClean WC: Nutritional management of acute diarrhea. An appraisal of the alternatives. *Pediatrics* 73:119–125, 1984.

156. Nelson JD, Kusmiesz H, Jackson LH: Comparison of trimethoprim/sulfamethoxazole and ampicillin therapy for shigellosis in ambulatory patients. *J Pediatr* 89:491–493, 1976.

157. Nelson JD, Kusmiesz H, Jackson LH, Woodman E: Trimethoprim/sulfamethoxazole therapy for shigellosis. *JAMA* 235:1239–1244, 1976.

158. Nelson JD, Haltalin KC: Amoxicillin less effective than ampicillin against Shigella *in vitro* and *in vivo*. Relationship of efficacy to activity in serum. *J Infect Dis* 129(suppl):222–227, 1974.

159. Snyder MJ, Perroni J, Gonzalez O, Woodward WE, Palomino C, Gonzalez C, Musie SI, DuPont HL, Hornick RB, Woodward TE: Comparative efficacy of chloramphenicol, ampicillin and cotrimoxazole in the treatment of typhoid fever. *Lancet* 2:1155–1157, 1976.

160. Bryan JP, Rocha H, Scheld WM, Lowe B, Chang T: Problems in salmonellosis: Rationale for clinical trials with newer β-lactam agents and quinolones. *Rev Infect Dis* 8:189–207, 1986.

161. Bartlett JG, Tedesdo FJ, Shull S, Lowe B, Chang T: Symptomatic relapse after oral vancomycin therapy of antibiotic-associated pseudomembranous colitis. *Gastroenterology* 78:431–434, 1980.

162. *Medical Letter*. Drugs for parasitic infections: 26:27–34, 1984.

163. Davidson RA: Issues in clinical parasitology: The treatment of giardiasis. *Am J Gastroenter* 79:256–261, 1984.

164. Garner JS, Simmons BP: Guideline for isolation precautions in hospitals. *Infect Control* 4 (suppl):245–325, 1983.

6

Viral Respiratory Infection

Ronald B. Turner, M.D. and J. Owen Hendley, M.D.

INTRODUCTION

The respiratory viruses are an important cause of nosocomial infection in pediatric patients. A recent study reported 0.97 nosocomial respiratory infections in a children's hospital for every 100 patients discharged (1). Viral pathogens were responsible for 61% of the infections for which an etiologic diagnosis was established. Wenzel, et al. (2), reported that 17% of preschool children who were hospitalized for at least 1 week during the winter or spring seasons developed a nosocomial viral respiratory infection. Although viral respiratory infections are not generally associated with serious morbidity or mortality, these infections may have important implications for the hospitalized patient. Some patients, including those with congenital heart disease, neonates, and immunocompromised hosts, appear to be at risk for serious illness and increased mortality if they acquire a viral respiratory infection in the hospital (3–5). Although these serious infections do not occur in most patients, the development of a minor febrile illness in a hospitalized patient can result in unnecessary diagnostic studies and/or administration of antibiotics. Overall, nosocomial viral respiratory infections have been estimated to prolong hospitalization 5–7 days (6,7).

The viral pathogens that cause respiratory infection include rhinovirus, coronavirus, adenovirus, parainfluenza virus, respiratory syncytial virus (RSV), and influenza virus. Infection with these viruses may produce the common cold, pharyngitis, croup, bronchiolitis, or pneumonia as a result of infection at different levels of the respiratory tract. Viruses spread via the respiratory tract, but which produce prominent symptoms in other organ systems (i.e., measles, varicella-zoster) are not considered in this chapter.

POPULATION

Nosocomial respiratory infections with a particular virus are temporally related to the presence of the virus in the community (8–12). Thus, the incidence of hospital-acquired viral respiratory disease is seasonal, and the risk of infection is greatest during community epidemics.

Virtually all patients and hospital personnel are at risk of infection with nosocomial respiratory pathogens. A large pool of susceptible individuals is insured for these viruses by two different mechanisms. One mechanism is illustrated by the parainfluenza viruses and RSV, which are capable of reinfecting the same individual multiple times (13,14). Although there are only four different parainfluenza serotypes and only one RSV serotype, the ability to reinfect allows transmission of these viruses to a large number of individuals. Reinfection usually results in an attenuated illness, which is less likely to be associated with lower respiratory symptoms. In the hospital, however, patients or staff with mild or asymptomatic infection provide an important reservoir of infection. The rhinoviruses and adenoviruses illustrate a second mechanism by which a population susceptible to infection is assured. These viruses produce solid immunity in response to infection (15,16), but each has multiple antigenically distinct serotypes. Large proportions of the population remain susceptible to each serotype. Similarly, the influenza viruses have the ability to change the antigens presented on the surface of the virus (17) and thus behave as though there were multiple serotypes. The interaction of the coronaviruses with host immunity is not well-defined. Recent evidence suggests that there are multiple distinct immunotypes of coronavirus that are capable of inducing protective immunity (18).

In contrast to other nosocomial infections,

specific risk factors, such as intravascular lines or immunosuppression, are not associated with an increased incidence of viral respiratory infection. An apparent exception to this general rule has been observed in premature infants. In two outbreaks involving RSV, parainfluenza virus, and rhinovirus, infants who had feeding tubes or orotracheal tubes were at increased risk of infection (19,20). In one of these outbreaks, mechanical ventilation also appeared to increase the risk of infection (20).

Although risk factors are not important for the acquisition of viral respiratory infection, the severity of the illness produced by the infection may depend upon the patient's underlying disease. RSV infection has been found to be associated with particularly high mortality rates in hospitalized patients with congenital heart disease. MacDonald, et al. (3), reported that 37% of these patients died compared with 1.5% of hospitalized patients with RSV infection but with no underlying heart disease. Other populations of hospitalized patients in which RSV infection is associated with increased mortality rates include patients with compromised immune function and patients in newborn intensive care units (4,5). Although the published information is limited to RSV infection, it is likely that the same patient populations are at increased risk from lower respiratory tract infection with any of the viral respiratory pathogens. Asthmatic children may have exacerbations of their pulmonary disease during infection with any of the respiratory viruses (21,22).

DIAGNOSIS

Epidemiologic and clinical information can provide important clues to the specific etiology of viral respiratory infections. The occurrence of viral respiratory disease in a community is the result of sequential and relatively discreet epidemics of individual pathogens (23,24). Knowledge of which viruses are prevalent in the community at a given time provides valuable information for making an etiologic diagnosis in an individual patient. Furthermore, although any of the viral respiratory syndromes may be caused by any of the pathogens, specific pathogens are frequently associated with particular clinical syndromes (Table 6.1). When a patient presents with a clinical syndrome characteristic of a virus known to be present in the community, the etiologic diagnosis can be predicted with reasonable assurance.

Laboratory confirmation of the etiologic diagnosis is usually not necessary for management of viral respiratory infections. When it is necessary to know the specific etiology of an infection, the methods available for viral diagnosis are virus isolation, viral antigen detection in respiratory secretions, or detection of specific antiviral antibodies in acute and convalescent sera (Table 6.2). Virus isolation in cell cultures is the standard method for diagnosis of the respiratory pathogens. Isolation of these viruses in cell culture, however, generally requires several days, and in some cases, may take more than 2 weeks (25,26). The need for more timely

Table 6.1
Clinical Syndromes Associated with Viral Respiratory Pathogens

Virus	Characteristic Clinical Syndrome	Other Clinical Syndromes
Rhinovirus	Common cold	
Coronavirus 229E	Common cold	Pneumonia (?)
Adenovirus	Pharyngoconjunctival fever	Bronchiolitis Pneumonia
Parainfluenza	Croup	Bronchiolitis Pneumonia
RSV	Bronchiolitis	Pneumonia Croup Common cold
Influenza	Pneumonia	Pharyngitis Croup Bronchiolitis Common cold

Table 6.2
Methods for Etiologic Diagnosis of Viral Respiratory Disease

Virus	Standard Method	Antigen Detection	Serology
Rhinovirus	Virus isolation	No	No
Coronavirus	None	Yes[a]	Yes[a]
Adenovirus	Virus isolation	Yes[a]	Yes
Parainfluenza	Virus isolation	Yes[a]	Yes
RSV	Virus isolation	Yes	Yes
Influenza	Virus isolation	Yes[a]	Yes

[a]Research procedure not generally available in clinical diagnostic laboratories.

information has prompted an interest in rapid diagnostic methods. Detection of viral antigen in respiratory secretions, which allows a diagnosis within hours, has been reported for many of the respiratory viruses (27,28) but is commercially available only for RSV. Serologic assays are available for most of the respiratory pathogens; however, the need for a convalescent serum limits the usefulness of the serologic tests in the clinical setting.

Collection of Specimens

Virus Isolation. Specimens for virus isolation should be obtained as early as possible in the course of the patient's illness. Although some individuals may shed virus for weeks (29,30), virus is most consistently recovered in the first few days after the onset of symptoms (29,31). Respiratory pathogens are most readily isolated from specimens collected by nasal wash (32,33). A nasal wash is done in infants by drawing approximately 5 ml of normal saline into a clean suction bulb. With the child's head at a 45° angle, the tip of the suction bulb is placed into the nostril, and the saline is expelled. The saline is then recovered by immediate aspiration of the nose with the suction bulb. The recovered saline is then placed into a clean container and is tightly capped. If a nasal wash specimen cannot be collected, a nasopharyngeal swab and a throat swab should both be done. The swabs should be placed immediately into a vial of viral-collecting broth. Specimens for virus isolation should be kept at refrigerator temperature (4°C) and transported to the laboratory as quickly as possible.

Viral Antigen Detection. Specimens collected by nasal wash for virus isolation are also suitable for antigen detection methods. Since specimen requirements vary for the different antigen detection methods, the laboratory should be consulted prior to collection of specimens for antigen detection.

Viral Serology. Acute serum specimens should be obtained as soon as possible after onset of symptoms, and convalescent sera should be collected 2–3 weeks later. Sera may be stored at 4°C for short periods and may be stored at −20°C indefinitely. Hemolyzed specimens may not be acceptable for some serologic assays.

Interpretation of Laboratory Results

Virus Isolation. The isolation of a viral pathogen from the upper respiratory tract of a patient with respiratory symptoms is generally considered diagnostic. Virus isolation is absolutely specific if the laboratory confirms the identity of virus by immunologic methods. Two potential problems should be considered, however, when attributing respiratory symptoms to a virus isolated from the upper respiratory tract. First, although true asymptomatic carriage of viral pathogens in the respiratory tract does not occur, some viruses, particularly adenovirus, may be shed in respiratory secretions for many weeks after infection. Adenovirus can be isolated from the upper respiratory tract in approximately 5% of healthy children (34,35). Isolation of adenovirus from the respiratory tract of an ill child may therefore be unrelated to the acute illness.

The second problem with attributing respiratory symptoms to a virus isolated from the upper respiratory tract is the possibility that upper respiratory isolates may not accurately reflect the pathogens in the lower respiratory tract. In a study of hospitalized infants, 25% of patients with documented viral upper respiratory infection had evidence of a concurrent bacterial infection (36).

The sensitivity of virus isolation for detection of viral respiratory pathogens is not known. The time of collection in relation to onset of symptoms, the method of specimen collection, and the handling of the specimen prior to inoculation into cell culture all affect the recovery of virus from infected individuals. Even under optimal conditions, viral cultures from the respiratory tract may be falsely negative. Multiple cultures or confirmation by serology increase the reliability of the culture results.

Viral Antigen Detection.   Detection of viral antigen in respiratory secretions allows more rapid diagnosis of viral infection. The commercially available reagents for detection of RSV infection have a sensitivity and specificity of 85–95% compared with virus isolation in cell culture (37,38). Antigen detection may be more sensitive than virus isolation in some situations since viral antigen can be detected in specimens which do not contain infectious virus particles.

Viral Serology.   Interpretation of serologic results is dependent upon comparison of antibody levels in acute and convalescent sera. Antibody levels in a single serum specimen are generally not helpful for diagnosis of viral infection. A 4-fold increase in antibody titer in a convalescent serum compared with the titer in an acute serum drawn early in the illness is evidence of infection with the virus. Unfortunately, a 4-fold increase in antibody does not occur in response to all infections. The antibody response is particularly unreliable in young infants and in patients who are reinfected with a virus in spite of preexisting antibody.

TREATMENT

The illnesses caused by respiratory viral pathogens are generally self-limited and are treated symptomatically. Two antiviral agents that may be useful for specific treatment in some patients are currently available.

Ribavirin (Virazole®) has recently been approved for use in patients infected with RSV. Although statistically significant improvement in symptoms has been reported in ribavirin-treated infants in controlled trials, the clinical benefit of treatment is modest (39,40). Previously healthy patients with uncomplicated disease are not candidates for ribavirin therapy. Patients in the high-risk groups for serious illness associated with RSV may benefit from treatment. Ribavirin is administered as an aerosol in a tent, head box, or face mask for 12–18 hours each day for 3–7 days. The drug is not approved for use in patients on ventilators; however, administration of the drug through the ventilator has been done safely under carefully controlled conditions (41).

Amantadine (Symmetrel®) is an effective antiviral agent for the treatment or prevention of influenza A infections (42–46). Although the drug has a modest clinical benefit, it is inexpensive and its use can be justified in patients with underlying cardiac or pulmonary disease who may be at risk for increased morbidity from influenza. Administration of amantadine has been associated with insomnia, dizziness, or inability to concentrate in some patients (44). These side effects can generally be controlled by reducing the dose of the drug and are resolved promptly when treatment is discontinued. Amantadine has no effect on influenza B infections.

Treatment with either of these antiviral agents would ideally follow definitive identification of the viral pathogen responsible for the infection. The availability of rapid diagnostic techniques for RSV allows an etiologic diagnosis prior to the use of ribavirin in most patients. Rapid diagnostic techniques are not generally available for the detection of influenza A, and treatment is usually started on the basis of a consistent clinical syndrome during a time when influenza A is prevalent in the community.

PREVENTION

Vaccines.   The influenza vaccine is the only vaccine available for the prevention of infection with the respiratory viruses. Adenovirus vaccines are produced for use in military personnel, but are not available to the civilian population. Attempts to develop vaccines to other respiratory viruses have been unsuccessful.

The influenza vaccine usually contains one or more type A strains and one type B strain selected to provide immunity to the virus expected in the following influenza season. The strains of virus in the vaccine are changed as necessary in response to the changing epidemiology of the influenza viruses. The vaccine viruses are produced in eggs, then inactivated and purified so that the vaccine contains no infectious material. Some vaccines are treated with lipid solvents, which produce a "split virus" vaccine. These preparations produce fewer side effects than "whole virus" vaccine and are the recommended vaccine for children under 12 years of age. Pediatric patients older than 12 years may be given either the whole virus or the split virus vaccine (47).

Patients for whom the influenza vaccine is indicated include patients with chronic cardiac or pulmonary disease (47). Children with diabetes mellitus, chronic renal disease, or compromised immune function, and patients who are receiving long-term aspirin therapy are also candidates for the vaccine. Administration of the vaccine simultaneously with immunosuppressive therapy will decrease the response to the vaccine. Others who should be considered potential candidates for the vaccine include health care workers who are responsible for the care of patients in the high-risk groups. Some have suggested that family members of these high-risk patients should also be immunized (48). Patients under 6 months of age are generally not immunized, unless they are in a high-risk group.

The side effects of the vaccine are generally mild, although some patients will develop influenza-like symptoms, such as fever, myalgia, and headache. These symptoms are readily controlled with analgesics and generally persist for less than 48 hours. The vaccine contains small amounts of egg protein and should not be given to patients who are allergic to eggs.

Antivirals.   Amantadine is an effective agent for prophylaxis of influenza A infections (44–46). Use of amantadine is recommended for high-risk patients who have not been immunized (47). Patients who are immunized after influenza is present in the community may be given amantadine for several weeks after immunization to prevent infection prior to development of a protective antibody response. Rimantadine, an analogue of amantadine, is also effective for prophylaxis and treatment of influenza A infections, but has not yet been licensed for use in the United States (44,49).

Recombinant human alpha-interferon given intranasally has been shown to be effective for prophylaxis of rhinovirus and coronavirus colds (50–52). The use of interferon is associated with an unacceptable incidence of side effects, however, and the role of this product in the prevention of viral respiratory illness remains to be determined.

Isolation.   Patients who have symptoms of viral respiratory illness should be placed in contact isolation (53). Other recommended measures during community epidemics include cohorting of patients, cohorting of staff, if possible, and restriction of visitors with respiratory symptoms.

The measures necessary to interrupt transmission of infection are dependent to some extent upon the mechanism of spread of the pathogen (Table 6.3). Respiratory viruses can be transmitted from person-to-person by aerosols or by hand contact with the virus followed by self-inoculation. Aerosols are readily produced by coughing, sneezing, and nose-blowing (54,55). Some aerosolized particles have also been detected during normal speech (54).

Small-particle aerosols, composed of droplet nuclei 2–3 μm in diameter, comprise approximately 95% of the total number of particles and 25% of the total volume of coughs and sneezes (54). The small particle aerosol fraction is slightly higher for coughs than for sneezes. These particles remain suspended in the air and can be transmitted over extended distances. Once an air space is contaminated by virus suspended in a small-particle aerosol, the length of time infection can be transmitted is limited only by the circulation of the air and the ability of the virus to survive in the environment. Small-particle aerosols are not filtered by the nose and are inhaled into the lungs.

Table 6.3
Mechanism of Transmission of Respiratory Viruses[a]

Route	Virus	Interruption Techniques
Aerosols		
Small-particle	Influenza Coronavirus 229E	Negative pressure airflow Masks U-V radiation (?)
Large-particle	RSV (?)	Spatial separation Masks (?)
Direct contact	RSV Rhinovirus	Handwashing Environmental decontamination Eye/nose goggles

[a]No information is available which describes the route of transmission of adenovirus or parainfluenza virus.

Large-particle aerosols are composed of particles larger than 10 μm in diameter. These particles settle quickly and are transmitted only a few feet. For this reason, transmission of infection by large-particle aerosol requires relatively close contact between infected and susceptible individuals. Large-particle aerosols are effectively filtered in the nose and do not reach the lower respiratory tract.

Transmission of viral respiratory infections by direct contact requires that susceptible individuals contaminate their hands with virus by contact with either the patient or fomites. The virus is then inoculated onto the mucous membranes by hand-to-nose or hand-to-eye contact. Respiratory viruses can conceivably be spread from infected to susceptible individuals by an uninfected intermediate person, but this has not been conclusively established. Spread of infection by direct contact is limited only by the ability of viruses to survive on skin and environmental surfaces.

Information about the mechanisms of spread of different viral pathogens under natural conditions is limited. While it is likely that any of the different mechanisms of transmission may be involved in the spread of respiratory infection, studies in controlled settings suggest that for some viruses, one route may be more efficient than another (56–59; Table 6.3).

Special Precautions

Respiratory Syncytial Virus (RSV). RSV is spread by close contact with an infected individual (56). Patients with RSV infection should be placed in contact isolation. Health care personnel should be careful to practice good handwashing and to avoid hand-to-eye or hand-to-nose contact while working with the patient. The use of gowns and masks by hospital staff has not consistently been shown to have a beneficial effect on the spread of RSV in the hospital (60–62). Recent studies have suggested that using goggles or gloves to prevent inoculation of the eyes or nose with contaminated hands reduces the spread of infection to both hospital staff and hospitalized patients (63,64). The mechanisms of spread and recommended isolation procedures are described in detail in Chapter 15 of this text.

Influenza A and B. Transmission of influenza A and B appears to occur by small-particle aerosols (57). Respiratory isolation utilizing a negative pressure airflow room is useful for interruption of small-particle aerosol spread of infection. The use of masks by either infected or susceptible individuals may reduce the transmission of small-particle aerosols. Ultraviolet radiation has been reported to reduce the incidence of influenza infections in the hospital setting (65); however, carefully controlled studies of U–V radiation for disinfection in the general hospital setting have not been conducted.

REFERENCES

1. Welliver RC, McLaughlin S: Unique epidemiology of nosocomial infection in a children's hospital. *Am J Dis Child* 138:131–135, 1984.
2. Wenzel RP, Deal EC, Hendley JO: Hospital-acquired illness on a pediatric ward. *Pediatrics* 60:367–371, 1977.
3. MacDonald NE, Hall CB, Suffin SC, Alexson C, Harris PJ, Manning JA: Respiratory syncytial viral infection in infants with congenital heart disease. *New Engl J Med* 307:397–400, 1982.
4. Hall CB, Kopelman AE, Douglas RG Jr., Geiman JM, Meagher MP: Neonatal respiratory syncytial virus infection. *New Engl J Med* 300:393–396, 1979.
5. Hall CB, Powell KR, MacDonald NE, Gala CL, Menegus ME, Suffin SC, Cohen HJ: Respiratory syncytial viral infection in children with compromised immune function. *New Engl J Med* 315:77–81, 1986.
6. Roy TE, McDonald S, Patrick ML, Keddy JA: A survey of hospital infection in a pediatric hospital. II. The distribution of hospital infections in different areas of the hospital, postoperative wound infections, and the consequences of infection. *Can Med Assoc J* 87:592–599, 1962.
7. Valenti WM, Hall CB, Douglas RG Jr., Menegus MA, Pincus PH: Nosocomial viral infections: I. Epidemiology and significance. *Infect Control* 1:33–37, 1980.
8. Ditchburn RK, McQuillin J, Gardner PS, Court SDM: Respiratory syncytial virus in hospital cross-infection. *Br Med J* 3:671–673, 1971.
9. Gardner PS, Court SDM, Brocklebank JT, Downham MAPS, Weightman D: Virus cross-infection in paediatric wards. *Br Med J* 2:571–575, 1973.
10. Brocklebank JT, Court SDM, McQuillin J, Gardner PS: Influenza A infection in children. *Lancet* 2:497–500, 1972.
11. Hall CB, Douglas RG Jr., Geiman JM, Messner MK: Nosocomial respiratory syncytial virus infections. *New Engl J Med* 293:1343–1346, 1975.
12. Hall CB, Douglas RG Jr.: Nosocomial influenza infection as a cause of intercurrent fevers in infants. *Pediatrics* 55:673–677, 1975.
13. Henderson FW, Collier AM, Clyde WA Jr., Denny FW: Respiratory syncytial virus infections, reinfections and immunity: A prospective, longitudinal study in young children. *New Engl J Med* 300:530–534, 1979.
14. Glezen WP, Frank AL, Taber LH, Kasel JA: Parainfluenza virus type 3: Seasonality and risk of infection and reinfection in young children. *J Infect Dis* 150:851–857, 1984.
15. Hendley JO, Edmondson WP Jr., Gwaltney JM Jr.: Relation between naturally acquired immunity and infectivity of two rhinoviruses in volunteers. *J Infect Dis* 125:243–248, 1972.
16. Top FH Jr., Buescher EL, Bancroft WH, Russell PK: Immunization with live types 7 and 4 adenovirus vaccines. II. Antibody response and protective effect against acute respiratory disease due to adenovirus type 7. *J Infect Dis* 124:155–160, 1971.
17. Webster RG, Laver WG: Antigenic variation of influenza viruses. In Kilbourne ED (ed): *The Influenza Viruses and Influenza.* New York, Academic Press, 1975, p. 270.

18. Reed SE: The behaviour of recent isolates of human respiratory coronavirus in vitro and in volunteers: Evidence of heterogeneity among 229E-related strains. *J Med Virol* 13:179–192, 1984.

19. Meissner HC, Murray SA, Kiernan MA, Snyderman DR, McIntosh K: A simultaneous outbreak of respiratory syncytial virus and parainfluenza virus type 3 in a newborn nursery. *J Pediatr* 104:680–684, 1984.

20. Valenti WM, Clarke TA, Hall CB, Menegus MA, Shapiro DL: Concurrent outbreaks of rhinovirus and respiratory syncytial virus in an intensive care nursery: Epidemiology and associated risk factors. *J Pediatr* 100:722–726, 1982.

21. McIntosh K, Ellis EF, Hoffman LS, Lybass TG, Eller JJ, Fulginiti VA: The association of viral and bacterial respiratory infections with exacerbations of wheezing in young asthmatic children. *J Pediatr* 82:578–590, 1973.

22. Minor TE, Dick EC, DeMeo AN, Ouellette JJ, Cohen M, Reed CE: Viruses as precipitants of asthmatic attacks in children. *J Am Med Assoc* 227:292–298, 1974.

23. Frost WH, Gover M: The incidence and time distribution of common colds in several groups kept under continuous observation. In Maxcy KF (ed): *Papers of Wade Hampton Frost*. New York, The Commonwealth Fund, 1941, p 359.

24. Monto AS, Cavallaro JJ: The Tecumseh study of respiratory illness. II. Patterns of occurrence of infection with respiratory pathogens, 1965–1969. *Am J Epidemiol* 94:280–289, 1971.

25. Herrmann EC Jr.: Experience in providing a viral diagnostic laboratory compatible with medical practice. *Mayo Clin Proc* 42:112–123, 1967.

26. Menegus MA, Douglas RG Jr.: Viruses, rickettsiae, chlamydiae, and mycoplasmas. In Mandell GL, Douglas RG Jr., Bennett JE (eds): *Principles and Practice of Infectious Diseases*, ed 2. New York, John Wiley & Sons, 1985, p 138.

27. Fulton RE, Middleton PJ: Comparison of immunofluorescence and isolation techniques in the diagnosis of respiratory viral infections of children. *Infect Immun* 10:92–101, 1974.

28. Sarkkinen HK, Halonen PE, Arstila PP, Salmi AA: Detection of respiratory syncytial, parainfluenza type 2, and adenovirus antigens by radioimmunoassay and enzyme immuno-assay on nasopharyngeal secretions from children with acute respiratory disease. *J Clin Microbiol* 13:258–265, 1981.

29. Hall CB, Douglas RG Jr., Geiman JM: Respiratory syncytial virus infections in infants: Quantitation and duration of shedding. *J Pediatr* 89:11–15, 1976.

30. Winther B, Gwaltney JM Jr., Mygind N, Turner RB, Hendley JO: Sites of rhinovirus recovery after point inoculation of the upper airway. *JAMA* 256:1763–1767, 1986.

31. Gwaltney JM Jr., Hendley JO, Simon G, Jordan WS Jr.: Rhinovirus infections in an industrial population. I. The occurrence of illness. *New Engl J Med* 275:1261–1268, 1966.

32. Cate TR, Couch RB, Johnson KM: Studies with rhinoviruses in volunteers: Production of illness, effect of naturally acquired antibody, and demonstration of a protective effect not associated with serum antibody. *J Clin Invest* 43:56–67, 1964.

33. Hall CB, Douglas RG Jr.: Clinically useful method for the isolation of respiratory syncytial virus. *J Infect Dis* 131:1–5, 1975.

34. Brandt CD, Kim HW, Jeffries BC, Pyles G, Christmas EE, Reid JL, Chanock RM, Parrott RH: Infections in 18,000 infants and children in a controlled study of respiratory tract disease. II. Variation in adenovirus infections by year and season. *Am J Epidemiol* 95:218–227, 1972.

35. Fox JP, Hall CE, Cooney MK: The Seattle virus watch. VII. Observations of adenovirus infections. *Am J Epidemiol* 105:362–386, 1977.

36. Paisley JW, Lauer BA, McIntosh K, Glode MP, Schachter J, Rumack C: Pathogens associated with acute lower respiratory tract infection in young children. *Pediatr Infect Dis* 3:14–19, 1984.

37. Cheeseman SH, Pierik LT, Leombruno D, Spinos KE, McIntosh K: Evaluation of a commercially available direct immunofluorescent staining reagent for the detection of respiratory syncytial virus in respiratory secretions. *J Clin Microbiol* 24:155–156, 1986.

38. Lauer BA, Masters HA, Wren CG, Levin MJ: Rapid detection of respiratory syncytial virus in nasopharyngeal secretions by enzyme-linked immunosorbent assay. *J Clin Microbiol* 22:782–785, 1985.

39. Taber LH, Knight V, Gilbert BE, McClung HW, Wilson SZ, Norton HJ, Thurson JM, Gordon WH, Atmar RL, Schiaudt WR: Ribavirin aerosol treatment of bronchiolitis associated with respiratory syncytial virus infection in infants. *Pediatrics* 72:613–618, 1983.

40. Hall CB, McBride JT, Walsh EE, Bell DM, Gala CL, Hildreth S, Ten Eyck LG, Hall WJ: Aerosolized ribavirin treatment of infants with respiratory syncytial viral infection: A randomized double-blind study. *New Engl J Med* 308:1443–1447, 1983.

41. Demers RR, Parker J, Frankel LR, Smith DW: Administration of ribavirin to neonatal and pediatric patients during mechanical ventilation. *Respir Care* 31:1188–1195, 1986.

42. Knight V, Fedson D, Baldini J, Douglas RG, Couch RB: Amantadine therapy of epidemic influenza A2 (Hong Kong). *Infect Immunol* 1:200–204, 1970.

43. Younkin SW, Betts RF, Roth FK, Douglas RG Jr.: Reduction in fever and symptoms in young adults with influenza A/Brazil/78 H1N1 infection after treatment with aspirin or amantadine. *Antimicrob Agents Chemother* 23:577–582, 1983.

44. LaMontagne JR, Galasso GJ: Report of a workshop on clinical studies of the efficacy of amantadine and rimantadine against influenza virus. *J Infect Dis* 138:928–931, 1978.

45. Stanley ED, Muldoon RE, Akers LW, Jackson GG: Evaluation of antiviral drugs: The effect of amantadine on influenza in volunteers. *Ann NY Acad Sci* 130:44–51, 1965.

46. Togo Y, Hornick RB, Dawkins AT Jr.: Studies on induced influenza in man. 1. Double-blind studies designed to assess prophylactic efficacy of amantadine hydrochloride against A2/Rockville/1/65 strain. *JAMA* 203:1089–1094, 1968.

47. ACIP: Prevention and control of influenza. *MMWR* 35:317–326, 331, 1986.

48. Glezen WP: The pediatrician's role in influenza control. *Pediatr Infect Dis* 5:615–618, 1986.

49. Clover RD, Crawford SA, Abell TD, Ramsey CN, Glezen WP, Couch RB: Effectiveness of rimantadine prophylaxis of children within families. *Am J Dis Child* 140:706–709, 1986.

50. Hayden FG, Albrecht JK, Kaiser DL, Gwaltney JM Jr.: Prevention of natural colds by contact prophylaxis with intranasal alpha2-interferon. *New Engl J Med* 314:71–75, 1986.

51. Monto AS, Shope TC, Schwartz SA, Albrecht JA: Intranasal interferon-alpha 2b for seasonal prophylaxis of respiratory infection. *J Infect Dis* 154:128–133, 1986.

52. Turner RB, Felton A, Kosak K, Kelsey DK, Meschievitz CK: Prevention of coronavirus colds with intranasal alpha-2b interferon. *J Infect Dis* 154:443–447, 1986.

53. Valenti WM, Betts RF, Hall CB, Hruska JF, Douglas RG Jr.: Nosocomial viral infections: II. Guidelines for prevention and control of respiratory viruses, herpes viruses, and hepatitis viruses. *Infect Control* 1:165–178, 1980.

54. Buckland FE, Tyrrell DAJ: Experiments on the spread of colds. I. Laboratory studies on the dispersal of nasal secretion. *J Hyg Camb* 62:365–377, 1964.

55. Gerone PJ, Couch RB, Keefer GV, Douglas RG, Derrenbacher EB, Knight V: Assessment of experimental and natural viral aerosols. *Bacteriol Rev* 30:576–584, 1966.

56. Hall CB, Douglas RG Jr.: Modes of transmission of respiratory syncytial virus. *J Pediatr* 99:100–103, 1981.

57. Moser MR, Bender TR, Margolis HS, Noble GR, Kendal AP, Ritter DG: An outbreak of influenza aboard a commercial airliner. *Am J Epidemiol* 110:1–6, 1979.

58. Gwaltney JM Jr., Moskalski PB, Hendley JO; Hand-to-hand transmission of rhinovirus colds. *Ann Intern Med* 88:463–467, 1978.

59. Turner RB, Meschievitz CK, Streisand AC, Kelsey DK: Mechanism of transmission of coronavirus 229E in human volunteers. *Clin Res* 35:145A, 1987.

60. Hall CB, Douglas RG Jr.: Nosocomial respiratory syncytial viral infections: Should gowns and masks be used? *Am J Dis Child* 135:512–515, 1981.

61. Hall CB, Geiman JM, Douglas RG Jr., Meagher MP: Control of nosocomial respiratory syncytial viral infections. *Pediatrics* 62:728–732, 1978.
62. Murphy D, Todd JK, Chao RK, Orr I, McIntosh K: The use of gowns and masks to control respiratory illness in pediatric hospital personnel. *J Pediatr* 99:746–750, 1981.
63. Gala CL, Hall CB, Schnabel KC, Pincus PH, Blossom P, Hildreth SW, Betts RF, Douglas RG Jr.: The use of eye-nose goggles to control nosocomial respiratory syncytial virus infection. *JAMA* 256:2706–2708, 1986.
64. Leclair JM, Freeman J, Sullivan BF, Crowley CM, Goldmann DA: Prevention of nosocomial respiratory syncytial virus infections through compliance with glove and gown isolation precautions. *New Engl J Med* 317:329–334, 1987.
65. McLean RL: General discussion of the mechanism of spread of Asian influenza. *Am Rev Respir Dis* 83 (part 2):36–38, 1960.

7

Dermatitis

George B. Fisher, Jr., M.D.

A large number of organisms can produce nosocomial skin disease. Three of these—*Staphylococcus aureus*, *Streptococcus pyogenes*, and *Sarcoptes scabiei*—are important causes of hospital epidemics and outbreaks. These organisms will be discussed here.

STAPHYLOCOCCUS AUREUS

Background

Staphylococcus aureus is a Gram-positive coccus which forms clusters of organisms as it multiplies. It is a formidable pathogen with a variety of attributes which make prevention, control, and eradication a difficult task. *S. aureus* has the ability to survive desiccation and is relatively heat-resistant (1). During the antibiotic era, it has developed resistance to penicillin and, more recently, many strains have acquired resistance to the penicillinase-resistant antibiotics. Clinically, *S. aureus* enjoys a privileged position, with approximately 11–33% of normal individuals harboring the organism in the nares in a carrier state (2,3), from whence the bacteria have easy access to cutaneous surfaces. Once it becomes a pathogen, *S. aureus* produces a wide spectrum of cutaneous and systemic syndromes, mediated through both direct invasion as well as through the release of several toxins (4).

Infections with *S. aureus* produce significant morbidity and mortality. A survey found the incidence of hospital-acquired infections caused by *S. aureus* to be exceeded only by the number produced by *Escherichia coli*, and *S. aureus* was cultured from ⅓ of all cutaneous nosocomial infections (5). Hospital epidemics are often the result of *S. aureus*, with methicillin-resistant *S. aureus* (MRSA) assuming more importance in recent years (3).

The early diagnosis and treatment of cutaneous staphylococcal infections, therefore, becomes paramount in preventing more serious complications for the affected patient and possible spread to other susceptible individuals.

Cutaneous infections with *S. aureus* can be manifest in a variety of appearances. Most patients acquire the organism from another person through direct contact or transmit it to the skin from their own nasal reservoir (4,6). Clinically apparent infection results when the organism penetrates through minor breaks in the skin. A brief review of several types of cutaneous staphylococcal processes follows.

Folliculitis

Infection of the hair follicle produces a pustule with an erythematous base surrounding the involved hair. This is frequently superficial and asymptomatic but may progress to a deeper process.

Furuncles and Carbuncles

These abscesses are deeper, painful staphylococcal infections. They commonly originate in follicles and spread into the surrounding tissue, creating indurated, tender, erythematous nodules which often progress to fluctuance and suppuration.

Carbuncles are larger lesions which spread through the dermis and subcutaneous fat to produce several interconnected sites of drainage. Characteristic locations are the posterior neck, the back, and thighs, whereas furuncles commonly involve the face, neck, buttock, extremities, and axillae.

Bullous Impetigo

Impetigo caused by *S. aureus* is usually due to phage group II, Type 71, which produces an exfoliative exotoxin (exfoliatin), causing a localized flaccid blister (7). The bullae are larger than the small vesicles seen with streptococcal impetigo and contain a yellowish fluid (Fig. 7.1). The bullae are easily ruptured, and *S. aureus* can be cultured from intact blisters.

Omphalitis

The umbilical stump is one of the first sites of colonization by *S. aureus* in neonates (8). Frank infection can develop, evidenced by purulent drainage from the umbilicus with surrounding erythema and induration.

Cellulitis

Staphylococcus aureus is a common cause of cellulitis in pediatric patients. Spreading areas of erythema, edema, tenderness, and warmth are seen, usually with an indistinct border. Blistering, lymphangitis, and regional adenopathy may also be found.

Staphylococcal Scalded Skin Syndrome (SSSS)

Staphylococcal scalded skin syndrome is caused by an exfoliative exotoxin (exfoliatin) produced by a localized staphylococcal infection, frequently in the conjunctiva or upper respiratory tract. Children under 5 years of age are generally affected. Onset is rapid with fever and the de-velopment of widespread painful erythema progressing to edema and blisters. These flaccid bullae are easily ruptured, and the skin is readily denuded by gentle shearing pressure (Fig. 7.2). Mucous membranes are spared.

The intact bullae are sterile, but staphylococci can be isolated from the localized source of infection. As in bullous impetigo, phage group II staphylococci are usually found.

Population

Humans are the major reservoir of staphylococci and similarly are primarily involved in the transmission of staphylococci to susceptible individuals (1). Therefore, identification of an at-risk population requires knowledge of which patients are prone to acquire staphylococcal infections and persons who are likely to carry the organism.

Carrier States

At any time, a significant percentage of persons carries *S. aureus* in an asymptomatic form. This is usually confined to the anterior nares, although the throat, perineum, and skin folds may be involved in a lesser number. Positive nasal cultures of normal individuals have ranged from 11–33% (2,3). Hospital personnel, including

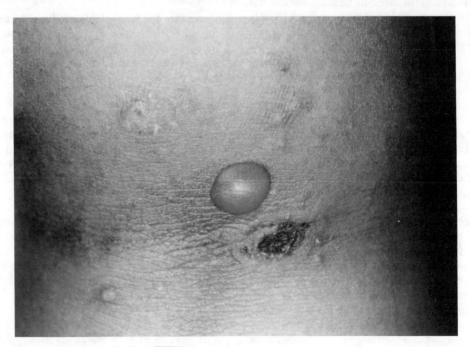

Figure 7.1. Staphylococcal bullous impetigo.

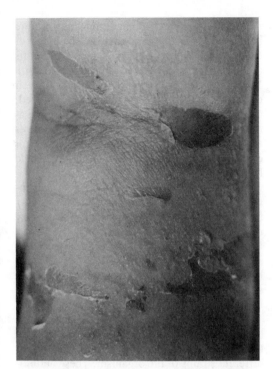

Figure 7.2 Erythema and early desquamation of staphylococcal scalded skin syndrome.

doctors and nurses, generally have higher rates of carriage (9). Carrier states are more commonly found among individuals whose medical condition or lifestyle necessitates the use of needles. These include parenteral drug abusers (2), hemodialysis patients (10), insulin-dependent diabetics (11), and otherwise healthy patients receiving allergy injections (12). The mechanism of this increased rate of carriage is unclear. Small breaks in the skin may lead to transient cutaneous colonization with subsequent spread to the nares where the staphylococci tend to persist. The reverse pathway is known to be important, as the more serious staphylococcal infections seen with drug abusers and dialysis patients are caused by organisms of the same phage type and antibiotic sensitivity as the staphylococci residing in the nares of the respective patient.

Carriage of *S. aureus* on the skin of normal individuals is much less common than nasal carriage. Although evidence of colonization may be obtained more frequently from intertriginous areas, the percentage of positive staphylococcal cultures from nonintertriginous sites is usually less than 5% (12,13). It has been repeatedly demonstrated that patients with atopic dermatitis are extremely predisposed to staphylococcal skin colonization, involving both lesional and apparently normal skin. Greater than 90% of cultures taken from lesional skin have been positive, while approximately 75% from clinically normal skin have grown *S. aureus* (13–15). Rates of positive nasal cultures from the same patients were also markedly elevated (14,15).

The skin of psoriatic patients has also been evaluated (16). While lesions produced a higher incidence of positive staphylococcal cultures, nonlesional skin and nasal cultures were comparable to normal individuals.

Several inferences can be made from the aforementioned data. Although the risks posed by nasal carriage in drug abusers and dialysis patients seem greatest to themselves, the increased possibility of transmission of *S. aureus* to personnel and other patients must be noted. Similarly, insulin-dependent diabetics and patients receiving allergy injections are common in the pediatric population, and their increased carriage rate may pose a significant problem. Atopic dermatitis patients almost universally harbor *S. aureus*. When hospitalized, their care usually includes the application of topical preparations, exposing hospital staff and providing an opportunity for indirect transmittal to other patients. Psoriatic patients, while less often colonized with *S. aureus*, produce considerable desquamating scale, which may spread staphylococci.

Increased Susceptibility

All patients are susceptible to staphylococcal infections. Certain subgroups have increased difficulty controlling and eradicating this organism. Previous mention has been made of patients with atopic dermatitis as well as the increased carriage rate of persons using needles. Immunocompromised patients are generally predisposed to infections, including *S. aureus*.

Less common conditions with special susceptibility to staphylococcal infections should also be included. Patients with chronic granulomatous disease are unable to kill staphylococci within phagocytic vacuoles and experience chronic and recurrent staphylococcal infections. The hyperimmunoglobulin E syndrome has recurrent, frequent staphylococcal infections as one of its characteristics. Similarly, patients with

Wiskott-Aldrich syndrome, Chédiak-Higashi syndrome, and Down's syndrome may have an increased incidence of staphylococcal infections.

Neonates deserve special mention in regard to staphylococcal infections, since many hospital epidemics in the past have occurred in newborn nurseries. The immaturity of their immune system, combined with exposure to hospital personnel involved in the care of numerous other neonates and an open wound (umbilical stump), make these infants especially susceptible to staphylococcal colonization and subsequent infection. The umbilicus or groin is usually the first area colonized with later spread to the nares (8). The staphylococcal strain is contracted from both hospital personnel (17) and mothers (18). The incidence of clinical infections depends upon the virulence of the strain involved, but a variety of presentations, including omphalitis, folliculitis, furuncles, mastitis, paronychia, conjunctivitis, bullous impetigo, staphylococcal scalded skin syndrome, and toxic-shock syndrome have been observed (19). Even the milder cutaneous infections can rapidly progress to more serious, life-threatening conditions in this age group. The unique proximity of neonates to other newborns in most nurseries, along with the necessity for nursing and medical staffs to closely handle many infants, can lead to staphylococcal epidemics if appropriate preventive measures are not followed.

Diagnosis

It is axiomatic that the hallmark in the control of nosocomial staphylococcal infection is early diagnosis and treatment with simultaneous institution of measures to prevent the spread of the organism. As noted above, all patients can be affected by staphylococci. Pustules, blisters, abscesses, cellulitis, and clinically infected wounds (surgical or traumatic) should prompt cultures of appropriate tissue and Gram strains. In certain situations, such as fever, hypotension, cellulitis or signs of other more serious sites of infection, blood and cerebrospinal fluid cultures may be warranted. *Staphylococcus aureus* is typically not found on the skin in staphylococcal scalded skin syndrome and toxic-shock syndrome since these conditions are related to staphylococcal toxins. A search for a localized focus of infection should follow, however.

Specific patients and conditions may require heightened suspicions of possible staphylococcal disease. Individuals with atopic dermatitis are commonly colonized and infected with *S. aureus*, which may precipitate flares of their dermatitis. When such patients are hospitalized, cultures may be necessary along with segregation from other susceptible patients. Neonates are another group in which the threshold for evaluating and culturing cutaneous lesions should be low.

As discussed previously, staphylococcal infections may progress rapidly in some newborns; plus, an involved infant may initiate many new cases in a nursery.

If there have been a cluster of staphylococcal infections, the threshold for cultures should again be lowered in an attempt to diagnose new cases and to control spread to other patients. This will be discussed further under *Prevention*.

When cultures are positive for *S. aureus*, antibiotic sensitivities are important not only in the choice of antibiotics but also as markers for different strains of the organism. These antibiograms, with or without phage typing of the isolated bacteria, are extremely useful in the epidemiologic tracing and unraveling of hospital outbreaks.

Treatment

Essentially, all hospital-acquired cutaneous *S. aureus* infections will require antibiotics. Although it may be possible to control superficial staphylococcal lesions in the outpatient with good hygiene and topical antibiotics, the risk of transmitting the process to many other susceptible individuals dictates that systemic antibiotic therapy be employed for inpatients. The presence of an abscess necessitates concomitant drainage.

Even in the community setting, almost all strains of *S. aureus* are now resistant to penicillin (20). Recently, the emergence of *S. aureus* resistant to penicillinase-resistant antibiotics has altered the treatment of hospital-acquired infections. The choice of drugs is eventually determined by antibiotic sensitivities, but the initial therapy must depend on the type of infection, the individual host, and the past experience of the hospital in regard to *S. aureus*, specifically methicillin-resistant *S. aureus* (MRSA).

Oral versus parenteral antibiotics is usually dictated by the severity of the infection. If MRSA has not been or is not a current problem, then the institution of a penicillinase-resistant penicillin, first generation cephalosporin, erythromycin, trimethoprim/sulfamethoxazole, or clindamycin is a reasonable initial therapy. It is important to remember that a small percentage of patients who are allergic to penicillin will have a cross-reacting allergic reaction with the cephalosporins, and that a significant percentage of S. aureus strains are resistant to erythromycin and clindamycin, even if sensitive to methicillin.

In hospitals where MRSA has become a factor, vancomycin is the drug of choice for serious infections (21). Trimethoprim/sulfamethoxazole also appears to retain its effectiveness in the treatment of MRSA. Rifampin has been useful against MRSA but must be administered in conjunction with a second antibiotic, since resistance develops rapidly when used as a single agent (20).

Therapy of asymptomatic nasal carriers is not routinely undertaken, but selected patients and hospital staff who are shown to be transmitters of S. aureus infection may be likely candidates. In the past, recurrent courses of oral and topical antibiotics have been unsuccessful at more than transiently decreasing the bacterial count. After such a reduction, however, bacterial interference has been successfully employed with the introduction of nonpathogenic strain 502A of S. aureus (22). It must be noted, though, that the 502A strain has occasionally produced serious and fatal infections (23), and this approach is now used less frequently.

Rifampin is secreted into the nares in high concentrations and is quite effective against S. aureus (24). Again, a concomitant antibiotic must be employed to avoid the development of resistance. A 10-day course of 600 mg of rifampin per day and 500 mg of cloxacillin every 6 hours eradicated nasal carriage in 80% of those treated (25).

A new topical antibiotic under investigation in the United States is mupirocin. When used intranasally, this drug has shown excellent results as a single agent in eradicating S. aureus carriage (3,26).

Prevention

Recommendations intended to prevent nosocomial staphylococcal disease are based upon the known pathways this organism travels between patients. The three major sources of cutaneous infection are:

1. From the patient's own nasal carriage to his skin;
2. From a hospital staff member's nasal carriage to his hands and then to the patient's skin; and
3. From an infected lesion of one patient to the hands of a staff member and then to the skin of a second patient (4,6).

Fomites appear to transmit S. aureus relatively infrequently (27), although they may be important in selected instances (28).

Along with antimicrobials, handwashing and isolation are keys to the control and prevention of staphylococcal infections. Effective handwashing between patients is essential. Cleansing with soap and water appears to be acceptable in most instances, but antiseptic agents may be indicated in high-risk procedures and in dealing with susceptible individuals (29). Appropriate isolation of infected patients is required. Contact isolation is indicated for those with major wound or skin infections, including the staphylococcal scalded skin syndrome. For lesser degrees of cutaneous involvement drainage/secretion precautions suffice (30) (Table 7.1). Restrictions should apply until the process has cleared.

Since hospital personnel are commonly involved in hospital-acquired staphylococcal infections, appropriate attention must be paid to this group as well as to patients. Staff with symptomatic lesions are likely to transmit the organism to patients and must, therefore, be treated and relieved from patient contact until the infection has cleared (31) (Table 7.2). Asymptomatic nasal carriage is not unusual in personnel, but routine cultures are not advised, and therapy is generally not indicated unless the individual has been linked epidemiologically to cases of staphylococcal infections.

When a cluster of hospital-acquired S. aureus infections develops, a coordinated systematic course must be adopted to limit its spread. The approach must be tailored to the outbreak based on the individual hospital and the extent of the problem, but the following measures are useful as guidelines. Education of involved personnel with an emphasis on good handwashing should be initiated. Simultaneously, a search for an

Table 7.1
Isolation Precautions for Cutaneous Infections (30)

Disease	Category	Private Room	Masks	Gowns	Gloves	Duration	Comments
Staphylococcus aureus							
Major	Contact Isolation	Yes	No	If soiling likely	For touching infective material	Duration of illness	Major: draining and pus not covered or contained by dressing
Minor	Drainage/ Secretion Precautions	No	No	If soiling likely	For touching infective material	Duration of illness	Minor: dressing covers and contains the pus or infected area is very small
Scalded Skin Syndrome	Contact Isolation	Yes	No	If soiling likely	For touching infective material	Duration of illness	
Streptococcus pyogenes skin infection							
Major	Contact Isolation	Yes	No	If soiling likely	For touching infective material	For 24 hours after start of effective treatment	Major: draining and pus not covered or contained by dressing
Minor	Drainage/ Secretion Precautions	No	No	If soiling likely	For touching infective material	For 24 hours after start of effective treatment	Minor: dressing covers and contains the pus or infected area is very small
Scabies	Contact Isolation	Yes, if patient hygiene is poor	No	For close contact	For close contact	For 24 hours after start of effective therapy	

active staphylococcal lesion in these staff members should be undertaken with appropriate treatment and restrictions instituted as necessary. Affected patients must be isolated according to their disease (Table 7.1). It may be advisable to restrict the movement of fomites, e.g., blood pressure cuffs, tourniquets, etc., from this room.

If the source of the staphylococcal infections still remains unclear, surveillance cultures of personnel and other patients are warranted. Any possible infected site should be cultured along with the nares, and possibly, the perineum of personnel who may be linked with the outbreak.

Determination of phage types and antibiotic sensitivities is critical in distinguishing between nasal carriage of a particular pathogenic strain and one unrelated to the hospital outbreak. Treatment aimed at eradicating the carrier state is indicated in personnel harboring a pathogen implicated in a hospital epidemic.

Cohort nursing may be implemented for infected patients and those colonized, but not infected, with the same strain. Although therapy is not usually advised for asymptomatic colonized patients, quarantining them with infected patients is worthwhile. The nurses who care for such patients should not be in contact with other

Table 7.2
Work Restrictions for Infected Hospital Personnel (31)

Disease	Relieved from patient contact	Duration
Staphylococcus aureus (cutaneous lesions)	Yes	Until lesions resolved
Streptococcus pyogenes	Yes	Until 24 hours after treatment started
Scabies	Yes	Until adequately treated

noncolonized patients. The closure of or restriction of access to wards may be necessary to eradicate persistent outbreaks. Such measures prohibit admission of patients to a ward unless they are already colonized or infected with the epidemic strain. Conversely, no patient is transferred from the ward except via discharge, and only when all patients are discharged and the ward is cleaned are new admissions permitted and the ward reopened.

Newborn nurseries are the most susceptible pediatric areas to epidemics of staphylococcal infection. Although the aformentioned guidelines apply to nurseries as well, a few additional comments should be made. To help combat the increased risk in nurseries, the routine use of antimicrobial soaps for handwashing has been advised (29), along with attempts to reduce the incidence of colonization of the umbilicus. Triple dye, bacitracin (32), and chlorhexidine (33) have been used to decrease colonization and subsequent infection in this area. When staphylococcal outbreaks do arise in the nursery, it may become necessary to resume limited hexachlorophene baths. Daily bathing of the diaper area and umbilical stump has been beneficial in eradicating outbreaks (34), although routine use of hexachlorophene has been discontinued in neonates due to its potential neurotoxicity. Because of the rapid turnover of patients in nurseries, surveillance cultures must include recently discharged neonates who may not manifest any disease process until well after arrival at home. Cultures must also be taken from the umbilicus rather than from just the nares or perineum, since the umbilicus is generally the initial site of neonatal colonization (8).

STREPTOCOCCUS PYOGENES

Although *Streptococcus pyogenes* has been supplanted by *Streptococcus agalactiae* (group B streptococcus) as the usual pathogen producing serious neonatal infections, it remains a commonly detected organism with potentially severe sequelae. It is involved in a variety of infectious processes and still can create hospital epidemics, especially in newborn nurseries.

Background

Streptococcus pyogenes, commonly known as group A streptococcus, is a Gram-positive facultatively anaerobic coccus which forms chains. Almost all strains produce beta hemolysis. Various constituents of group A streptococci are useful in the epidemiologic classification of strains. M protein is an important component of the cell wall. This protein provides virulence to the streptococcus, and the variable types of M protein are used to categorize group A streptococci. Some streptococcal strains lack M proteins, or their M proteins have not been adequately described. These organisms, therefore, have nontypable M proteins. Other cell wall constituents, T protein and serum opacity factor, are also employed in the classification of group A streptococcal strains (35,36).

Although a few strains of *S. pyogenes* are capable of producing both pharyngitis and pyoderma, the majority of types preferentially affect only one site. However, the cutaneous strains frequently may colonize the pharynx without producing symptomatic disease (37).

The acquisition of cutaneous streptococcal pyoderma in outpatients has been well-studied. Colonization of the normal skin by streptococci occurs approximately 10 days prior to the onset of infection (38). Invasion presumably occurs through sites of minor skin trauma. The incidence of infection is enhanced by crowding, lower socioeconomic living conditions (39,40), poor hygiene, and warmer, humid climates (41). Hospital-acquired cutaneous streptococcal infections are more likely to be transmitted directly from contaminated hands (6,42), although at times, other pathways may be important.

A variety of clinical syndromes can be seen with group A streptococci, ranging from an indolent omphalitis in neonates (19) to life-threatening necrotizing fasciitis (43). Streptococcal pyoderma or impetigo presents with the appearance of small vesicopustules which rapidly rupture, creating a thick honey-colored crust with a "stuck-on" (Fig. 7.3) appearance. Regional adenopathy is characteristically found.

Surgical patients and newborns appear to be most frequently affected by nosocomial streptococci. Infected wounds may become erythematous and tender with increased drainage, and patients may have associated fever.

The umbilical stump is typically the first site to be colonized in neonates (44), and an indolent omphalitis characterized by a moist stump with drainage and surrounding erythema is often the initial sign of infection (19,34,44–47). This can progress to impetiginization of periumbilical skin or even to a more serious systemic illness, but it typically remains localized.

Other types of nosocomial group A streptococcal infections that may be encountered include lymphangitis, paronychia, erysipelas, and cellulitis, as well as meningitis, sepsis, peritonitis, and pneumonia. Poststreptococcal glomerulonephritis has followed cutaneous infections, but acute rheumatic fever is not seen.

Population

In the pediatric population, neonates are the most susceptible to the acquisition of group A streptococci. Nursery epidemics have become less common, but still occur (44–48). Although the organism can be carried in the vagina and rectum, as well as the nose and pharynx, transmission from hospital personnel appears to be more frequent than acquisition from the birth canal at the time of delivery (44,48).

Patients with cutaneous wounds, especially surgical, are also at increased risk for the development of secondary streptococcal infections. Epidemics of wound infections caused by *S. pyogenes* have been linked to anal and vaginal carriage by health care workers (49,50).

Diagnosis

When hospitalized patients develop cutaneous lesions suggestive of group A streptococcal infection, investigation with appropriate cultures and Gram stains should be initiated. Depending upon the circumstances of the infection and the involved host, blood, cerebrospinal fluid, and other cultures may be indicated.

In the setting of an epidemic, typing of cultured streptococci may be necessary to trace the progression of the outbreak. Many strains involving the skin have nontypable M proteins, and classifying T proteins and serum opacity factor is useful (35).

Although of no benefit in the early detection of cutaneous streptococcal infections, the measurement of antibody titers to extracellular prod-

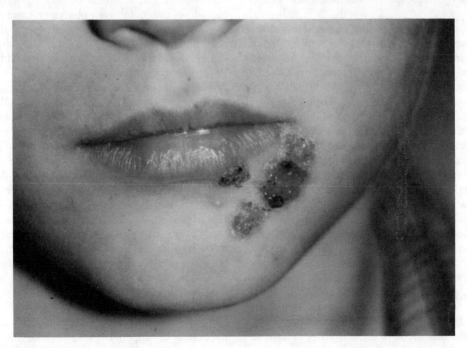

Figure 7.3. Streptococcal impetigo.

ucts of group A streptococci may reveal evidence of recent infection. These data may be important in epidemiologic investigations. The most important antibody responses seen with cutaneous involvement are anti-DNase B and antihyaluronidase, whereas the antistreptolysin O (ASO) response is muted and is a less sensitive marker (51).

Treatment

Many cases of streptococcal impetigo appear to be self-limited, and most do not progress to more serious infections. Antibiotics have not been demonstrated to prevent acute glomerulonephritis. However, in both the hospital and outpatient setting, systemic antibiotics are indicated in the treatment of cutaneous streptococcal infections.

Eradication of the streptococci serves to reduce spread to other susceptible individuals and to prevent extension of the infection to a serious systemic illness. The two classes of inpatients typically affected by group A streptococci are predisposed to both of these events. Neonates are at an increased risk to develop complications, such as meningitis or sepsis, and their close proximity to many other similarly susceptible patients accentuates the risk of transmission. Surgical patients likewise have an increased potential for complications and may also be a source of infection for other postoperative patients on a surgical ward.

Group A streptococci have retained their sensitivity to penicillin, and treatment is usually oral or parenteral penicillin, depending upon the type of infection and the host. Erythromycin, cephalosporins, and clindamycin are also effective agents.

In the past, topical antibiotics have been comparatively less effective than systemic antibiotics in the treatment of streptococcal pyoderma. Moreover, the addition of topical antibiotics to oral antibiotics has not improved results when compared with oral antibiotics alone (36). As mentioned earlier, a new topical antibiotic, mupirocin, has been quite effective in eliminating both streptococci and staphylococci from impetigo lesions (52). Whether this antibiotic will serve a primary or adjunctive treatment role in the future will depend upon further studies.

Prevention

The approach to preventing the development of cutaneous nosocomial streptococcal infections as well as isolating and controlling the spread of established cases is similar to that employed for staphylococcal pyoderma. Good handwashing practices by personnel are essential if new cases are to be eliminated. Antiseptic cleansing agents are indicated when dealing with high-risk procedures or susceptible groups of patients, such as neonates (29).

Isolation of infected individuals is required. Major cutaneous involvement necessitates contact isolation, whereas minor disease can be handled with drainage/secretion precautions. Precautions need to be maintained until 24 hours after the institution of treatment (30) (Table 7.1).

If an epidemic or cluster of cases of streptococcus arises, a regimen aimed at identifying and eliminating sources and pathways of infection must be instituted. Education of personnel with emphasis on appropriate handwashing between patients is necessary. A search for staff or patients with active infection should be undertaken. Any personnel with pharyngitis or pyoderma should be cultured, treated, and relieved from patient care (31) (Table 7.2). Asymptomatic personnel epidemiologically linked to an outbreak should have cultures taken from the pharynx, rectum, and vagina—areas of frequent carriage (31). The streptococcal carrier state usually responds to a single course of antibiotics and is more easily eradicated than staphylococcal nasal carriage.

Surveillance cultures are worthwhile to define the extent of the epidemic and to evaluate the efficacy of control procedures. Those cultured should include at-risk patients and epidemiologically important personnel. When the outbreak is located in a nursery, umbilical cultures are the most productive, since this site appears to be the initial area of colonization (44). It is also important to assess and culture recently discharged infants, since clinical disease often does not appear until after discharge from the nursery (45).

Several approaches have been beneficial in controlling nursery epidemics. Cohort nursing of infants has reduced transmission to unaffected neonates (46–48). Routine prophylactic treatment of the umbilical stump with triple dye (46,48) and bacitracin ointment (44) has been felt to be effective adjunctive therapy to help prevent colonization of the umbilicus. Treatment of infected individuals, isolation or cohort nursing of these infants, a search for and treatment of symptomatic or asymptomatic carriers, and prophylactic cord care is usually an effective approach. However, in some epidemics, eradication of streptococcal infection has been achieved only by instituting prophylactic penicillin for all infants (34,44–46).

SCABIES

During the 1950s, scabies was an uncommon dermatosis, but over the past 2 decades it has again reached epidemic proportions. Although scabies has not been a common cause of nosocomial dermatitis, it remains a serious threat because of its frequently missed or delayed diagnosis, its infectivity, and its prolonged incubation period, which allows ample opportunity for spread of disease before symptoms arise.

Background

Scabies is produced by *Sarcoptes scabiei*, a mite with a rounded body measuring approximately 400 μm in length and 4 pairs of legs (53). The entire life cycle is spent on human skin. Female mites create burrows in the stratum corneum and deposit eggs there. These ova hatch, and the larvae mature on the skin surface, where they spread to other sites. An infested person harbors from 3–50 mites at one time (54).

Mites can survive for several days off the human host, especially if protected from dessication and temperature extremes (55). However, close personal contact is felt to be the predominant method of transmission with spread via fomites being uncommon. Because of the vast number of mites in Norwegian (crusted) scabies, however, fomites probably play a more important role in this variant.

Scabies is highly contagious. In one study, spread was detected in 38% of family contacts (56). Several hospital epidemics have been related to extremely infectious Norwegian scabies (57–59), with attack rates of exposed staff as high as 69%.

A delayed hypersensitivity response appears to be important in producing the symptoms and signs of scabies infestation. It is usually 4–6 weeks before lesions and pruritus appear, although with reinfestation in a previously sensitized person, this incubation period may be shortened to a few days (54). In epidemics in which the index case was one of crusted scabies, incubation periods were frequently shortened (57–60), possibly related to the large number of infecting mites (58).

The clinical picture of scabies is polymorphous, but symptoms are usually consistent, with pruritus, especially nocturnal, almost invariably being present. The hands, especially the fingerwebs (Fig. 7.4), along with the wrists, elbows, anterior axillary folds, buttock, abdomen, umbilicus, female breasts, and male genitalia are common sites of involvement. Lesions ranging from excoriations to vesicles and pustules, to eczematous scaly patches, to papules and nodules, as well as the characteristic burrows can be observed. The typical burrow is a short dirty line which may contain darker matter within. Burrows are most commonly found on fingerwebs, wrists, ankles, and the sides of hands and feet. The penis and scrotum are particularly prone to developing nodular lesions.

In infants and young children, the appearance may differ. Whereas scabies classically spares the head and neck, in this young age group, these areas may be involved along with the palms and soles. Vesicular lesions are more common than in older patients.

Norwegian, or crusted, scabies is a rare condition but is important epidemiologically because of its extreme infectivity. These patients often exhibit minimal pruritus, although they are infested with thousands of mites. They manifest a widespread crusted scaly dermatosis with accentuation on the hands, feet and dystrophic nails.

Population

All patients in all age groups are potentially susceptible to scabies. An increased incidence has been noted in adopted foreign-born children (53). Crusted scabies has a propensity to affect mentally retarded, institutionalized individuals, physically debilitated patients, and immunosuppressed persons (53).

Diagnosis

Because the clinical manifestations of scabies may be so protean, a high index of suspicion must be maintained for any patient with a pruritic dermatosis. Several historical clues may be useful in evaluating these individuals. Pruritus is almost always found except in the rare crusted form of scabies. Nocturnal accentuation of pruritus is characteristic. Most patients have an insidious onset of both pruritus and rash as their sensitivity to the mite develops. An abrupt, explosive appearance is unusual. Involvement of other family members or intimate contacts is common if the patient's case has been present

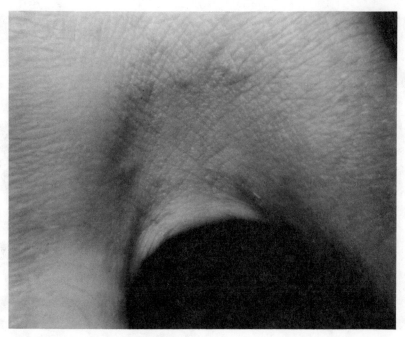

Figure 7.4.   Small fingerweb papules in scabies.

for any length of time. Finally, an eruption consistent with scabies should be seen (61).

Confirmative diagnosis is usually based upon microscopic examination of skin scrapings. A fresh, nonexcoriated burrow provides the best site for such scrapings, and various techniques aimed at enhancing localization of the burrows have been described (61). The obtained specimen is placed in mineral oil and examined for mites, eggs, and feces (Fig. 7.5).

Occasionally, scabies is diagnosed by skin biopsy. This is usually serendipitous, as biopsy is a very low-yield procedure for finding organisms.

Treatment

Lindane (gamme benzene hexachloride) in a 1% formulation is the most commonly used treatment for scabies. It is simple and effective, but concerns regarding its use have been raised (62). When used excessively and inappropriately, lindane may be neurotoxic, but problems following correct usage have been extremely rare (63). However, because of these potential side effects, revisions of treatment regimens have been made. Limiting the time of application to 8 hours, avoiding lindane in pregnant women, infants, young children, and severely excoriated indi-

viduals, and retreating only after a week are reasonable restrictions (63,64).

While the avoidance of potential therapeutic complications is a necessity, it is equally important to treat patients correctly to achieve a cure. Application to the entire body surface below the neck is essential, not just to affected areas. In small children, the head may be involved, and it must also be treated. Although transmission of scabies via formites is infrequent, laundering of the individual's clothing and linen is a worthwhile recommendation. Since the scabicidal agents have not been demonstrated to be ovicidal, a repeat application in 1 week appears warranted.

Crotamiton is another scabicide which is probably less toxic than lindane. Unfortunately, it is also less effective (65) and requires successive daily applications for 2–5 days (63).

Precipitated sulfur in a 5–10% concentration in petrolatum is another alternative to lindane. While this has been safely employed in infants and other patients for many years, it is messy, smelly, and cosmetically unappealing. This treatment is usually applied daily for 3 consecutive days.

Permethrin cream is another agent that has shown great promise in a recent study (66). This

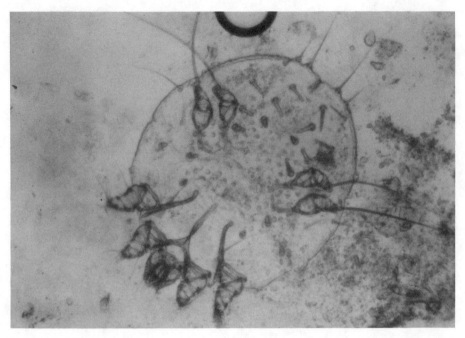

Figure 7.5.   Adult scabies mite.

new product has been demonstrated to be both effective and safe, but is not yet commercially available.

Modification of treatment is necessary for crusted scabies. Because of the thick scale and crust in these patients, adjunctive use of a keratolytic agent is necessary so that the scabicide can adequately reach the mites. Retreatment may be required several times and should be directed by frequent repeat scrapings looking for live mites. Careful cleansing of fomites is also needed, since the huge number of mites makes this method of transmission more significant.

Even with curative treatment with any of these agents, total relief of pruritus is not achieved for days to weeks. Explanation of this to patients may prevent overuse of these products.

Prevention

Numerous hospital epidemics of scabies have been documented (57–60,67–68). The infectivity and potentially long incubation period for asymptomatic contacts who may unwittingly transmit the disease to other patients and staff makes aggressive, coordinated treatment and isolation the key to controlling these outbreaks. Patients identified as having scabies should be placed on contact isolation precautions until 24 hours after institution of appropriate therapy (30) (Table 7.1). The recalcitrant nature of crusted scabies dictates that precautions be continued until a cure is apparent.

Although close personal contact is generally required to transmit scabies, staff involved in direct patient care have ample opportunity to contract this mite. It is quite possible that prior to the establishment of the correct diagnosis, these individuals applied a variety of topical treatments. Infested staff should be relieved from patient care until after effective treatment (31) (Table 7.2).

Treating asymptomatic contacts of infested patients may be necessary to arrest an outbreak (58,59,68). Asymptomatic family members of affected patients and staff shoud also be included in such a treatment program. Incubation periods can range from a few days to 6 weeks, and awaiting the appearance of symptoms provides too great an opportunity for further spread. Educational material and free scabicides have been provided as part of the control measures in an attempt to improve compliance (57–59). Ideally, it is best to treat everyone simultaneously to prevent reinfestation, the so-called ''ping-pong'' effect. This may be impossible when large numbers of people are involved, but adherence to this approach as closely as possible is preferred. If compliance or reinfestation is a problem, the routine use of gowns and gloves when administering care to all patients may be needed to prevent spread by asymptomatic carriers (59).

REFERENCES

1. Waldvogel FA: *Staphylococcus aureus* (including toxic shock syndrome). In Mandell GL, Douglas RG Jr, Bennett JE (eds): *Principles and Practice of Infectious Diseases*, ed 2. New York, John Wiley & Sons, 1985, p. 1097.
2. Tuazon CU, Sheagren JN: Increased rate of carriage of Staphylococcus aureus among narcotic addicts. *J Infect Dis* 129:725–727, 1974.
3. Casewell MW, Hill RLR: The carrier state: methicillin-resistant *Staphylococcus aureus. J Antimicrob Chemother* 18 (Suppl. A):1–12, 1986.
4. Sheagren JN: *Staphylococcus aureus*. The persistent pathogen (Part I). *N Engl J Med* 310:1368–1373, 1984.
5. National nosocomial infections study—United States, 1975–76. MMWR 26:377–378, 383, 1977.
6. Rammelkamp CH Jr, Mortimer EA Jr, Wolinsky E: Transmission of streptococcal and staphylococcal infections. *Ann Intern Med* 60:753–758, 1964.
7. Tunnessen WW: Practical aspects of bacterial skin infections in children. *Pediatr Dermatol* 2:255–265, 1985.
8. Hurst V: Transmission of hospital staphylococci among newborn infants. II. Colonization of the skin and mucous membranes of the infants. *Pediatrics* 25:204–214, 1960.
9. Waldvogel FA: *Staphylococcus aureus* (including toxic shock syndrome). In Mandell GL, Douglas RG Jr, Bennett JE (eds): *Principles and Practice of Infectious Diseases*, ed 2. New York, John Wiley & Sons, 1985, p. 1099.
10. Kirmani N, Tuazon CU, Murray HW, Parrish AE, Sheagren JN: *Staphylococcus aureus* carriage rate of patients receiving long-term hemodialysis. *Arch Intern Med* 138:1657–1659, 1978.
11. Tuazon CU, Perez A, Kishaba T, Sheagren JN: *Staphylococcus aureus* among insulin-injecting diabetic patients. An increased carrier rate. *JAMA* 231:1272, 1975.
12. Kirmani N, Tuazon CU, Alling D: Carriage rate of *Staphylococcus aureus* among patients receiving allergy injections. *Ann Allergy* 45:235–237, 1980.
13. Dahl MV: *Staphylococcus aureus* and atopic dermatitis. *Arch Dermatol* 119:840–846, 1983.
14. Aly R, Maibach HI, Shinefield HR: Microbial flora of atopic dermatitis. *Arch Dermatol* 113:780–782, 1977.
15. White MI, Noble WC: Consequences of colonization and infection by *Staphylococcus aureus* in atopic dermatitis. *Clin Exp Dermatol* 11:34–40, 1986.
16. Aly R, Maibach HI, Mandel A: Bacterial flora in psoriasis. *Br J Dermatol* 95:603–606, 1976.
17. Mortimer EA Jr, Lipsitz PJ, Wolinsky E, Gonzaga AJ, Rammelkamp CH Jr: Transmission of staphylococci between newborns. Importance of the hands of personnel. *Am J Dis Child* 104:289–295, 1962.
18. Wolinsky E, Gonzaga AJ, Mortimer EA Jr: The mother as a source of neonatal staphylococci. *N Engl J Med* 267:535–538, 1962.
19. Hebert AA, Esterly NB: Bacterial and candidal cutaneous infections in the neonate. *Dermatol Clin* 4:3–21, 1986.
20. Sheagren JN: *Staphylococcus aureus*. The persistent pathogen (Part II). *N Engl J Med* 310:1437–1442, 1984.
21. Watanakunakorn C: Treatment of infections due to methicillin-resistant *Staphylococcus aureus. Ann Intern Med* 97:376–378, 1982.
22. Steele RW: Recurrent staphylococcal infection in families. *Arch Dermatol* 116:189–190, 1980.

23. Houck PW, Nelson JD, Kay JL: Fatal septicemia due to *Staphylococcus aureus* 502A. *Am J Dis Child* 123:45–48, 1972.
24. Sande MA, Mandell GL: Effect of rifampin on nasal carriage of *Staphylococcus aureus. Antimicrob Agents Chemother* 7:294–297, 1975.
25. Wheat LJ, Kohler RB, White AL, White A: Effect of rifampin on nasal carriers of coagulase-positive staphylococci. *J Infect Dis* 144:177, 1981.
26. Dacre JE, Emmerson AM, Jenner EA: Nasal carriage of gentamicin and methicillin resistant *Staphylococcus aureus* treated with topical pseudomonic acid. *Lancet* 2:1036, 1983.
27. Gonzaga AJ, Mortimer EA Jr, Wolinksy E, Rammelkamp CH Jr: Transmission of staphylococci by fomites. *JAMA* 189:711–715, 1964.
28. Berman DS, Schaefler S, Simberkoff MS, Rahal JJ: Tourniquets and nosocomial methicillin-resistant *Staphylococcus aureus* infections. *N Engl J Med* 315:514–515, 1986.
29. Steere AC, Mallison GF: Handwashing practices for the prevention of nosocomial infections. *Ann Intern Med* 83:683–690, 1975.
30. Garner JS, Simmons BP: CDC guidelines for the prevention and control of nosocomial infections. Guideline for isolation precautions in hospitals. *Am J Infect Control* 12:103–163, 1984.
31. Williams WW: CDC guidelines for the prevention and control of nosocomial infections. Guideline for infection control in hospital personnel. *Am J Infect Control* 12:34–57, 1984.
32. Klainer LM, Agrawal HS, Mortimer EA Jr, Wolinsky E: Bacitracin ointment and neonatal staphylococci. *Am J Dis Child* 103:564–568, 1962.
33. Seeberg S, Brinkhoff B: Epidemiology and control of staphylococcal pyoderma among newborn infants: evaluation of a method for routine cord care with 4 per cent chlorhexidine-detergent solution. *J Hosp Infect* 5:121–136, 1984.
34. Gezon HM, Schaberg MJ, Klein JO: Concurrent epidemics of *Staphylococcus aureus* and group A streptococcus disease in a newborn nursery—control with penicillin G and hexachlorophene bathing. *Pediatrics* 51:383–390, 1973.
35. Bisno AL: Streptococcus pyogenes. In Mandell GL, Douglas RG Jr, Bennett JE (eds): *Principles and Practice of Infectious Diseases*, ed 2. New York, John Wiley & Sons, 1985, pp. 1125–1126.
36. Peter G, Smith AL: Group A streptococcal infections of the skin and pharynx (Part I). *N Engl J Med* 297:311–317, 1977.
37. Bisno AL: *Streptococcus pyogenes*. In Mandell GL, Douglas RG Jr, Bennett JE (eds): *Principles and Practice of Infectious Diseases*, ed 2. New York, John Wiley & Sons, 1985, p. 1131.
38. Ferrieri P, Dajani AS, Wannamaker LW, Chapman SS: Natural history of impetigo. I. Site sequence of acquisition and familial patterns of spread of cutaneous streptococci. *J Clin Invest* 51:2851–2862, 1972.
39. Nelson KE, Bisno AL, Waytz P, Brunt J, Moses VK, Haque R: The epidemiology and natural history of streptococcal pyoderma: An endemic disease of the rural southern United States. *Am J Epidemiol* 103:270–283, 1976.
40. Sharrett AR, Finklea JF, Potter EV, Poon-King T, Earle DP: The control of streptococcal skin infections in South Trinidad. *Am J Epidemiol* 99:408–413, 1974.
41. Taplin D, Lansdell L, Allen AM, Rodriguez R, Cortes A: Prevalence of streptococcal pyoderma in relation to climate and hygiene. *Lancet* 1:501–503, 1973.
42. Lannigan R, Hussain Z, Austin TW: *Streptococcus pyogenes* as a cause of nosocomial infection in a critical care unit. *Diagn Microbiol Infect Dis* 3:337–341, 1985.
43. Goldberg GN, Hansen RC, Lynch PJ: Necrotizing fasciitis in infancy: Report of three cases and review of the literature. *Pediatr Dermatol* 2:55–63, 1984.
44. Geil CC, Castle WK, Mortimer EA Jr: Group A streptococcal infections in newborn nurseries. *Pediatrics* 46:849–854, 1970.
45. Dillon HC Jr: Group A type 12 streptococcal infection in a newborn nursery. *Am J Dis Child* 112:177–184, 1966.
46. Nelson JD, Dillon HC Jr, Howard JB: A prolonged nursery epidemic associated with a newly recognized type of group A streptococcus. *J Pediatr* 89:792–796, 1976.

47. Isenberg HD, Tucci V, Lipsitz P, Facklam RR: Clinical laboratory and epidemiological investigations of a *Streptococcus pyogenes* cluster epidemic in a newborn nursery. *J Clin Microbiol* 19:366–370, 1984.

48. Wiesenthal AM: A maternal-neonatal outbreak of infections due to an unusual group A B-hemolytic streptococcus. *Infect Control* 5:271–274, 1984.

49. Richman DD, Breton SJ, Goldmann DA: Scarlet fever and group A streptococcal surgical wound infection traced to an anal carrier. *J Pediatr* 90:387–390, 1977.

50. Stamm WE, Feeley JC, Facklam RR: Wound infections due to a group A streptococcus traced to a vaginal carrier. *J Infect Dis* 138:287–292, 1978.

51. Bisno AL, Nelson KE, Waytz P, Brunt J: Factors influencing serum antibody response in streptococcal pyoderma. *J Lab Clin Med* 81:410–420, 1973.

52. Eells LD, Mertz PM, Piovanetti Y, Pekoe GM, Eaglstein WH: Topical antibiotic treatment of impetigo with mupirocin. *Arch Dermatol* 122:1273–1276, 1986.

53. Orkin M, Maibach HI: Scabies in children. *Pediatr Clin North Am* 25:371–386, 1978.

54. Burkhart CG: Scabies: An epidemiologic reassessment. *Ann Intern Med* 98:498–503, 1983.

55. Arlian LG, Runyan RA, Achar S, Estes SA: Survival and infestivity of *Sarcoptes scabiei var. canis and var. hominis*. *J Am Acad Dermatol* 11:210–215, 1984.

56. Church RE, Knowelden J: Scabies in Sheffield: A family infestation. *Br Med J* 1:761–763, 1978.

57. Gooch JJ, Strasius SR, Beamer B, Reiter MD, Correll GW: Nosocomial outbreak of scabies. *Arch Dermatol* 114:897–898, 1978.

58. Lerche NW, Currier RW, Juranek DD, Baer W, Dubay NJ: Atypical crusted "Norwegian" scabies: Report of nosocomial transmission in a community hospital and an approach to control. *Cutis* 31:637–639, 641–642, 668, 684, 1983.

59. Cooper CL, Jackson MM: Outbreak of scabies in a small community hospital. *Am J Infect Control* 14:173–179, 1986.

60. Haydon JR Jr, Caplan RM: Epidemic scabies. *Arch Dermatol* 103:168–173, 1971.

61. Estes SA: Diagnosis and management of scabies. *Med Clin North Am* 66:955–963, 1982.

62. Pramanik AK, Hansen RC: Transcutaneous gamma benzene hexachloride absorption and toxicity in infants and children. *Arch Dermatol* 115:1224–1225, 1979.

63. Rasmussen JE: The problem of lindane. *J Am Acad Dermatol* 5:507–516, 1981.

64. Shacter B: Treatment of scabies and pediculosis with lindane preparations: An evaluation. *J Am Acad Dermatol* 5:517–527, 1981.

65. Cubela V, Yawalkar SJ: Clinical experience with crotamiton cream and lotion in treatment of infants with scabies. *Br J Clin Pract* 32:229–231, 1978.

66. Taplin D, Meinking TL, Porcelain SL, Castillero PM, Chen JA: Permethrin 5% dermal cream: A new treatment for scabies. *J Am Acad Dermatol* 15:995–1001, 1986.

67. Bernstein B, Mihan R: Hospital epidemic of scabies. *J Pediatr* 83:1086–1087, 1973.

68. Belle EA, D'Souza TJ, Zarzour JY, Lemieux M, Wong CC: Hospital epidemic of scabies: Diagnosis and control. *Can J Public Health* 70:133–135, 1979.

8

Infections Associated with Intravascular Catheters and Cerebrospinal Fluid Shunts

Carla M. Odio, M.D.

Infections Associated with Intravascular Devices

A significant number of hospitalized and ambulatory patients receive intravenous therapy either through an intravenous cannula or an indwelling venous device. The latter (e.g., Hickman or Broviac) has facilitated the management of patients undergoing cancer therapy, short bowel syndrome, and related conditions that require home hyperalimentation for chronic bowel disorders. These catheters have also facilitated the home care of patients undergoing extended courses of intravenous antibiotic treatment.

Despite the benefits they offer, indwelling intravenous catheters pose risks for significant infection. Also, their placement can be complicated by bleeding, pneumo- or hemothorax, and thrombosis. Suppurative thrombophlebitis in children is the most severe form of infection caused by intravenous cannulation (1). This severe infection can present after either percutaneous or cutdown insertion of an intravenous cannulae, but it is more likely to complicate the latter (2).

Indwelling long-term venous-access devices have alleviated some of the problems associated with poor venous access in cancer, short bowel syndrome, and bone marrow transplantation patients. However, use of these devices is associated with an inherent risk of infection. Proper prevention, early recognition and adequate treatment of catheter-related bacteremia are important determinants of outcome in such patients.

HISTORY

Suppurative thrombophlebitis secondary to indwelling venous catheters was described by Neuhof and Seley in 1947 in a report of 54 cases (3). In 1958, Phillips and Eyre (4) reported three additional cases of staphylococcal sepsis related to intravenous catheters. O'Neill et al. reported 35 cases of life-threatening suppurative thrombophlebitis in burn patients (5). Pruitt et al. reviewed the experience at the United States Army Surgical Research Unit from 1960–1968 and showed that 4% of 778 burn patients developed life-threatening suppurative thrombophlebitis complicating intravenous cannulation (6). These same investigators showed that in 521 burn patients admitted to this unit from 1967–1968, 24 (4.6%) developed suppurative thrombophlebitis, but the diagnosis was made antemortem in only 11 (45.8%) of these patients (7).

In 1973, Broviac (8) developed the first indwelling right atrial catheter. It was an all-Silastic (silicone rubber) catheter measuring approximately 90 cm in length with a 55 cm intravascular segment. The internal diameter of the Broviac catheters measures 0.6–1 mm. It is inserted by venous cutdown into either the cephalic, subclavian, or jugular vein, and its tip is located in the chest cavity below the clavicles, above the waist, and anterior to the shoulder. The correct tip position is at the superior vena cava-right atrial junction. After placement in the vessel, it is tunneled subcutaneously, and the thicker extravascular segment is then externalized, but remains attached to the chest wall by a Dacron cuff. The success of these catheters in the supportive management of cancer and short bowel syndrome or bone marrow transplant patients led to modifications of the original Broviac catheter. In 1975, Hickman (9) widened the internal diameter from 0.6–1.0 mm to 1.6 mm, allowing blood sampling, and the infusion of chemotherapeutics and blood products. Further advances or modifications of the structure of these types of catheters have included percutaneous placement without cutdown, multipurpose catheters, double and triple lumen catheters, thus further expanding the application of these devices to patients undergoing intensive treatment regimens in whom continuous intravenous access route is essential. Modifications in surgical technique now permit subcutaneous implantation of these catheters without the need of a cutdown (e.g., Port-A-Cath, Infusaport, Medi-Port) thus avoiding the ligation of veins. Also, subcutaneously implanted reservoir-type catheters have been introduced recently with the advantage of requiring less care and maintenance. They are more aesthetically pleasing to the patient; however, the experience with those implantable-type devices is limited, and their type and incidence of complications is unknown (10,11).

RISK FACTORS AND INCIDENCE

The estimated risk of infection related to intravenous devices ranges from 3–60%. O'Neill et al. (5) and Pruitt et al. (6,7) found a 4% incidence of suppurative thrombophlebitis with nearly 50% of the cases diagnosed postmortem. Moran et al. (12) found that the rate of infection of indwelling catheters increased directly with the duration of time the catheter remained in place, with a sharp rise at 72 hours. Another determinant of the risk of catheter-related infections is the material they are made of. Polyethylene catheters are the most irritating to the vein, followed by the Teflon catheters, which are moderately reactive, and Silastic catheters, which are least reactive. However, septic thrombophlebitis has also been observed in association with metal needles (13). The third and most important determinant of catheter-related infections is the type of host and immunologic competency. In cancer patients, the incidence of infections associated with the Hickman-Broviac catheters has ranged from 9–80%. These are the results of the works published by Broviac, Riella, Hickman, and Shapiro (8,14–29). The range of incidence rates of catheter-associated infection is extremely wide, since the majority of these studies were retrospective. In addition, there were multiple variables, such as the frequency of treatment-related complications (e.g., neutropenia, guidelines for catheter insertion, maintenance, and longevity) and the different definitions that were employed. Hiemenz et al. found that 39% of cancer patients with catheters had a "catheter associated" bacteremia, and of these, 60% occurred while the patient was granulocytopenic (30).

Other risk factors for development of catheter-related infections are disruption of natural barriers against infection, such as skin by either puncture or venous cutdown; intrinsic factors related to the characteristics of the foreign body; the administration of drugs that are irritating and favor sclerosis, red blood cells, and platelet adhesion to the catheter wall or to the endothelial wall with thrombus formation with the increased likelihood of bacteria nesting within it. To assess the impact of catheters on the risk of developing a bacteremia, Hiemenz et al. compared the frequency of bloodstream infections in patients with and without catheters in place (30). In neutropenic patients who developed fever, the risk of having an associated bacteremia was increased 4-fold if the patient had an intravascular catheter in place. The risk of having a bacteremia was increased nearly 40-fold in non-neutropenic patients if they had a catheter. Thus, simply placing a catheter in the cancer patient significantly increases the risk for developing a bacteremia.

It is important to ascertain the role of this increased risk on the real morbidity and mortality of the patients. In other words, one must assess whether the risks of a catheter-associated bacteremia outweigh the benefits of ready venous access. This will depend on how easily and successfully catheter-associated infections can be treated and whether the infection necessitates removal of the catheter for control.

Intravenous cannulae infection secondary to intravenous therapy presents in 0.1–6.5% of the cases (2,31). Berkowitz et al. (32) reported that 2% of all bacteremias are related to intravenous therapy. He and his colleagues reported eight cases (32) of suppurative thrombophlebitis in children, and 12.5% of the patients with suppurative thrombophlebitis died. Burn patients are at particularly high risk of developing suppurative thrombophlebitis with a 4.2–8.1% incidence (7,33). The overall incidence of suppurative thrombophlebitis based on data from the National Nosocomial Infection Study (2) is 76 per 100,000 discharges. As mentioned earlier, the incidence of both phlebitis and positivity of cannula cultures rises significantly with increasing duration of cannulation (31,34–36).

PATHOGENESIS

Indwelling venous catheters may become contaminated with bacteria from the skin surrounding the exit site, from transient bacteremia or via the gastrointestinal tract. This results in potentially lethal complications, such as septic or suppurative thrombophlebitis or catheter-related bacteremia. Septic thrombophlebitis may result from infection of the intraluminal thrombus by bacteria or fungi from direct contamination of the indwelling catheter or needle or from hematogenous spread from distant sites. Usually, the same bacteria isolated from the skin surrounding the exit site are isolated from the bloodstream of patients with catheter-related septicemia. However, in a study from the University of Pittsburgh (26) where 14 of 21 catheters in place had associated bacteremia and six were removed for persistent bacteremia, five of them were sterile when cultured. In only one case was the catheter tip, when removed, positive for the same organism which had been grown from the bloodstream.

Some investigators have attributed the source of *Staphylococcus epidermidis* to a gastrointestinal (instead of a cutaneous) focus (37). The type of underlying disease has been associated with the source of infection of patients with an indwelling venous catheter. For example, short bowel syndrome patients develop infection secondary to seeding from the gastrointestinal tract. There may be other factors that explain the pathogenesis of infection related to intravascular devices. First, of course, is the possibility of direct contact of the foreign body with an in-

fected surface, such as the skin. One should also consider the type of underlying disease. Finally, there are unique properties intrinsic to the infecting microorganism. *S. epidermidis* species, which is the most common cause of catheter-related sepsis, is known for its ability to adhere and to colonize plastic tubing. Many strains produce a slime that acts as a barrier to phagocytosis and to antibiotic contact (38). The source of other organisms such as *Klebsiella species* and *Escherichia coli* can be the skin. They have been found at the catheter exit sites (39). When microorganisms such as *Streptococcus pneumoniae*, which have no predilection for catheters, are isolated from the bloodstream of febrile patients with a central venous catheter, they usually do not represent catheter involvement with nitching of the microorganism in the tube walls. Rather, they reflect transient bacteremia diagnosed by a blood culture sampled through a central catheter (39).

In conclusion, most of the pathogenesis of infection related to intravascular devices is that of foreign body infection. Zimmerli (40) used an animal model involving the subcutaneous implantation of tissue cages into guinea pigs and documented subsequent infection with *S. aureus*. This model was used to study factors pertinent to foreign body infection. Whereas 10^8 colony-forming units did not produce abscesses in the absence of foreign material, 10^2 was enough to infect 95% of the tissue cages despite the presence of polymorphonuclear leukocytes. Opsonic coating of the organism was decreased, and the polymorphonuclear leukocytes from sterile tissue cages showed decreased phagocytic and bactericidal activities when compared with polymorphonuclear leukocytes from either blood or peritoneal exudate obtained after short- or long-term stimulation.

ETIOLOGY

Most catheter-related infections are caused by Gram-positive microorganisms, mainly coagulase-negative staphylococci. However, *S. aureus*, *Corynebacterium*, *Bacillus species*, Gram-negative bacteria, and fungi have all been implicated in catheter-associated infections. Until recently, *Staphylococcus* was the most common organism isolated in septic or suppurative thrombophlebitis. In recent years, however, an increase in infections due to enteric Gram-negative organisms has been recognized (13). In the study by Sears et al., both staphylococci and *Klebsiella species* were implicated in the infectious process. When granulocytopenic, the immunocompromised patient is at increased risk for infection. The isolation of organisms, such as *Serratia marcescens*, *Escherichia coli*, and *Klebsiella pneumoniae*, from blood samples drawn through the patient's catheter may constitute a catheter-associated complication or may simply be a coincidental systemic infection. Hiemenz et al. found that regardless of whether the patient was neutropenic or non-neutropenic, the predominant isolate associated with bacteremia was *S. epidermidis* (30). In neutropenic patients, nearly one-third of the isolates were Gram-negative bacteria and, less frequently, *Candida spp.* During the last several years, the number of non-neutropenic patients who present with mixed Gram-positive and Gram-negative infections has increased (30). Prince et al. (39) found that *S. epidermidis* species was the most common cause of catheter-related sepsis.

The etiology of suppurative thrombophlebitis has been reported to be due to enteric bacilli, *Candida spp.*, when patients were receiving broad-spectrum antimicrobial therapy. However, in those not receiving antibiotics, *S. aureus* is generally the causative organism (32). The microorganisms most commonly involved in cannula-related infection or suppurative thrombophlebitis are staphylococci, Gram-negative, and fungi (1,2,7,33–35,41,42).

CLINICAL PRESENTATION

Suppurative thrombophlebitis is an infectious complication of indwelling intravenous catheters. The clinical spectrum of thrombophlebitis includes:

1. *Nonseptic, nonsuppurative thrombophlebitis*, manifested by local pain, tenderness, and redness over the course of the vein;
2. *Septic, nonsuppurative inflammation* due to infection of an intraluminal thrombus; and
3. *Suppurative thrombophlebitis*, characterized by clot liquefaction, intraluminal purulent exudate, vein necrosis, and periphlebitic abscess.

The septic forms of thrombophlebitis generally manifest with systemic symptoms, such as fever and malaise, and septic emboli to distant sites (especially the lungs) may occur (13). Nonseptic thrombophlebitis is related to injury involving the vein endothelium resulting in intimal inflammation (6,13).

The clinical forms of infection associated with the indwelling Hickman-Broviac catheters are catheter-associated bacteremia, local cellulitis around the exit site of the catheter, or infection along its subcutaneous tunnel. Local signs can be absent, and symptoms may develop several days after removal of the central line or the intravenous cannula (5,7,33). The most common clinical manifestations of catheter-related infection are fever and purulent exudate at the cannula entry site (5,7,33,41,42). Berkowitz et al. (41) found that 62.5% of patients with fever in whom a central line was in place had a positive blood culture. Others have observed that randomly drawn blood cultures from Hickman catheters can sometimes be positive in completely asymptomatic patients (43).

The clinical presentation of suppurative thrombophlebitis includes fever, swelling along the vein, edema of the affected area with or without crepitus, pustules at the affected site, and phlebitis, all present with fever and local signs, such as either phlebitis and swelling along the vein or edema of the affected vein (41). The clinical diagnosis can be difficult and many of these cases are diagnosed at autopsy (7).

DIAGNOSIS

The diagnosis of catheter-related sepsis is based primarily on the clinical presentation. However, according to Maki, a precise definition of catheter-related sepsis cannot be made without catheter removal (44). For the definitive diagnosis of bacteremia, a blood culture obtained by venipuncture of a noncannulated vein after the overlying skin has been sterilely prepped should always be performed. The isolation of the same organisms from the blood as those isolated from the skin surrounding the exit site of the catheter does not clearly indicate a cause and effect in the etiology of the catheter-related infection. One would need to perform a plasmid profile determination (45) to ensure that it is the same microorganism. The yield of *S. epidermidis* from blood cultures has increased by newer blood culture techniques [e.g., lysis-centrifugation system (DuPont Isolator)], making the potential for false-positive isolates greater (46).

In clinical practice, it is most important to determine whether an isolate obtained from a catheter is a contaminant or a true pathogen. It can be difficult, if not impossible, to ascertain whether isolated Staphylococci represent infection or contamination when isolated from blood obtained through a catheter or from the skin surrounding the exit site. In some instances, quantitative blood cultures may assist in distinguishing false- from true positives. Raucher (47) ascribed the bacteremia to the catheter if the number of bacterial colonies obtained from blood drawn through the catheter exceeded those which were obtained from a peripheral vein. One could extrapolate results of quantitative blood cultures obtained from a catheter to those of a peripheral vein.

Hiemenz et al. have found that when there are greater than 25 colonies per plate from a catheter blood culture, the peripheral venous samples are virtually always positive, even though it may take several days for these cultures to grow (30). Obtaining regular skin surveillance cultures from patients with a central line to predict the risk of catheter-related infection has been suggested by some authors (48). However, one can find potentially infecting organisms around the catheter exit site or on the patient's skin and may still be unable to ascertain what the finding means. The chance of false-positive cultures is high, and the interpretation of these cultures is uncertain.

MANAGEMENT

For management of septic thrombophlebitis, rest, elevation, local heat, and, occasionally, anticoagulant therapy are used. Since 1947, when septic thrombophlebitis was described, surgical intervention has been an important part of therapy (3). Antibiotic therapy alone failed to improve the local infection or to sterilize the blood in the reports of Sears et al. (1) and O'Neill et al. (5). The latter showed that 12 adults with suppurative thrombophlebitis treated with conventional medical management died from secondary problems of this disease, whereas 23 patients treated by surgical measures survived. Zinner et al. (13) reported 11 cases of septic thrombophlebitis that did not respond to conservative management but were resolved promptly after local excision of the involved venous segment in conjunction with antibiotic therapy. It is clear that local venous excision with primary skin closure is an efficacious method of treat-

ment for septic thrombophlebitis. In cases of suppurative thrombophlebitis and an associated periphlebitis abscess, however, a more radical venous excision and delayed wound closure are recommended (1,5). When the infection subsides and the open wound displays granulation tissue, delayed closure can be safely performed.

With the initial reports of the infectious complications associated with the Hickman-Broviac catheter it became apparent that the catheter-associated bacteremias could, in some patients, be treated successfully with antibiotics alone, without the necessity of catheter removal (9,16,17). This defies one of the classic principles of treatment of foreign body-related infection (40) i.e., if the infection is to be treated successfully, the foreign body must be removed. In a study from the University of Pennsylvania, 93% (14/15) of catheter-related septicemia were successfully treated with antibiotics without catheter removal (23). At the University of Pittsburgh, five of six catheters removed for persistent bacteremia while on antibiotics were sterile when removed (26). However, electron microscopy scanning of the catheter wall to visualize adhered microorganisms was not performed. Hiemenz et al. (30) outlined guidelines for managing catheter-associated infection according to their definition categories:

1. *Exit site tenderness or cellulitis.* If the patient is non-neutropenic, afebrile, and found to have tenderness or erythema around the Hickman-Broviac exit site, one should look for a discharge from around the exit port. Gram-stained smear of the material and culture should help to tailor antibiotic therapy. If the area of local tenderness is limited and not progressing rapidly, a trial of oral antibiotics active against Staphylococci can be attempted. However, keep in mind that *S. epidermidis*, which is the most common etiologic agent, is not susceptible to most oral antistaphylococcal drugs, and parenteral therapy with vancomycin will be necessary. In neutropenic patients, exit site infection is an indication for hospitalization. Antibiotics should be administered intravenously after the patient has been properly cultured. The ideal initial antibiotic coverage is vancomycin plus either an aminoglycoside or a 3rd-generation cephalosporin. Exit site infection can be caused by unusual organisms, including fungi and atypical mycobacteria. The failure to respond to

standard antibiotics should prompt reevaluation with culture or biopsy and aspiration and a broader antibiotic coverage that includes amphotericin B.

2. *Tunnel infection*. Catheter tunnel infection can be associated with exit site drainage, cellulitis, or bacteremia. In such cases, the patients should be managed with parenterally administered antibiotics plus removal of the catheter. Removal of the catheter is required in this setting because of the inability to attain significant antibiotic concentration in that area.

3. *Suspected bacteremia*. A new episode of fever in the cancer patient with an indwelling intravenous catheter should raise the suspicion of catheter-related bacteremia. Neutropenic patients should always be hospitalized, cultured, and started on vancomycin plus an aminoglycoside or a third-generation cephalosporin. If the patient was already on broad spectrum antibiotics, amphotericin B should be added after the patient is properly cultured and reevaluation of the Gram-negative enteric coverage is undertaken. Antibiotics should be continued for at least 10–14 days. If the patient is non-neutropenic and there is no obvious cause of fever, the patient should be hospitalized, cultured, and started empirically on the aforementioned antibiotic combination. If after 48–72 hours of antibiotic therapy the patient is asymptomatic, there is no obvious focus of catheter-related infection, and both central and peripheral blood cultures are sterile, antibiotics can be safely discontinued and the patient closely observed and recultured 48–72 hours later. If the cultures are positive, patients should receive a full course (i.e., 10–14 days) of specific antibiotic therapy. Whether or not non-neutropenic patients should be treated in such an aggressive way has not been established. Until more data are available, Hiemenz et al. consider this approach to be the safest (30).

4. *Proven bacteremia*. If the preantibiotic cultures are positive, the question of whether the catheter should be removed will depend on the type of microorganism. Staphylococci can be safely treated with antibiotics alone, without catheter removal. However, when the infection is caused by fungi, mainly *Candida spp.* or by *Bacillus spp.*, the catheter should be removed and specific antibiotic therapy administered for 10–14 days. When cultures are positive for enteric Gram-negative bacilli, the infection can be successfully treated with antibiotics alone, without catheter removal in only 50% of the cases (39). One should follow these patients closely and remove the catheter if after 48 hours of antibiotic therapy, cultures remain positive or there is lack of clinical improvement or clinical deterioration. Patients with double- or triple-lumen catheters should have separate cultures drawn through each port, and antibiotics rotated and administered through each lumen. Failure to clear the infection in patients with double- or triple-lumen catheter may occur unless antibiotics are administered into each of the ports. Rotating antibiotics from one lumen port to the next avoids the possibility of one of them serving as a "reservoir," which can set the stage for a subsequent treatment failure, thus prolonging morbidity and increasing the risk of seeding the infection to distant sites. Withholding antibiotic treatment is undesirable for a potentially septic patient with significant underlying disease in whom the infection may be related to an indwelling venous catheter.

Antibiotic therapy alone without catheter removal *should not* be attempted when fungal, *Bacillus spp.*, tunnel infection, or Gram-negative coliform bacilli infection of the bloodstream is documented. In patients in whom the catheter is not essential, the catheter should be removed when a catheter-related infection is suspected. Febrile patients with a central venous catheter should be promptly evaluated, cultured, and empirically started on broad spectrum antibiotic therapy. This approach is warranted to control bacterial multiplication, thus diminishing the inoculum size within the catheter and the bloodstream.

PREVENTION

Careful handwashing and preparation of the anticipated intravenous site with an antibacterial solution, such as iodophor or ethanol 70%, and meticulous aseptic technique are important in reducing catheter-related infection. Indwelling venous catheters should optimally be Silastic or Teflon, and the dressing, if present, should be changed every 2–3 days. Intravenous cannulae should be removed and changed every 48–72 hours. Modifications of intravenous infusions with low-dose heparin and, when possible, a neutral pH may be useful adjunctive methods to decrease the sclerosing properties of the solution being administered.

The value of applying an antibiotic ointment to the exit site or to the cannula entry site is controversial (2,35,49), and the local application of povidone-iodine is of no proven value (50,51). Until local antibiotics or antibacterial solutions prove to be useful—and even then—rigorous aseptic technique with strict hand-washing is the best method of preventing bacterial entry into the intravascular device.

Infections Associated with Cerebrospinal Fluid Shunt Catheters

---

Refinement of surgical techniques and improved devices in cerebrospinal fluid (CSF) shunt procedures have improved survival and the quality of life of infants with hydrocephalus (52–54). Currently, the most frequent and disabling complication of these procedures is CSF-shunt (CSF-S) infection. The reported incidence of CSF-shunt infection varies from 4–20% (52–58).

HISTORY

CSF-shunts are devices that relieve hydrocephalus and increased intracranial pressure resulting from a variety of lesions which cause obstruction of the intracranial cerebrospinal fluid pathways. Miculicz is described in historical reviews as the individual who designed the first CSF catheter in the 1890s (59). This catheter consisted of an elongated mass of glass wool inserted into the lateral ventricle. This was followed by gold, silver, glass, linen, and rubber catheters. The first CSF ventriculoperitoneal (VP) shunt was placed in 1908, and in 1948 Matson (60) began using shunts made from polyethylene tubing. The extracranial drainage sites have included heart, peritoneal cavity, bone marrow, mastoid, pleural cavity, and genitourinary tract (61,62). Three decades ago, peritoneal drainage was frequently used but was abandoned by many surgeons because the peritoneal catheter frequently became occluded with fibrous and/or omental tissue (63,64). With the introduction of silicone rubber and silastic drainage tubes, long-term success has been attained. During the last 15 years, ventriculoperitoneal shunts (VP-S) have been more widely used. The ventriculoatrial shunts (VA-S) have been less satisfactory than the VP-S because there are multiple complications related to its position in the right atrium.

Besides meningitis and infections in and out of the CNS, additional complications related to CSF-VA and CSF-VP shunts have been noted. These include septic pulmonary embolus and infected cardiac catheters, both of which have been reported in a higher number of patients with VA-S than in those with VP-S. Blockage, requiring revision of the system at a shorter period of time after placement, and shunt nephritis have been reported more frequently in patients with VA-S. The lower incidence of serious infections, need for revisions, and overall morbidity related to CSF-VP shunts make them the first choice in managing most forms of hydrocephalus in children.

RISK FACTORS AND INCIDENCE

Conditions associated with a higher incidence of CSF-S infection are age less than 1 year, myelomeningocele, more than three previous procedures per patient, type of procedure, higher incidence of infection related to total replacement versus revision, type of catheter and operation time (65–68). Approximately three-fourths of the infections are diagnosed within the first 2 months after surgery (56,65). The reported incidence of shunt infection is 10–35% in patients with CSF-VA shunts and 2–20% (64,69–71) in patients with CSF-VP shunts. Shunt infections can present at any age, although they are more common in infants.

PATHOGENESIS

The pathogenesis of CSF-shunt infection is determined by the characteristics of the infecting microorganism and those of the foreign body. Many infections of staphylococci are producers of "slime," which gives the microorganism an adhesive factor to the foreign material and promotes the formation of true nitches in the tubes of the catheter (72). In addition, irregularities, such as indentations and protrusions of the luminal surface of the valve and the catheter, make adherence of microorganisms to the CSF-shunt system more likely (73). Although antiseptic agents are bactericidal to microorganisms of the skin and scalp, they fail to reach bacteria lying deep in the sebaceous glands, sweat glands, and hair follicles. Gram-negative coliform bacillary infection, especially when found in mixed culture with anaerobes and/or enterococci, have been associated with ulcerated myelomeningocele wounds or perforation of an abdominal viscus by the distal end of the catheter (74).

CSF-shunt infections can occur secondary to intraoperative contamination of the wound and/or shunt. This results in early postoperative infection of the surgical wound or the catheter tunnel. Perforation of an abdominal viscus by the distal catheter can also result in early catheter colonization and infection (75). In patients with CSF-VA shunts, the infection can also occur secondary to the seeding of the intrauricular catheter during episodes of bacteremia (75). Urinary tract infections (UTI) have rarely been implicated as a cause of CSF-shunt infection (65). Bacterial contamination of the surgical wound leading to catheter colonization accounts for the majority of catheter-associated infection. This has been supported by demonstrating that organisms present in the wound at the time of surgery are of the same species and have the same plasmid profile as those causing catheter-related infection (76).

ETIOLOGY

The bacteriology of CSF-shunt infections reflects the normal skin and scalp flora. In one series of 297 patients followed over 7 years, 75% of the infectious episodes were caused by coagulase-negative staphylococci and *Staphylococcus aureus* (65). Nineteen percent of the infectious episodes were caused either solely or in mixed infection by Gram-negative coliform bacillary microorganisms. Other miscellaneous organisms, such as enterococcus, viridans streptococci, and diphtheroids were noted to coexist with anaerobes and coliform bacilli in patients with VP-shunt infections.

CLINICAL PRESENTATION

The clinical presentation of CSF-shunt infections will depend on the type of shunt, the offending pathogen, and the age of the patient. The time of onset of symptomatology will vary according to the size of the inocula and the type of pathogen. Gram-negative coliform bacilli are more virulent and cause overwhelming disease. Infections caused by *Staphylococcus aureus* often present with surgical wound infections or subcutaneous abscess formation (65). Coagulase-negative staphylococcal infections usually present in a less virulent and more insidious manner. In patients with CSF-VA shunts, there are three recognized forms of presentation of clinical shunt infection:

1. *Acute sepsis*. The onset is from 2–7 days after surgery; there is usually erythema with purulence at the surgical wound site, which is culture-positive; patients present with high fever, shunt malfunction, anemia, CSF pleocytosis greater than 500 leukocytes/mm^3, and a predominance of neutrophils in the differential white blood count. The putative agent is generally staphylococci and is isolated from blood and cerebrospinal fluid in the majority of cases; Gram-negative coliform bacilli are isolated in approximately 19% of cases (65).

2. *Indolent infection*. The onset of infection is usually from 3–8 months following surgery. Erythema of the surgical wound is mild or absent; patients present with low-grade fever; repetitive episodes of shunt malfunction which resolve spontaneously; anemia is mild or absent; and CSF pleocytosis is generally less than 500 leukocytes/mm^3. The microorganism is recovered from CSF in approximately 60% of the patients and very seldom from the blood.

3. *Clinically inapparent infection*. This entity has been recognized by routinely culturing all shunts at the time of elective revision. There are no local signs or symptoms of infection; the CSF cellularity ranges from 0–50 leukocytes/mm^3. The transoperative CSF culture is positive in approximately 30% of cases. However, the cultures of the shunt and catheter are invariably positive (65).

In patients with CSF-VP shunt infection, the clinical presentation is nonspecific; most of the patients present with fever, vomiting, lethargy, irritability, and anorexia. Patients who present with wound infection generally have high-grade fever, changes in the sensorium, and are irritable. Patients without wound infection usually present with shunt malfunction and gastrointestinal symptoms such as vomiting, abdominal pain, diarrhea, and peritonitis. The time of onset of infection after the surgical procedure has been associated with the type of microorganism involved. Patients infected with *Staphylococcus aureus* have early onset (within the first 15 days after surgery), whereas those infected with coagulase-negative staphylococci have delayed (after 15 days of the surgical procedure) infection.

DIAGNOSIS

The diagnosis of CSF shunt infection will primarily rely on the index of clinical suspicion of the attending physician. When a child who has a CSF shunt presents with any of the aforementioned symptoms, and there is no other apparent focus of infection, the physician must be aggressive in making a diagnosis and formulating a treatment plan. A CSF sample of the shunt obtained via a sterile tap of the shunt tubing or reservoir should be obtained for culture and analysis. Patients with documented CSF-shunt infection have a mean leukocyte count of 156/mm^3 with a wide range from 0–2.623/mm^3. The highest white blood counts in the CSF have been observed in patients with Gram-negative coliform bacillary infections. The mean percentage of segmented forms is 63% (range 20–100%). The protein content is usually elevated, mean 136 mg/dl (range 40–375 mg/dl). Patients with hypertensive hydrocephalus have CSF leukocytosis and elevated protein content in the absence of infection.

The degree of hypoglycorrhachia and the percentage of segmented neutrophils may help differentiate between patients with shunt malfunction with and without infection when the Gram-stained smear does not show microorganisms. The glycorrhachia in patients with CSF-shunt infection is usually below 40 mg/dl (mean 23 mg/dl), and the percentage of segmented neutrophils is usually above 60% (mean 67 mg %/dl) (65).

MANAGEMENT

The management of CSF-shunt related infections is controversial. There are different approaches, depending on the type of shunt, the infecting microorganism, and the presence or absence of wound or soft tissue infection. The two major approaches include a conservative one, without surgical intervention, and a more aggressive one, which depends on the removal of the shunt system. Removal of the shunt can be followed by immediate replacement in the contralateral site or by ventricular external drainage until sterilization of the CSF is attained and subsequent placement of another system (77). For CSF-ventriculoatrial shunt infections, the most successful method of treatment is antibiotics with removal of the system with immediate or delayed shunt placement. Immediate removal of the infected foreign body in CSF-VA shunts is important because of the high incidence of bacteremia and shunt nephritis associated with these systems (56,65,78). Other conditions requiring removal of the foreign body are infections caused by Gram-negative coliform bacilli because of the greater morbidity and mortality associated with infection with these organisms (65).

When the system is exposed, and there is wound infection or infection of the skin overlying the system, sterilization of the CSF is practically unattainable because of the large inoculum size in the CSF and in the foreign body (79). Conservative management leaving the shunt in place can be attempted in the case of staphylococcal infections when there is no soft tissue infection or external exposure of the system. Dr. Yogev (79) compiled the experience of many authors in the management of CSF-shunt infection with different treatment modalities. The higher success rates of 96% were attained with shunt removal plus systemic antibiotic therapy, followed by a 65% success rate with immediate shunt replacement plus systemic antibiotics. The poorest outcome was attained when the shunt was left in place. However, most of these studies were retrospective in design, and the authors do not show in a consistent manner the etiology of the infection, the type of antibiotics employed, and the susceptibility of the causative organisms to the administered antibiotics. Other authors in similar retrospective reviews have found a success rate of 62% when patients were treated with vancomycin alone without removal of the shunt (65). Preliminary results of an ongoing study conducted at the Hospital Nacional de Niños in San Jose, Costa Rica have shown cure rates of 69–73% in patients with CSF-VP shunt infections treated conservatively with either vancomycin, vancomycin plus rifampin, or vancomycin plus rifampin plus intrareservoir vancomycin (80).

Initial empiric antibiotic therapy for CSF-shunt infection should include a drug active against all staphylococci, such as vancomycin, and a drug active against Gram-negative coliform bacilli. For Gram-negative coliform bacilli, third-generation cephalosporins such as ceftriaxone, cefotaxime, ceftazidime, with or without aminoglycoside is adequate, and for staphylococci, vancomycin would be the drug of choice. The addition of rifampin to enhance the antistaphylococcal therapy may be efficacious. The instillation of antibiotics into the ventricle or reservoir has not been shown to be superior to the use of systemic antibiotic therapy alone. Since CSF-shunt infection is the major complication in hydrocephalic patients (81), familiarity with the type of clinical presentation and the etiology should be the key to ideal management of these patients when they do become infected. The most important method in the prevention of these infections is strict adherence to good aseptic technique prior to, during, and after the surgical procedure. The value of the prophylactic administration of antibiotics to prevent infection related to CSF-shunt procedures is still an unanswered question. Many studies looking at the value of prophylactic antibiotics have been performed. Most have been retrospective and sequential, and others have utilized historical controls from the literature from their prophylactic trials (77,79–85). Of the published studies that have been prospective and controlled, only the one performed by Dr. Yogev, using nafcillin or nafcillin plus rifampin, showed a statistically significant beneficial effect for prevention of early CSF-shunt postoperative infection (85).

PREVENTION

One should suspect a CSF-shunt infection in children with recent prior CSF-shunt surgery who present with fever, neurologic abnormalities, irritability, and or evidence of shunt malfunction. Analysis and culture of CSF from the shunt is essential for diagnosis. Empiric antibiotic therapy should include vancomycin and a third-generation cephalosporin. If the cultured pathogen is a Gram-negative coliform bacilli or

a fungus, such as *Candida species*, or the shunt is exposed independent of the causative pathogen, the shunt should be removed and appropriate antibiotic coverage should be administered. In up to 66% of the patients with staphylococcal CSF-VP-shunt infections, the infection can be treated without removing the shunt. In such cases, the duration of days with positive CSF cultures should not exceed seven, and the CSF's bactericidal activity should be equal or greater to three dilutions. Prophylaxis with nafcillin or nafcillin plus rifampin administered one or two doses prior to surgery, one transoperative dose, and two to three postoperative doses can reduce the incidence of early CSF-shunt infection. Careful aseptic technique prior to, after, and throughout the surgical procedure is the most important method of preventing CSF-shunt-related infections.

REFERENCES

1. Sears N, Grosfeld JL, Weber TR, Kleiman MB: Suppurative thrombophlebitis in childhood. *Pediatrics* 68:630–632, 1981.
2. Rhame FS, Maki DG, Bennett JV: Intravenous cannula-associated infections. In Bennett JV, Brachman PS (eds): *Hospital Infection*. Boston, Little, Brown & Co, 1979, p 433–442.
3. Neuhof H, Seley GP: Acute suppurative phlebitis complicated by septicemia. *Surgery* 21:831–842, 1947.
4. Phillips RW, Eyre JD Jr: Septic thrombophlebitis with septicemia: a report of three cases due to *Staphylococcus aureus* infection after the intravenous use of polyethylene catheters for parenteral therapy. *N Engl J Med* 259:729–731, 1958.
5. O'Neill JA Jr, Pruitt BA Jr, Foley FD, Moncrief JA: Suppurative thrombophlebitis: a lethal complication of intravenous therapy. *J Trauma* 8:256–267, 1968.
6. Pruitt BA Jr, Stein JM, Foley FD, Moncrief JA, O'Neill JA Jr: Intravenous therapy in burn patients. Suppurative thrombophlebitis and other life threatening complications. *Arch Surg* 100:399–404, 1970.
7. Stein JM, Pruitt BA Jr: Suppurative thrombophlebitis. *N Engl J Med* 282:1452–1455, 1970.
8. Broviac JW, Cole JJ, Scribner BH: A silicone rubber atrial catheter for prolonged parenteral alimentation. *Surg Gynecol Obstet* 136:602–606, 1973.
9. Hickman RO, Buckner CD, Clift RA, Sanders JE, Stewart P, Thomas ED: A modified right atrial catheter for access to the venous system in marrow transplant recipients. *Surg Gynecol Obstet* 148:871–875, 1979.
10. Gyves JW, Ensminger WD, Niederhuber JE, Dent T, Walker S, Gilbertson S, Cozzi E, Saran P: A totally implanted injection port system for blood sampling and chemotherapy administration. *JAMA* 251:2538–2541, 1984.
11. Schuman E, Brady AM, Galen WP, Winters V: Implanted venous access ports have significantly fewer complications than Hickman catheters. *Proc Am Soc Clin Oncol* 3:95, 1984.
12. Moran JM, Atwood RP, Rowe MI: A clinical and bacteriologic study of infections associated with venous cutdowns. *N Engl J Med* 272:554–560, 1965.
13. Zinner MJ, Zuidema GD, Lowery BD: Septic nonsuppurative thrombophlebitis. *Arch Surg* 111:122–125, 1976.
14. Broviac JW, Scribner BH: Prolonged parenteral nutrition in the home. *Surg Gynecol Obstet* 139:24–28, 1974.
15. Riella MC, Scribner BH: Five years' experience with a right atrial catheter for prolonged parenteral nutrition at home. *Surg Gynecol Obstet* 143:205–208, 1976.

16. Byrne WJ, Halpin TC, Asch MJ, Fonkalsrud EW, Ament ME: Home total parenteral nutrition: an alternative approach to the management of children with severe chronic small bowel disease. *J Pediatr Surg* 12:359–366, 1977.

17. Abrahm J, Mullen JL, Jacobson N, Polomano R: Continuous central venous access in patients with acute leukemia. *Cancer Treat Rep* 63:2099–2100, 1979.

18. Thomas JH, MacArthur RI, Pierce GE, Hermreck AS: Hickman-Broviac catheters. Indications and results. *Am J Surg* 140:791–796, 1980.

19. Blacklock HA, Pillai MV, Hill RS, Matthews JR, Clarke AG, Wade JF: Use of modified subcutaneous right-atrial catheter for venous access in leukaemic patients. *Lancet* 1:993–994, 1980.

20. Pollack PF, Kadden M, Byrne WJ, Fonkalsrud EW, Ament ME: 100 patient years' experience with the Broviac silastic catheter for central venous nutrition. *JPEN* 5:32–36, 1981.

21. Merritt RJ, Ennis CE, Andrassy RJ, Hays DM, Sinatra FR, Thomas DW, Siegel SE: Use of Hickman right atrial catheter in pediatric oncology patients. *JPEN* 5:83–85, 1981.

22. Shapiro ED, Spiegelman KN, Wald ER, Nelson KA: Catheter-related bacteremia in oncology patients with indwelling Broviac catheters. *Pediatr Res* 15:587, 1981.

23. Abrahm JL, Mullen JL: A prospective study of prolonged central venous access in leukemia. *JAMA* 248:2868–2873, 1982.

24. Shapiro ED, Wald ER, Nelson KA, Spiegelman KN: Broviac catheter related bacteremia in oncology patients. *Am J Dis Child* 136:679–681, 1982.

25. Hiemenz JW, Robichaud KJ, Johnston MR, Pizzo PA: Bacteremia in patients with indwelling silastic catheters. *Proc Am Soc Clin Oncol* 1:57, 1982.

26. Reilly JJ Jr, Steed DL, Ritter PS: Indwelling venous access catheters in patients with acute leukemia. *Cancer* 53:219–223, 1984.

27. Press OW, Ramsey PG, Larson EB, Fefer A, Hickman RO: Hickman catheter infections in patients with malignancies. *Medicine (Baltimore)* 63:189–200, 1984.

28. Houston G, Maher J, Vance R: Infectious complications associated with the Broviac catheter (CATH). *Proc Am Soc Clin Oncol* 2:86, 1983.

29. Brady AM, Schuman E, Winters V: Successful chronic intravenous access via right atrial catheters. *Proc Am Soc Clin Oncol* 3:95, 1984.

30. Hiemenz J, Skelton J, Pizzo PA: Perspective on the management of catheter-related infections in cancer patients. *Pediatr Infect Dis* 5:6–11, 1986.

31. Tager IB, Ginsberg MB, Ellis SE, Walsh NE, Dupont I, Simchen E, Faich GA: An epidemiologic study of the risks associated with peripheral intravenous catheters. *Am J Epidemiol* 118:839–851, 1983.

32. Berkowitz FE, Argent AC, Baise T: Suppurative thrombophlebitis: a serious nosocomial infection. *Pediatr Infect Dis* 6:64–67, 1987.

33. Pruitt BA Jr, McManus WF, Kim SH, Treat RC: Diagnosis and treatment of cannula-related intravenous sepsis in burn patients. *Ann Surg* 191:546–554, 1980.

34. Bentley DW, Lepper MH: Septicemia related to indwelling venous catheter. *JAMA* 206:1749–1752, 1968.

35. Maki DG, Goldmann DA, Rhame FS: Infection control in intravenous therapy. *Ann Intern Med* 79:867–887, 1973.

36. Collin J, Collin C, Constable FL, Johnston ID: Infusion thrombophlebitis and infection with various cannulae. *Lancet* 2:150–153, 1975.

37. Wade JC, Schimpff SC, Newman KA, Wiernik PH: *Staphylococcus epidermidis*: an increasing cause of infection in patients with granulocytopenia. *Ann Intern Med* 97:503–508, 1982.

38. Diaz-Mitoma F, Harding GKM, Hammond GW, Hoban N, MacFarlane R, Malazdrewicz R, Low DE: Ventriculoperitoneal shunt infections due to coagulase-negative staphylococci: correlation between slime production and clinical outcome. Presented at the 23rd Interscience Conference on Antimicrobial Agents on Chemotherapy (ICAAC), Las Vegas, NV, October 24–26, 1983, Abstract No. 665, pp 206.

39. Prince A, Heller B, Levy J, Heird WC: Management of fever in patients with central vein catheters. *Pediatr Infect Dis* 5:20–24, 1986.

40. Zimmerli W, Waldvogel FA, Vaudaux P, Nydegger UE: Pathogenesis of foreign body infection: description and characteristics of an animal model. *J Infect Dis* 146:487–497, 1982.

41. Berkowitz FE: Bacteremia in hospitalized black South African children. A one-year study emphasizing nosocomial bacteremia and bacteremia in severely malnourished children. *Am J Dis Child* 138:551–556, 1984.

42. Munster AM: Septic thrombophlebitis. A surgical disorder. *JAMA* 230:1010–1011, 1974.

43. Cohen J, Donnelly JP, Goldman JM: Bacteremia in neutropenic patients with indwelling venous catheters. Presented at the Third International Symposium on Infections in the Immunocompromised Host, Toronto, Ontario, Canada, June, 1984.

44. Maki DG, Weise CE, Sarafin HW: A semiquantitative culture method for identifying intravenous catheter-related infection. *N Engl J Med* 296:1305–1309, 1977.

45. Archer GL, Karchmer AW, Vishniavsky N, Johnston JL: Plasmid-pattern analysis for the differentiation of infecting from noninfecting *Staphylococcus epidermidis*. *J Infect Dis* 149:913–920, 1984.

46. Gill VJ, Zierdt CH, Wu TC, Stock F, Pizzo PA, MacLowry JD: Comparison of lysis centrifugation with lysis filtration and a conventional unvented bottle for blood cultures. *J Clin Microbiol* 20:927–932, 1984.

47. Raucher HS, Hyatt AC, Barzilai A, Harris MB, Weiner MA, LeLeiko NS, Hodes DS: Quantitative blood cultures in the evaluation of septicemia in children with Broviac catheters. *J Pediatr* 104:29–33, 1984.

48. Bjornson HS, Colley R, Bower RH, Duty VP, Schwartz-Fulton JT, Fischer JE: Association between microorganism growth at the catheter insertion site and colonization of the catheter in patients receiving total parenteral nutrition. *Surgery* 92:720–727, 1982.

49. Zinner SH, Denny-Brown BC, Braun P, Burke JP, Toala P, Kass EH: Risk of infection with intravenous indwelling catheters: effect of application of antibiotic ointment. *J Infect Dis* 120:616–619, 1969.

50. Noble CJ, Morgan-Capner P, Hammer M, Sivyer C, Wagstaff P, Pattison JR: A trial of povidone iodine dry powder spray for the prevention of infusion thrombophlebitis. *J Hosp Infect* 1:47–51, 1980.

51. Thompson DR, Jones GR, Sutton TW: A trial of povidone-iodine ointment for the prevention of cannula thrombophlebitis. *J Hosp Infect* 4:285–289, 1983.

52. Robertson JS, Maraqa MI, Jennett B: Ventriculoperitoneal shunting for hydrocephalus. *Br Med J* 2:289–292, 1973.

53. Schoenbaum SC, Gardner P, Shillito J: Infections of cerebrospinal fluid shunts: epidemiology, clinical manifestations, and therapy. *J Infect Dis* 131:543–552, 1975.

54. Raimondi AJ, Robinson JS, Juwawura K: Complications of ventriculoperitoneal shunting and a critical comparison of the three-piece and one-piece systems. *Childs Brain* 3:321–342, 1977.

55. Yogev R, Davis AT: Neurosurgical shunt infections. A review. *Childs Brain* 6:74–81, 1980.

56. George R, Leibrock L, Epstein M: Long-term analysis of cerebrospinal fluid shunt infections. A 25 year experience. *J Neurosurg* 51:804–811, 1979.

57. McCullough DC, Kane JG, Presper JH, Wells M: Antibiotic prophylaxis in ventricular shunt surgery. I. Reduction of operative infection rates with methicillin. *Childs Brain* 7:182–189, 1980.

58. Nelson JD: Cerebrospinal fluid shunt infections. *Pediatr Infect Dis* 3(Suppl):S30–S32, 1984.

59. Davidoff LM: Treatment of hydrocephalus. Historical review and description of a new method. *Arch Surg* 18:1737–1762, 1929.

60. Matson DD: A new operation for the treatment of communicating hydrocephalus; Report of a case secondary to generalized meningitis. *J Neurosurg* 6:238–247, 1949.

61. Naito H, Toya S, Shizawa H, Iizaka Y, Tsukumo D: High incidence of acute postoperative meningitis and septicemia in patients undergoing craniotomy with ventriculoatrial shunt. *Surg Gynecol Obstet* 137:810–812, 1973.
62. Scarff TB, Nelson PB, Reigel DH: External drainage for ventricular infection following cerebrospinal fluid shunts. *Childs Brain* 4:129–136, 1978.
63. Bayston R, Penny SR: Excessive production of mucoid substance in staphylococcus SIIA: a possible factor in colonization of Holter shunts. *Dev Med Child Neurol* 27(Suppl):25–28, 1972.
64. Strife CF, McDonald BM, Ruley EJ, McAdams AJ, West CD: Shunt nephritis: the nature of the serum cryoglobulins and their relation to the complement profile. *J Pediatr* 88:403–413, 1976.
65. Odio C, McCracken GH, Jr, Nelson JD: CSF shunt infections in pediatrics. A seven year experience. *Am J Dis Child* 138:1103–1108, 1984.
66. Rekate HL, Yonas H, White RJ, Nulsen FE: The acute abdomen in patients with ventriculoperitoneal shunts. *Surg Neurol* 11:442–445, 1979.
67. Hammond WM: Evaluation and use of the ventriculoperitoneal shunt in hydrocephalus. *J Neurosurg* 34:792–795, 1971.
68. Anderson FM: Ventriculocardiac shunts. Identification and control of practical problems in 143 cases. *J Pediatr* 82:222–227, 1973.
69. Hubschmann OR, Countee RW: Gram-positive peritonitis in patients with infected ventriculoperitoneal shunts. *Surg Gynecol Obstet* 149:69–71, 1979.
70. Hubschmann OR, Countee RW: Acute abdomen in children with infected ventriculoperitoneal shunts. *Arch Surg* 115:305–307, 1980.
71. Sells CJ, Shurtleff DB, Loeser JD: Gram-negative cerebrospinal fluid shunt associated infections. *Pediatrics* 59:614–618, 1977.
72. Peters G, Locci R, Pulverer G: Adherence and growth of coagulase-negative staphylococci on surfaces of intravenous catheters. *J Infect Dis* 146:479–482, 1982.
73. O'Brien M, Parent A, Davis B: Management of ventricular shunt infections. *Childs Brain* 5:304–309, 1979.
74. James HE, Walsh JW, Wilson HD, Conner JD, Bean JR, Tibbs PA: Prospective randomized study of therapy in cerebrospinal fluid shunt infection. *Neurosurgery* 7:459–463, 1980.
75. Holt RJ: Bacteriological studies on colonized ventriculoatrial shunts. *Dev Med Child Neurol* 22(Suppl):83–87, 1970.
76. Archer GL, Karchmer AW, Vishniavsky N, Johnston JL: Plasmid-pattern analysis for the differentiation of infecting from noninfecting *Staphylococcus epidermidis*. *J Infect Dis* 149:913–920, 1984.
77. Fokes EC Jr: Occult infections of ventriculoatrial shunts. *J Neurosurg* 33:517–523, 1970.
78. Bruce AM, Lorber J, Shedden WIH, Zachary RB: Persistent bacteraemia following ventriculo-caval shunt operations for hydrocephalus in infants. *Dev Med Child Neurol* 5:461–470, 1963.
79. Yogev R: Cerebrospinal fluid shunt infections: a personal view. *Pediatr Infect Dis* 4:113–118, 1985.
80. Odio C, Umana M, Salas J, McCracken GH: Treatment (Tx) of CSF shunt infections (CSF-SI). Presented at the 26th Interscience Conference on Antimicrobial Agents and Chemotherapy (ICAAC), New Orleans, LA, September 28–October 1, 1986. Abstract No. 867, pp 256.
81. Sekhar LN, Moossy J, Guthkelch AN: Malfunctioning ventriculoperitoneal shunts. Clinical and pathological features. *J Neurosurg* 56:411–416, 1982.
82. Venes JL: Control of shunt infection. Report of 150 consecutive cases. *J Neurosurg* 45:311–314, 1976.
83. Yu HC, Patterson RH Jr: Prophylactic antimicrobial agents after ventriculo-atriostomy for hydrocephalus. *J Pediatr Surg* 8:881–885, 1973.
84. Malis LI: Prevention of neurosurgical infection by intraoperative antibiotics. *Neurosurgery* 5:339–343, 1979.
85. Yogev R, Shinco F, McLone D: Prophylaxis for ventriculoperitoneal shunt surgery with nafcillin alone or in combination with rifampin. Presented at the 23rd Interscience Conference on Antimicrobial Agents and Chemotherapy (ICAAC), Las Vegas, NV, October 24–26, 1983. Abstract No. 664, pp 206.

9

Transfusion-Associated Infection

Naomi L.C. Luban, M.D.

INTRODUCTION

The transfusion of stored blood has been made possible by the development of methods to anticoagulate blood, by classification of donor and recipient groups and types, by cross-matching of blood, and more recently, by improvement in anticoagulants to prolong the shelf life of stored blood. These advances have resulted in a serologically and metabolically safe product for the recipient. Despite these advances, we have a new problem to deal with; that is, transfusion-transmitted diseases. In the 1940s, posttransfusion syphilis was a major worry; in the 1950s, "serum" hepatitis was further classified, and in the 1960s, etiological agents for hepatitis were identified. While significant advances in characterizing hepatitis A and B continued through the 1970s, non-A/non-B hepatitis as a transfusion-transmitted disease was described by default and continues to be an enigma that defies identification and prevention. The 1980s is the decade of cytomegalovirus (CMV) and human immunodeficiency virus (HTLV III/LAV/HIV). In this chapter, diseases transmitted by blood transfusion will be reviewed with an emphasis on donor screening and the use of different types of products to decrease morbidity and mortality from transfusion-transmitted disease.

BACKGROUND

Bacteria

The pathogenesis of transfusion-transmitted disease covers a wide range of organisms, including bacteria, viruses [hepatitis A, hepatitis B, non-A/non-B hepatitis (NANB), Epstein-Barr Virus (EBV), cytomegalovirus (CMV), human immunodeficiency virus (HIV], malarial, and nonmalarial parasites.

Bacterial infections secondary to blood transfusion are uncommon in the United States for several reasons. These include the careful cleansing of the donor's intravenous site with bacteriostatic agents, use of closed systems of blood collection, i.e., the use of sterile, disposable plastic blood bags with integral needles and tubing, and the storage of blood in precisely temperature-controlled refrigerators. Breaks in the protocol of collection, storage, or administration can result in bacterial contamination of blood and blood products, and can produce sepsis in the transfusion recipient. Examples of sources of contamination include inadequate preparation of the donor venipuncture site, contact contamination of the needle or tubing, prolonged storage at temperatures greater than 6°, or manipulation of the product. Examples of this latter phenomena include pooling of platelets or reconstitution of packed cells, wherein bacteria may be introduced during the preparation despite the sterility of the initial product.

The prevalence of bacterial-induced transfusion-transmitted disease is thought to be very low; 0.1% or less of all transfusions will result in clinically recognized bacterial disease (1). However, some cases may go unrecognized secondary to difficulty in diagnosis, and to the concomitant administration of antibiotics in patients also receiving contaminated blood. In 1980, Myhre reported on fatalities induced by transfusion: only 2 of 77 deaths in a 3-year period were attributable to bacterial contamination (2). The case fatality rate from bacterial contamination increased dramatically from 1985–1986 (3) due predominantly to contaminated platelets. Data by Buchholz et al. in the early 1970s demonstrated a 2.4% incidence of contaminated single donor platelets, and the frequency of bacterial recovery in platelet concentrates stored at 22° increased with increasing storage time (4). These data and those of others refuting it (5,6) were considered with new data provided by manufacturers when the Food and Drug Administration (FDA) agreed to license 22° stored platelet concentrates for 7-day storage in 1984. Following an increase in case fatality reports and growing published accounts of fatal and nonfatal sepsis secondary to platelet transfusion, (7–11) only 5-day storage is currently allowed. Sepsis from platelet contamination has also been reported in products collected by plateletpheresis. Four cases occurred in patients receiving plateletpheresis-collected platelets from one donor; two of these cases were in children (8). Pooling of platelets was not a source of contamination in this study. Further investigation revealed that the pheresis donor had dimpling at the site of repetitive venipuncture; coagulase-negative staphylococci grew repeatedly in blood samples obtained from the dimpling site, but not from the other antecubital fossa. Four additional donors with dimpling were cultured through the dimpling site which had been prepared with Iodaphore, and bacterial growth was observed in 5 of 7 occasions (8). Pediatric cases of sepsis from platelet concentrates are reviewed in Table 9.1.

Other sources of contamination of blood products may occur during storage and handling. These include failure to change intravenous lines, inadequate preparation of the *recipient* venipuncture site, use of unrefrigerated or inadequately refrigerated blood, and contaminated pumps or transfusion devices. The standards set by the American Association of Blood Banks for transfusion of previously refrigerated products are based on the concept that bacteria will proliferate in blood when warmed over time even when closed, plastic bag systems are used (12). Thus, established standards state that blood must be maintained at between 1–6°C continuously, and must not be warmed and recooled; blood should not be reused if it has been out of a controlled refrigerator for more than 30 minutes. When it is anticipated that multiple units of blood will be transfused, adequate cold storage must be assured. In a pediatric setting, this might involve use of one of several integrally attached bags from a quadruple or triple pack.

A series of transfusion-transmitted bacterial septicemias demonstrate the difficulty in evaluating the cause of the contamination. Five cases of pseudomonas sepsis (*Ps. fluorescence* in four and *Ps. putida* in one) were fully evaluated by the FDA. Despite the fact that the units of blood causing these episodes (two of which were fatal) were collected at the same regional blood collection facility, no specific etiology could be defined (13). In a second series, *Yersinia enterocolitica* was isolated post-transfusion from two recipients (14). Donor testing revealed titers to the H and O antigens of *Yersinia*, but no organisms grew in the one donor cultured. Manipulation of a unit to simulate bacteremia was done; in addition, experiments performed to make antisera to the H and O antigens produced a temperature-dependent growth curve, implying that the length of time the organism is held at 22° may determine the virulence of the organism when it is later stored and transfused (14).

Brucellosis has also been reported as a transfusion-transmitted organism. Interestingly, 7 of

Table 9.1
Pediatric Cases of Bacteremia from Platelet Concentrates[a]

Case No.	Ages (yr)	Product	Underlying Disease	Organism	Outcome	Reference
1	6	Plt	ALL	Salmonella Cholera suis	Bacteremia recurrent	7
2	3	Plt	Wiscott-Aldrich	Salmonella Cholera suis	Bacteremia recurrent	7
3	10	Plt	Aplastic anemia	*Serratia marcescens*	Bacteremia	10
4	5	Pheresis	Neuroblastoma	*S. aureus*	Bacteremia	9
5	6	Pheresis	Aplastic anemia	*Enterococcus*	Bacteremia	9
6	13	Plt	ALL, marrow transplant	*S. epidermidis*	Bacteremia septic shock	11

[a]Age under 13 years.
Plt, platelet concentrate; ALL, acute lymphoblastic leukemia; pheresis, plateletpheresis unit.

the 10 reported cases have been in children. Two carefully reported cases were in splenectomized children with Thalassemia major who were being maintained on regular transfusion programs. The asymptomatic donor was a farmer who had contact with goats and cattle (15). Although rarely reported in the United States, the potential for transmission, especially in areas endemic for brucella, warrants concern, especially in view of a study from the University of Minnesota, where almost 2% of acceptable blood donors had brucella agglutinins of 1:160 or higher, titers which are diagnostic for active brucellosis (16).

The spirochete *Treponema pallidum* does not survive in blood that has been refrigerated at 4° for 72 hours. Thus, no cases of *T. pallidum* have been reported following transfusion of stored blood (1). *T. pallidum* can, however, survive in unrefrigerated blood products, such as platelet and granulocyte concentrates, fresh unrefrigerated, or short-term refrigerated blood; use of such products may occur in neonatal or pediatric patients requiring open-heart surgery, infants with sepsis, older immunocompromised children, or those with traumatic injuries where fresh blood and platelet concentrates might be used. Frozen blood and frozen plasma do not appear to transmit *T. pallidum* (1). Most cases of transmission are historical in nature; they have occurred in individuals who were asymptomatic, prior to appearance of a chancre and prior to positive serological testing. The donor usually had active primary syphilis, although rare cases of donors with latent-stage infection were documented in the 1930s.

A number of additional bacterial organisms have been reported to produce post-transfusion morbidity. Some may be inactivated or removed by the reticuloendothelial system or by the transfusion recipient's own immunological response. In other cases, the immunological status of the recipient may be compromised, permitting fatal sepsis despite modest bacterial growth in the product. Because blood (but not platelets) is stored in the cold, psychrophilic organisms are more common. Because citrate is used as one component of the anticoagulant solution, those organisms that can use citrate as a carbon source are more likely to be isolated (17). Table 9.2 reviews bacterial organisms that have been reported to be transmitted by blood with their associated clinical infection.

Two pediatric circumstances require special comment in regard to bacteria and transfusion. Neonatal patients in extremis may be administered placental transfusions in the delivery room. Blood is removed from the umbilical vein of the placenta into a heparinized syringe, filtered and infused directly into the infant (18). Evaluation of sterility of the "autologous" placental blood has been done by two investigators aware of the potential for contamination. One study demonstrated a 9.7% incidence of bacterial growth, with mixed aerobic and anaerobic species and was conservative in its endorsement of this practice (19). In another study, the use of two bacteriostatic cleansing agents to prepare the vessels were compared: a 2.9% contamination rate was observed with one agent, while 5.8% was noted with another (20). The primary organisms isolated were Gaffkya species, *Staphylococcus epidermidis*, and another unclassifiable anaerobic organism.

Necrotizing enterocolitis (NEC) is a disease of multifactorial etiology and pathogenesis, usually affecting the newborn. There are 2000–4000 newborns diagnosed with NEC each year in the United States (21), many of whom are of low birthweight. Gastrointestinal mucosal injury may result in or occur because of bacterial overgrowth. The result is an enterocolitis with or without sepsis, which may require surgical intervention to remove the diseased bowel. Certain bacteria that have been isolated in cases of NEC, specifically pneumococcus and certain isolates of clostridium, are known to produce an extracellular neuraminidase that can remove N-acetylneuraminic acid from the red blood cell surface and expose the Thomsen-Friedenreich cryptantigen. This phenomena is called T activation. Antibodies to this antigen are naturally occurring, IgM antibodies to an oligosaccharide determinant and are found routinely in human adult plasma. Several investigators have described hemolysis following transfusion of plasma and plasma-containing products to infants (22–25) and older children (22) who have T activation. Despite a well-defined etiology for this syndrome, its exact incidence is unknown.

Parasites

Two major groups of parasites have been responsible for transfusion-transmitted diseases: babesiosis and malaria. Although other parasites and helminthic disease have been reported to

Table 9.2.
Bacteria, Viruses, and Parasites Known to be Transmitted by Blood[a]

Class	Products Involved	Incubation	Clinical Highlights
Bacteria			
Gram-negative and Gram-positive	RBC PLT stored greater than 80 hours	hours—1 day	Rapid onset fever, malaise, chills, circulatory collapse, DIC
Brucellosis	WB RBC	6 days–4 months	Headache, muscle pain, malaise, remitting fever, LAD, HSP, arthritis
Treponema pallidum	PLT WBC Unrefrigerated WB, RBC	4–14 weeks	Skin lesion
Parasites			
Babesia microti	PLT RBC Frozen RBC	4–6 weeks	Fever, malaise, myalgia, DIC
Malaria	RBC PLT WBC Fresh plasma Frozen RBC	8 days–3 months	Fever (paroxysmal or periodic), malaise, myalgia, abdominal pain
Viruses			
Hepatitis A	WB/RBC/FFP	22–30 days	Fever, malaise, jaundice myalgia, arthralgia
Hepatitis B	All products ?All products	14–280 days	Fever, malaise, jaundice, myalgia, arthralgia,
Non-A/non-B	?All products	6–8 weeks	Fever, malaise, hepatic necrosis, acute icteric hepatitis, acute and chronic hepatitis, chronic carrier state, cirrhosis
CMV	WB/RBC/PLT/WBC	2–6 weeks	"Mono-like" illness
EBV	WB/RBC/PLT/WBC	3—7 weeks	Fever, anorexia, fatigue, pharyngitis, malaise; hepatitis; LAD; HSP
HIV	WB/RBC/PLT/WRBC/FFP	2–8 weeks	Fever, malaise, "mono-like" illness; Late onset with LAD, HSP, FUO, thrombocytopenia, FTT, diarrhea

ALT, alanine aminotransferase; CF, complement fixation; CMV, cytomegalovirus; DIC, disseminated intravascular coagulation; EA, early antigen to Epstein-Barr; anti-EBNA, Epstein-Barr nuclear antigen; FFP, fresh frozen plasma; Frozen RBC, frozen deglycerolized red blood cells; FTA, fluorescent treponema antibody; FTT, failure to thrive; FUO, fever of unknown origin; HAVAB, hepatitis A virus antibody; anti-HBcore, antibody to hepatitis B core antigen; HBsAG, hepatitis B surface antigen; HIV, human immunode-

Table 9.2
cont.

Treatment	Detection	Prevention
Antibiotics, fluids, Shock protocol	1. Gram stain and culture unit with 10 ml or more in anaerobic and aerobic media 2. Culture patient	1. Sterility of collection processing and administration 2. Strict donor exclusion criteria
Cotrimoxazol-streptomycin-tetracycline	1. Culture donor and recipient 2. IFA, CF, or tube agglutination antibody titer	1. Screen donor and exclude if 1:1000 agglutination titer 2. Donor exclusion for endemic area
Penicillin	1. Darkfield examination spirochetes 2. STS + FTA-ABS in serum of donor and recipient	1. Use refrigerated products in cold for 3 days or more 2. STS or FTA testing, of all blood products
Exchange transfusion Clindamycin phosphatequinine Pentamidine	1. Microscopic exam for intraerythrocytic forms 2. Indirect IFA assay 3. Hamster inoculation	1. Use donors from nonendemic areas 2. Screen blood microscopically or by antibody test
Chloroquine-primaquine	1. Microscopic exam for parasites, q 8 h, thick and thin, Wrights' and Giemsa 2. IFA for persistent or cured infection	1. Strict donor exclusion criteria based on travel, medication history
No definitive therapies available	HAVAB IgG, HAVAB IgM	1. Donor exclusion for history travel, prodromal disease
	HBsAg, anti-HBc	1. Donor exclusion by history 2. Voluntary blood only 3. HBsAg testing of all blood products
	Exclusion of other causes	1. Donor exclusion with surrogate testing (anti-HBc and ALT)
	1. CMV-IgM, CMV-IgG 2. Culture of urine, blood, buffy coat, multiple times	1. CMV seronegative product 2. Deglycerolization of RBC 3. Leukodepletion techniques
	1. Microscopic exam for atypical lymphs 2. IgM-anti-VCA, IgG-EA, anti-EBNA 3. Culture	1. Donor exclusion for history and prodomal disease
	1. Anti-HIV, Western blot 2. Immunological testing	1. Donor exclusion for risk factors and medical history 2. Anti-HIV testing of all blood products 3. Surrogate tests

ficiency virus; IFA, immunofluorescence; LAD, lymphadenopathy; PLT, platelet concentrates; RBC, red blood cells; STS, serological test for syphilis; anti-VCA, antiviral capsid antigen; WB, whole blood; WBC, white blood cell concentrates; WRBC, washed red blood cells.

cause disease, including species of filariae, toxoplasmosis, *Borrelia*, and others, they are highly unlikely to occur in the United States with current donor screening (26).

In contrast to the bacteria *T. pallidum*, *Babesia microti* withstands refrigeration in stored blood. In the United States, babesiosis is transmitted by *Ixodes dammini* ticks, which are endemic to the Northeastern coastal region. The first transfusion-transmitted case was reported in 1980 following platelet transfusion into an elderly man who had been splenectomized and was receiving steroids; the donor of one of the platelet units had an anti-B microti titer of 1:256 (27). Four additional cases have now been reported, (28–31) including one premature infant (28) and a young woman with Thalassemia major (29) who received frozen-thawed, deglycerolized red blood cells. In both reports, the donors had vacationed on Fire Island and had experienced tick bites. In each case, red blood cell transfusions were implicated, and there was difficulty in making the diagnosis. Transfusion-induced malaria was the most frequently considered diagnosis.

Transfusion-transmitted malaria presenting from infection with the intraerythrocyte plasmodia has been recognized since 1911. The increase in emigration and air travel from areas with endemic malaria might lead to greater numbers of expected cases (26). A comparison of the epidemiology of transfusion malaria in two different time periods reveals that differences in U.S. donor sources are responsible for the increase in transfusion-related disease. From 1967–1971, 6.4 transfusion-transmitted cases per year were reported, reflecting donors who were returning military personnel from Southeast Asia, who accounted for 66% of the cases. From 1972–1981, 2.6 cases per year were reported; most of these donors were foreign-born. For all years, there was an equal distribution of the three major *Plasmodium* species, although two of the four fatal cases were due to *P. malariae* (32). Transfusional malaria has most frequently been reported following red blood cell transfusion, but platelets, white blood cells, and fresh plasma have also been implicated (33–36). Platelets and granulocyte concentrates are known to have red blood cell contamination and may account for the source, although plasmodia have also been seen inside platelets, suggesting that the platelets themselves might be capable of transmitting the disease (33). Frozen plasma has not been implicated, but frozen red blood cells have been (34). Of the 26 cases reported in a case control study, two were infants and two were children. Two additional premature infants (35) and seven transfusion-dependent Thalassemic patients have also been reported (34).

Other parasites known to be transmitted by blood transfusion, but which are rare in the United States, include *Trypanosoma cruzi*, *Wuchereria bancrofti*, *Loa loa*, and *Toxoplasma gondii*. Transfusion-transmitted disease from these organisms are not at all uncommon in certain parts of the world and have been recently reviewed (26).

Viruses

The greatest source of mortality and morbidity from transfusion is from viruses contained in blood and blood products. Changes in medical practice have exacerbated viral transfusion-transmitted diseases in recent years. These include the use of blood products from plasma pools obtained from thousands of donors and the treatment of highly immunosuppressed patients. The use of plasma pools for the manufacture of factor concentrate has resulted in dramatically improved care for the hemophiliac community. By virtue of manufacturing processes, however, one contaminated pool may produce disease in hundreds of recipients of a single lot. Treatment of patients with malignancy, aplastic and hypoplastic anemia, and the increase in solid organ and bone marrow transplants has resulted in a useful albeit dangerous therapeutic approach to these patients: extensive immunosuppression- and/or chemotherapy-induced aplasia followed by supportive care from the blood bank by replacement of cellular components. When exposed to viruses in blood and blood components, many of these patients develop overwhelming and occasionally fatal viral diseases. Historically, perhaps the greatest donor factor accounting for viral transmitted disease was the use of commercial blood donors. In most areas of the United States, this is now a defunct practice. Current donor factors predisposing to viral carriage are less clearly defined, as donors are usually healthy, asymptomatic, and give their blood voluntarily. The viral agents usually have the characteristics of long incubation periods and prolonged, high level of viremia. They also produce mild subclinical infection in the donor. Latent infection in certain peripheral blood cells e.g., lymphocytes, which are stable during processing of the stored blood product, or viruses, which are present in plasma or sera alone, are both capable of transmitting viral transmitted diseases.

Cell-Free or Plasma Viruses: Hepatitis B Virus, Hepatitis A Virus, and Non-A/Non-B

Hepatitis B virus (HBV) infection following the inoculation of contaminated human blood or plasma has been recognized since the late 19th century (37). In 1964, the etiological agent for hepatitis B was discovered. Hepatitis B surface antigen or HBsAg, and additional surface antigens and serum antibodies to this 42 nm virus and its determinants have been characterized in Chapter 14. In 1970, it was demonstrated that a major risk for acquisition of hepatitis B was receipt of a HBsAg-positive unit of blood (38). Shortly thereafter, Alter and colleagues demonstrated an 85% reduction in post-transfusion hepatitis when both HBsAg-positive and commercial blood doors were excluded (39). Federal requirements mandate that all blood and blood products be tested for HBsAg by a sensitive third-generation test, capable of detecting weakly positive samples. Thus, the only cases of post-transfusion hepatitis B would result from an asymptomatic, chronically infected donor who has HBs antigenemia at a level too low for detection with current methodology. The exact number of such individuals is unknown, but is estimated by one study to be about 0.6% (40). Several factors increase the seroprevalence rate among individuals who might be blood donors. These include sexual promiscuity, lower socioeconomic class, employment in an occupation where contact with body fluids is likely, and presence in the household of an HBsAg-positive individual, regardless of the relationship between them (1).

Tests for detection of hepatitis A virus (HAV) were developed in 1973 (41). Shortly thereafter, it was recognized that most cases of post-transfusion hepatitis not caused by hepatitis B were also not caused by hepatitis A (42,43). A newly recognized post-transfusion hepatitis, non-A/non-B (NANB) was defined. Using voluntary donor blood, negative for HBsAg, several investigators (40,43,45) described a post-transfusion hepatitis incidence between 7–17%, and 90% of these cases were attributable to NANB. Since 1980, most prospective NANB studies have been done outside of the United States, where hepatitis incidences between 3–44% have been reported, again with the majority being due to NANB (37). NANB has been transmitted by transfusion of blood, blood products, and by plasma derivatives (46); formalin heat treatment destroys infectivity, while lyophilization and freezing do not (47). Nonparenteral transmission is thought to account for the high prevalence among healthy blood donors. In contrast to hepatitis A or B, close contact with an infected person does not transmit clinically significant disease (48).

The etiology of NANB may be one or more agents. This is based on differences in clinical presentation and presumed incubation periods. Both short incubation (1–5 weeks) and long incubation (7–12 weeks) disease has been described, and more than one virus has been suggested by studies performed in both hemophiliac patients and monkeys. The candidate serological assays for the elusive virus(es) have been reviewed extensively (49–51). A diagnosis of NANB can be made only after serological studies have excluded hepatitis A, hepatitis B, cytomegalovirus, Epstein-Barr virus, varicella-zoster, and herpes-simplex as infectious causes, and the exclusion of disease and drug-related etiologies for the usually mild increase in liver function abnormalities. Although mild disease is seen in most cases, in greater than 50% of cases there may be chronic alanine aminotransferase (ALT) elevations. Some 10% of these individuals may develop cirrhosis (37).

A large, unique, and often-quoted national study reported that between 5–15% of recipients of 1–5 units of blood transfused in the United States may develop NANB hepatitis (38,40). This study involved recipients 16 years or older. Another large study of Veterans Administration hospitals similarly had no pediatric cases. Thus, the incidence of post-transfusion NANB, HBV, and HAV has not been evaluated in pediatric patients, despite the fact that sick premature and older hospitalized children frequently receive greater than five donor exposures per hospitalization (52,53).

Data do exist for some viral-induced post-transfusion complications in selected pediatric populations and are usually reported as single case reports. These include Thalassemic patients, hemophiliacs, and infants in intensive care units. A case of a 10-year-old girl who received one unit of packed cells during open-heart surgery provided the first clear evidence of transmission of HAV from donor to a pediatric recipient (54); this was based on electron microscopic and HAV antigen isolation from the donor's liver. Chimpanzee studies (54) suggested the cause to be transmission via plasma. One case of transmission by fresh frozen plasma in an older individual (55) supported the concept that hepatitis can be transmitted via a number of blood derivatives. Since then, a total of 20 infants in five studies have been reported with post-transfusion HAV occurring secondary to whole blood exchange (56), and packed cell transfusions (55–58).

Serological studies in Thalassemic patients have most frequently come from Europe (59–63) and one each from Singapore and Saudi Arabia (64,65), with only two major U.S. studies (66,67). In the largest and most comprehensive serological study of 128 children evaluated over 4 years, all children age 12 and older had evidence of HBV infection, and 23 episodes of NANB hepatitis were observed (59). Based on biopsies performed for chronic alanine aminotransferase elevations in another study, chronic liver disease was present in 32% of Thalassemic children, likely due to NANB (62).

Most recently, a study of 25 American Thalassemic patients failed to demonstrate seroconversion to anti-HBs (67). This outcome stands in direct contrast to a previous U.S. study where 48% of Thalassemic patients had anti-HBs or HBsAg (66). The use of exclusively volunteer blood in the current study and a higher prevalence of HBsAg in foreign communities probably account for the differences described in different studies. Unfortunately, the Pearson study did not evaluate either HAV serology or chronic ALT elevations; thus a current assessment of HAV or NANB status in the U.S. Thalassemics receiving voluntary blood has not yet been performed.

There is extensive literature on the development of HBV and NANB in hemophiliac patients. Greater than 70% of patients with hemophilia who have received transfusions, especially with pooled products, have antibody against HBsAG, and 40–50% have elevated alanine aminotransferase concentrations (68,69). Between 5–7% of patients with hemophilia are chronic carriers of HBsAg (68,70,71). In a study by Spero and associates, of 13 hemophiliac children who underwent liver biopsy because of chronic alanine aminotransferase elevations, 8 had clinically persistent hepatitis; 2 had chronic active hepatitis; and 2 had postnecrotic cirrhosis (70). In an effort to protect children from acquisition of HBs antigenemia, the National Hemophilia Foundation recommends that patients with only anti-HBs or who are HBsAg-negative, receive passive immunization with hepatitis B vaccine (personal communication).

Even young hemophiliac children exposed to factor concentrate have a higher incidence of liver function abnormalities (70%) than do children treated with cryoprecipitate alone (40%). At least 50% of these children had liver function abnormalities, but only 30% had serological evidence of HBV, suggesting that other agents might be responsible (72). Those family members living in a household with a young hemophiliac child with evidence of prior hepatitis B infection are also at risk for developing positive hepatitis markers and may be infectious to others (73,74).

Cell-Associated Viruses: Cytomegalovirus, Epstein-Barr Virus, Human Immunodeficiency Virus

Cytomegalovirus and Epstein-Barr Virus

There are five herpes virus family agents: herpes simplex I and II, varicella-zoster virus, Epstein-Barr virus (EBV), and cytomegalovirus (CMV). All four viruses are spread by cell-to-cell association and may result in virus in the extracellular phase. Antibody is present, despite the presence of intracellular virus.

Both CMV and EBV are widely distributed in mammalian species and are presumed to produce latent infection. While EBV is known to produce latent infection of B lymphocytes, the cells harboring CMV are less well-characterized, but are likely to be peripheral blood elements, most likely in the white blood cell line. Both CMV and EBV are difficult to isolate from banked blood (75–77). Because active CMV infection can result from the transfusion of CMV seropositive blood from which virus cannot be uncovered, CMV meets the criteria for latency. Additional studies in CMV antibody-positive transplant patients and other patients requiring immunosuppression support the concept that reactivation of latent virus can occur (78). CMV has also been transmitted by transplantation of the liver, heart, and bone marrow. One group has suggested that rather than an immature or infective immune system, allogeneic stimulation of latently infected blood into allogeneic and syngeneic recipients results in reactivation of the virus (79). This theory, based on a murine model, has not been reproduced in human in vitro experiments (80,81).

There is a high prevalence of CMV seropositivity which varies geographically; in addition, exposure to the virus as evidenced by CMV seropositivity increases with age and lower socioeconomic conditions. In some studies, seroprevalence rates in healthy blood donors of 70% have been reported for CMV (82). Similarly, EBV antibody prevalence increases with age, and more than 90% of blood donors have antibodies to EBV (83). With such a high rate of antibody prevalence, and the fact that latent virus has the ability to actively infect the host, there must be several factors to attenuate this infectivity in stored blood. These include the viability of the infected lymphocyte (or other white blood cells) during storage (84); the immune status of the recipient—both cellular and humoral immune status; and the presence of immune or neutralizing antibody along with the virus containing lymphocyte in the transfusion product. Despite these caveats, the risk of transmission of CMV has been estimated to range from 2.7–12% per unit in one study (85).

The risk of transmission for EBV has not been studied by number of units transfused or by product. Certain data are, however, available on EBV transmission. Following transfusion to patients without pre-existing antibody to EBV, 33–46% of individuals may develop evidence of transfusion-transmitted infection (84,86). In those individuals having pre-existing antibody who then receive blood, approximately 5% may develop an elevation of antibody titer, suggesting either reinfection or reactivation (87).

Transfusion-transmitted EBV has rarely been reported in pediatric patients. Twenty-five seronegative pediatric open-heart surgery patients were serially followed for 6–12 months postoperatively. Twenty-three patients had evidence of passively transferred antibody, which subsequently declined in titer; one patient with Down's syndrome demonstrated what was felt to be true seroconversion 63 days following exposure, but with only an IgG and no IgM response (83). Two additional pediatric cardiac patients were reported by Kääriäinen as part of a study of five seronegative patients; one of the two children had asymptomatic serologically definable disease (86). Papaevangelou et al. documented a 76.4% frequency of antiviral capsid antigen (anti-VCA) in 149 polytransfused Thalassemic children, as compared with 69.8% in age matched controls. There was no evidence of acute mononucleosis-like illness in their patient population or matched controls; they concluded that the incidence of post-transfusion EBV was very low (63). Pearson et al. also evaluated anti-VCA in 25 Thalassemic children and found an incidence of 82%; the prevalence of anti-VCA was felt to be age-appropriate and unrelated to transfusion (67). One report is of a putatively infected donor who developed mononucleosis 3 days after donation and whose red cells were frozen, deglycerolized, and eventually transfused to three neonates. The neonates demonstrated no serological evidence of disease when studied acutely and at 3 months post-transfusion (88). An EBV-like disease without serological markers for EBV was reported in five patients with leukemia receiving granulocyte concentrates. CMV was excluded in these children (89).

Transfusion-associated CMV has been observed among heart surgery patients, infants, and children with chemotherapy-induced immunosuppression and those with congenital immunosuppression, children receiving kidney and marrow transplantation, and a subgroup of neonates. Post-transfusion CMV has been reported with the use of whole blood, packed cells, platelets, and white blood cells. It has not been seen when frozen deglycerolized red cells were used (90–92), with one exception (93). There is controversy over whether washed red blood cells will prevent post-transfusion CMV (see below) (94,95).

Post-transfusion CMV may be asymptomatic, may result in a mild, self-limited febrile illness or may result in an infectious, mononucleosis-like syndrome. CMV may also produce pneumonia, pericarditis, hepatitis, and encephalitis; the more severe symptoms occur more frequently in the immunosuppressed patient. Some authors have hypothesized that CMV may also *produce* immunosuppression and result in increased susceptibility to other bacterial and viral diseases. This is primarily based on the data demonstrating absolute decrease in T-helper cells and the increase in T-suppressor cells for as long as 10 months following acute primary CMV infection (92) and the association between CMV and AIDS (96).

The association between transfusion and CMV was first reported in 1960 by Kreel and associates, who described a "postperfusion" syndrome in patients who underwent cardiopulmonary bypass with fever, lymphocytosis, and splenomegaly occurring 3–8 weeks following the procedure (97). Prince et al. and many others reported that blood transfusion was the cause of the CMV infection (98). This has been further supported by large numbers of studies (reviewed in 78, 99, 100).

Three basic types of CMV infection can occur. These include primary infection, reactivation, and secondary infection. Primary infection occurs in the seronegative individual who is exposed to the virus for the first time. Reactivation occurs in individuals who are seropositive but who are not actively shedding virus when studied initially. Reactivation is demonstrated by resumption of active viral replication and may be associated with a rise in titers to IgG antibodies. Secondary infection occurs in seropositive individuals who become reinfected with a different strain of virus. It is demonstrated by a clear-cut increase in IgG antibody titer, isolation of shed virus, and more importantly, by demonstrating differences in DNA genome or the presence of more than one strain of CMV by restriction endonuclease analysis. There are no adequate estimates of the frequency of reinfection or reactivation in post-transfusion CMV, but the estimates for primary infection range from 2.5–12% per transfused unit (85, 90, 99).

CMV as a post-transfusion complication in pediatrics was first suggested by McCracken and McEnery in infants who underwent exchange transfusion and developed a post-transfusion syndrome with fever, respiratory distress, hepatosplenomegaly, and CMV viruria; one infant had disseminated CMV on autopsy (101, 102). In another study, seronegative mothers who underwent multiple intrauterine transfusions, some of which were from seropositive donors, delivered infants who developed CMV viruria. This was the first study to establish a causal link between exchange transfusion and acquisition of CMV in seronegative mothers and infants (103). Additional observations by Kumar, Pass, Tobin, and others in infants who received exchange transfusions from seropositive donors supports seroconversion CMV in infants, but there is little associated morbidity or mortality (104–106). The incidence of seroconversion in premature infants receiving unscreened blood and blood products is between 10–30%, based on the several studies published to date, while estimates of infectivity of a seropositive unit vary between 3–15% (78).

In contrast to full-term infants and children, premature infants have a higher likelihood of excreting CMV. It should be noted that premature infants are likely to receive multiple small transfusions from many donors. An early study by Yeager reported on acquisition of postnatal CMV disease in six preterm infants where transfusion was thought to be the cause (107). This prompted a large prospective study of 164 seronegative infants; 0 of 90 seronegative infants receiving seronegative blood shed CMV, while 10 of 74 seronegative infants receiving at least one seropositive unit shed CMV and seroconverted (13.5%). Factors associated with acquisition of CMV were weight less than 1250 g, receipt of greater than 50 ml of seropositive blood, and lack of maternal antibody (108). Similar conclusions were reached by Adler (90).

In the studies published to date, the symptoms and signs of post-transfusion CMV are difficult to attribute to CMV alone and not to complications of prematurity. To attribute respiratory distress, pneumonia, and hepatosplenomegaly to CMV alone requires demonstration of the virus in the tissue in question—an infrequent occurrence, unless autopsy has been obtained. Thus, the extent of morbidity from post-transfusion CMV is difficult to obtain. Mortality data are similarly sketchy. In one study of eight seronegative infants of less than 1200 g, three deaths occurred, and one was autopsied; CMV was demonstrated in lung and liver (109). In another study, four deaths in seven low-birthweight infants occurred, and CMV was thought to be causative in two of the deaths; CMV was recovered in the lungs of one infant (91). Nevertheless, the concurrence of CMV viruria and seroconversion in transfused, seronegative infants is felt to be of sufficient concern. Indeed, the American Association of Blood Banks has mandated the processing of transfusion products to ameliorate this circumstance in seronegative infants or those of unknown serological status (12). Those infants who are seropositive and are made seronegative by repetitive transfusion of seronegative products are at risk for symptomatic CMV disease acquired from their seropositive mothers. This suggests that passively transferred antibody from mother to infant is protective and may attenuate or prevent perinatally acquired CMV (110). Importantly, those low-birthweight infants who were seropositive and those of birthweight greater than 1250 g have not demonstrated morbidity or mortality following receipt of seropositive units, unless they receive exclusively seronegative products. Transfusing infants with exclusively seronegative products may produce an essentially seronegative infant who is then at risk for nosocomial acquisition of CMV (110).

Organ transplant recipients are another group at risk for acquisition of post-transfusion CMV. Studies evaluating pediatric recipients alone have not been performed, so one must extrapolate from adult data. Seronegative recipients who receive kidneys from seronegative donors rarely develop CMV (111), while those seronegative recipients receiving seropositive kidneys frequently develop symptoms. The disease is most likely to be severe because of the recipients' immunosuppressed condition. The impact of pretransplant transfusion on CMV antibody status and degree of clinical disease is not clear (112–114). Cardiac transplantation has been more easily studied. Again, CMV infection was not demonstrated in seronegative individuals receiving seronegative hearts. Seronegative recipients receiving seropositive hearts became infected (115) and in a different study had an increased risk of infection with bacteria and fungi. Of five seronegative recipients receiving seronegative hearts but unscreened blood, one became infected (116). In bone marrow transplant recipients, CMV is the major cause of morbidity and the most common infectious cause of death. While most seropositive patients develop reactivation of their latent virus, seronegative patients may acquire it from bone marrow or blood products, with an incidence of 40% (117). In a recent study by Bowden and associates, 97 seronegative individuals prior to transplant received either intravenous (i.v.) CMV immunoglobulin (CMV i.v. IgG) and seronegative blood and blood

products, seronegative products alone, CMV i.v. IgG alone, or neither treatment. The incidence of infection as determined by virological culture and weekly serologic determinations was 5%, 13%, 24%, and 40% respectively. The use of seronegative blood did not prevent CMV infection among patients who received a seropositive marrow donor (118).

There are a few studies that address posttransfusion CMV in the child with leukemia and cancer. Seroconversion rates of 13–16% were reported in leukemic children given a mean of three random transfusions (119). In another study, children with acute lymphoblastic leukemia (ALL) who were viremic and viruric were more heavily transfused than those who were not viremic. An overall prevalence rate of 30% for CMV antibody was reported (120). Because units of blood were not tested and because not all of the children were seronegative prior to transfusion it is difficult to know how much of the viremia was reactivation of latent virus and how much was truly transfusion transmitted. Based on the much greater numbers of adult leukemia and solid tumor patients who are transfused and remain asymptomatic for CMV, post-transfusion CMV has no or limited associated morbidity or mortality. Splenectomy added to immunosuppression, however, may place an individual at greater risk (121). Five splenectomized young men who had traumatic injuries in two separate studies all acquired post-transfusion CMV with significant mortality (20%) and morbidity (40%) (121, 122).

Human immunodeficiency virus

Human immunodeficiency virus (HIV) is a human retrovirus now considered to be the etiologic agent causing acquired immunodeficiency disease (AIDS), aids related complex (ARC), and asymptomatic HIV infection. As of March 9, 1987, the Centers for Disease Control (CDC) had reported 31,526 total cases of AIDS, of which 602 (2%) were related to HIV-contaminated blood, and 266 were in adult hemophiliacs. An additional 51 transfusion-related and 24 hemophiliac cases have been reported in children. When compared with the 364 children who acquired the disease from infected parents, the percentage of children with transfusion-transmitted AIDS is small. The stringent CDC classification system has likely excluded large numbers of children who would otherwise be accepted. For example, children with primary immunodeficiency, malignancy, or malnutrition who received blood and blood products contaminated with HIV would be excluded based on the CDC case definition of pediatric AIDS (123). There are also no published estimates of the number of children who are HIV-positive and asymptomatic, who have ARC, or who may be excluded based on the stringent CDC criteria.

Post-transfusion HIV has been reported following the transfusion of red blood cells, frozen deglycerolized red blood cells, fresh frozen plasma, cryoprecipitate, platelets, and pooled plasma products to neonates, children receiving few or many transfusions, those who have normal immunity, and those who are immunocompromised. Passive acquisition of positive antibody status has been demonstrated following transfusion of i.v. immunoglobulin prepared by either reduction and alkylation or by acid and pepsin treatment (124). Both enzyme-linked immunosorbent assay (ELISA) and Western blot positivity were demonstrated in 15 out of 45 paired samples. By 28 days postinfusion, ELISA and blots became negative (124). The safety of other immunoglobulin preparations was addressed in an *MMWR* publication which reviewed serological data on 938 individuals enrolled in a needle-stick study, 183 of whom had received either hepatitis B immune globulin (HBIG), intramuscular immunoglobulin, or both preparations. One of 183 HBIG recipients was HIV-antibody positive, but no pretransfusion sample was available for analysis of seroconversion (125).In a separate part of that report, no virus could be cultured from 38 lots of HBIG, intramuscular or intravenous immunoglobulin (124), despite high titer of antibody.

Although the data are sketchy, certain characteristic features of pediatric post-transfusion HIV disease became evident after review of the available literature (126–139). The incidence of transfusion-associated AIDS in infants was 2.43 per 100,000, greater than 0.40 per 100,000 population reported in adults (140). When the data were recalculated based on the number of transfusions received, those infants who received 10 or more units had an incidence rate of 22.4% compared with the adult rate of 4.83%. In another study, infants accounted for 10% of all transfusion-related cases, but received only 2% of the whole blood or red blood cells according to U.S. statistics collected in 1980. Of the 194 cases reported, 21 were in children, and 14 of the 21 were in premature infants. Infants differed from adults in the mean incubation period, which was defined as time from exposure to diagnosis of AIDS. The interval from time of exposure to onset of symptoms was shorter in the children (15 months) versus the adults (27 months) (141). The incubation time from viral exposure to antibody production is thought to be 6 weeks to 2 months. Thus, considerable time may elapse before the patient presents for evaluation. The full natural history of the transfused-associated AIDS is still unknown, and the nature of the clinical presentation and how it may differ in children who have in utero infection versus postnatally acquired HIV remains to be seen. Certain factors that appear to contribute to increased pathogenicity of the virus in transfusion recipients include prematurity, male sex, concomitant viral infections (128), certain immunosuppressive events, such as anesthesia and surgery, or repetitive episodes of septicemia (135).

The Transfusion Safety Study (TSS), a multicenter cooperative study to evaluate the extent to which blood and blood products transmit HIV and other viruses, has presented timely data in abstract form (142). Donors and recipients in selected institutions in four regions of the country where there is a high prevalence of HIV have been followed since September 1984, permitting prospective study of transfusion recipients prior to the onset of HIV screening of donor blood. Although 75% of recipients of HIV-positive units have died of causes unrelated to AIDS, 48 of these 53 recipients or 91% were positive for HIV antibody when reported in July 1986 (142).

The hemophiliac population appears to be uniquely different from those patients receiving blood products other than pooled concentrates. Prior to the growing concern and knowledge about HIV, the immunological dysfunction present in pediatric hemophiliacs has been documented amply since 1983 (143-146) and is now felt to be secondary to chronic antigenic stimulation (147). More recently, 80–90% of adult hemophiliacs and 59% of pediatric cases have been found to be HIV-positive (148), and a progressive immunological deterioration has been reported in some hemophiliacs (149), with 1–4% of all hemophiliacs now fitting criteria for AIDS. Because of the large number of antibody-positive individuals with the relatively small number of chronically diseased patients, certain investigators feel that the antibody is the result of exposure to the virus, disrupted or attenuated by the processes used to make factor concentrate, and that this antibody is protective (149). Only time will permit us to fully assess the extent of HIV disease in HIV antibody-positive individuals.

Human T-lymphotropic virus (HTLV-I) is another retrovirus that was initially isolated from a patient with an aggressive T cell lymphoma. It is thought to be the cause of a unique adult T cell leukemia/lymphoma (ATLL) that is endemic in southwestern Japan and the Caribbean basin. Antibodies to HTLV-I are present in 3–25% of healthy individuals in these endemic areas. In one study of healthy Japanese blood donors, between 0.5–13% of donors were positive, depending on their age, and the location of the donor facility, with the highest rates in areas where ATLL is endemic (150). In a study of recipients of blood positive for HTLV-I, anti-HTLV-I developed in 62.4% of those individuals receiving blood containing cells, but not in those receiving only fresh frozen plasma. Antibody positivity developed from 3–6 weeks post-transfusion and was identical in specificity to the viral polypeptides that persist in patients with individuals with ATLL. Past studies (151) have demonstrated that those individuals with antibody have type C retrovirus particles in their peripheral blood lymphocytes. In a more recent study, peripheral blood lymphocytes from healthy HTLV-I antibody-positive carriers had abnormal blast transformation and increased expression of the HLA class II antigens termed Ia and DR (152). The atypical blast transformation and presence of retroviral particles in post-transfusion recipients raises concerns over whether individuals positive for antibody should be allowed as blood donors (153). Pooled plasma products can also probably transmit HTLV-I (154). The clinical presentation of post-transfusion HTLV-I is to date one of a myelopathy, and maternal infant transmission has also been reported (155).

DIAGNOSIS

Bacteria

The diagnosis of bacterial infection secondary to transfusion is based on the clinical presentation of temperature elevation 2° greater than pretransfusion temperature, coupled with a variety of clinical manifestations. These may include chills, headache, malaise, vomiting, diarrhea, abdominal pain, or flushing. Symptoms may be so severe as to produce shock with circulatory collapse, disseminated intravascular coagulation, and death. The symptoms may occur within a few minutes of the transfusion or may occur a short time thereafter. In the fatal transfusion deaths, two-thirds of the deaths occurred within the first 24 hours following transfusion, while the remaining one-third occurred from 2–10 days after transfusion (1).

Laboratory confirmation of infection should include inspection of the bag for hemolysis, Gram stain and culture of the transfused product, and blood culture and Gram stain from the patient. A positive Gram stain indicates greater than or equal to 10^6 organisms per milliliter of blood. Bacterial culture of the bag specimen, however, will be positive with as few as 24 organisms per milliliter (1). If the blood bag is empty, swabbing of the bag following addition of a small amount of sterile water should provide a sufficient culture inoculation. If the blood bag is unavailable for culture segments, one can use tubing from the units that are routinely saved in all blood banks. If these are not available, the donor tube that is saved by the blood collection facility could be utilized. Culturing should be performed at 4°, 20–26°, and 37°, in both aerobic and anaerobic media and maintained for at least 7 days to assure a true-negative culture result. The only true proof that a contaminated unit produced transfusion-transmitted disease is to identify identical organisms in both the bag and the patient.

Parasites

Because of the rarity of malaria in the general population, it is infrequently considered as a post-transfusion disease. Findings are nonspecific and include fever and malaise. Diagnosis depends upon identification of the parasites in the peripheral blood smear of the transfusion recipient and should be performed on thin smears stained with Wright's stain and thick smears stained with both Wright's and Giemsa. If identification of the species is difficult, or if mixed infection is suspected, patients should be treated as if they had a chloroquine-resistant parasitemia until adequate identification can be made.

Identification of the donor can be made by two methods: examination of the smear and immunofluorescence antibody (IFA) titer, using multispecies antigens. The titer rises 1–2 weeks after onset of fever and persists until 6 months after adequate treatment of the infection. The diagnostic positive titer is defined as 1:20 or greater. The smear may be negative if there are less than 100 parasites/μl of blood; thus, low-grade parasitemia may be missed by visual inspection (26). Titers of 1:64 in IFA tests have been obtained in immune but noninfected donors (26). In individuals on chemoprophylaxis, development of a positive IFA titer in the face of infection may be delayed. Only a negative IFA assay indicates a high probability of no malaria.

The diagnosis of post-transfusion babesiosis should be made when the constellation of fever, malaise, and hemolytic anemia follow transfusion. Subclinical disease has not been reported as a post-transfusion event. Peripheral blood smear should demonstrate small intracellular ring form parasites that may be confused with malaria. IFA titers to *Babesia* are considered positive at a titer of 1:20. Infection can be confirmed only by intraperitoneal inoculation of putatively infected blood into hamsters, and observation for ring forms in the peripheral blood of the hamsters. The donor should be traced, and IFA titers and inoculation of the donor blood into hamsters performed as well. In one study, the donor blood was traced 1 year following tick bite, and grew *Babesia* in the hamster.

Viruses

Hepatitis A and Hepatitis B

The diagnoses of hepatitis A (HAV) and B (HBV) are now made easy by virtue of commercially available, standardized, sensitive immunological testing kits. Identification of a variety of markers permit one to classify the disease as acute, acute infectious, convalescent, or chronic. These are more fully reviewed in Chapter 14. The clinical presentation of HBV is very broad and may include subclinical elevation of liver enzymes or fulminant hepatic necrosis, which may be fatal. Malaise, fatigue, anorexia, vomiting, jaundice, and scleral icterus with hepatosplenomegaly may be present and may develop as early as 2 weeks following transfusion. Immune complex-mediated syndromes have also

been described and include serum-sickness, pruritic urticaria, polyarthritis, and polyarteritis nodosa. These may develop from a few days to 6 weeks prior to the onset of clinical hepatitis and are likely due to circulating HBsAg-anti HBs immune complexes (1). Immune complex disease is seen in hemophiliacs, but is likely due to nonspecific immune complex-mediated deposition; this is supported by a high prevalence of antinuclear factor and anti-smooth-muscle antibodies.

Post-transfusion hepatitis A is a rare event, but should be suspected in an individual who presents with anorexia, fatigue, malaise, jaundice, elevation in liver enzymes, and hepatosplenomegaly. The incubation period of HAV is 28 days, shorter than both post-transfusion NANB and HBV and the viremic period is very short. HAV differs from other viruses in a few respects: Diarrhea is more common, chronic hepatitis is rare, and fulminant and fatal hepatitis from HAV is very rare (156). Tracking of the donor is necessary, and a history of donation at the peak of a presumed viremia will usually be elicited in a relatively asymptomatic individual.

Non-A/Non-B Hepatitis

Post-transfusion hepatitis due to NANB is the most frequent post-transfusion hepatitis and should be considered whenever HBV, HAV, CMV, and EBV have been excluded and/or when paid or untested donor blood has been used. NANB hepatitis is usually anicteric and symptomatically mild, although rare, acute, fulminant cases have been reported. The alanine aminotransferase (ALT) levels fluctuate widely from normal to abnormal through the acute and chronic phase of the disease, making the diagnosis of recovery difficult. Fatigue may be present, but anorexia, weight loss, jaundice, and hepatosplenomegaly are rare. At least three prospective studies in small numbers of adult patients utilizing liver biopsy have demonstrated that approximately 60% of those individuals with NANB had chronic active hepatitis and 3–12% had cirrhosis. Of those with chronic active hepatitis, an additional 10% will progress to cirrhosis (37). Diagnosis of NANB will be especially difficult in children because of the following:

1. There is no historical foundation on which to base incidence figures or populations at risk, except for Thalassemic and hemophiliac children.

2. Those multiply transfused children at risk for NANB may be on chemotherapeutic agents, antibiotics, or hyperalimentation, all known to cause elevation of the ALT.
3. Children may be less clinically affected (although likely not less infected) because of the regenerating capability of their livers.

There is no serological test or surrogate test that will define NANB. Nevertheless, such cases should be reported to the blood collection agency, and donors recalled for repeat serological analysis, anti-core antibody to HBV, and ALT testing.

Cytomegalovirus

The diagnosis of post-transfusion cytomegalovirus (CMV) is frequently difficult because active CMV infection may or may not coexist with recognizable CMV disease. The clinical spectrum of disease will vary in different patient populations. Post-transfusion recipients of CMV-infected units who are asymptomatic will likely be diagnosed when seroepidemiological studies are in progress; they are most likely to be immunocompetent. Those who are immunoincompetent may present with clinical disease. Postnatal, post-transfusion CMV presents with pneumonia, lymphadenopathy, rash, and hepatosplenomegaly, hepatitis, and ascites. For some infants with pre-existing respiratory distress, worsening blood gases, apnea and increased ventilatory needs have been reported. One study of premature infants demonstrated severe neurological handicaps in those who excreted CMV at less than 8 weeks of age (157). Infants with late-onset CMV excretion had significantly less cardiopulmonary disease and no neurological handicaps (157). The older child who is severely immunosuppressed and who develops post-transfusion CMV would likely develop the multisystem disease, similar to that seen in adults. This includes interstitial pneumonia, hepatitis, arthralgia, meningoencephalitis, retinitis, and gastrointestinal ulceration (100). Actually, few studies performed to date on transfused children with malignancy fail to demonstrate clinically significant post-transfusion CMV disease. Bone marrow or solid organ graft survival may be compromised when CMV-positive organs are transfused into CMV-negative recipients (see above), and the signs and symptoms of graft rejection may complicate the diagnosis.

Several different methods may be used to diagnose infection with CMV. These include the use of viral culture of urine, blood, saliva, buffy-coat, or other body fluid. Because shedding is intermittent, and viremia is transient, multiple cultures preferably from multiple sites will increase the yield of culture positivity. Serial cultures or weekly cultures from multiple sites are most effective. The aliquot is inoculated onto human fibroblast lines or human foreskin fibroblasts, and the cultures are examined for focal cytopathic effect in 1–2 weeks or on second passage. The virus is notoriously slow-growing, and 4–6 weeks of observation are needed until cultures are considered negative. DNA hybridization techniques are established and have proved to be instructive in individual laboratories for sorting out the epidemiology of different subtypes of CMV as a cause of infection (158, 159), but the probes are not routinely available and have not been used in clinical laboratories for diagnosis. Serodiagnosis can be used to distinguish congenital, perinatal, acquired, and carrier states, but remain imperfect because of the lack of sensitive and specific assays for IgM CMV and antibody to early antigen. There are many assays used for detecting IgG anti-CMV. These include complement fixation, indirect hemagglutination, indirect immunofluorescence, latex agglutination, radioimmunoassay (RIA), and ELISA, and what is considered to be a positive titer will depend on the methodology used. Four-fold or greater titer rise is usually considered diagnostic for reactivation. Lamberson suggests use of a battery of these tests to establish the type of post-transfusion infection (Table 9.3) (78). True proof of the relationship between symptoms and post-transfusion CMV requires either biopsy or autopsy for examination of intranuclear inclusions in tissue or tissue culture.

Human Immunodeficiency Virus

The diagnosis of post-transfusion HIV should be suspected in any individual who presents with nonspecific findings of fever of unknown origin, weight loss, fatigue, lymphadenopathy, cough, and hepatosplenomegaly who has been transfused with blood or blood products collected in the United States from 1978 to the spring of 1985. This coincides with the time interval from the initial description of AIDS as an infectious disease to the onset of testing of and destruction

Table 9.3
Different Serological and Virological Tests and Their Interpretation in Post-Transfusion and Congenital Cytomegalovirus

		IgM[b]	Anti-EA	IgG or Total[c]			Viral Culture
				IFA	IHA	CF	
Congenital:	Infant	+					+
	cord blood	+	+	+	+R	+R	+
Perinatal:	Infant	+	+(R)	+(R)	(R)	+(R)	+ after
	cord blood	−					exposure
		−					−
Acquired		+(R)	+(R)	+(R)	+(R)	+(R)	variable
Latent		−	−	+	+	+	variable

[a]Adapted from Reference 78.
[b]Commercially available as IFA, ELISA.
[c]Commercially available as IHA, IFA, ELISA, Latex.
CF, complement fixation; ELISA, enzyme-linked immunofluorescence assay; IFA, immunofluorescence, IHA, immunohemagglutinin; R, rising titer; +, positive, present; −, negative, not present.

of blood and blood products positive for anti-HIV antibody.

Children with congenital and acquired bleeding disorders who received clotting concentrates from any source, regardless of the year in which the product was manufactured, should be evaluated for serological status, especially if they are symptomatic. The continued availability and use of concentrates from unscreened donors through the spring of 1987, despite what was thought to be adequate processing to inactivated viruses, makes this group of patients at risk. Children of hemophiliacs may also be at risk for acquisition via a perinatal route: father to mother to infant (160). To adequately classify an individual as having transfusion-transmitted HIV, the parents, especially the mother, should be tested. Several children with perinatal transmission who have also been transfused have been reported (161). Conversely, children born to mothers who were transfused and acquired disease through HIV-positive blood and blood products may acquire HIV from their mothers (162).

There are no specific clinical signs or symptoms of post-transfusion HIV that distinguish it from perinatal HIV.

Children with transfusion HIV may present or be traced via one of three routes:

1. Clinical presentation with nonspecific findings, repetitive infection, e.g., chronic otitis media, pneumonitis, or opportunistic infection.

2. Referral via a "Look Back" program, wherein the blood of a donor now testing positive for antibody is identified and recipients of previous donor blood of unknown serological status at time of transfusion are recalled and tested.

3. Physician request because of a history of transfusion in a child without other obvious risks.

The presence of a seronegative, viremic state poses a special problem in the serological diagnosis of HIV disease in both the recipient and the donor. In the donor, it is likely that there is viremia, but testing is done before antibody is positive. Two other reasons for failure of antibody response are also possible. These include B cell dysfunction with subsequent lack of antibody production to HIV antigen or the possibility that virus variants are not being picked up by currently available testing methodologies. Both may be possible in either the donor or the recipient and require consideration by the diagnostician.

The diagnosis of post-transfusion HIV is made by obtaining a positive test for antibody to HIV in the recipient. Seroconversion is thought to occur 6–8 weeks following infection, although antigenemia is likely to occur 2–3 weeks postinfection in the recipient. Tests for HIV antibody measure IgG or total antibody (163) and include enzyme-linked immunoassay (ELISA), radioimmunoassay (RIA), radioimmunoprecipitation (RIP), and immunoelectrophoresis (IEP).

The enzyme immunoassay (EIA or ELISA) for HIV is licensed for use in blood donors and is manufactured by at least four different companies. The source of antigen is inactivated virus which is frequently grown in human lymphoid cell lines. False-positive tests can occur when there is cross-reactivity between human antibody and antigens on the cell line (164,165). False-negatives can occur when the test lacks sensitivity for viral proteins. For example, one assay system may identify certain antibodies more than others: antibody to gp 41 envelope protein, which is thought to occur later in the disease, is more often identified than p 24 or core protein, which occurs in early stages of the disease. Western blot methodology is most often used to confirm a positive ELISA. This method uses electrophoretic separation of viral proteins and glycoprotein on sodium sulfate polyacrylamide gel electrophoresis (SDS-PAGE), followed by nitrocellulose blotting and fixation. Patient sera is applied and incubated with peroxidase conjugated goat anti-human IgG, followed by staining. Certain bands are specifically recognized, and include p 15–18, p 24–25 (core antibody), gp 51–45 (envelope antibody), p 53–55, p 64–65, gp 120, and gp 160. Seropositivity is considered in the presence of the gp 41 band, or in its absence, in the presence of both p 24 and p 55 (165).

Radioimmunoprecipitation (RIP) is frequently used as a confirmatory test for HIV in place of or concomitant with Western blot. Virus present in the supernatant of labeled lymphocytes is concentrated by ultracentrifugation and used with protein-A-sepharose. Immune complexes of supernatant virus with patient specimen containing antibody are electrophoresed and autoradiographed for identification. Specific banding patterns can thus be identified (166). More sensitive and specific assays for both IgG and IgM antibody are being developed utilizing recombinant DNA protein methods, but are not yet licensed as of this writing. One competitive immunoassay employs as the antigen recombinant DNA-produced proteins to envelope and core antibodies.

Several methods for detection of virus in cultivated lymphocytes allow a more secure diagnosis of infection and are particularly valuable in two settings: the infant with passive maternal antibody to HIV, and the infant or child who is profoundly hypogammaglobulinemic. The classical viral culture methodology measures reverse transcriptase in culture supernatants of infected cell clones; electron microscopy (EM) for viral particles or other specific DNA probe assays of the supernatant may also be obtained.

Several newer methods utilize other techniques. One method amplifies viral nucleic acid sequences in HIV in cells by a technique called polymerase chain reaction (PCR), which is followed by rapid detection of the sequence by enzyme restriction analysis. Two viral nucleic acid sequences that are invariant throughout the different strains of HIV have been sequenced and their restriction enzyme sites have been identified. PCR amplifies the number of copies of the sequence. A labeled DNA probe that is complementary to the sequence with the restriction site is applied. If the sequence for HIV is present in the sample, the probe will hybridize with it. Digestion with an appropriate restriction enzyme generates a short, single strand of labeled DNA which can be detected by gel electrophoresis. Another company has manufactured an enzyme immunoassay to detect HIV antigens in serum, plasma, or tissue culture. In this assay system, polystyrene beads coated with HIV antibody are incubated with either a specimen or control. Antigen will bind to the bead, and rabbit anti-HIV antibody is added. Goat anti-rabbit IgG conjugated with horseradish peroxidase is added and then o-phenylene diamine is added to develop the reaction which is read in a spectrophotometer. Two studies demonstrate the usefulness of these assays in CSF and in surveillance studies (167,168).

Additional diagnostic tests that may assist in defining the degree of immunological dysfunction include quantitation of lymphocytes, subclass analysis of T cells, in vitro mitogenic response to phytohemagglutinin (PHA), conconavalin A (conA), and poke weed mitogen (PWM), quantitative immunoglobulins, skin test reactivity, antibodies to diphtheria, tetanus, and measles in children who have been previously immunized. Other studies have included thymulin quantitation, alpha or gamma interferon quantitation, antibodies to other viruses, especially EBV-VCA, CMV, and HSV, and serum lactate dehydrogenase as a marker of B cell proliferation (169–171). A recent evaluation of 18 children studied prospectively demonstrated that nonsurvivors belonged to a group of patients who had negative antigen-induced mitogenic responses, and that absence or disappearance of HIV proteins, p 25 and p 18, was correlated with poor survival (170).

TREATMENT

Bacteria

Broad spectrum antibiotics and supportive care of the patient should be instituted immediately. If the patient is immunocompromised and already on antibiotics, one should add to or change the coverage based on preliminary identification from Gram stain.

Parasites

Adequate treatment for malaria will depend on the identification of the kind of malaria and the area of the world where it was acquired. In the past, chloroquine was the drug of choice for malaria, but cannot be used exclusively due to chloroquine-resistant stains. Currently, sulfadiazine, pyrimethamine, and/or quinine can be used, but it is important to constantly review World Health Organization recommendations and to use suggested medications based on changing parasite sensitivities. *Babesia microti* infections have in the past responded well to clindamycin-quinine sulphate combination. One recent treatment failure (31) may portend the changing sensitivity of this organism.

In other areas of the world, concern over transmission of parasitic diseases in blood is higher than in the U.S., where these are rare post-transfusion events. Different treatment and preventive measures may be required where the disease is pandemic. They include addition of 0.25% gentian violet to stored blood for Chagas' disease and pretreatment of the donor and recipient with chloroquine for malaria.

Viruses

There are no specific treatments for virally transmitted post-transfusion disease. The reader is referred to chapters in which experimental treatment modalities and supportive care for hepatitis A, hepatitis B, CMV, and HIV are discussed.

Several treatment modalities for HIV have been attempted in small-scale clinical trials in adults. These include the use of ribavarin, azidothymidine (AZT), HPA-23, toscarnet, ∝-interferon and dideoxycytidine (DDC). Ribavirin use in infants with AIDS demonstrated no clinical, immunological, or virological improve-

ment (168). AZT appears to be the most promising in adults, and clinical trials are underway at NIH in children. Twin-to-twin bone marrow transplantation and lymphocyte infusions and cultured thymic fragment implantation have also been tried in adults, with discouraging results (171). Treatment with Thymosin and ∝-interferon has likewise been disappointing (172).

Other than supportive care, the primary method of treating pediatric HIV has been the use of i.v. immunoglobulin (i.v. IgG). Modification of in vitro suppressor cell function, improvement in poke weed mitogen-driven gamma-globulin secretion (173), and decline in serum lactate dehydrogenase quantitation have been reported following use of i.v. IgG in pediatric HIV infection (169). Clinical trials comparing placebo, high HIV titer i.v. IgG serum lactate dehydrogenase quantitation have been reported following use of i.v. IgG in pediatric HIV infection (169). Clinical trials comparing placebo, high HIV titer i.v. IgG, and standard i.v. IgG are underway.

PREVENTION

Bacteria

The use of closed, plastic, sterile blood-bag systems with integral needles has all but eliminated bacterial infection as a major cause of transfusion-transmitted bacterial disease. Other measures must include adequate donor selection with specific exclusion of donors with recent dental procedures and/extractions and the very careful observation of and preparation of the donor venipuncture sites rotated to prevent dimpling as a source of occult infection. Most other prevention measures are all part of standard, routine blood banking procedures, which are detailed in *Standards and Technical Manual of the American Association of Blood Banks* (12). Nevertheless, a few highlights can be stressed.

Blood must be stored in quality controlled refrigerators with alarm systems that permit only a minimal variability in temperature (1–6°). While platelets are stored at ambient room temperatures (20–22°), the temperature should be monitored. When products such as platelets or cryoprecipitate are pooled, this should be done by trained personnel and according to established protocols. Plasma must be thawed in plastic overwraps in water that is changed frequently or in which a bacteriostatic and/or fungistatic agent is added. Blood and blood products should not be transfused if the following guidelines have been exceeded:

Red Blood Cells
1. Stored at 1–6° and older than:
   Citrate phosphate dextrose anticoagulant (CPD) 21 days;
   Citrate phosphate dextrose adenine anticoagulant (CPDA1) 35 days;
   Adsol/Nutracell anticoagulant 42 days.
2. Out of refrigerator for greater than 20 minutes if unentered.
3. Washed, stored for greater than 24 hours.
4. Spiked and infusing into patient greater than 4 hours.

Fresh Frozen Plasma
1. Stored at −18° and older than 1 year from phlebotomy;
2. Thawed greater than 24 hours;
3. Thawed and spiked greater than 4 hours.

Cryoprecipitate
1. Stored at −30° and older than 1 year from phlebotomy;
2. Thawed greater than 6 hours;
3. Thawed and infusing greater than 4 hours.

Platelets
1. Age from collection variable depending on bag and source of platelets;
2. Variable, depending on bag and source of platelets;
3. Spiked and infusing greater than 4 hours.

Plateletpheresis
1. Twenty-four hours or 5 days single donor platelets;
2. Spiked and infusing greater than 4 hours.

Deglycerolyzed Red Blood Cells
1. Stored at −65°C or colder for greater than 1 year, except for rare antigen blood;
2. Defrosted, washed, and stored greater than 24 hours.

No medication or substance should be added to blood or blood products. Only sterile spiking or docking devices should be used in conjunction with the plastic spiking parts.

Recipients of other components made from the contaminated unit should be cultured and any as yet untransfused component should be cultured and then destroyed.

Current regulations for screening of donors for syphilis with VDRL and refrigeration of most blood products which kills the treponema has resulted in no post-transfusion *T. pallidum* in-fection reported lately. If unrefrigerated blood is to be used, VDRL screening should be performed prior to transfusion.

Parasites

Prevention of malaria in the United States is based on stringent donor exclusion criteria. Individuals may be accepted if they

1. Have had confirmed malaria and have been asymptomatic for and/or completed antimalarial therapy 3 years prior to donation;
2. Are immigrants or visitors from endemic areas, and have shown no symptoms of malaria for 3 years after departure from that area;
3. Have traveled to an endemic area and have taken malarial prophylaxis for 6 months following their return and are free from unexplained febrile illnesses.

Prevention of babesiosis is more difficult to assure because the parasite is normally confined to domestic animals, and the carrier state is difficult to confirm in the immunologically competent adult. Although donor questionnaires frequently include tick bite and use it as an exclusion criteria, the problem of long-term carriers is not addressed. Some areas of the U.S. will exclude donors from endemic areas regardless of history or IFA titer. The use of ELISA or IFA testing of donor samples for either parasite and for Chagas' disease does not seem to be cost-effective, unless the post-transfusion incidence of these diseases were to increase.

Viruses

Preventive management strategies for transfusion-transmitted viral disease center around donor exclusion criteria. These may take the form of donor history, specific immunological tests to evaluate the presence of antibody to specific viral antigens, or nonspecific tests known to be aberrant when an individual harbors the virus. Virological culture of donor blood is currently impractical due to the length of time required for viral cultures, although new methods of dot-blot hybridization may change our ability to screen for potentially infective samples in the future. Preventive techniques using immunization with pooled immune serum globulin and active immunization with vaccines are appropriate for selected patient populations, and will be discussed with each virus.

Hepatitis A and Hepatitis B

The cornerstone of HBV prevention is based on three factors: voluntary deferral of those individuals with a history of any kind of hepatitis, the use of exclusively volunteer rather than paid donors, and the introduction of sensitive, specific assays for HBsAg antigen. In a recent review of five studies comparing paid with voluntary blood donors, the risk of acquisition of hepatitis (not B specifically) was 6.9% when volunteer blood was used as compared with 27.5% for paid blood (37). Screening of all blood and blood products for HBsAg was mandated by federal law in 1972, and post-transfusion HBV has virtually disappeared. Most blood banks utilize volunteer blood, but its use is not mandated by law or by inspection/accreditation agencies.

Passive immunization to HBV using immunoglobulin prepared from individuals with high titer to hepatitis B surface antigen (HBIG) was initiated in the 1970s in individuals at high risk for needle-stick injuries or bloody fluid contact and was and is still used for some specific clinical indications. However, two prospective double-blind studies have failed to demonstrate any decrease in the incidence of post-transfusion hepatitis (174,175). Hepatitis B vaccine prepared with formalin, urea, pepsin, and heat treatment inactivation steps has replaced the use of HBIG for many clinical situations, and vaccine efficacy and strategies for vaccination and development are beyond the scope of this chapter. There are, however, two highly transfused groups where hepatitis B vaccine provides preventive protection. These include dialysis patients, staff, and hemophiliac children. Clinical trials are now underway to evaluate the dosage and timing of vaccine administration in very young hemophiliacs who do not yet have anti-HBs antibody.

Non-A/Non-B Hepatitis

Because testing for HBsAg is not 100% effective and because post-transfusion hepatitis occurs despite HBsAg testing, screening for anti-HBc has been suggested as a means to assure removal of potentially infectious blood from being used. The Transfusion-Transmitted Viruses Study Group (TVS) demonstrated that the risk of NM-HBV post-transfusion hepatitis is greater among recipients of anti-HBc-positive units (19%) as compared with anti-HBc-negative blood (7%)

(40). Because of concerns over methodology, loss of donors, and cost-effectiveness, anti-HBc testing was not implemented after this publication. However, the continued concern over post-transfusion viral disease in the 1980s has mandated the collection agencies and government to assure the safest blood supply possible. Thus, anti-HBc testing of donor units has been recommended by several investigators, and by the end of 1987, anti-HBc testing will be performed by most blood collection facilities (12). The TVS similarly demonstrated that recipients of blood with elevated alanine aminotransferase (ALT) had a 39% incidence of hepatitis compared with 3.4% for those receiving blood with normal ALT (40). These data were confirmed in later studies by Alter (43). Based on the work of Stevens, it must be pointed out that ALT and anti-HBc tests probably delineate two separate NANB carrier populations. In this study of 121 donors with ALT greater than 45 I.U., only 15% were anti-HBc-positive, while of 220 donors who were anti-HBc positive, only 8% had elevated ALT (176). The use of ALT to further exclude donors at risk for transmission of NANB has received much attention. Problems with ALT screening include the fact that it is a surrogate test and therefore is not specific, and the cost of testing measured in dollars and in units of blood discarded is very high. In addition, there are several different established methodologies for performing the test, and no knowledge as to which one is better, no uniform laboratory determination which defines a significant elevation, and no guidelines for donor deferral. Despite these concerns, ALT testing of donor units has begun in many donor collection facilities and is now required along with anti-HBc according to American Association of Blood Banks standards (12). Continued observations in blood recipients by Alter and by the new NIH sponsored multi-institutional Transfusion Safety Group will permit us to judge the efficacy of these new screening procedures. Subsequently, federal mandates will likely be established.

Cytomegalovirus

Control of post-transfusion CMV should be directed to those individuals who are at highest risk. Our current understanding is that these individuals include seronegative preterm infants, seronegative transplant patients who may receive organs from seronegative donors, and seronegative recipients of granulocyte concentrates. Other groups for whom none, insufficient, or conflicting data exist, and who do not therefore have clear-cut indications include all infants, regardless of birthweight or serological status, children with solid tumors or leukemia receiving ablative chemotherapy, infants and children with AIDS, neonates of unknown or seronegative status receiving granulocyte transfusions, and children undergoing cardiopulmonary bypass. As additional data accumulate on these groups of children, the indications may expand or contract.

Several approaches to the prevention of post-transfusion CMV have been utilized. These include provision of CMV seronegative blood and blood products, processing of blood and blood products to leukodeplete them, passive immunization of high-risk groups, and active immunization using CMV vaccine. Because both retrospective and prospective analysis have demonstrated that CMV seronegative blood carries a low risk of transmitting CMV, this has been the mainstay of prevention. Tests to measure total or IgG-specific CMV are most often used. Prevalences of CMV antibody positivity vary widely, with significant regional variations in the U.S. Provision of CMV-negative products may not be feasible in those areas with high seroprevalence rates. Based on prospective studies, it is unlikely that all seropositive donors who test with CMV antibodies by current testing can transmit disease. Three studies to date have attempted to evaluate IgM CMV-positive donors as a source of truly infective units capable of transmitting post-transfusion CMV. Although preliminary in nature, these studies suggest that use of IgM CMV-negative products should substantially reduce the risk of CMV infection (177–179).

Because CMV is likely harbored in white blood cells, the use of leukodepleted products has been suggested as a mechanism to reduce post-transfusion CMV. Several studies to date support the use of frozen deglycerolized red blood cells, regardless of donor serological status in reducing the risk of post-transfusion CMV in cardiac surgery and dialysis patients and in multiply transfused neonates (85, 90, 91, 93). Two studies have addressed the use of saline-washed packed cells to reduce CMV risk. Demmler and coworkers identified IgG CMV seroconversion in 6 of 54 infants who received washed red blood cell products, of whom four became symptomatic. They concluded that washed cells were ineffective. However, review of their data demonstrates significance between uninfected and infected infants only for those who received platelets and IgM-CMV antibody-positive washed red blood cells (94). Another study confirmed that use of seronegative products prevents seroconversion in the seronegative infant, and also demonstrated that the use of saline-washed red blood cells of unknown serological status, including IgM-positive blood, prevented post-transfusion CMV (95). In those areas of the U.S. where provision of CMV seronegative products is difficult, the use of saline-washed red blood cells and CMV-negative platelet and white blood cell products may be the most efficacious until sensitive, specific tests of donor infectivity are developed.

Passively acquired CMV antibody from the mother or by transfusion to the infant is protective against CMV. This fact was utilized by bone marrow transplantationists who administered high-titer immune plasma transfusions, CMV immune globulin, and, most recently, i.v. CMV immune globulin with variable success to reduce the incidence and severity of interstitial pneumonitis and other sequelae of CMV. A recent study utilizing CMV-negative blood and blood products and specially prepared CMV immunoglobulin failed to demonstrate protection against the acquisition of CMV in bone marrow transplant patients, and additional studies were recommended (118). Controlled studies in neonates and recipients of solid organs and additional studies in bone marrow transplant recipients should help in evaluating this potentially favorable modality. Active immunization for high-risk populations is reviewed in Chapter 12. To date, no published trials in transfusion recipients have been performed.

Human Immunodeficiency Virus

Following U.S. Public Health Service recommendations in March of 1983, blood banks adopted voluntary self-deferral and direct donor questioning, which would allow for identification of an at-risk donor and removal of that blood from use. Certain blood donor centers implemented phone number call-back systems and other confidential systems to allow donors to donate, but have their blood removed from use (178). Two centers utilizing voluntary deferral reported reduction in numbers of young male donors following implementation of these systems (180, 181).

In March of 1985, testing of blood and blood components for antibody to HIV was implemented in many collection facilities in the U.S. It was mandated by the American Association of Blood Banks to be in place by July 1985 and became a recommendation from the Centers for Disease Control in January 1985 (182). We believe this has effectively eliminated HIV antibody-positive blood from the system. Donor education, specific questions, and options for postdonation notification are still utilized as an added safeguard. There is a theoretic possibility that a viremic seronegative donor who does not consider himself at risk, who answers all questions truthfully and negatively, or who lies, may donate a unit which eventually is transfused. The NIH Consensus Panel estimates that despite screening transfusion of HIV-positive blood may occur in less than 1 in 10,000 transfusions, with an estimated potential for approximately 100 post-transfusion AIDS cases to occur in the U.S. per year.

Certain surrogate tests may be utilized alone or in combination to further exclude donors who may be seronegative. These include quantitative T cell subsets, β_2-microglobulin, acid labile interferon, immune complex assays, anti-HBc, and anti-CMV. These nonspecific tests are not cost-effective, many are cumbersome to perform, and discussion of their use was more appropriate when specific tests for HIV antibody were not possible. The potential for even more specific antigen screening or DNA probe tests makes discussion of surrogate tests unnecessary.

Preventive strategies for hemophiliacs who depend on long-term use of factor concentrates prepared from pools of thousands of plasma donors is a much more complex issue. Several factors determine whether these concentrates will harbor transmissible virus. These include the viremic state of the donor at the time of donation, whether the virus is intracellular, extracellular, or both; its concentration in the plasma, whether neutralization antibody is present in the plasma pool; and what happens to the virus during the fractionation and lyophilization process. HIV and NANB can withstand fractionation and produce clinical disease in recipients. HTLV-I and parvovirus may also withstand fractionation (153,183). Manufacturers have utilized several

different methodologies to stabilize proteins and then allow them to withstand heat for prolonged periods of time (60°C for 10 or more hours); the methods are proprietary and thus unknown. What is now known is that use of heat-treated concentrates prepared from unscreened or HIV antibody-positive plasma pools is capable of transmitting both HIV and NANB (182, 184). Inactivation of virus in plasma pools using pepsin, trypsin, β-propriolactone, ultraviolet irradiation, or other chemicals in combination may produce products with less potential for viral transmission (185,186). At the very least, no plasma containing HIV antibody will be used to manufacture factor concentrates by spring of 1987.

Other preventive measures for hemophiliacs will depend upon the severity of their hemophilia, which determines their transfusion requirements. Young hemophiliacs can be treated with plasma or cryoprecipitate in place of factor concentrates. One can further decrease the number of donors to whom a hemophiliac is exposed by increasing the yield of factor VIII per donor. This can be accomplished by pretreating plasma donors with DDAVP, which releases endothelial stores of factor VIII, and by using heparin rather than citrate as an anticoagulant for plasma collections. Cryoprecipitate and plasma prepared in this way has 2- to 5-fold more factor VIII than standard products (187, 188). In a further effort to decrease donor exposure, donors can have plasmapheresis performed and cryoprecipitate made from their donations to "stockpile" for use by one specific recipient (189). Biotechnology may bring us a recombinant factor VIII that is bioactive. This will certainly replace plasma-derived products, no matter how they are inactivated, (190) once safety and efficacy have been established.

REFERENCES

1. Tabor E: Bacterial infections transmitted by blood. In Tabor E (ed): *Infectious Complications of Blood Transfusion*. New York, Academic Press. 1982, pp 147–163.
2. Myhre PA: Fatalities from blood transfusion. *JAMA* 244:1333–1335, 1980.
3. Braine HG: Bacterial contamination of platelet concentrates. NIH Consensus Conference: *Platelet Transfusion Therapy*. Bethesda, MD, National Institutes of Health, 1986, p 88.
4. Buchholz DH, Young VM, Friedman NR, Reilly JA, Mardiney MR: Bacterial proliferation in platelet products stored at room temperature. *N Engl J Med* 285:429–433, 1971.
5. Katz AJ, Tilton RC: Sterility of platelet concentrates stored at 25°C. *Transfusion* 10: 329–330, 1970.

6. Schlicter SJ, Harker LA: Preparation and storage of platelet concentrates. *Br J Haem* 34:403–419, 1976.
7. Rahme FS, Root RK, MacLowry JD, Dadisman TA, Bennett JV: Salmonella septicemia from platelet transfusions: Study of an outbreak traced to a hematogenous carrier of Salmonella cholerae-suis. *Ann Intern Med* 78:633–641, 1973.
8. Heal JM, Singal S, Sardisco E, Mayer T. Bacterial proliferation in platelet concentrates. *Transfusion* 26: 388–389, 1986.
9. Anderson KC, Lew MA, Gorgone BC, Martel J, Leamy CB, Sullivan B: Transfusion related bacterial sepsis after prolonged platelet storage. *Am J Med* 81:405–410, 1986.
10. Van Lierde S, Fleisher GR, Plotkin SA, Campos JM: A case of platelet transfusion related *Serratia marcescens* sepsis. *Pediatr Infect Dis* 4:293–295, 1985.
11. Braine HG, Kickler TS, Charache P, Ness PM, Davis J, Reichart C, Fuller AK. Bacterial sepsis secondary to platelet transfusion: an adverse effect of extended storage at room temperature. *Transfusion* 26:391–392, 1986.
12. Widmann FK (ed): *Standards and Technical Manual of the American Association of Blood Banks.* ed 12. Arlington, VA, AABB, 1987.
13. Tabor E, Gerety R: Five cases of *Pseudomonas* sepsis transmitted by blood transfusion. *Lancet* 1:1403, 1984.
14. Stenhouse MAE, Milner LV: *Yersinia enterocolitica*: a hazard in blood transfusion. *Transfusion* 22:396–398, 1982.
15. Economidou P, Kalafatas P, Vatopoulou T, Petropoulou D, Kattamis C: Brucellosis in two thalassaemic patients infected by blood transfusion from the same donor. *Acta Haematol* 55:244–249, 1976.
16. Spink WW, Anderson O: *Brucella* studies in bank blood in a general hospital; agglutinins; survival of *Brucella*. *J Lab Clin Med* 35:440–445, 1950.
17. Pittman M: A study of bacteria implicated in transfusion reactions and of bacteria isolated from blood products. *J Lab Clin Med* 42:273–288, 1953.
18. Paxson CL: Collection and use of autologous fetal blood. *Am J Obstet Gynecol* 134:708–710, 1979.
19. Golden SM, O'Brien WF, Lissner C, Cefalo RC, Monaghan W, Schumacher H. Hematological and bacteriological assessment of autologous cord blood for neonatal transfusion. *J Pediatr* 97:810–812, 1980.
20. Golden SM, Petit N, Mapes T, Davis SE, Monaghan W: Bacteriologic assessment of autologous cord blood for neonatal transfusion. *Am J Obstet Gynecol* 149:907–908, 1984.
21. Kliegman RM, Fanaroff AA: Necrotizing enterocolitis. *N Engl J Med* 310:1093–1103, 1984.
22. Seges RA, Kinney A, Bird GWG, Wingham J, Baals H, Stauffer UG: Pediatric surgical patients with severe anaerobic infection: report of 16 T antigen positive cases and possible hazard of blood transfusion. *J Pediatr Surg* 16:905–910, 1981.
23. Novak RW: Bacterial induced RBC alterations complicating NEC. *Am J Dis Child* 138:183–185, 1984.
24. Cohen DH, Moncrieff RE, Silvergleid AJ: Neonatal Th activation. *Transfusion* 25:81–82, 1985.
25. Mullard GW, Thompson IH, Lee D, Owen WG: Strong T-transformation associated with a severe hemolytic reaction in a young infant transfused with packed red cells. *Clin Lab Haemat* 3: 357–364, 1981.
26. Bruce-Chwatt L: Transfusion-associated parasitic infections. In Dodd RY, Barker LF (eds): *Infection, Immunity and Blood Transfusion.* New York, Alan R Liss, 1985, pp 101–125.
27. Jacoby GA, Hunt JA, Kosinski KS, Demirjian ZN, Huggins C, Etkind P, Marcus LC, Spielman A: Treatment of transfusion-transmitted babesiosis by exchange transfusion. *N Engl J Med* 303:1098–1100. 1980.
28. Wittner M, Rowin KS, Tanowitz HB, Hobbs JF, Saltzman S, Wenz B, Hirsch R, Chisolm E, Healy GR. Successful chemotherapy of transfusion babesiosis. *Ann Int Med* 96:601–604, 1982.
29. Grabowski EF, Giardina RJV, Goldberg D, Masur H, Read SE, Hirsch RL, Benach JL: Babesiosis transmitted by a transfusion of frozen thawed blood. *Ann Int Med* 96:466–467, 1982.
30. Marcus LC, Valigorsky JM, Fanning WL, Joseph T, Glick B. A case of report of transfusion-induced babesiosis. *JAMA* 248:465–467, 1982.
31. Smith RP, Evans AT, Popovsky M, Mills L, Spielman A: Transfusion-acquired babesiosis and failure of antibiotic treatment. *JAMA* 256:2726–2727, 1986.
32. Guerrero IC, Weniger BC, Schultz MG: Transfusion malaria in the United States 1972–1981. *Ann Int Med* 99:221–226, 1983.
33. Fajardo LF: The role of platelets in infections. I. Observations in human and murine malaria. *Arch Pathol Lab Med* 103:131–134, 1979.
34. De Virgiliis S, Galanello R, Cao A: *Plasmodium malariae* transfusion malaria in splenectomized patients with thalassemia major. *J Pediatr* 98:584–585, 1981.
35. Piccoli DA, Perlman S, Ephros M: Transfusion-acquired *Plasmodium malariae* infection in two premature infants. *Pediatrics* 72:560–562, 1983.
36. Najem GR, Sulzer AJ: Transfusion-induced malaria from an asymptomatic carrier. *Transfusion* 16:473–476, 1976.
37. Alter H: Post-transfusion hepatitis. In Dodd RY, Barker LA (eds): *Infection, Immunity, and Blood Transfusion*, New York, Alan R Liss, 1985, pp 47–61.
38. Blumberg BS, Gerstley BJ, Hungerford DA, London WT, Sutnick AL: A serum antigen (Australian antigen) in Down's syndrome, leukemia and hepatitis. *Ann Intern Med* 66:924–931, 1967.
39. Alter HJ, Holland PV, Purcell RH, Lander JJ, Feinstone SM, Morrow AG, Schmidt PJ: Post-transfusion hepatitis after exclusion of the commercial and hepatitis B antigen positive donor. *Ann Intern Med* 77:691–699, 1972.
40. Aach RD, Szmuness W, Mosley JW, Hollinger FB, Kahn RA, Stevens CE, Edwards VM, Werch J: Serum alanine aminotransferase of donors in relation to the risk of non-A, non-B hepatitis in recipients: the transfusion transmitted viruses study. *N Engl J Med* 304:989–994, 1981.
41. Feinstone SM, Kapikian AZ, Purcell RH: Hepatitis A: detection by immune electron microscopy of a viruslike antigen associated with acute illness. *Science* 182:1026–1028, 1973.
42. Feinstone SM, Kapikian AZ, Purcell RH, Alter HJ, Holland PV: Transfusion-associated hepatitis not due to viral hepatitis type A or B. *N Engl J Med* 292:767–770, 1975.
43. Alter HJ, Purcell RH, Holland PV, Feinstone SM, Morrow AG, Moritsugu Y: Clinical and serological analysis of transfusion-associated hepatitis. *Lancet* 2:838–841, 1975.
44. Knodell RG, Conrad ME, Dienstag JL, Bell CJ: Etiologic spectrum of post-transfusion hepatitis. *Gastroenterology* 69: 1278–1285, 1975.
45. Seef LB, Wright EC, Zimmerman HJ, Hoofnagle JH, Dietz AA, Felsher BF, Garcia-Pont PH, Gerety RJ, Greenlee HB, Kiernan T, Leevy CM, Nath N, Schiff ER, Schwartz C, Tabor E, Tamburo C, Vlahcevic Z, Zemel R, Zimmerman DS: Post-transfusion hepatitis. 1973–1975: A Veterans Administration cooperative study. In Vyas GN, Cohen SN, Schmid R (eds): *Viral Hepatitis: A Contemporary Assessment of Etiology, Epidemiology, Pathogenesis and Prevention.* Philadelphia, Franklin Institute Press, 1978, pp 371–382.
46. Craske J, Dilling N, Stern D: An outbreak of hepatitis associated with intravenous injection of factor VIII concentrate. *Lancet* 2: 221–223, 1975.
47. Tabor E, Gerety RJ: Inactivation of an agent of human nonA, nonB hepatitis by formalin. *J Infec Dis* 142:767–770, 1980.
48. Dienstag JL, Alaama A, Mosley JW. Redeker AG, Purcell RH: Etiology of sporadic hepatitis B surface antigen-negative hepatitis. *Ann Intern Med* 87:1–6, 1977.
49. Bayer WL, Tegtmeir GE, Barbara JA: The significance of non-A, non-B hepatitis, cytomegalovirus and the acquired immune deficiency disease in transfusion practice. *Clin Haematol* 13:253–269, 1984.
50. Gerety RJ (ed): *Non A-non B Hepatitis.* New York, Academic Press, 1981.
51. Bradley DW: Research perspectives in post-transfusion nonA-nonB hepatitis. In Dodd RY and Barker LF (eds): *Infection,*

Immunity and Blood Transfusion. New York, Alan R Liss, 1985, pp 81–87.

52. Luban, NLC: Neonatal transfusion medicine: HTLV-III implications. In *NIH Consensus Conference: Impact of Routine HTLV-III Antibody Testing on Public Health.* Bethesda, MD, National Institutes of Health, 1986, pp 88–97.

53. Kim HC: Red blood cell transfusions in the neonate. *Semin Perinatol* 7:159–174, 1983.

54. Hollinger FB, Khan NC, Oefinger PE, Yawn DH, Schmulen AC, Dressman GR, Melnick JL: Post-transfusion hepatitis A. *JAMA* 250:2313–2317, 1983.

55. Sherertz RS, Russell BA, Reuman PD: Transmission of hepatitis A by transfusion of blood products. *Arch Intern Med* 144:1579–1580, 1984.

56. Seesberg S, Brandberg A, Hermodsson S, Larsson P, Lundgren S: Hospital outbreak of hepatitis A secondary to blood exchange in a body. *Lancet* 1:1155–1156, 1981.

57. Azimi PH, Roberto RR, Gurlnick J, Livermore T, Hoag S, Hagens S, Lugo N: Transfusion acquired hepatitis A in a premature infant with secondary nosocomial spread in an intensive care unit. *Am J Dis Child* 140:23–27, 1986.

58. Noble RC, Kane MA, Reeves SA, Roeckel I: Post-transfusion hepatitis A in a neonatal intensive care unit. *JAMA* 252:2711–2715, 1984.

59. Moroni GA, Piaceotini G, Teizdi S, Jean G: Hepatitis B or nonA-nonB virus infection in multitransfused thalassaemic patients. *Arch Dis Child* 59:1127–1130, 1984.

60. Baraldini M, Miglio F, Pirillo H, Cursaro C, Meliconi R, Stefanini GF, Gasbarrini G: Hepatitis B virus markers in hematologic patients: relation to transfusion treatment and hospitalization. *Vox Sang* 45:112–120, 1983.

61. Economidou J: Problems related to treatment of beta-Thalassaemia major. *Paediatrician* 11:157–177, 1982.

62. DeVirgiliis S, Fiorelli G, Forgion S, Cornacchia G, Sanna G, Cossu P, Murgia V, Cao A: Chronic liver disease in transfusion dependent Thalassaemia: hepatitis B virus marker studies. *J Clin Pathol* 33:949–953, 1980.

63. Papaevangelou G, Economidou J, Roumetiotou A, Adrachta D, Parchas, S: Epstein-Barr infection in polytransfused patients with homozygous B-Thalassaemia. *Vox Sang* 37:305–309, 1979.

64. Babiker MA, Bahakim HM, el-Hazmi MA: Hepatitis B and A markers in children with Thalassaemia and sickle-cell disease in Riyadh. *Ann Trop Paediatr* 6:59–62, 1986.

65. Quak SH, Doi, Tan KP, Chio LF, Aw SE: Repeated transfusions and serological markers of hepatitis A and hepatitis B. *J Surg Pediatr Soc* 26:94–97, 1984.

66. Stevens CE, Silbert JA, Miller DR, Dienstag JL, Purcell RH, Szmuness W: Serologic evidence of hepatitis A and B virus infections in thalassaemia patients: a retrospective study. *Transfusion* 18:356–360, 1978.

67. Pearson HA, Wood C, Andeman W, Bove J, Rink L: Low risk of hepatitis B from blood transfusions in Thalassaemic patients in Connecticut. *J Pediatr* 108:252–253, 1986.

68. Cederbaum AI, Blatt PM, Levine PH: Abnormal serum transaminase levels in patients with hemophilia A. *Arch Intern Med* 142:481–484, 1982.

69. Spero JA, Lewis JH, Fisher SE, Hasiba U, Van Thiel DH: The high risk of chronic liver disease in multitransfused juvenile hemophiliac patients. *J Pediatr* 94:875–878, 1979.

70. Spero JA, Lewis JH, Van Thiel DH, Robin BS: Asymptomatic structural liver disease in hemophiliacs. *N Engl J Med* 298:1371–1378, 1978.

71. Mannucci PM, Capitanio A, Del Dinno E: Asymptomatic liver disease in hemophiliacs. *J Clin Pathol* 28:620–24, 1975.

72. Gomperts ED, Lazerson J, Berg D, Lockhart D, Sergis-Deavenport E: Hepatocellular enzyme patterns and hepatitis B virus exposure in multitransfused young and very young hemophilia patients. *Am J Hematol* 11:55–59, 1981.

73. Buchanan GR, Richards N, Hottkamp CA, Rutledye J: Hepatitis in household contacts of patients with hemophilia who have received multiple blood transfusions. *J Pediatr* 108:937–939, 1986.

74. Kashiwagi S, Hayashi I, Ikematsu H, Romura H, Kajiyama

W, Shingu T, Hayashida K, Kaji M: Transmission of hepatitis B virus among siblings. *J Epidemiol* 120:617–625, 1984.

75. Kane RC, Rousseau WE, Noble GR, Tegtmeier GE, Wulff H, Herndon HB, Chin TDY, Bayer WL: Cytomegalovirus infection in a volunteer blood donor population. *Infect Immunol* 17:719–723, 1975.

76. Perham TGM, Carl EW, Conway PJ, Mott MG: Cytomegalovirus infection in blood donors—a prospective study. *Br J Haematol* 20:307–320, 1971.

77. Mirkovic R, Werch J, South MA, Beyesh-Melnick N: Incidence of cytomegaloviremia in blood bank donors and in infants with congenital cytomegalic inclusion disease. *Infect Immunol* 3:45–50, 1971.

78. Lamberson HV: Cytomegalovirus (CMV): The agent, its pathogenesis and its epidemiology. In Dodd RY and Barker LF (eds): *Infection, Immunity, and Blood Transfusion.* New York, Alan R Liss, 1985 pp 149–173.

79. Cheung KS, Lang DJ: Transmission and activation of cytomegalovirus with blood transfusion: a mouse model. *J Infect Dis* 135:841–845, 1977.

80. Olding LB, Jensen FC, Oldstone MBA: Pathogenesis of cytomegalovirus infection: I. Activation of virus from bone marrow-derived lymphocytes by in vitro allogenic reaction. *J Exp Med* 141:561–572, 1975.

81. Purtillo DT, Linder J: Oncological consequences of impaired immune surveillance against ubiquitous viruses. *J Clin Immunol* 3:197–206, 1983.

82. Williams AE, Luban NLC, MacDonald M, Sacher R, Mikesell J, Hoffman-Panetta K, Williams K, Dodd RY: Low incidence of neonatal post-transfusion cytomegalovirus infection associated with the use of washed red blood cell products. *Transfusion* 24:430, 1984.

83. Henle W, Henle G: Immunology of Epstein-Barr virus. In Roizman B (ed): *Comprehensive Virology Series: The Herpes Viruses.* New York, Plenum Press, 1982, vol. 1, p. 209.

84. Paloheimo JA, von Essen R, Klemola E, Kaariainen L, Siltanen P: Subclinical cytomegalovirus infections and cytomegalovirus mononucleosis after open heart surgery. *Am J Cardiol* 22:624–630, 1968.

85. Tolkoff-Rubin NE, Rubin RH, Keller EE, Baker GP, Stewart JA, Hirsch MS. Cytomegalovirus infection in dialysis patients and personnel. *Ann Intern Med* 89:625–628, 1978.

86. Kääriäinen L, Klemola E, Paloheimo J: Rise of cytomegalovirus antibodies in an infectious-mononucleosis-like syndrome after transfusion. *Br Med J* 1:1270–1278, 1966.

87. Henle W, Henle G, Scriba M, Joyner CR, Harrison FS, von Essen R, Paloheimo J, Klemola E: Antibody responses to the Epstein-Barr virus and cytomegaloviruses after open-heart and other surgery. *N Engl J Med* 282:1068–1074, 1970.

88. Jacobs RF: Frozen deglycerolized blood and transmission of Epstein-Barr virus. *J Infect Dis* 153:800, 1986.

89. Ritchey KA, Andiman W, McIntosh S, Berman B, Luce D: Mononucleosis syndrome following granulocyte transfusion in patients with leukemia. *J Pediatr* 97:267–269, 1980.

90. Adler SP, Lawrence LT, Baggett J, Biro V, Sharp DE: Prevention of transfusion-associated cytomegalovirus infection in very low-birthweight infants using frozen blood and donors seronegative for cytomegalovirus. *Transfusion* 24:333–335, 1984.

91. Taylor BJ, Jacobs RF, Baker RL, Moses EB, McSwain BE, Shulman G: Frozen deglycerolized blood prevents transfusion acquired cytomegalovirus infections in neonates. *Pediatr Infect Dis J* 188–191, 1986.

92. Rubin RH, Carney WP, Schooley RT, Colvin RB, Burton RC, Hoffman RA, Hansen WP, Cosimi AZ, Russell PS, Hirsch MS: The effect of infection on T lymphocyte subpopulations: a preliminary report. *Int J Immunopharmacol* 3:307–312, 1981.

93. Lang DJ, Ebert PA, Rodgers BM: Reduction of postperfusion cytomegalovirus infections following the use of leukocyte depleted blood. *Transfusion* 17:391–395, 1977.

94. Demmler GT, Brady MT, Bijou H, Speer ME, Milam JD, Hawkins EP, Anderson DC, Six H, Yow MD: Post-transfusion

cytomegalovirus infection in neonates: role of saline-washed red blood cells. *J Pediatr* 108:762–765, 1986.

95. Luban NLC, Williams AE, MacDonald MG, Mikesell G, Williams K, Sacher RA: Low incidence of acquired cytomegalovirus infections in neonates transfused with washed red blood cells. *Am J Dis Child* 141:416–419, 1987.

96. Gottleib MS, Schroff R, Schanker HM, Weisman JD, Fan PT, Wolf RA, Saxan A: Pneumocystis carinii pneumonia and mucosal candidiasis in previously healthy homosexual men: evidence of a new acquired cellular immunodeficiency. *N Engl J Med* 305:1425–1431, 1981.

97. Kreel I, Zaroff LI, Canter JW: A syndrome following total body perfusion. *Surg Gynecol Obstet* 111:317–321, 1960.

98. Prince AM, Szmuness W, Millian SJ, David DS: A serologic study of cytomegalovirus infections associated with blood transfusions. *N Engl J Med* 284:1125–1131, 1971.

99. Tegtmeier GE: Cytomegalovirus infection as a complication of blood transfusion. *Semin Liver Dis* 6:82–95, 1986.

100. Adler SP: Neonatal cytomegalovirus infections due to blood. *Crit Rev Clin Lab Sci* 23:1–14, 1985.

101. McCracken GH, Shinefield HR, Cobb K, Rausen AR, Dische MR, Eichenwald HF: Congenital cytomegalic inclusion disease. *Am J Dis Child* 117:522–539, 1969.

102. McEnery G, Stern H: Cytomegalovirus infection in early infancy: five atypical cases. *Arch Dis Child* 45:669–673, 1970.

103. King-Lewis PA, Gardner SD: Congenital cytomegalic inclusion disease following intrauterine transfusion. *Br Med J* 2:603–605, 1969.

104. Kumar A, Nankervis GA, Cooper RA, Gold E, Kumar ML: Acquisition of cytomegalovirus infection in infants following exchange transfusion: a prospective study. *Transfusion* 20:327–331, 1980.

105. Pass MA, Johnson JD, Schulman IA, Grumet CF, Hafleigh EB, Malachowski NC, Sunshine P: Evaluation of a walking-donor blood transfusion program with intensive care nursery. *J Pediatr* 89:646–651, 1976.

106. Tobin JOH, MacDonald H, Brayshay M: Cytomegalovirus infection and exchange transfusion. *Br Med J* 4:404, 1975.

107. Yeager AS: Transfusion-acquired cytomegalovirus infection in newborn infants. *Am J Dis Child* 128:478–483, 1974.

108. Yeager AS, Grumet FC, Hafleigh EB, Arvin AM, Bradley JS, Prober CG: Prevention of transfusion-acquired cytomegalovirus infections in newborn infants. *J Pediatr* 98:281–287, 1981.

109. Adler SP: Transfusion-associated cytomegalovirus infections. *Rev Infect Dis* 5:977–993, 1983.

110. Yeager AS, Palumbo PE, Malachowski N, Ariagno RL, Stevenson DK: Sequelae of maternally derived cytomegalovirus infections in premature infants. *J Pediatr* 102:918–922, 1983.

111. Betts RF, Freeman RB, Douglas RG, Talley TE: Clinical manifestations of renal allograft derived primary cytomegalovirus infection. *Am J Dis Child* 131:759–763, 1977.

112. Betts RF, Freeman RB, Douglas RG, Talley TE, Rundell B: Transmission of cytomegalovirus infection with renal allograft. *Kidney Int* 8:385–392, 1975.

113. Ho M, Suwansirikul S, Dowling JN, Youngblood LA, Armstrong JA: The transplanted kidney as a source of cytomegalovirus infection. *N Engl J Med* 293:1109–1112, 1975.

114. Pass RF, Long WK, Whitley RJ, Soong SJ, Diethelm AG, Reynolds DW, Alford CA: Productive infection with cytomegalovirus and herpes simplex virus in renal transplant recipients: role of source of kidney. *J Infect Dis* 137:556–563, 1978.

115. Preiksaitis JK, Rosno S, Grumet C, Merigan TC: Infections due to herpes viruses in cardiac transplant recipients: role of the donor heart and immunosuppressive therapy. *J Infect Dis* 147:974–981, 1983.

116. Rand KH, Pollard RB, Merigan TC: Increased pulmonary superinfections in cardiac transplant patients undergoing primary cytomegalovirus infection. *N Engl J Med* 297:951–953, 1978.

117. Meyers JD, Flournoy N, Thomas ED: Risk factors for cytomegalovirus infection after human marrow transplantation. *J Infect Dis* 153:478–488, 1986.

118. Bowden RA, Sayers M, Flournoy N, Newton B, Banaji M, Thomas ED, Meyers JD: Cytomegalovirus immune globulin and seronegative blood products to prevent primary cytomegalovirus infection after marrow transplantation. *N Engl J Med* 314:1006–1010, 1986.

119. Cox F, Hughes WT: Cytomegaloviremia in children with acute lymphocytic leukemia. *J Pediatr* 87:190–194, 1975.

120. Cox F, Hughes WT: The value of isolation procedures for cytomegalovirus infection in children with leukemia. *Cancer* 36:1158–1161, 1975.

121. Drew NL, Minor RC: Transfusion-related cytomegalovirus infection following noncardiac surgery. *JAMA* 247:2389–2391, 1982.

122. Baumgartner JD, Glauser MP, Burgo-Black AL, Black RD, Pyndiah N, Chiolero R: Severe cytomegalovirus infection in multiply transfused, splenectomized, trauma patients. *Lancet* 2:63–66, 1982.

123. CDC: Current trends: Revision of the case definition of acquired immunodeficiency for national reporting. *MMWR* 34:373–375, 1985.

124. Woods CC, Williams AE, McNamara JG, Annunziata JA, Feorino PM, Conway CO: Antibody against the human immunodeficiency virus in commercial intravenous gammaglobulin preparations. *Ann Intern Med* 105:536–538, 1986.

125. CDC: Safety of therapeutic immunoglobulin preparations with respect to transmission of human T-lymphotropic virus type III/lymphadenopathy-associated virus infection. *MMWR* 35:231–233, 1986.

126. Ammann AJ, Cowan MJ, Wara DW, Weintrub P, Dritz S, Goldman H, Perkins HA: Acquired immunodeficiency in an infant: possible transmission by means of blood products. *Lancet* 30:956–958, 1983.

127. Church JA, Lewis J, Spotkov JM: IgG subclass deficiencies in children with suspected AIDS. *Lancet* 1:279, 1984.

128. Church JA, Isaacs H: Transfusion-associated acquired immune deficiency syndrome in infants. *J Pediatr* 105:731–737, 1984.

129. Tong TK, Andrew LR, Albert A, Mickell JJ: Childhood acquired immune deficiency syndrome manifesting as acrodermatitis enteropathica. *J Pediatr* 108:426–428, 1986.

130. Shannon K, Ball E, Wasserman RL, Murphy FK, Luby J, Buchanan GR: Transfusion-associated cytomegalovirus infection and acquired immune deficiency syndrome in an infant. *J Pediatr* 103:859–863, 1983.

131. Maloney MJ, Cox F, Wray BB, Guill MF, Hagler J, Williams D: AIDS in a child 5½ years after a transfusion. *N Engl J Med* 312:1256, 1985.

132. Berkowitz CD, Seidel JS: Spontaneous resolution of cryptosporidiosis in a child with acquired immunodeficiency syndrome. *Am J Dis Child* 139:967, 1985.

133. Wykoff RF, Pearl ER, Saulsbury FT: Immunologic dysfunction in infants infected through transfusion with HTLV-III. *N Engl J Med* 312:294–296, 1985.

134. Cox F, Wray B, Chaudhary T, Karlson K, Sherwood B, Greenberg M: Transfusion-associated acquired immunodeficiency syndrome in a twin infant. *Pediatr Infect Dis* 4:106–108, 1985.

135. Luban NLC, Williams SE, Josephs S, Edwards M, Reaman GH: Spectrum of illness in eight children receiving washed RBCs from two HTLV-III infected donors. *Blood* 66:114a, 1985.

136. Lange JMA, vandenBerg H, Dooren LJ, Vossen JMJ, Kuis W, Goudsmit J: HTLV-III/LAV infection in nine children infected by a single plasma donor: clinical outcome and recognition patterns of viral proteins. *J Infect Dis* 154:171–174, 1986.

137. Saulsbury FT, Boyle RJ, Wykoff RF, Howard TH: Thrombocytopenia as the presenting manifestation of human T-lymphotropic virus type III infection in infants. *J Pediatr* 109:30–34, 1986.

138. Groopman JE, Hammer SM, Sallan SE, Allan JD: Human T-lymphotropic virus type III infection in previously immunocompromised hosts. *J Clin Oncol* 4:540–543, 1986.

139. Anderson KC, Gorgone BC, Marlink RG, Ferriani R, Essex ME, Benz PM, Groopman JE: Transfusion-acquired human

immunodeficiency virus infection among immunocompromised persons. *Ann Intern Med* 105:519–527, 1986.

140. Hardy AM, Allen JR, Morgan WM, Curran JW: The incidence rate of acquired immunodeficiency syndrome in selected populations. *JAMA* 253:215–220, 1985.

141. Peterman TA, Jaffe HW, Feorino PM, Getchell JP, Warfield DT, Haverkos HW, Stoneburner RL, Curran JW: Transfusion-associated acquired immunodeficiency syndrome in the United States. *JAMA* 254:2913–2917, 1985.

142. Moseley JW: Transfusion-transmitted HTLV-III (abstracts). In NIH Consensus Development Conference: Impact of Routine HTLV III Antibody Testing on Public Health, July 7–9, 1986.

143. Luban NLC, Kelleher JF, Reaman GH: Altered distribution of T-lymphocyte subpopulations in children and adolescents with haemophilia. *Lancet* 1:503–505, 1983.

144. Gill JC, Menitove JE, Wheeler D, Aster RN, Montgomery RR: Generalized lymphadenopathy and T-cell abnormalities in hemophilia A. *J Pediatr* 103:18–22, 1983.

145. Menitove JE, Aster RH, Casper JT, Lauer SJ, Gottschall JL, Williams JE, Gill JC, Wheeler DV, Piaskowski V, Kirchner P, Montgomery RR: T-lymphocyte subpopulations in patients with classic hemophilia treated with cryoprecipitate and lyophilized concentrates. *N Engl J Med* 208:83–86, 1983.

146. Lederman MM, Ratnoff OD, Scillian JJ, Jones PK, Schacter B: Impaired cell-mediated immunity in patients with classic hemophilia. *N Engl J Med* 308:79–83, 1983.

147. Sullivan JL, Brewster FE, Brettler DB, Forsberg AD, Cheeseman SH, Byron KS, Baker SM, Willitts DL, Lew RA, Levine PH: Hemophiliac immunodeficiency: influence of exposure to factor VIII concentrate, LAV/HTLV-III, and herpes viruses. *J Pediatr* 108:504–510, 1986.

148. Hilgartner M: AIDS in the transfused patient. *Am J Dis Child* 141:194–198, 1987.

149. Eyster ME, Whitehurst DA, Calatano PM, McMilan CW, Goodnight SH, Kasper CK, Gill JC, Aledort LM, Hilgartner MW, Levine PH, Edson JR, Hathaway WE, Lusher JM, Gill FM, Poole K, Shapiro S: Longterm follow-up of hemophiliacs with lymphocytopenia and thrombocytopenia. *Blood* 66:1317–1320, 1985.

150. Okochi K, Sato H: Adult T-cell leukemia virus, blood donors and transfusion: experience in Japan. In Dodd RY and Barker LA (eds): *Infection, Immunity and Blood Transfusion.* New York, Alan R Liss, 1985, pp 245–256.

151. Okochi K, Sato H, Hinum Y: A retrospective study on transmission of adult T-cell leukemia virus by blood transfusion: seroconversion in recipients. *Vox Sang* 46:245–253, 1984.

152. Yasuda K, Sei Y, Yokoyama MM, Tanaka K, Hara A: Healthy HTLV-I carriers in Japan: the haematological and immunological characteristics. *Br J Haematol* 64: 195–203, 1986.

153. Sato H, Okochi K: Transmission of human T-cell leukemia virus (HTLV-I) by blood transfusion: demonstration of proviral DNA in recipients' blood lymphocytes. *Int J Cancer* 37:395–400, 1986.

154. Goudsmit J, Breederveld K, Terpstra F, Melief CJM: Antibodies to T-cell leukemia lymphoma virus type I in Dutch hemophiliacs. *Vox Sang* (in press).

155. Osame M, Igatur A, Usuku K, Rosales RL: Mother-to-child transmission in HTLV-I associated myelopathy. *Lancet* 2:106, 1987.

156. Lemon SM: Type A viral hepatitis: new developments in an old disease. *N Engl J Med* 313:1059–1067, 1985.

157. Paryari SG, Yeager AS, Hosford-Dunn H, Johnson SJ, Ariagno RL, Stevenson DK: Sequelae of acquired cytomegalovirus infection in premature and sick term infants. *J Pediatr* 107:451–456, 1985.

158. Spector SA: Transmission of cytomegalovirus among infants in hospital documented by restriction-endonuclease digestion analysis. *Lancet* 1:378–381, 1983.

159. Tolpin MD, Stewart JA, Warren D, Mojica BA, Collins MA, Doveikis SA, Cabradilla C, Schauf V, Raju TNK, Nelson K: Transfusion transmission of cytomegalovirus confirmed by restriction endonuclease analysis. *J Pediatr* 107:953–956, 1985.

160. Ragni MV, Spero JA, Bontemp FA, Lewis JA: Recurrent infections and lymphadenopathy in the child of a hemophiliac: a survey of children of hemophiliacs positive for human immunodeficiency virus antibody. *Ann Intern Med* 105:886–887, 1986.

161. Rosner F, Forgel M, Telsey A, Cuterman S, Charyton M, Rubinstein A: Acquired immunodeficiency syndrome in infants and children: report of nine cases. *Biomed Pharmacother* 39:350–355, 1985.

162. Centers for Disease Control: Human immunodeficiency virus infection in transfusion recipients and their family members. *MMWR* 36:137–140, 1987.

163. Allain JP, Laurian Y, Paul DA, Senn D: Serological markers in early stages of human immunodeficiency virus infection in haemophiliacs. *Lancet* 1:1233–1236, 1986.

164. Peterman TA, Lang GR, Mikos NJ, Soloman SL, Schable CA, Feorino PM, Britz JA, Allen JR: HTLV-III/LAV infection in hemodialysis patients. *JAMA* 255:2324–2326, 1986.

165. Burke DS, Redfield RR: False positive Western blot tests for antibodies to HTLV III. *JAMA* 256:347, 1986.

166. Barre-Sinoussi F, Chermann JC, Rey F, Nugeyre MT, Chamaret S, Gruest J, Dauguet C, Axler-Blin C, Vezinet-Brun F, Rouzioux C, Rozenbaum W, Montagnier L: Isolation of a T-lymphotrophic retrovirus from a patient at risk for acquired immune deficiency syndrome (AIDS). *Science* 220:868–870, 1983.

167. Goudsmit J, Paul DA, Lange JMA, Speelman H, Van Der Moordaa J, Van Der Helm HJ, DeWolf F, Epstein LG, Krone WJA, Wolters EC, Oleske JM, Courtinho RA: Expression of human immunodeficiency virus antigen (HIV-Ag) serum and cerebrospinal fluid during acute and chronic infection. *Lancet* 2:177–180, 1986.

168. Blanche S, Fischer A, LeDeist F, Griscelli C, Guetard D, Favier V, Montagnier L: Ribavirin in HTLV III/LAV infection of infants. *Lancet* 1:863, 1986.

169. Silverman BA, Rubinstein A: Serum lactate dehydrogenase levels in adults and children with acquired immune deficiency syndrome (AIDS) and AIDS-related complex: possible indicator of B cell lymphoproliferation and disease activity. *Am J Med* 78:728–736, 1985.

170. Blanche S, LeDeist F, Fischer A, Verber F, Devre M, Chamaret S, Montagnier L, Griscelli C: Longitudinal study of 18 children with perinatal LAV/HTLV III infection: attempt at prognostic evaluation. *J Pediatr* 109:965–970, 1986.

171. Danner SA, Schurrman HJ, Lange JMA, Meylin FHJG, Schellekens PTA, Hubo J, Kater L: Implantation of cultured thymic fragments immunodeficiency syndrome. *Arch Intern Med* 146:1133–1136, 1986.

172. Rubinstein A, Novick B, Sicklick MJ, Bernstein L, Incefy G, Naylor PH, Goldstein AC: Circulating thymulin and thymosin 21, activity in pediatric acquired immune deficiency syndrome: in vivo and in vitro studies. *J Pediatr* 109:422–427, 1986.

173. Gupta A, Novick BE, Rubinstein A: Restoration of suppressor T-cell functions in children with AIDS following intravenous gamma globulin treatment. *Am J Dis Child* 140:143–146, 1986.

174. Kuhns WJ, Prince AM, Brotman B, Hazzi C, Grady GF: A clinical and laboratory evaluation of immune serum globulin from donors with a history of hepatitis: attempted prevention of post-transfusion hepatitis. *Am J Med Sci* 272, 255–261, 1976.

175. Seeff LB, Zimmerman HJ, Wright EC, Finkelstein JD, Garcia-Pont P, Greenlee HB, Dietz A, Levy CM, Tamburro CH, Schiff ER, Schimmel EM, Zemel R, Zimmon DS, McCollum RW: A randomized, double blind controlled trial of the efficacy of immune serum globulin for the prevention of post-transfusion hepatitis. *Gastroenterology* 72:111–121, 1977.

176. Stevens CE, Aach RD, Hollinger FB, Mosley JW, Szmuness W, Kahn R, Werrch J, Edwards V: Hepatitis B virus antibody in blood donors and the occurrence of non-A, non-B hepatitis in transfusion recipients: an analysis of the transfusion-transmitted viruses study. *Ann Int Med* 101:733–738, 1984.

177. Beneke JS, Tegtmeier GE, Alter HJ, Luetkemeyer RB, Solomon R, Bayer WL: Relation of titers of antibodies to CMV

in blood donors to the transmission of cytomegalovirus infection. *J Infect Dis* 150:883–888, 1984.

178. Lamberson H, McMillan J, Weiner L, Williams M, Clark D, McMahon C, Bousman E, Patti A: Nursery-acquired cytomegalovirus infection. *Transfusion* 23:418a, 1983.

179. Lamberson H, McMillan J, Weiner L, Williams M, Clark D, McMahon C, Bousman E, Patti A: Nursery acquired CMV infection in transfused neonates. *Transfusion* 24:430a, 1984.

180. Pindyck J: Psychosocial impact of anti-HTLV III notification: the New York experience. In NIH Consensus Conference: Impact of Routine HTLV III Antibody Testing on Public Health Bethesda, MD, NIH, July 6, 1986, pp 77–78.

181. Kaplan HS, Kleinman SH: AIDS: Blood donor studies and screening programs. In Dodd RY, Barker LA (ed): *Infection, Immunity and Blood Transfusion*. New York, Alan R Liss, 1985, 297–308.

182. CDC: Provisional Public Health Service inter-agency recommendations for screening donated blood and plasma for antibody to the virus causing acquired immunodeficiency syndrome. *MMWR* 34:1–5, 1985.

183. Mortimer PP, Luban NLC, Kelleher JF, Cohen BJ: Transmission of serum parvovirus-like virus by clotting factor concentrate. *Lancet* 2:482–483, 1983.

184. VandenBerg W. TenCate JW, Breederveld, C, Goudsmit J: Seroconversion to HTLV-III in hemophiliac given heat-treated factor VIII concentrate. *Lancet* 2:803–804, 1986.

185. Kernoff PBA, Miller EJ, Savidge GF, Machin SJ, Dewar MS, Preston FE: Wet heating for safer factor VIII concentrate? *Lancet* 2:721, 1985.

186. Hollinger FB, Dolana G, Thomas W, Gyorkey F: Reduction in risk of hepatitis transmission by heat treatment of a human factor VIII concentrate. *J Infect Dis* 150:250–262, 1984.

187. Mikaelsson M, Nilsson IM, Vilhardt H, Wiechel B: Factor VIII concentrate prepared from blood donors stimulated by intranasal administration of a vasopressin analogue. *Transfusion* 22:229–233, 1982.

188. Rock G, Palmer AS: Accumulative effect of DDAVP and heparin in increasing plasma factor VIII levels. *Vox Sang* 41:56–60, 1981.

189. McLeod BC, Scott JP: Transfusion studies of "single donor" factor VIII derived from plasma exchange donation. *JAMA* 252:2726–2729, 1984.

190. Wells MA, Wittek AE, Epstein JS, Marcus-Sekura C, Daniel S, Tawkersley DL, Preston MJ, Quinnan GV: Inactivation and partition of human T-cell virus type III during ethanol fractionation of plasma. *Transfusion* 26:210–213, 1986.

2
PATHOGENS

10

Varicella-Zoster Virus

Anne A. Gershon, M.D. and Philip S. LaRussa, M.D.

BACKGROUND

Varicella (chickenpox) and zoster (shingles) are caused by the same agent, the varicella-zoster virus (VZV), a member of the herpes virus group. Morphologically, herpes viruses have a diameter of about 180 nm, a core of nucleic acid (DNA), surrounded by an icosahedral (20-sided) protein capsid covered by a tegument, and an outermost envelope containing lipids and glycoproteins. Virally specified glycoproteins appear not only on the surface of the virion but also on the membrane of the infected cell (1). These glycoproteins are of special importance, since they seem to play a role in viral infectivity, and as antigens, they are responsible for stimulation of immune responses, which ultimately can enable the host to control the organism. While it is possible to infect certain animals such as guinea pigs and patas monkeys with VZV, there is no practical animal model for study of infections caused by this virus.

As with the other herpes viruses, VZV has the potential to cause latent infection during the first encounter with the agent. Following primary infection with VZV, varicella, patients are at risk to develop reactivation of latent VZV resulting in secondary infection, zoster.

Varicella

This is a disease largely of children. In the United States, about 80% of children beyond the age of 10 have had varicella; subclinical infection probably occurs in about 5% of the population, and about 95% of adults are immune. Clinically, varicella is characterized by a pruritic rash concentrated on the head and trunk (Fig. 10.1). The lesions are initially maculopapular; they quickly progress to vesicles, followed by pustulation and crusting. Most children have a low-to-moderate grade fever accompanying the rash. Complications are unusual in otherwise healthy children, but they include bacterial superinfection, especially of the skin, but also of the lung, and various encephalopathies (cerebellar ataxia, cerebral encephalitis, and Reye's syndrome). In addition, viral arthritis, glomerulonephritis, transverse myelitis, and other bacterial superinfections, such as osteomyelitis, may follow varicella, but they are rare. Most otherwise healthy children with varicella are ill for 5–7 days. As will be discussed below, varicella may be particularly severe when it occurs in persons deficient in cell-mediated immunity, newborn infants whose mothers have active varicella at delivery, and adults.

The proposed pathogenesis of varicella is shown in Figure 10.2. The virus is believed to infect by the respiratory tract and then to invade the regional lymph nodes, where further replication takes place, resulting in a low-grade viremia (2). Virus then invades certain viscera: the liver, spleen, and perhaps other organs; subsequently, a secondary viremia of greater magnitude occurs, delivering VZV to the skin, and resulting in the characteristic generalized rash. Usually, this takes about 14 days, although the incubation period can range from 10–21 days. Only subsequent to development of the rash can specific antibody and cell-mediated immunity to VZV be detected. Antibodies may be measured by a variety of methods (see below); cellular immunity can be assessed by an intradermal skin test with VZV antigen, and by in vitro analysis of lymphoid cells obtained from peripheral blood. The latter includes stimulation of lymphocytes by exposure to VZV antigen, and the ability of various lymphoid cells to lyse tissue culture cells infected with VZV, when blood cells from varicella immune donors are utilized.

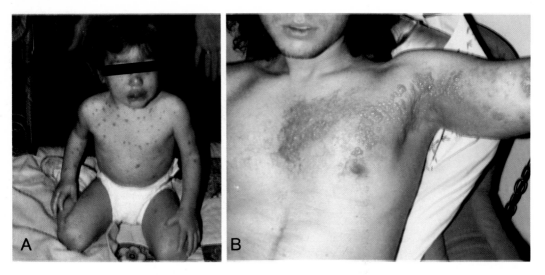

Figure 10.1.   *A*, Varicella, day 5 in an otherwise healthy 2-year-old boy. *B*, Zoster in an immunocompromised 23-year-old male.

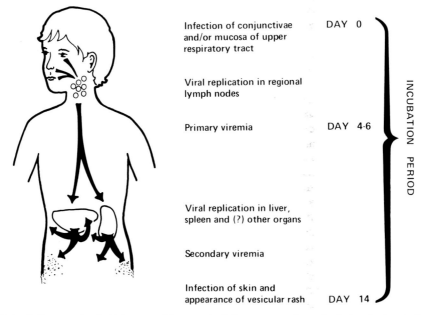

Infection of conjunctivae and/or mucosa of upper respiratory tract — DAY 0

Viral replication in regional lymph nodes

Primary viremia — DAY 4-6

Viral replication in liver, spleen and (?) other organs

Secondary viremia

Infection of skin and appearance of vesicular rash — DAY 14

INCUBATION PERIOD

Figure 10.2.   Pathogenesis of chickenpox. Diagram depicting proposed events during the incubation period of varicella. (From Gross CH: Variation on a theme by Fenner: the pathogenesis of chickenpox. *Pediatrics* 68:735–737, 1981.)

After varicella, these responses can be detected in most persons for life, although after the age of about 50 years, cell-mediated immune responses to VZV seem to decline.

Zoster

Since zoster is due to reactivation of latent VZV, the first prerequisite for its development is prior infection with the virus, usually an episode of clinical varicella. Zoster occurs mainly in immunosuppressed patients and in adults over the age of 50. (Fig. 10.1*B*). Infants who have experienced varicella while in utero (due to maternal chickenpox) are also at increased risk to develop zoster at a young age. In one classic study, the rate of zoster per year in children age 0–9 years was 0.74 per 1000, but in adults between the ages of 50–59 years, it was 5.09 (3). The rate of zoster is highest in the 9th decade of life (about 10 per 1000 persons per year), and it has been estimated that if a cohort of 1000 persons were to be followed until the age of 85, ½ would have experienced one attack of zoster and 10 would have experienced two attacks (3).

Zoster may be thought of as a localized form of varicella; the individual lesions are very similar, except that zoster vesicles have a greater tendency toward confluence than do those of varicella. The rash of zoster is unilateral, affecting 1–3 dermatomes (Fig. 10.3). In contrast to chickenpox, the lesions tend to be painful rather than pruritic. In addition to the acute pain associated with the rash of zoster, the elderly in particular may experience a persistent, often severe, and disabling syndrome of postherpetic pain lasting for as long as a year, long after the skin lesions may have healed. Postherpetic pain is almost unheard of in the pediatric population. Some patients with zoster, particularly those who are immunocompromised, may also develop dissemination of the rash to more distant skin areas. Dissemination of a mild nature, with less than 25 lesions out of the dermatomal distribution, is not uncommon and does not necessarily herald a poor prognosis. In contrast, disseminated zoster of greater magnitude may be serious and may require specific therapy (see below).

During varicella, VZV becomes latent in dorsal root ganglia (Fig. 10.3). It probably reaches the ganglia by traveling from the skin along sensory nerves during varicella. Zoster is most commonly seen on the trunk and face, reflecting the distribution of the rash of varicella. While viral DNA and messenger RNA have been detected in sensory ganglia at autopsy (4,5), it is not possible to determine whether latent infection is present during life. Presumably, most or all persons who have had chickenpox have latent VZV. Containment of latent VZV is probably dependent to a great extent upon the immune system, since zoster is most common in severely immunocompromised patients such as those with advanced Hodgkin's disease and those who have undergone bone marrow transplantation. Clinical zoster is probably the result of a two-step process: (*a*) reactivation of latent VZV, and (*b*) a defective cellular immune response to the virus, resulting in development of rash. Reactivation of VZV in the absence of skin lesions (zoster sine herpete) with an increase in the VZV antibody response has been recorded. Moreover, by no means will all persons with decreased cell-mediated immunity to VZV develop zoster, suggesting that at least two major factors are involved in pathogenesis.

Second clinical attacks of varicella are unusual but have been described; boosting of specific immune responses after reexposure to VZV has also been described and may be of importance in long-term maintenance of immunity (6–8). A diagram showing the natural history of VZV infection and illustrating some of these concepts is presented in Figure 10.4.

POPULATION AT RISK

Immunocompromised patients and severe varicella. VZV infections may be severe in immunocompromised patients of all ages. Immunocompromised children are prone to develop severe varicella, but they may also develop severe zoster if they have already had chickenpox. Severe varicella may take two forms; a prolonged disease known as progressive varicella, and a more rapidly fatal illness in which disseminated intravascular coagulation develops within a few days after onset. Hemorrhagic skin lesions may be seen in both forms. Serious disease may be preceded by severe abdominal pain. In progressive varicella, new lesions develop for up to 2 weeks; during this time, repeated episodes of viremia are believed to occur. Development of primary viral pneumonia with bilateral fluffy infiltrates appearing on x-ray is an ominous sign, although antiviral drugs have im-

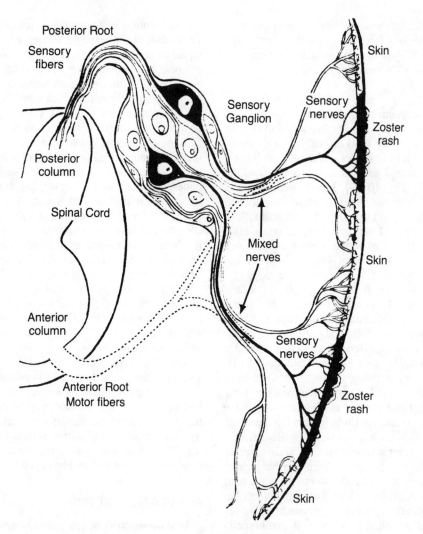

Figure 10.3. Diagram of the proposed pathogenesis of zoster. From Hope-Simpson RE: The nature of herpes zoster: a long-term study and a new hypothesis. *Proc R Soc Med* 58:9–20, 1965.

proved the prognosis of this complication (see below).

It was recognized that varicella could be severe or fatal in children with an underlying malignancy in the 1950s (8). As more children with malignant disease have survived due to more intense chemotherapy and radiotherapy, varicella has become a greater problem for them. Children with acute leukemia and lymphoma are at greatest risk; untreated, about 30% develop severe infections, with 21% mortality (7% of the total) (9). Children with solid tumors may also develop severe varicella, but it seems to be less life threatening for them than it is for leukemics. Usually, one case of varicella provides lifelong protection; however second cases seem to be more common in immunocompromised patients than in normal individuals. Second attacks of varicella have been described particularly in patients with an underlying malignancy and in renal transplant recipients (7,10,11). Immunocompromised children who develop varicella should be treated promptly with antiviral drugs as soon as the disease is diagnosed, unless they have been passively or actively immunized against varicella (see below).

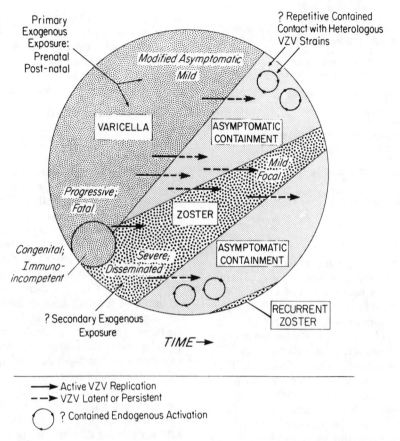

Figure 10.4. Diagrammatic summary of the natural history of infection with varicella-zoster virus. Two variables are depicted: time and clinical severity. In the competent host the containment period is on the order of decades; however, in the immunocompromised person the two clinical processes may merge without an intervening asymptomatic interval. The containment period after congenital varicella is typically of short duration. During the asymptomatic containment period episodes of endogenous viral replication probably occur, and contact with heterologous exogenous strains may stimulate host defenses, usually in the absence of overt disease. (Reprinted by permission of the publisher. From Weller TH: Varicella and herpes zoster: Changing concepts of the natural history, control, and importance of not-so-benign virus. *N Eng J Med*, 309:1364, 1983.)

Varicella in pregnancy. Pregnant women who contract varicella may experience a severe infection that can be fatal. A recent prospective study of 43 consecutive pregnant women with varicella found that 9% developed pneumonia; there was one fatality (2% of the total) (12). While it has been thought that there is no increased risk of abortion in such women (13), in this same study, 10% had premature labor temporally related to chickenpox (12).

Congenital varicella syndrome following maternal varicella. Infants whose mothers have gestational varicella are also at increased risk from the infection. It is thought that VZV crosses the placenta to the infant during the maternal viremia, which occurs just prior to the onset of the maternal rash. A rare congenital varicella syndrome of anomalies in infants whose mothers developed varicella in the 1st or 2nd trimester of pregnancy has been described, with an estimated incidence of less than 5% (12,13). Infants with this syndrome usually have a hypoplastic limb with cicatricial scarring of the skin, evidence of brain damage, and various eye defects, such as chorioretinitis, and cataracts (Table 10.1). The pathogenesis of the syndrome is not known, although reactivation of VZV in

Table 10.1.
**Fetal Abnormalities Associated with Maternal
VZV Infection (Distribution and Type of Defects)[a]**

37 Reported Cases 86% following maternal varicella; 14% following maternal zoster 8–28 weeks of pregnancy (median 12 weeks)	
Cicatricial skin lesions	70%
Ocular abnormalities	62%
cataract, chorioretinitis, Horner's syndrome, microphthalmia, nystagmus	
Hypoplastic limb	46%
Cortical atrophy/mental retardation	30%
Early death	24%

[a]Modified from reference 13.

utero may be involved and would explain a hypoplastic limb and skin scarring that resemble zoster. There is no evidence of chronic VZV infection, and it has not been possible to isolate VZV from tissues of any affected infants. Studies of VZV antibody and cellular immunity, when performed, however, have indicated that VZV infection has occured in the infant (13). There is no known way to diagnose the congenital varicella syndrome in utero. There are no data concerning the utility of amniocentesis, but it is unlikely to be helpful, since many infants infected in utero would not be expected to manifest anomalies. Ultrasound has been suggested as a means for identification of a damaged fetus with, for example, a limb or other deformity after maternal chickenpox, although its successful use in this situation has been reported only once (14). The disease is so unusual (about 30 cases having been reported in the world literature since the 1940s), that it is difficult to make firm recommendations concerning whether or not to terminate pregnancy in the absence of obvious fetal defects. Consideration is often given to maternal age and ease of conception in addition to varicella when making a decision regarding abortion.

Early development of zoster. Most infants whose mothers have varicella during pregnancy (except near term) are perfectly well at birth. In utero infection with VZV becomes apparent, however, when the patient develops zoster within the first few years of life and has no history of ever having had varicella. It has been suggested that the immune response to VZV in utero is immature, resulting in occurrence of zoster at

an early age (15,16). Infants who develop varicella in the 1st year of life are also at increased risk to develop zoster compared with children who develop chickenpox at a later age (17). Fortunately, these cases of zoster in young children are almost always mild and self-limited.

Severe neonatal infections. Infants born to women who develop varicella close to term are at risk to develop severe or fatal varicella; attack rates ranging between 17%–45% have been reported, and untreated, about 30% of cases are fatal (13,18,19). Infants born to women whose onset of varicella is less than 5 days prior to delivery are at greatest risk, due to transmission of virus from mother to fetus prior to development of specific maternal antibodies. Infants born to women whose onset of varicella was earlier than 5 days before delivery may transmit VZV to their child, but there will have been enough time for antibodies to the virus to have developed, resulting in a modified infection in the baby. Thus, infants actually born with varicella have very mild disease, in contrast to those who develop it at 5–10 days of age (13). Relationships between maternal varicella, development of maternal IgG to VZV, and birth of the infant are diagrammed in Figure 10.5. Passive immunization of infants born to women with varicella at delivery has nearly eradicated infant mortality in this situation (see below for specific recommendations).

Patients at high risk to develop severe zoster. Zoster occurs in an older age group than does varicella; one reason is that previous chickenpox is a prerequisite for developing zoster. In addition, older persons are relatively more immunocompromised than are the young. Zoster may be an especially difficult problem for patients with malignant disease and for those who have undergone organ transplantation (20). This population has a higher incidence of zoster than do age-matched controls. Also, the illness tends to be more severe. Presumably, these increased risks are directly related to the degree of deficiency of cell-mediated immunity to VZV (21,22). It has long been thought that cellular immunity plays the major role in host defense against VZV, since patients with agammaglobulinemia respond normally to VZV infections, and they do not have a higher than usual incidence of zoster than normal persons of the same age. In contrast, patients being treated for lym-

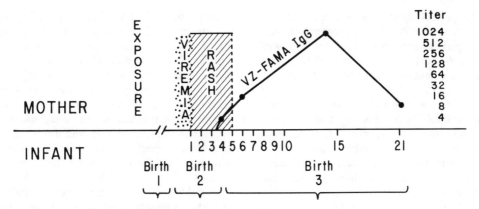

Figure 10.5. The relationship between transmission of VZV and VZV antibodies from mother to infant during maternal varicella near term. Babies born at 1 will not acquire congenital varicella, but may be exposed postnatally. Babies born at 2 may have been congenitally infected but will not have received transplacental maternal antibody to VZV and may develop severe varicella. Babies born at 3 have detectable transplacental VZV antibodies and, if infected with VZV, develop a modified infection. From Krugman S, & Gershon A (eds): *Infections of the Fetus and Newborn Infant.* New York, Alan R. Liss, 1975, p 90.

phoma and those who have had transplantation have decreased cellular immunity to VZV and a higher incidence of zoster than controls. It has become customary to administer antiviral chemotherapy early in the illness to many immunocompromised patients who develop zoster (see below). As will be discussed, passive immunization with high titer-specific antiserum does not seem to either prevent or modify zoster, probably because most zoster patients have detectable VZV antibodies, although their cellular immune responses are abnormal.

Epidemiologic data suggest that zoster is caused by reactivation of latent infection rather than by a second infection with VZV (3,8). The incidence of zoster is not seasonal as is varicella, which is most common in the winter and spring. Moreover, the incidence of varicella in young adults who are frequently exposed to children with chickenpox is low. If zoster were due to reinfection with VZV, one would expect the incidence of both diseases to parallel each other. Recently, more concrete data which support the epidemiologic observations have become available. VZV was isolated in both instances from a boy with Wiscott-Aldrich syndrome who developed varicella, followed by zoster, within a few months' time. Virus isolates from his episode of varicella and of zoster were identical by analysis of the DNA with four restriction enzymes (23). Analysis with four enzymes has

been found to be sufficient to distinguish between epidemiologically different VZV isolates (24). Therefore, both isolates from this boy can be said to have been similar, indicating that zoster was due to reactivation of latent VZV. In another instance, a child with leukemia in remission developed zoster about 2 years after immunization with live attenuated varicella vaccine. With a similar restriction enzyme analysis, it was found that viral DNA obtained from his zoster rash was identical to the DNA of the varicella vaccine virus with which he had been immunized (25).

Zoster in pregnancy. Zoster in a pregnant woman does not result in severe varicella in the infant. In zoster there is a marked anamnestic antibody response in the mother so that the infant is well-endowed with specific antibodies to VZV. This situation may be thought of as a natural form of passive immunization of the baby.

Congenital varicella syndrome following maternal zoster. In contrast to maternal varicella, transmission of VZV from a mother with zoster to her fetus is probably lower than the transmission rates of about 20%–50% observed for maternal varicella. For example, in 14 reported consecutive cases of maternal zoster, there was no evidence of fetal infection (12). This phenomenon is probably due to the presence of maternal VZV antibodies during zoster which help to protect most infants from infection. However, several cases of the congenital varicella syndrome have been recorded following maternal zoster (13). It is known that in some patients, a viremia may accompany zoster. This may account for dissemination of lesions beyond the dermatomal distribution and the rare case of fetal infection following maternal zoster. While no large or prospective study has been performed, it seems reasonable to conclude that the risk of transmission of VZV to the fetus is lower after maternal zoster than it is after maternal varicella.

Nosocomial varicella. Spread of varicella in hospitals has long been a significant problem. The disease is highly contagious, with 80%–90% of susceptibles who have an intimate, household-type exposure becoming infected (26), although transmission rates after hospital exposures may not necessarily be so high. Several factors contribute to the highly infectious nature of VZV. While the specifics of viral spread are still unknown, the moist skin lesions of both varicella and zoster, particularly in the early stage of the illness, are full of infectious virions. Although it is almost impossible to isolate VZV from throat cultures in patients with varicella, there is epidemiologic evidence that these patients are infectious for 1–2 days prior to the onset of the rash; therefore, respiratory transmission of varicella almost certainly occurs. The virus spreads to others by the airborne route; this has been well-documented in at least two hospital studies (27,28). Since both zoster and varicella are caused by the same virus, patients with either disease may transmit chickenpox to persons with whom they have close contact who have never had varicella. Finally, no population is ever completely protected from VZV, since those who are immune to varicella may develop zoster and reintroduce the virus into the population again, perhaps an evolutionary mechanism for perpetuation of VZV and other latent viruses.

Outbreaks of varicella in hospitals that have lasted many weeks and have involved numerous immunocompromised patients and hospital employees have been well-described (29). Such outbreaks may be exceedingly costly, since in many hospitals personnel with no history of disease are furloughed during their potential period of contagion. Varicella also tends to be more severe in adults than in children, and occasional

fatalities in adults have been reported. Therefore, many hospitals now require serologic testing of employees for immunity to varicella. A number of sensitive antibody tests are now commercially available for this purpose (see below). Since varicella rarely occurs more than once in the same person, hospital employees with no past history of varicella but with detectable serum VZV antibodies, measured with a reliable test, may come in contact with varicella and zoster with essentially no risk to themselves or to patients.

About 5% of healthy adults are susceptible to varicella. A history of previous varicella is often a good indicator of immunity to the disease, but the lack of knowledge of previous varicella does not necessarily mean susceptibility. In most studies, only about 25% of adults with no history of varicella are actually susceptible (30,31). Presumably, in the remaining 75%, varicella was subclinical or so mild that it went unnoticed or was misdiagnosed. The risk for susceptibility is higher in adults reared in tropical or semitropical countries and has been reported to be as high as about 50% (32). Determination of whether or not serum antibodies are present, therefore, is necessary before concluding that an adult with no history of varicella is susceptible. Those with positive VZV antibody tests may be considered immune. No serologic assay is perfect, but most of the commercially available assays are acceptable. Fortunately, for practical control of nosocomial varicella, false-negativity of these assays seems to be more of a problem than false-positivity.

It seems reasonable, particularly in pediatric hospital settings, where there are often large numbers of varicella susceptibles, to have a logically developed plan in mind for dealing prospectively with prevention of nosocomial transmission of VZV. One possibility is the use of an algorithm such as that shown in Figure 10.6 (33). This strategy is useful for example, when considering admission of any child to a hospital. The following factors are taken into account: whether the child had varicella previously, whether any recent exposure to varicella has occurred, and if so, when, and whether the child is at high risk to develop severe varicella. Use of such an algorithm plus serologic testing of hospital employees who have never had varicella could potentially avert a great deal of nosocomial VZV infection. Hopefully, use of the live attenuated varicella vaccine, when it is li-

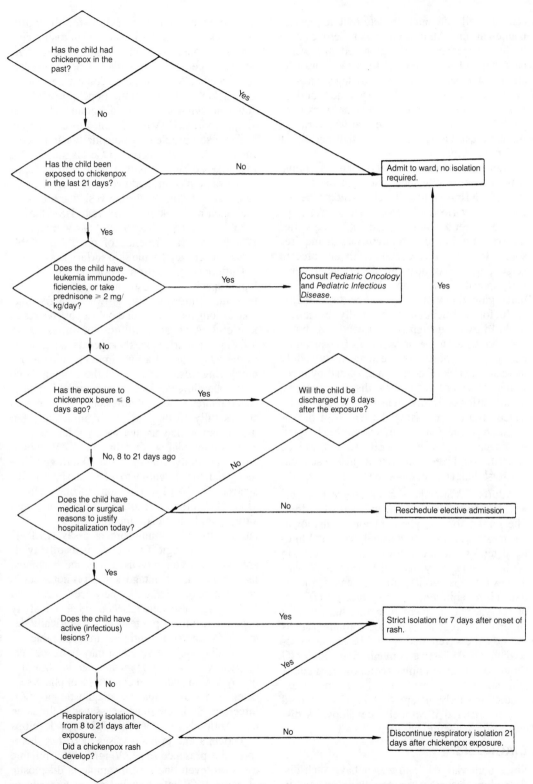

Figure 10.6.   An algorithm for chickenpox exposure. From Brawley RL, Wenzel RP: An algorithm for chickenpox. *Pediatr Infect Dis* 3:502–504, 1984.

censed, will add another deterrent to our armamentarium. At present, when seronegative hospital employees working on pediatric wards have been closely exposed to VZV, consideration should be given to the following strategies. Employees should either be furloughed for days 8–21 after the exposure, or they can work temporarily in an area where there are no varicella susceptibles during their potential period of communicability.

Transmission requires contact of a susceptible with an overtly infected person, so there is no risk of transmission until 24–48 hours before the rash of varicella develops. Therefore, these steps need not be implemented until 8 days after the exposure. Fortunately, transmission requires some type of direct contact with an infected person; there has been no documented third-party spread of chickenpox. Varicella-zoster immune globulin (VZIG), as will be discussed, is useful for modification of potentially severe varicella in exposed high-risk susceptibles, but it is of no value in the prevention of nosocomial chickenpox. In fact, its use may inadvertently increase the risk of nosocomial spread by modifying the severity of clinical disease, allowing mildly affected individuals to remain undetected, and by increasing the length of the incubation period. Therefore, susceptible hospital employees who receive VZIG should still be either furloughed or cohorted as just described, but for a longer interval—28 days.

Adults. Varicella is more severe in otherwise healthy adults than it is in healthy children. The reason for this phenomenon is unknown, but most viral diseases normally seen in childhood tend to be more severe if they occur in adults. Interestingly, as will be discussed, varicella vaccine is also less immunogenic for adults than it is for children, and the protective efficacy of the vaccine is lower in adults than it is in children. Varicella in immunocompromised adults can be quite severe and should be managed accordingly (34). Passive immunization with VZIG should be given to immunocompromised adults with no history of varicella at the time of exposure, and early therapy with acyclovir should be administered if varicella develops, as discussed for leukemic children.

DIAGNOSIS

Since both varicella and zoster have such distinct clinical characteristics, laboratory confirmation is often not necessary for diagnostic purposes. It is helpful in certain confusing clinical situations, however, to utilize rapid diagnostic procedures. Varicella has been mistaken for rickettsial pox, scabies, contact dermatitis, Coxsackie virus infection, impetigo, Stevens-Johnson syndrome, and disseminated herpes simplex virus (HSV) infection. Zoster is less of a diagnostic problem; it potentially can be confused with HSV infection. One diagnostic clue that may be helpful is that zoster rarely recurs in the same patient, and even more rarely in the same area of skin. Recurrent vesicular eruptions are much more likely to be due to HSV than to VZV. Laboratory diagnosis of VZV infections is aided by the presence of readily available virus concentrated at the skin surface in vesicles.

Culture of virus from vesicular fluid is the major specific diagnostic test available in most hospitals; unfortunately, growth of VZV may take as long as a week, and only a positive result is useful. A negative culture does not rule out VZV, particularly since this agent is rather labile in the laboratory. Various immunologic assays employing vesicular fluid as the antigen, such as immunofluorescence, countercurrent immunoelectrophoresis, and gel diffusion have been used successfully to diagnose VZV infections, but unfortunately, they are not widely available (35). The commercial availability of VZV monoclonal antibody conjugated to fluorescein has increased the potential to make a specific diagnosis. Dot-blot hybridization utilizing a cloned viral DNA probe also offers promise of a sensitive, rapid diagnostic method (36) as does an enzyme-linked immunosorbent assay (ELISA) (37). The cytologic Tzanck test is readily available and is frequently used in some hospitals; its principal disadvantage is that it is not specific and it cannot distinguish betweeen VZV and HSV. It may also yield falsely positive and falsely negative results; rapid tests that specifically detect VZV and/or its antigens are preferable.

The diagnosis of varicella may be made serologically. A 4-fold or greater rise in VZV antibody titer in acute and convalescent phase sera taken 7–10 days apart is diagnostic of VZV infection. Both sera must be assayed in the same test. Antibody to VZV of the IgM type develops in varicella and in many cases of zoster; therefore, the presence of VZV IgM (by a reliable assay) in even one serum sample is diagnostic of acute VZV infection but not necessarily of primary infection. IgM may be detected using immunofluorescence, but it is not a simple assay to interpret since false-positive reactions due to rheumatoid factor may occur. Antibody titers of a certain magnitude may be seen only in active disease, so that in some instances, a diagnosis of acute infection may be made on only one serum specimen. This latter approach would apply only to laboratories with great experience in serodiagnosis of VZV infections, where the upper limit of VZV antibody titers seen in healthy varicella immune individuals is known.

The laboratory must be utilized to identify adults with no history of chickenpox who are actually immune. Methods that have been successfully employed for this purpose include indirect immunofluorescence, including the very sensitive fluorescent antibody to membrane antigen (FAMA) test (38); ELISA (39–41); immune adherence hemagglutination assay (IAHA) (42); radioimmunoassay (RIA) (43); and anti-complement immunofluorescence test (ACIF) (44). The complement fixation (CF) test is not sensitive enough for the purpose of identifying varicella immunes, although it may be used to analyze acute and convalescent serum specimens to document acute VZV infection. The other tests mentioned are more sensitive than CF. Each laboratory performing assays for the purpose of identifying varicella immunes should assume the responsibility for quality control of the test. Serologic testing for VZV antibodies is difficult, and especially with a commercial kit, it is important to standardize values for known positive and negative sera before interpreting values of random sera.

A skin test provides another approach to determining susceptibility to varicella. This test utilizes heat inactivated VZV antigen, which is injected intradermally; the reaction detects cell-mediated immunity to VZV (30,45). Some VZV skin test antigens require a control uninfected antigen (injected into the opposite forearm) (30), and others do not (46). The test is read after 48 hours; a positive test is indicated by at least 5 mm diameter of erythema at the site of the VZV antigen. Tests that are negative after 24 hours are very unlikely to become positive (30). Unfortunately, this test is not now commercially available in the United States, although it may become so in the future. This test provides an excellent means for any physician at any time to determine whether his or her patient is immune to varicella. There have been no side effects associated with VZV skin testing. Unfortunately, persons above the age of 50 may no longer manifest a positive VZV skin test, although they continue to maintain humoral immunity to VZV (47). However, it is so unusual for a person beyond the age of 50 to be susceptible to varicella that there is very little need to perform skin tests on this population. In young adults, in contrast, the skin test is an excellent indicator of immunity to varicella (30).

TREATMENT

Most VZV infections, especially those seen in normal hosts, require no specific therapy. The itching of varicella may be controlled with calamine lotion and/or antihistamines. Aspirin should not be administered to children or adolescents with chickenpox because both aspirin and varicella have been linked to Reye's syndrome. Zoster may also be treated locally with calamine lotion or Burrows solution.

Whether or not to administer steroids to patients with zoster is a controversial issue that has not yet been resolved. The aim of such treatment is to lessen the chances of developing postherpetic neuralgia. Since this complication is so rare in children, use of steroids in children is usually not an issue. Double-blind placebo controlled studies in small numbers of patients with zoster suggest that steroid therapy is associated with a decrease in postherpetic pain without interfering with healing of vesicles in patients who are over the age of 60 (48). While specific adverse effects of steroid therapy have not been described, the argument against the use of steroids has been that they may predispose to other, more severe infections. Other nonspecific therapies of zoster, such as tranquilizers, narcotic analgesics, and vitamins are not recommended for children with zoster.

Acyclovir (ACV) is now the preferred specific antiviral therapy for VZV infections, although at this time it is not licensed for this purpose, but rather for treatment of HSV infections. ACV is mainly indicated for treatment of immunocompromised patients who are likely to have severe VZV infections. Published data regarding the efficacy of ACV for varicella in immunocompromised patients are scant, involving only about 40 treated patients; some of these experiences, moreover, were uncontrolled. In one study involving 12 children who received ACV and eight who received placebo, there was no mortality or serious morbidity from chickenpox in ACV recipients, but 45% of those who received placebo developed varicella pneumonia. There was no mortality in the untreated group (49). The interpretation of these data, however, is clouded by the fact that several of the children had also been passively immunized with VZIG. In another study, ACV was given to seven children with varicella and an underlying malignancy (50). Those treated within 1–2 days after onset did well; those treated 5–9 days after onset had increased morbidity, and two died. An additional randomized placebo-controlled study by this same group (51) found that eight immunosuppressed children who received ACV had less VZV pulmonary involvement than 12 who were given placebo. There was no difference in the time for healing of skin lesions in treated and control children. A final study compared the efficacy of ACV with that of vidarabine against varicella in 22 children with underlying cancer (52). Children who received ACV had similar rates of duration of new lesion formation and continued isolation of VZV from vesicular fluid. However the incidence of dissemination of VZV to the lungs was lower in children who received ACV for their varicella than in those who received vidarabine. In addition, there was more frequent and severe drug toxicity in children treated with vidarabine, especially of a neurologic nature. Similar results were obtained in 20 children with zoster also included in this study (52). These data and the experience of many experts in the field of pediatric infectious diseases suggest that ACV is very well-tolerated and effective for treatment of varicella, and that fatalities due to this disease have become less common since its introduction. Given the overall impression that ACV is effective therapy for varicella, it seems unlikely that a large placebo-controlled study in children with malignant disease will ever be performed. It is possible, however, that a large study comparing the efficacy of ACV with vidarabine for varicella may yet emerge.

The efficacy of intravenous ACV for zoster is well-documented. In one double-blind placebo-controlled study of 94 immunocompromised zoster patients, there was less progression of disease, and there were fewer treatment failures in those receiving ACV than in controls (53). In another study, ACV was compared with vidarabine in 22 immunocompromised patients with zoster; most had undergone bone marrow transplantation. In this study, there was no dissemination in ACV-treated patients, but 55% of those on vidarabine had dissemination. In addition, the time for healing was shorter in patients on ACV (54). In neither of these studies, nor in any other studies or ACV, has there been any effect on the incidence of severity of postherpetic pain, although the pain of *acute* zoster has been less in patients who received antiviral therapy.

VZV is several times less sensitive to ACV than are HSV I and II. There is, in addition, considerable variability of the sensitivity of different strains of VZV to ACV, ranging from about 0.5–11 μg/ml (55). In contrast, the mean sensitivity of clinical isolates of HSV I and II are 0.13–0.22 μg/ml respectively (55). An intravenous dose of 250 or 500 mg/m^2 will result in blood levels that are about 15–25 μg/ml, significantly above levels required to treat VZV. Oral administration of ACV at the usual dosage for HSV (200 mg 5 times a day), however, probably will not. Only 15–30% of orally administered ACV is absorbed; in adults, blood levels of 0.25–1 μg/ml follow oral administration of this dose (55). Therefore, it is not surprising that treatment of VZV infections with oral ACV in a few published studies has met with mixed success. The exact importance of blood levels of the drug is furthermore debatable since intracellular levels might be of greater importance against a cell-associated virus such as VZV. Drug levels in vesicular fluid may be more important than blood levels (56). Theoretical considerations aside, however, patients needing therapy for severe VZV infection are likely to be immunodeficient, and to maximize the chances for successful treatment, ACV is best given intravenously, at a dose of 500 mg/m^2 three times a day (1500 mg/m^2/day). This is the dose that was employed in the successful studies described above. There is no indication for use of oral ACV in patients with VZV infections at this time, even at higher doses than those used for HSV, except on an experimental basis, because the efficacy of this approach is not yet known. It is hoped that such information is forthcoming. Intravenous ACV is usually given for 5–10 days, although in some instances, a shorter or a longer interval may seem more appropriate.

Immunocompromised patients with varicella who have not been passively immunized or who have not received varicella vaccine previously should be admitted to the hospital as soon as the diagnosis of varicella is made. Treatment with intravenous ACV should be started immediately, even if the patient has only a few skin lesions. Successful antiviral therapy has been associated with administration of the drug within the first 3 days after onset of infection. One should not wait for such a patient to develop severe symptoms before beginning antiviral therapy, although this approach means that in order to save one child, many will be treated unnecessarily. Whether treatment was really necessary or not can be difficult to decide, even if judged in retrospect. It is rarely possible early in the course of varicella, to identify the child who will do poorly if untreated; therefore, early treatment, even of children who may not require therapy seems to be the safest approach. Baseline chest x-ray, blood gases, and transaminase levels should be obtained on the patient prior to starting therapy. Consideration should be given to temporary postponement of chemotherapy for the underlying illness. The dose of steroids should be lowered to physiologic levels if possible, unless, because of the severity of clinical VZV infection, stress doses seem indicated. Steroids should not be stopped abruptly. It is reasonable to consider discontinuing ACV in patients who cease developing new lesions for a period of at least 4 days, who have become afebrile, and who are clearly recovering. It is not uncommon, however, for patients in the early stages of severe varicella to appear to be stable for 1 or 2 days and then to begin to manifest new lesions, presumably secondary to another bout of viremia. Therefore, care should be taken not to stop ACV too soon.

Even fewer potentially high-risk patients with zoster will develop severe disseminated infection than similar patients with varicella. Furthermore, even those with zoster who disseminate may have a self-limited infection. Presumably, since zoster is a secondary infection rather than a primary one, the prognosis is better for zoster in the immunocompromised patient than it is for

varicella. Whether or not to begin ACV therapy in zoster patients can therefore be a difficult decision, since it involves hospitalization. Although ACV is so well-tolerated, however, it is still prudent to treat most if not all zoster patients with an underlying illness causing poor immune function. The goal of therapy in such patients is to prevent dissemination (or further dissemination) of VZV. ACV should be viewed not only as a lifesaving drug, but also as one that can decrease morbidity. Zoster patients who are treated have more rapid healing, less acute pain, and fewer days of vesiculation than untreated patients, although postherpetic pain is not prevented. Latent infection with VZV is also not prevented or cured with any currently available antiviral drug. To date, VZV isolates have not been observed to become resistant to ACV following a course of therapy (57).

It is difficult to make recommendations concerning antiviral therapy for patients with CNS involvement with VZV, since the underlying pathogenesis of this complication is unknown and no controlled studies of the efficacy of antiviral therapy have been performed. Often, clinicians will elect to treat immunocompromised patients with VZV infections and CNS involvement but not to administer antivirals to immunologically normal patients with VZV CNS complications. This rationale is based on the likelihood that at least part of the problem in immunocompromised patients is due to viral multiplication; this would be unlikely in immunologically normal patients. It is quite unusual to isolate VZV from cerebrospinal fluid in patients with CNS complications of VZV infection (58). On the other hand, some physicians will try a course of ACV in all patients with CNS complications of VZV, since the issue is controversial and ACV is unlikely to cause harm.

Relatively common adverse effects of ACV include the following: dose-dependent phlebitis due to the high pH of the intravenous solution (expected in about 15% of patients), reversible elevation of the serum creatinine (expected in about 5%), hive-like rash (expected in about 5%), and nausea and vomiting (expected in about 1%). The elevation of serum creatinine is due to precipitation of the drug when it is administered at high concentration in the renal tubules. This may be prevented by avoidance of bolus administration, allowing at least 1 hour for infusion of each dose, and providing maintenance volumes of fluids during and just preceding each infusion. Rare toxicity of ACV includes encephalopathic manifestations such as tremors, confusion, and agitation. The dosage of ACV used in patients with abnormal renal function (creatinine clearance less than 50 ml/min/1.73 m²) should be decreased by ⅓–½ to prevent development of toxic concentrations of the drug, according to the manufacturer.

Vidarabine is now the second line drug for treatment of VZV infections. Zoster patients treated with vidarabine fared less well than those who were given ACV, as already noted (54). Not only did ACV therapy result in more rapid recovery; vidarabine treatment was associated with a higher incidence of CNS toxicity. In addition to the usual side effects of nausea, vomiting, and skin rash, zoster patients treated with vidarabine have developed severe tremors and, at times, psychosis. Similar neurotoxicity has been described in immunocompromised children with severe varicella who were treated with vidarabine. In one instance, a study comparing the efficacy of ACV and vidarabine had to be terminated when a child developed severe permanent brain damage that was ascribed to vidarabine (52).

Despite its higher rate of toxicity, administration of vidarabine has been associated with more rapid healing and lower mortality than placebo treatment, both for varicella and zoster (59,60). If, for some reason, ACV cannot be given, vidarabine should be used for high-risk patients. There are no data concerning the simultaneous use of both drugs for VZV infections, but because of potential toxicity, this approach is not recommended.

PREVENTION

Varicella-Zoster Immune Globulin

This material, originally termed zoster immune globulin (ZIG), was shown to be effective for prevention of clinical varicella in healthy children exposed to a sibling with chickenpox (61). ZIG was prepared by cold fractionation of plasma collected from patients convalescing from zoster. In the original double-blind study (61), either 0.5 ml of ZIG or placebo was administered within 72 hours of exposure to siblings of children who developed varicella. Twelve children

were studied, and six cases of clinical varicella were observed. When the code was broken, it was apparent that all the children who had received ZIG were protected. When a similar dose of ZIG was given to a leukemic child who had been exposed to varicella, a mild case of varicella occurred (Brunell, unpublished). Therefore, a larger dose of ZIG, 2 ml, was administered within 3 days of household exposure to varicella in a study of the efficacy of ZIG for prevention of varicella in immunocompromised children (62). In this study, involving 15 leukemic children receiving maintenance chemotherapy who were susceptible to varicella, mild to moderate chickenpox developed in 67%, and no clinical disease occurred in 33%. All the children who appeared to be protected, however, had been subclinically infected with VZV, based on development of IgM antibodies to VZV and persistence of IgG antibodies to the virus for up to 2 years after ZIG had been given (62). Since all of these children were receiving chemotherapy, about 30% would have been expected to develop severe varicella without passive immunization (9). Subsequent studies on ZIG to prevent severe varicella in immunocompromised children and involving larger numbers of children yielded similar results (63). In these studies, a dose of 125 units of ZIG for every 10 kg of body weight was used.

Since ZIG was prepared from plasma of patients recovering from zoster, it was always in short supply, and it was often unavailable for children who needed it. Therefore, in the late 1970s, the efficacy of a new preparation, varicella-zoster immune globulin (VZIG) was compared with that of ZIG in a double-blind randomized fashion. VZIG was prepared not from blood of convalescent zoster patients, but rather from outdated plasma that had been screened for high titers of VZV antibodies. Units of plasma with titers of 1:25 or greater, measured by complement fixation, were used to prepare VZIG. While the titers of VZV antibody measured by various methods were somewhat lower in VZIG than they were in ZIG, both preparations were found to be equally effective in preventing severe varicella in immunocompromised children (64).

VZIG was licensed in 1981. Since VZIG is prepared from blood from healthy donors, it is readily available. It is produced and distributed in Massachusetts by the Massachusetts Public

Health Biologic Laboratory and distributed else-where by the American Red Cross through local blood centers (65,66). Although VZIG is effec-tive when administered up to 3 days after ex-posure, it should be given as soon as possible. Even though optimal results cannot be expected, VZIG may also provide benefit if given as long as 5 days after exposure. The dose is 125 units for every 10 kg of body weight, with a maxi-mum of 625 units.

The most important use of VZIG today is for prevention of severe varicella in immunocom-promised children who have been closely ex-posed to varicella or zoster. This includes children with primary immune deficiency disorders, those with neoplastic diseases for which immunosup-pressive therapy is being given, children re-ceiving large doses of steroids for any reason, and newborn infants whose mothers have active varicella at the time of delivery. Candidates for whom VZIG is recommended by the Centers for Disease Control (CDC) in Atlanta, Georgia, are listed in Table 10.2.

Infants and children who are listed in the high-risk group should receive VZIG if they have had a close exposure to varicella or zoster, as in-dicated in Table 10.3. They should be consid-ered to be susceptible to varicella if they have either no history of having had the illness or are uncertain as to whether they have had it in the past. It is potentially hazardous to base the de-cision to withhold VZIG on a positive antibody titer in a child who has no history of the clinical illness. Many high-risk children have been transfused with blood products, which may lead to a transiently positive VZV antibody test; this effect can occur with plasma, platelets, and even

Table 10.2.
Candidates for Whom VZIG is Indicated[a]

1. No previous history of clinical varicella, *and*
2. Underlying condition:
   Leukemia, lymphoma
   Congenital or acquired immunodeficiency
   Immunosuppressive therapy (including
     prednisone 1.5 mg/kg/day or greater)
   Newborn infant of mother with onset of varicella
     within 5 days before delivery and 2 days after
     delivery
   Premature infant more than 28 weeks gestation
     whose mother has no prior history of varicella
   Premature infant less than 28 weeks gestation,
     and
3. Significant exposure (see Table 10.3).

[a]Modified from reference 65.

Table 10.3.
Indications for Use of VZIG[a]

1. Continuous household contact, *or*
2. Playmate contact, greater than 1 hour indoors, *or*
3. Hospital contact: in same 2 or 4 bedroom or adjacent beds in large ward; face-to-face contact with an infectious employee or patient, *or*
4. Newborn contact with infected mother, *and*
   Within 3 days of contact (preferably given sooner; in some cases may give up to 5 days after exposure), *and*
   High risk to develop severe varicella (see Table 10.2).

[a]Modified from reference 65.

packed red blood cells. In addition, false-pos-itive VZV antibody tests can occur, due to cross-reactions to HSV or even secondary to a labo-ratory error. Therefore, the best indication of immunity to varicella for high-risk children is a past history of chickenpox. Additional infor-mation concerning the source of the illness and transmission of chickenpox to others may be helpful in being more certain that the clinical illness was indeed chickenpox. When uncertain, it is best to administer VZIG rather than to with-hold it in a child at high risk to develop severe varicella.

Since only about 25% of adults with no his-tory of varicella are truly susceptible, and since healthy adults are at substantially less risk to develop severe varicella than are immunocom-promised children, VZIG is not indicated for adults, unless they are proven to be susceptible by laboratory testing. It is therefore reasonable for adults with no past history of varicella who are likely to be closely exposed to VZV, such as medical personnel and parents of young chil-dren, to have their blood tested for VZV anti-bodies. Then, should a close exposure occur, VZIG could be given. This strategy is particu-larly important for pregnant women who have been reported to have serious morbidity and a mortality rate of 2% from varicella (12).

Immunocompromised adults with no history of varicella are somewhat more difficult to man-age with regard to an exposure to VZV. If, when tested repeatedly by a reliable serologic assay for VZV antibodies, a positive result occurs, and there has been no tranfusion of blood prod-ucts in the previous 3 months, VZIG may be withheld. If, on the other hand, there are no detectable VZV antibodies, or the validity of testing is in question, VZIG should be administered, given the potential risk of developing severe varicella.

Patients with AIDS and AIDS-related complex (ARC) constitute another potential high-risk group for varicella. Their management should be similar to that discussed above for immunocompromised children and adults. Children who have been receiving intravenous globulin for treatment of AIDS may well have detectable VZV antibodies. There are no data, however, to indicate whether these antibodies are always present or present in a high enough concentration to be protective. Therefore, a conservative approach seems warranted, and VZIG should be administered to children with AIDS or ARC if there is no past history of varicella and a close exposure has occurred.

Infants whose mothers have active varicella at delivery should also receive VZIG (13). This strategy is highly effective in prevention of severe varicella in neonates (66a). Specifically, infants whose mothers have the onset of chickenpox 5 days or less prior to delivery seem to be at highest risk and should therefore be passively immunized. A few of these infants have been described to develop severe varicella and require antiviral therapy despite administration of VZIG (67). Therefore, passively immunized infants warrant close watching; should they develop an extensive skin rash (over 500 vesicles) or evidence of pneumonia, ACV should be administered. It is controversial whether infants whose mothers develop varicella *after* delivery should be passively immunized. This policy is recommended by the CDC (65), but not enthusiastically by the American Academy of Pediatrics (66). The authors' personal preference is that of the CDC, to administer VZIG to infants whose mothers develop varicella during the first 48 hours after delivery. A 15-day-old infant with severe varicella whose mother developed chickenpox when he was 8 days old has been reported (68). The occurrence of severe varicella in an infant of this age, however, is extremely rare. Therefore, VZIG is not recommended for use in infants more than 48 hours old who are exposed to maternal varicella. Infants whose mothers have had varicella and who are exposed to siblings or others with chickenpox are probably at little risk to severe varicella since they are well-endowed with specific maternal antibody. Similarly, infants exposed to mothers with

zoster are not expected to develop severe varicella and therefore do not require prophylactic VZIG. While the reported mortality rate from varicella in children less than 1 year old is 4 times that seen in older children, both rates are exceedingly low—8 per 100,000 cases and 2 per 100,000 cases, respectively (69). In contrast, the mortality rate for adults is estimated to be 50 per 100,000 (65) and for leukemic children receiving chemotherapy, 7000 per 100,000 (7%) (9).

Antibody to VZV of the IgG class crosses the placenta. By 6 months of age, VZV antibody is no longer detectable in the serum of most infants (70). Even in some infants under 1500 g, VZV antibody may be detectable if there is a maternal history of varicella (71). Nevertheless, it is recommended that newborn infants weighing less than 1000 grams or of less than 28 weeks gestation who are exposed to VZV be passively immunized, even if the mother had varicella (Table 10.4) (65). A hospital outbreak of varicella in a premature nursery has been described, involving two infants whose mothers had previous varicella (72). Interestingly, varicella has also been observed in infants with preexisting maternal transplacental antibodies when exposed to VZV (73). Although this antibody may not necessarily have preventive value, it can usually be expected to modify chickenpox and it may be one reason why varicella in infants between 1–6 months of age is characteristically mild.

The practicing physician is frequently confronted with the problem posed when a newborn infant, ready for discharge from the hospital, has older siblings at home with active chickenpox. Delaying discharge or sending the siblings to another household seem to be extreme measures. One possible approach is to determine whether the mother has had varicella herself; if so, the infant can be safely discharged home. If chickenpox occurs, it can be expected to be modified in the infant by passively acquired maternal antibodies. If the mother has never had varicella or is uncertain, VZIG could be administered to the infant prior to discharge. In some situations, for example, if the mother is serologically proven to be susceptible, her older children have chickenpox, and she has not already been exposed or is within 3 days of an exposure to VZV, VZIG should also be administered to the mother.

Zoster occurs despite serum antibody to VZV, and patients with zoster manifest brisk increases in VZV antibody titer. Passive immunization has proven not to be useful to either treat or to prevent zoster in high-risk patients (74).

The dose of VZIG for infants is 125 units, administered intramuscularly. The cost of 125 units of VZIG is $75.

Varicella Vaccine

A live, attenuated varicella vaccine was developed in Japan about 15 years ago (75). While this vaccine is licensed in some European countries and in Japan, it is not yet licensed in the United States, although it is expected to be eventually. This vaccine, the Oka strain, was prepared from an isolate of VZV obtained from an otherwise healthy boy with chickenpox. Attenuation was achieved by passage in tissue culture. It was first tested in healthy populations and then in immunocompromised children (76).

When the vaccine was first introduced into the United States in the late 1970s, it was tested almost exclusively in immunocompromised children who could potentially derive the greatest benefit from it. The vaccine was highly protective in immunocompromised children (77–79). Thus, interest in the use of this vaccine in healthy populations has developed. At this time, there is great interest in vaccinating healthy children on a routine basis. Over 95% of vaccinated healthy children are protected by this vaccine (80). In contrast, only about 85% of leukemic children are entirely protected against varicella (77–79), and only about 50% of vaccinated healthy adults are completely protected (78). If it does not prevent infection, however, the vaccine dramatically modifies it so that those individuals who manifest a breakthrough illness after an exposure have very few skin lesions. Thus varicella vaccine has been 100% effective in preventing severe varicella in immunocompromised children and in healthy adults.

Leukemic children who are immunized have a 50% chance of developing a vaccine-associated rash if they are still receiving maintenance chemotherapy. It has become customary to suspend maintenance chemotherapy for 1 week before and 1 week after immunization. Nevertheless, about 5% of such vaccinated leukemic children will also require treatment with ACV for a vaccine-associated rash; fortunately, this therapy has not seemed to interfere with their immune response to VZV in the small numbers who have been studied. Vaccinees with a rash may also transmit the vaccine-type virus to other varicella susceptibles with whom they have close contact (77–79). While the potential for this transmission is low—only about 10%, in contrast to the transmission rate of 80–90% for wild-type virus infection—it is a potential problem. One would not wish for a vaccinee to transmit vaccine virus to another immunocompromised individual, especially one who might not tolerate the virus, such as another leukemic child receiving induction therapy. The vaccine has not been studied in leukemic children in remission for less than 9 months.

Varicella vaccine is best tolerated by healthy children; they have an incidence of a vaccine-associated rash of only about 5%. In addition, these rashes are much milder, rarely vesicular, and are very unlikely to result in transmission of vaccine virus to others. Healthy children require only 1 dose of vaccine to achieve a seroconversion rate of about 95% (80,81).

Varicella susceptible adults also tolerate the vaccine well with only about 5% incidence of rash, but their seroconversion rate after 1 dose of vaccine is only about 80%; if 2 doses are administered, 90% will seroconvert (78,82–84). Varicella vaccine has also been well-tolerated in the small number of renal transplant patients who have received it, but there are no available data concerning protection (85).

The potential influence of varicella vaccine on future control of hospital outbreaks of chickenpox is interesting to consider; it is anything but straightforward. Postexposure vaccination of healthy children within 3–5 days has been shown to prevent or modify varicella (83,86). Immunization of immunologically normal children has been shown to halt nosocomial varicella (75). This strategy has, however, not been tried in adults or leukemic children because their immune responses are more sluggish than are those of healthy children. It seems preferable to try to prevent or modify varicella in high-risk individuals who have been exposed by passive rather than by active immunization. Therefore, VZIG should be used.

It is possible that some control of nosocomial varicella can be achieved by elective immunization of varicella-susceptible hospital staff after the vaccine is licensed. However, since less than 50% of vaccinated adults with household exposures are protected, breakthrough varicella must be anticipated in some hospital workers vaccinated as adults. It is likely to develop, however, only in those adults who, following seroconversion, have lost detectable VZV FAMA antibodies after immunization. Breakthrough varicella even in immunized adults who have become seronegative, however, has been exceedingly mild, with only a few lesions (79). It is also possible that such individuals are less contagious to others than are those who develop hundreds of vesicles. There are no data as to whether there is spread of VZV by the respiratory route in vaccinees with breakthrough varicella.

There are some data available on long-term persistence of VZV antibodies following immunization. Studies involving small numbers of healthy children vaccinated up to 10 years previously have continued to demonstrate immune responses to VZV (87,88). The importance of boosting in maintenance of these long-term immune responses to VZV due to occasional exposure to the virus is also highly likely.

It is recognized that varicella virus, both wild and vaccine types, can become latent and later cause zoster, which is potentially a vehicle for further transmission of VZV (25,89,90). It is certain that varicella vaccine will not eliminate varicella or zoster, and therefore, the vaccine cannot be completely successful in eliminating varicella from hospital settings. However, its judicious use in the future may decrease transmission as well as provide a benefit to the individuals who receive it. Reexposure to VZV may also play a crucial role in boosting immunity of exposed individuals. Thus, breakthrough cases of varicella and zoster in some vaccinees may not be a total disadvantage. The incidence of zoster after vaccination is clearly not increased in comparison with the incidence following natural varicella (91,92).

Management of Nosocomial VZV Infections

Varicella outbreaks, especially in pediatric populations where the rate of susceptibility is high, may be exceedingly difficult to eradicate (93). A combination of testing for susceptibility, furloughing of susceptible personnel during potential incubation periods, cohorting exposed susceptible children and those with active varicella, and discharging exposed susceptibles is usually employed. Even using this strategy, however, hospital outbreaks lasting many weeks have been reported (29). Once varicella or herpes zoster has been introduced into a hospital setting, however, the following steps are recommended, as outlined in Tables 10.4 and 10.5.

1. The patient with varicella should be placed in strict isolation.
2. Serologic testing of all exposed staff with no prior history of varicella (if this has not been done previously). Seronegatives who have not received VZIG should be furloughed from days 8–21 after the exposure. Seronegatives who have received VZIG should be furloughed from days 8–28 after exposure. Alternatively, seronegatives may continue work in a setting where there are likely to be few varicella susceptibles. Seropositive staff may continue to work even if they have been exposed.
3. Every effort should be made to discharge hospitalized children with no history of var-

---

Table 10.4.
Strict Isolation for Varicella Infection

1. Infected patient should be placed in negative pressure private room.
2. Susceptibility of staff should be determined. Seronegative staff should not care for infected patients.
3. Exposed seronegative staff should be furloughed from days 8–21 following exposure *or* work in a setting where there are likely to be no varicella susceptibles. (If VZIG was given, risk period is extended to day 28 after exposure.)
4. Susceptibility of patients should be determined. Seronegative-exposed patients should be discharged *or* placed in strict isolation between days 8–21 following exposure.

Table 10.5.
Drainage Secretion Precautions for Herpes Zoster Infection

1. Patients with herpes zoster infection should be placed on drainage secretion precautions.
2. Immunocompromised patients with herpes zoster infection should be placed in strict isolation.
3. Susceptible staff should not care for patients with VZV infection.
4. Immunocompromised or susceptible patients should not be in close contact (playrooms, same patient room) with patients with VZV infection.

icella within 8 days of the exposure. If this is not feasible, they should be placed in a private room, utilizing strict isolation technique between days 8–21 after exposure. Two children with varicella may share a room, but exposed susceptibles should be kept apart if possible. If serologic testing is used to evaluate hospitalized children, attention should be given to whether they received transfusions in the past. History of previous varicella should be sought, and if positive, serology is unnecessary.

REFERENCES

1. Edson CM, Hosler BA, Poodry CA, Schooley RT, Waters DJ, Thorley-Lawson DA: Varicella-zoster virus envelope glycoproteins: biochemical characterization and identification in clinical material. *Virology* 145:62–71, 1985.
2. Grose CH: Variation on a theme by Fenner: the pathogenesis of chickenpox. *Pediatrics* 68:735–737, 1981.
3. Hope-Simpson RE: The nature of herpes zoster: A long term study and a new hypothesis. *Proc R Soc Med* 58:9–20, 1965.
4. Gilden D, Vafai A, Shtram Y, Becker Y, Devlin M, Wellish M: Varicella-zoster virus DNA in human sensory ganglia. *Nature* 306:478–480, 1983.
5. Hyman RW, Ecker JR, Tenser RB: Varicella-zoster virus RNA in human trigeminal ganglia. *Lancet* 2:814–816, 1983.
6. Arvin A, Koropchak CM, Wittek AE: Immunologic evidence of reinfection with varicella-zoster virus. *J Infect Dis* 148:881–885, 1982.
7. Gershon A, Steinberg S, Gelb L, and the NIAID Varicella Vaccine Collaborative Study Group: Clinical reinfection with varicella-zoster virus. *J Infect Dis* 149:137–142, 1984.
8. Weller TH: Varicella and herpes zoster: changing concepts of the natural history, control, and importance of a not-so-benign virus. *N Engl J Med* 309:1362–1368, 1983.
9. Feldman S, Hughes W, Daniel C: Varicella in children with cancer: 77 cases. *Pediatrics* 56:388–397, 1975.
10. Feldhoff C, Balfour H, Simmons SR, Najarian JS, Mauer M: Varicella in children with renal transplants. *J Pediatr* 98:25–31, 1981.
11. Morens DM, Bregman DJ, West M, Greene M, Mazur M, Dolin R, Fisher R: An outbreak of varicella-zoster virus infection among cancer patients. *Ann Int Med* 93:414–419, 1980.
12. Paryani S, Arvin A: Intrauterine infection with varicella-zoster virus after maternal varicella. *N Engl J Med* 314:1542–1546, 1986.
13. Young N, Gershon A: Chickenpox, measles, and mumps. In Remington J, Klein J (eds): *Infectious Diseases of the Fetus and Newborn Infant*. Philadelphia, Saunders, 1983, pp 375–427.
14. Essex-Cater A, Heggarty H: Fatal congenital varicella syndrome. *J Infect* 7:77–78, 1983.
15. Brunell PA, Kotchmar GS: Zoster in infancy: failure to maintain virus latency following intrauterine infection. *J Pediatr* 98:71–73, 1981.
16. Dworsky M, Whitley R, Alford C: Herpes zoster in early infancy. *Am J Dis Child* 134:618–619, 1980.
17. Guess H, Broughton D, Melton L, Kurland L: Epidemiology of herpes zoster in children and adolescents: a population-based study. *Pediatrics* 76:512–517, 1985.
18. Meyers JD: Congenital varicella in term infants: risk reconsidered. *J Infect Dis* 129:215–217, 1974.
19. Preblud S, Nelson WL, Levin MJ, Zaia JA: Modification of congenital varicella infection with VZIG. Abstract #317. Presented at 26th Interscience Conference on Antimicrobial Agents and Chemotherapy, New Orleans, 1986.
20. Locksley RM, Flornoy N, Sullivan KM, Meyers J: Infection with varicella-zoster virus after marrow transplantation. *J Infect Dis* 152:1172–1181, 1985.
21. Arvin AM, Pollard RB, Rasmussen LE, Merigan T: Cellular and humoral immunity in the pathogenesis of recurrent herpes viral infections in patients with lymphoma. *J Clin Investig* 65:869–878, 1980.
22. Arvin A, Pollard RB, Rasmussen L, Merigan T: Selective impairment in lymphocyte reactivity to varicella-zoster antigen among untreated lymphoma patients. *J Infect Dis* 137:531–540, 1978.
23. Straus SE, Reinhold W, Smith HA, Ruyechan W, Henderson D, Blaese RM, Hay J: Endonuclease analysis of viral DNA from varicella and subsequent zoster infections in the same patient. *N Engl J Med* 311:1362–1364, 1984.
24. Straus S, Hay J, Smith H, Owens J: Genome differences among varicella-zoster virus isolates. *J Gen Virol* 64:1031–1041, 1983.
25. Williams D, Gershon A, Gelb L, Spraker M, Steinberg S, Ragab A: Herpes zoster following varicella vaccine in a child with acute lymphocytic leukemia. *J Pediatr* 106:259–261, 1985.
26. Ross A, Lencher E, Reitman G: Modification of chickenpox in family contacts by administration of gamma globulin. *N Engl J Med* 267:369–376, 1962.
27. Gustafson TL, Lavely GB, Brawner ER, Hutcheson RH, Wright PF, Schaffner W: An outbreak of nosocomial varicella. *Pediatrics* 70:550–556, 1982.
28. Leclair JM, Zaia J, Levin MJ, Congdon RG, Goldmann DA: Airborne transmission of chickenpox in a hospital. *N Engl J Med* 302:450–453, 1980.
29. Krasinski K, Holzman R, LaCouture R, Florman AL: Hospital experience with varicella-zoster virus. *Infect Control* 7:312–316, 1986.
30. La Russa P, Steinberg S, Seeman M, Gershon A: Determination of immunity to varicella by means of an intradermal skin test. *J Infect Dis* 152:869–875, 1985.
31. Alter SJ, Hammond JA, McVey CJ, Myers M: Susceptibility to varicella-zoster virus among adults at high risk for exposure. *Infect Control* 7:448–451, 1986.
32. Nassar NT, Touma HC: Brief report: susceptibility of Filipino nurses to the varicella-zoster virus. *Infect Control* 7:71–72, 1986.
33. Brawley RL, Wenzel RP: An algorithm for chickenpox exposure. *Pediatr Infect Dis* 3:502–504, 1984.
34. Krugman S, Goodrich CH, Ward R: Primary varicella pneumonia. *N Engl J Med* 257:843–848, 1957.
35. Frey H, Steinberg S, Gershon A: Diagnosis of varicella-zoster infections. In Nahmias A, Dowdle W, Schinazi R (eds): *The Human Herpesviruses*. New York, Elsevier, 1981, pp 351–362.
36. Seidlin M, Takiff HE, Smith H, Hay J, Straus S: Detection of varicella-zoster virus by dot-blot hybridization using a molecularly cloned viral DNA probe. *J Med Virol* 13:53–61, 1984.
37. Zeigler T, Halonen PE: Rapid detection of herpes simplex and varicella-zoster virus antigens from clinical specimens by enzyme immunoassay. *Antiviral Res* 1985, Suppl 1:107–110.
38. Williams V, Gershon A, Brunell P: Serologic response to varicella-zoster membrane antigens measured by indirect immunofluorescence. *J Infect Dis* 1340:669–672, 1974.
39. Gershon A, Frey H, Steinberg S, Seeman M, Bidwell D, Voller A: Determination of immunity to varicella using an ELISA assay. *Arch Virol* 70:169–172, 1981.
40. Shehab Z, Brunell P: Enzyme-linked immunosorbent assay for susceptibility to varicella. *J Infect Dis* 148:472–476, 1983.
41. Shanley J, Myers M, Edmond B, Steele R: Enzyme-linked immunosorbent assay for detection of antibody to varicella-zoster virus. *J Clin Microbiol* 15:208–211, 1982.
42. Gershon A, Kalter Z, Steinberg S: Detection of antibody to varicella-zoster virus by immune adherence hemagglutination. *Proc Soc Exper Biol Med* 151:762–765, 1976.
43. Campbell-Benzie A, Heath RB, Ridehalgh M, Cradock-Wilson JE: A comparison of indirect immunofluorescence and radioimmunoassay for detecting antibody to varicella-zoster virus. *J Virol Meth* 6:135–140, 1983.

44. Preissner C, Steinberg S, Gershon A, Smith TF: Evaluation of the anticomplement immunofluorescence test for detection of antibody to varicella-zoster virus. *J Clin Micro* 16:373–376, 1982.

45. Kamiya H, Ihara T, Hattori A, Iwasa T, Sakurai M, Izawa T, Yamada A, Takahashi M: Diagnostic skin test reactions with varicella virus antigen and clinical application of the test. *J Infect Dis* 136:784–788, 1977.

46. Florman A, Umland E, Ballou D, Cushing A, McLaren L, Gribble J, Duncan M: Evaluation of a skin test for chicken pox. *Infect Control* 6:314–316, 1985.

47. Burke BL, Steele R, Beard OW, Wood JS, Cain TD, Marmer DJ: Immune responses to varicella zoster in the aged. *Arch Int Med* 142:291–293, 1982.

48. Dickinson JA: Should we treat herpes zoster with corticosteroid agents? *Med J Aust* 144:375–379, 1986.

49. Prober CG, Kirk LE, Keeney RE: Acyclovir therapy of chickenpox in immunosuppressed children—a collaborative study. *J Pediatr* 101:622–625, 1982.

50. Balfour H: Intravenous acyclovir therapy for varicella in immunocompromised children. *J Pediatr* 104:134–140, 1984.

51. Balfour H, McMonigal K, Bean B: Acyclovir therapy of varicella-zoster virus infections in immunocompromised patients. *J Antimicrob Chemo* 12 (Suppl) B:169–179, 1983.

52. Feldman S, Robertson P, Lott L, Thornton D: Neurotoxicity due to adenine arabinoside therapy during varicella-zoster virus infections in immunocompromised children. *J Infect Dis* 154:889–893, 1986.

53. Balfour HH Jr, Bean B, Laskin OL, Ambinder RF, Meyers JD, Wade JC, Zaia JA, Aeppli D, Kirk LE, Sefreti AC, Keeney RE, and the Burrows Wellcome Collaborative Acyclovir Study Group: Acyclovir halts progression of herpes zoster in immunocompromised patients. *N Engl J Med* 308:1448–53, 1983.

54. Shepp DH, Dandliker PS, Meyers JD: Treatment of varicella-zoster virus infection in severely immunocompromised patients: A randomized comparison of acyclovir and vidarabine. *N Engl J Med* 314:208–212, 1986.

55. Arvin A: Oral therapy with acyclovir in infants and children. *Pediatr Infect Dis* 6:56–58, 1987.

56. Peterslund NA, Esmann J, Christensen K, Peterson C: Oral and intravenous acyclovir are equally effective in herpes zoster. *J Antimicrob Chemother* 14:185–189, 1984.

57. Cole NL, Balfour HH: Varicella-zoster virus does not become more resistant to acyclovir during therapy. *J Infect Dis* 153:605–608, 1986.

58. Jemsek J, Greenberg S, Taber L, Harvey D, Gershon A, Couch R: Herpes-zoster associated encephalitis: clinicopathologic report of 12 cases and review of the literature. *Medicine* 62:81–87, 1983.

59. Whitley R, Hilty M, Haynes R, Bryson Y, Connor JD, Soong SJ, Alford CA, and the NIAID Collaborative Antiviral Study Group: Vidarabine therapy of varicella in immunosuppressed patients. *J Pediatr* 101:125–131, 1982.

60. Whitley R, Soong S, Dolin R, Betts R, Linnemann C, Alford C, and NIAID Collaborative Antiviral Study Group: Early vidarabine to control the complications of herpes zoster in immunosuppressed patients. *N Engl J Med* 307:971–975, 1982.

61. Brunell P, Ross A, Miller L, Kuo B: Prevention of varicella by zoster immune globulin. *N Engl J Med* 280:1191–1194, 1969.

62. Gershon A, Steinberg S, Brunell P: Zoster immune globulin: a further assessment. *N Engl J Med* 290:243–245, 1974.

63. Orenstein W, Heymann DL, Ellis RJ, Rosenberg R, Nakano J, Halsey N, Overturf G, Hayden G, Witte J: Prophylaxis of varicella in high risk children: dose response effect of zoster immune globulin. *J Pediatr* 98:368–373, 1981.

64. Zaia JA, Levin M, Preblud S, Leszczynski J, Wright G, Ellis RJ, Curtis AC, Valerio MA, LeGore J: Evaluation of varicella-zoster immune globulin: Protection of immunosuppressed children after household exposure to varicella. *J Infect Dis* 147:737–743, 1983.

65. Centers for Disease Control. Varicella-zoster immune globulin for the prevention of chickenpox. *MMWR* 33:84–100, 1984.

66. Committee on Infectious Diseases: Expanded guidelines for use of varicella-zoster immune globulin. *Pediatrics* 72:886–889, 1983.

66a. Hanngren K, Grandien M, Granström G: Effect of zoster immunoglobulin for varicella prophylaxis in the newborn. *Scand J Infect Dis* 17:343–347, 1985.

67. Bakshi S, Miller TC, Kaplan M, Hammerschlag M, Prince A, Gershon A: Failure of VZIG in modification of severe congenital varicella. *Pediatr Infect Dis* 5:699–702, 1986.

68. Rubin L, Leggiadro R, Elie MT, Lipsitz P: Disseminated varicella in a neonate: implications for immunoprophylaxis of neonates postnatally exposed to varicella. *Pediatr Infect Dis* 5:100–102, 1986.

69. Preblud S, Orenstein W, Bart K: Varicella: clinical manifestations, epidemiology, and health impact on children. *Pediatr Infect Dis* 3:505–509, 1984.

70. Gershon A, Raker R, Steinberg S, Topf-Olstein B, Drusin L: Antibody to varicella-zoster virus in parturient women and their offspring during the first year of life. *Pediatrics* 58:692–696, 1976.

71. Raker R, Steinberg S, Drusin L, Gershon A: Antibody to varicella-zoster virus in low-birth-weight newborn infants. *J Pediatr* 93:505–506, 1978.

72. Gustafson TL, Shehab Z, Brunell P: Outbreak of varicella in a newborn intensive care nursery. *Am J Dis Child* 138:548–550, 1984.

73. Baba K, Yabuuchi H, Takahashi M, Ogra R: Immunologic and epidemiologic aspects of varicella infection acquired during infancy and early childhood. *J Pediatr* 100:881–885, 1982.

74. Groth KE, McCullough J, Marker S, Howard R, Simmons R, Najarian J, Balfour H: Evaluation of zoster immune plasma: treatment of herpes zoster in patients with cancer. *JAMA* 239:1877–1879, 1978.

75. Takahashi M, Otsuka T, Okuno Y, Asano Y, Yazake T, Isomura S: Live attenuated varicella vaccine used to prevent the spread of varicella in hospital. *Lancet* 2:1288–1290, 1974.

76. Izawa T, Ihara T, Hattori A, Iwasa T, Kamiya H, Sakurai M, Takahashi M: Application of a live varicella vaccine with acute leukemia or other malignancies. *Pediatrics* 60:805–819, 1977.

77. Gershon A, Steinberg S, Gelb L, Galasso G, Borkowsky W, LaRussa P, Ferrara A, and the NIAID Varicella Vaccine Collaborative Study Group: Live attenuated varicella vaccine: efficacy for children with leukemia in remission. *JAMA* 252:355–362, 1984.

78. Gershon A, Steinberg S, Gelb L, and the NIAID Varicella Vaccine Collaborative Study Group: Live attenuated varicella vaccine: efficacy in immunocompromised children and adults. *Pediatrics* 78 (suppl):757–762, 1986.

79. Gershon A: Live attenuated varicella vaccine. *Ann Rev Med* (in press).

80. Weibel R, Neff B, Kuter B, Guess H, Rotherberger C, Fitzgerald A, Connor K, McLean A, Hilleman M, Buynak E, Scolnick E: Live attenuated varicella virus vaccine: efficacy trial in healthy children. *N Engl J Med* 310:1409–1415, 1984.

81. Arbeter A, Starr S, Preblud S, Ihara T, Paciorek PM, Miller DS, Zelson CM, Proctor EA, Plotkin SA: Varicella vaccine trials in healthy children. *Am J Dis Child* 138:434–438, 1984.

82. Alter SJ, McVey CJ, Jenski L, Myers MG: Varicella live virus vaccine in normal susceptible adults at high risk for exposure. Abstract #457, 25th Interscience Conference on Antimicrobial Agents and Chemotherapy, Minneapolis, MN, 1985.

83. Arbeter AM, Starr SE, Plotkin SA: Varicella vaccine studies in healthy children and adults. *Pediatrics* 78(suppl):748–756, 1986.

84. Ndumbe PM, Craddock-Watson JE, MacQueen S, Dunn H, Holzel H, Andre F, Davies EG, Dudgeon JA, Levinsky RJ: Immunization of nurses with a live varicella vaccine. *Lancet* 1:1144–1147, 1985.

85. Broyer M, Boudailliez B: Varicella vaccine in children with chronic renal insufficiency. *Postgrad Med J* 61 (Suppl 4):103–106, 1985.

86. Asano Y, Nakayama H, Yazaki T, Kato R, Hirose S, Tsuzuki K, Ito S, Isomura S, Takahashi M: Protection against varicella

in family contacts by immediate inoculation with live varicella vaccine. *Pediatrics* 59:3–7, 1977.

87. Asano Y, Albrecht P, Vujcic LK, Quinnan G, Kawakami K, Takahashi M: Five-year follow-up study of recipients of live attenuated varicella vaccine using enhanced neutralization and fluorescent antibody membrane antigen assays. *Pediatrics* 72:291–294, 1983.

88. Asano Y, Nagai T, Miyata T, Yazaki T, Ito S, Yamanishi K, Takahashi M: Long-term protective immunity of recipients of the OKA strain of live varicella vaccine. *Pediatrics* 75:667–671, 1985.

89. Hayakawa Y, Torigoe S, Shiraki K, Yamanishi K, Takahashi M: Biologic and biophysical markers of a live varicella vaccine strain (OKA): Identification of clinical isolates from vaccine recipients. *J Infect Dis* 149:956–963, 1984.

90. Gelb L, Dohner DE, Gershon A, Steinberg S, Waner J, Takahashi M, Dennehy P, Brown AE: The molecular epide-

miology of live attenuated varicella vaccine in children with leukemia and normal adults. *J Infect Dis* (in press).

91. Brunell PA, Taylor-Weidmann J, Geiser CF, Frierson L, Lydick E: The risk of zoster in children with leukemia who received varicella vaccine as compared to those who had chickenpox. *Pediatrics* 77:53–56, 1986.

92. Lawrence R, Gershon A, Steinberg S, Holzman R, and the NIAID Varicella Vaccine Collaborative Study Group: Incidence of zoster in leukemic children who received live attenuated varicella vaccine. Abstract #458, 25th Interscience Conference on Antimicrobial Agents and Chemotherapy, Minneapolis, MN, 1985.

93. Meyers JD, MacQuarrie MB, Merigan TC, Jennison H: Nosocomial varicella. I. Outbreak in oncology patients at a children's hospital. II. Suggested guidelines for management. *West J Med* 130:196–199, 300–303, 1979.

11

Herpes Simplex Virus

Richard J. Whitley, M.D.

BACKGROUND

Infections caused by herpes simplex viruses have been recognized since ancient Roman times when Herodotus associated mouth ulcers and lip vesicles with fever (1). Some 300 years later, genital herpetic infection was described by Astruc (2). Over an ensuing two centuries, the infectious nature of herpes simplex virus became clearly delineated, particularly as it related to the transmissibility of viruses associated with lip and genital lesions to the cornea of the rabbit (3). However, it was only recently that neonatal herpes simplex infection was identified as a distinct disease. Only 50 years ago, the first written descriptions of neonatal herpes simplex virus (HSV) infections were attributed nearly simultaneously to Hass, when he described the histopathologic findings of a fatal case, and to Batignani who described a newborn child with HSV keratitis (4,5). For several decades, our understanding of neonatal HSV infections was predicated upon histopathologic descriptions of the disease, which indicated a broad spectrum of involvement in infants. Such reports emanated from a variety of health care professionals, including pediatricians, pathologists, virologists, obstetricians, ophthalmologists, and dermatologists, among others. By the mid-1960s, Nahmias and Dowdle demonstrated two antigenic types of HSV; HSV-1 and HSV-2 (6). The recognition of two types of HSV prompted a rapid series of laboratory developments that led to a better understanding of the biochemistry of replication and molecular characteristics of HSV.

With the differentiation of two types of HSV, viral typing methods have been developed to define the epidemiology of these infections.

Herpes simplex virus infections "above the belt," primarily of the lip and oropharynx, were found, in most cases, to be associated with HSV-1. Those infections "below-the-belt," particularly genital infections, are usually caused by HSV-2. With the finding that both genital herpes infections and neonatal HSV infections are most often caused by HSV-2, a natural cause and effect relationship developed between these two entities. This causal relationship was strengthened by the finding of viral excretion in the maternal genital tract at the time of delivery, suggesting that acquisition of the virus by the infant occurs by contact with infected genital secretions during birth.

Over the past 15 years, a great deal has been learned about the epidemiology, natural history, and pathogenesis of neonatal HSV infections. The development of antiviral therapy represents a significant advance in the management of infected children, providing the opportunity to decrease the mortality and to improve the morbidity of these infections. Of all the herpesvirus infections, neonatal HSV infection represents the one that is most amenable to prevention and treatment because it is acquired most often at birth, rather than early in gestation. As our knowledge of the epidemiology of HSV infections has increased, it has become apparent that there are modes of infection other than contact with infected maternal genital infections. Postnatal acquisition of HSV, type 1, has been documented from nonmaternal sources. These issues, as well as the management of hospital personnel with HSV infections, will be the focus of this discussion. It should be recognized, however, that HSV infections are acquired by individuals of all ages and range from the totally asymptomatic to life threatening. Those HSV infections that are acquired beyond the neonatal age range and defined as nosocomially acquired will not be the subject of this review.

EPIDEMIOLOGY

The biologic, molecular, antigenic, and epidemiologic characteristics of HSV-1 and HSV-2 have been the subject of numerous publications. The most recent reviews highlight the importance of these organisms as models for viral replication and as pathogens in human infection (7,8). In order to evaluate the epidemiology of HSV infection as it relates to neonatal disease, viral replication will be considered.

Virus Structure and Replication

Our current understanding of HSV indicates that it consists of a genome of linear, double-stranded DNA with a molecular weight of approximately 100 million. The DNA will encode approximately 70 polypeptides, not all of which are understood biologically. The genome consists of a unique long and unique short segment that can invert upon itself, leading to four isomers (9). The viral DNA is packaged inside a protein structure, known as the capsid, which confers icosahedral symmetry to the virus. The capsid consists of 162 capsomers and is surrounded by a tightly adherent membrane known as the tegument. An envelope loosely surrounds the capsid and tegument, consisting of glycoproteins, lipids, and amines. The glycoproteins mediate attachment to cells and elicit host responses to the virus (10).

Herpes simplex viruses, types 1 and 2, are approximately 50% homologous. Of note, there is considerable overlap in the cross-reactivity between HSV-1 and HSV-2 glycoproteins, although unique ones do exist for each virus (10). Distinction between the two viral types can be demonstrated utilizing restriction enzyme analysis of viral DNA. This technique has been applied to epidemiologic investigations of HSV infections.

Replication of HSV is characterized by the expression of three gene classes, alpha, beta, and gamma genes, which are expressed in a cascade sequence. (7,11). Alpha proteins appear responsible for the initiation of replication. The beta gene products include enzymes necessary for replication and regulatory proteins. Structural proteins are usually of the gamma gene class (7,11). Replication of viral DNA occurs in the cell nucleus and results in the shut-down of cellular macromolecular protein synthesis, resulting in cell death. Assembly of the virus begins in the nucleus with acquisition of the envelope as the capsid buds through the inner lamella of the nuclear membrane.

A poorly understood phenomenon of HSV replication is the ability of the virus to establish a latent state and recur with the proper but as yet unidentified stimulus. Viral DNA can be detected in neuronal tissue of both animal models and humans (12–20). The mechanism(s) by which virus establishes a latent state and maintains it are not well-understood at this time.

Nature of Infection

Although many routes of infection have been suggested, transmission of HSV most often occurs in association with intimate, personal contact. Virus must come in contact with mucosal surfaces or abraded skin for infection to be initiated. With viral replication at the site of infection, either an intact virion or, more simply, the nucleocapsid is transported by neurons to the ganglia, where latency is established (21). Infection with HSV-1, generally limited to the oropharynx, is usually transmitted by respiratory droplets or through direct contact with infected secretions (such as virus-containing labial vesicular fluid). Acquisition often occurs during childhood. Like other herpesvirus infections, seroprevalence studies have demonstrated that transmission of HSV-1 infection is related to socioeconomic factors. Antibodies, indicative of past infection, are found earlier among individuals of lower socioeconomic groups compared with those in middle to upper socioeconomic groups. As many as 75–90% of individuals from lower socioeconomic populations develop antibodies by the end of the 1st decade of life compared with middle and upper middle socioeconomic groups in whom only 30–40% are seropositive by the middle of the 2nd decade of life (7,22–24). This observation of changing seroprevalence rates of HSV-1 is a recent observation and may account, in part, for the increased awareness of HSV-2 infections, since possibly protective antibodies are not present.

Because infections with HSV-2 are usually acquired through sexual contact, antibodies to this virus are rarely found until an age when sexual activity begins. There is a progressive increase in infection rates with HSV-2 in all populations beginning in adolescence. As with HSV-1 infections, the risk of acquisition of infection with HSV-2 appears related to socioeconomic factors. As many as 50–60% of lower socioeconomic groups will develop antibodies to HSV-2 in contrast to 10–20% of individuals in other socioeconomic groups (25–27). Until recently, the exact seroprevalence of antibodies to HSV-2 has been difficult to determine because of the cross-reactivity with HSV-1 antigens. Recently, seroepidemiologic studies performed by Dr. A. Nahmias in Atlanta have utilized type-specific antigen for HSV-2 (glycoprotein G-2), which identified antibodies to this virus in 35% of middle-class women receiving care through a health maintenance organization (28).

Maternal Infection

Genital HSV infection in the pregnant woman is not uncommon. The epidemiology and clinical nature of this infection does not appear to be influenced by pregnancy; however, this suggestion remains to be substantiated. Infection during gestation can manifest in innumerable ways. Prospective investigations utilizing cytologic and virologic screening indicate that genital herpes occurs with a frequency of about 1% at any time during gestation (29). Those factors that influence the frequency of both primary and recurrent infection are not well-defined. However, infection during gestation has been associated with fetal disease in utero, as summarized earlier (30). Specifically, it has been noted that after primary maternal infection, a proportion of women have a spontaneous abortion if infection occurred prior to 20 weeks in gestation. Infection that developed later in gestation did not lead to apparent neonatal disease.

The prevalence of genital herpes during gestation according to socioeconomic status is not defined. The frequency of HSV recurrences during gestation is of concern for women with a known history of infection, particularly at the time of delivery. Since HSV infection of the fetus is usually the consequence of contact with infected maternal genital secretions at the time of delivery, the incidence excretion data at this time are of utmost importance. The actual incidence of viral excretion at delivery has been suggested at 0.01–0.39% and was summarized by Nahmias (29,31,32); however, more representative studies remain to be performed. Without such precise data, recommendations for screening women with a history of HSV infection are meaningless. Regardless, given the seroprevalence of this infection, a significant degree of protection for the fetus must exist or the incidence of neonatal disease would be much higher. Importantly, most infants who develop neonatal disease are born to women who are completely asymptomatic for genital HSV infections at the time of delivery and have neither a past history of genital herpes nor a sexual partner reporting a genital vesicular rash (29,33,34). These women account for 60–80% of those delivering infected children.

The type of maternal genital infection probably influences the acquisition of infection. The duration of viral excretion and the time for total healing vary with primary, initial (first episode at the nonprimary site) and recurrent (HSV-1 or HSV-2) maternal genital infection (35,36). Primary infection is associated with larger quantities of virus replicating in the genital tract and a period of viral excretion, which may persist for an average of 3 weeks. In contrast, virus is shed for an average of 2–5 days and at lower quantities in recurrent genital infection. The difference in the natural history of primary and recurrent disease is most likely a major factor that influences the frequency of transmission and, perhaps, the severity of neonatal disease. A component of transmission, then, of virus from mother to fetus at the time of delivery is the maternal humoral antibody status. Transplacental maternal neutralizing antibodies appear to have a protective or at least an ameliorative effect on the acquisition of infection (31,32). Maternal primary infection late in gestation may not result in significant passage of maternal antibodies. It should be noted that the distinction between symptomatic and asymptomatic disease, whether primary, initial, or recurrent, remains poorly defined at present, especially in relation to the risks of transmission to the infant in such circumstances.

It should also be recognized that certain forms of medical intervention may increase the risk for neonatal HSV infection. Specifically, the utilization of fetal scalp monitors has created a site of infection. Such devices are contraindicated in women with a history of recurrent genital HSV infections.

Frequency and Transmission of Infection

Although centers caring for infants with neonatal HSV infections have observed fluctuations in incidence, the estimated rate of occurrence of neonatal HSV infection is approximately 1 in 2,000 to 1 in 5,000 deliveries per year (29). A progressive increase in the number of cases of neonatal HSV infection has been noted in some areas, with rates approaching 1 in 1,500 deliveries (37). Neonatal HSV infection occurs far less frequently than genital HSV infections in the adult childbearing population. Although underreporting of cases accounts in part for these differences, the existence of poorly understood inherent protective mechanisms, as noted above, that prevent the acquisition of infection or the absence of an active maternal infection at the time of delivery are possible explanations for these differences.

Herpes simplex virus infection of the newborn can be acquired at one of three times; in utero, intrapartum, or postnatally. Overwhelmingly, the most common time of transmission is intrapartum, accounting for 85–90% of cases. Still, the other two routes must be recognized and identified in a child with suspect disease. At each time of possible transmission, the consequences for the fetus or infant are invariably significant.

Information about in utero acquisition is increasingly available in the literature (30,38–40). Infection in this group of babies is characterized by disease that is apparent at birth, and is characterized by a triad of findings, including skin vesicles or scarring, eye disease, and the far more severe manifestations of microcephaly or hydranencephaly. Often, chorioretinitis alone or in combination with other eye findings, such as keratoconjunctivitis, is a component of the clinical presentation. The severity of this syndrome is linked directly to the time of acquisition of infection by the fetus. The frequency of occurrence of these manifestations has been estimated as between 1 in 100,000–200,000 deliveries (38). Factors associated with intrauterine transmission are not known; however, both primary and recurrent maternal infection as well as significantly prolonged rupture of membranes contribute to this disease. The recognition of in utero acquisition of HSV infection is relatively new,

considering that many students of the disease considered 1st trimester infection to be associated with spontaneous abortion (29). Acquisition of primary maternal infection late in gestation has been correlated with premature termination of gestation, a not unusual finding in babies with neonatal HSV infection in general. Since chorioretinitis alone can be a presenting sign, the pediatrician should be alerted to the possibility of this diagnosis, albeit a less common cause than other congenital infections.

As noted above, the most common route of infection is that of intrapartum contact with infected maternal genital secretions. Those factors that favor intrapartum transmission of infection include primary infection associated with large quantities of virus excreted for prolonged times, prolonged rupture of membranes, vaginal delivery, and perhaps, transplacental antibodies. The suggestion that one-third of women with primary infection during the 3rd trimester delivered a child who developed neonatal herpes in contrast to only 3% of women with recurrent disease provides credence for distinguishing between primary and recurrent infections as a risk factor for acquisition of disease in the newborn child (29,41,42). With recurrent HSV infection present at delivery, the possibility that transplacental antibodies as well as other factors, such as local genital immunity, which prevent infection must be considered, as noted above (29,43,44). Duration of ruptured membranes has also become an important indicator of risk for acquisition of neonatal infection. Observations by Nahmias and colleagues indicate that prolonged rupture of membranes (greater than 6 hours) increases the risk of acquisition of virus, probably the consequence of ascending infection (29,45). Based on this observation, it is recommended that women with active genital lesions at the time of onset of labor be delivered by cesarean section. The potential benefits of cesarean section may be demonstrated beyond 6 hours of ruptured membranes, but this has not yet been proven. Currently, our practice is to deliver women with genital herpes who are at term by cesarean section and, if possible, before the onset of labor. However, it should be recognized that infection of the newborn has occurred in spite of intervention by cesarean section (43,46).

Even though HSV-1 has been associated with genital lesions, postpartum transmission of HSV has been increasingly suggested because 15–20% of neonatal HSV infections are caused by HSV-1 (29). These data, in conjunction with recent documentation of postnatal transmission of HSV-1, have focused attention on other possible sources of virus for neonatal infection (47–49). These latter studies warrant special recognition, as hospital-acquired HSV infections are of increasing concern. Hammerberg et al. documented an identical virus by restriction endonuclease analyses of viral DNA, leaving little doubt as to the possibility of the spread of virus in a high-risk nursery. Nevertheless, the source of virus and vector of transmission have been inadequately studied. As a consequence, confusion exists in medical recommendations for isolation of these children. The potential legal implications for acquired HSV infection in a nursery are obvious. Maternal-infant postpartum transmission has been reported as a consequence of nursing on an infected breast (50). Relatives and hospital personnel with orolabial herpes may also be a reservoir of virus for newborns. In spite of reactivated labial herpes occurring in 1% of all individuals, including nursery personnel, postnatal transmission by this route is exceedingly low (51,52). Likely, vigorous handwashing procedures and continuing education of personnel in newborn nurseries have helped to maintain the low frequency of transmission in this environment. It should be recognized that the existence of a herpetic whitlow should preclude direct patient contact, irrespective of nursing unit.

Neonatal Infection

Following direct exposure, the newborn will either limit viral replication to the portal of entry, namely the skin, eye, or mouth (SEM), or viral replication will progress to more serious disease, including involvement of the central nervous system (CNS disease) or multiple organs (disseminated infection). Host mechanisms responsible for control or progression of viral replication at the site of entry are unknown. Although controversial, transplacental neutralizing antibodies do not appear to prevent the development of disseminated disease after intrapartum exposure to the virus (43,44). For CNS disease, it is possible that intraneuronal transmission of viral particles provides a privileged site that may be immune to circulating humoral defense mechanisms; thus, transpla-

cental maternal antibodies may be of less value under such circumstances. In contrast, disseminated infection can be the consequence of viremia or secondary to extensive cell-to-cell spread, as occurs with pneumonitis following aspiration of infected secretions.

Once virus has absorbed to cell membranes, and penetration has occurred, viral replication proceeds, leading to progeny virus as well as to cell death. It was noted previously that during the replication of HSV, the synthesis of cellular DNA and protein ceases as large quantities of HSV are produced. Cell death in critical organs of the newborn, such as the brain, can obviously result in devastating consequences, as reflected by long-term morbidity. Cellular swelling, the development of intranuclear inclusions, and cytolysis are all inherent components of the replicative process. When infected tissue stained with hematoxylin-eosin is viewed by microscopy, there is extensive evidence of hemorrhagic necrosis, clumping of nuclear chromatin, cell fusion leading to multinucleated giant cells and, ultimately, to a lymphocytic inflammatory response.

Clinical Findings. Clinical presentation of babies with neonatal HSV infection is a direct reflection of the site and extent of viral replication. Neonatal HSV infection is almost invariably symptomatic and frequently lethal. Although reported cases of asymptomatic infection in the newborn exist, they are most uncommon, and long-term follow-up of these children to document absence of subtle disease or sequelae has not been reported. Classification of newborns with HSV infection is mandatory for prognostic and therapeutic considerations. At present, babies with neonatal HSV infection can be divided into three categories, namely those with

1. Disease localized to the skin, eye, or mouth (SEM);
2. Encephalitis (CNS) with or without SEM involvement; and
3. Disseminated infection, which involves multiple organs, including CNS, lung, liver, adrenals, skin, eye, or mouth.

Historically, babies with neonatal HSV infection were classified as localized or disseminated, the former group being subdivided into those with SEM disease versus those with CNS infection; however, these classifications do not reflect the significant differences in outcome according to each category. The outcome of infection according to category varies significantly for both mortality and morbidity.

Table 11.1 summarizes disease classification in 95 babies with neonatal HSV from the NIAID Collaborative Antiviral Study Group. Babies with the worst prognosis both for mortality and morbidity have disseminated infection. Disseminated infection usually presents to tertiary care centers for therapy between 9–11 days of life; however, signs of infection are usually present on the average of 4 or 5 days earlier. This group of babies has historically accounted for approximately one-half to two-thirds of all children with neonatal HSV infection. Constitutional signs and symptoms include irritability, seizures, respiratory distress, jaundice, bleeding diatheses, shock, and frequently the characteristic vesicular exanthem that is often considered pathognomonic for infection. The vesicular rash, as described below, is particularly important in the diagnosis of HSV infection. However, 10% of children having disseminated infection will not develop skin vesicles during the course of their illness (53). In the absence of skin vesicles, the diagnosis becomes exceedingly difficult, since the other clinical signs are often vague and nonspecific, mimicking those of neonatal sepsis. Mortality in the absence of therapy exceeds 80%; all but a few survivors are impaired. The most common cause of death in babies with disseminated disease is either HSV pneumonitis or disseminated intravascular coagulopathy.

Evaluation of the extent of disease is imperative, as with all cases of neonatal HSV infection. The clinical laboratory should be utilized to define hepatic enzyme elevation, hyperbilirubinemia, neutropenia, thrombocytopenia, and bleeding diatheses, among others. In addition, chest roentgenograms, abdominal x-rays, electroencephalography, and computed tomography can all be serially and judiciously employed to determine the extent of disease. The radiographic picture of HSV lung disease is characterized by a diffuse, interstitial pattern that progresses to a hemorrhagic pneumonitis. Not infrequently, pneumonitosis intestinalis can be detected with gastrointestinal disease. Encephalitis appears to be a common component of this form of infection, occurring in about 60–75%. Cerebrospinal fluid examination and deployment of noninvasive neurodiagnostic tests, as defined below, will help assess brain disease.

Table 11.1
Demographic and Clinical Characteristics of Infants Enrolled in NIAID Collaborative Antiviral Study

	Disease Classification		
	Disseminated	CNS	SEM
No. Babies (%)	48 (50)	30 (32)	17 (18)
Male/Female	26/22	17/13	7/10
Race (Caucasian/Other)	27/21	22/8	10/7
Premature (<36 weeks)	22	10	6
Gestational Age: (Weeks ± SE)	35.9 ± 0.55	37.3 ± 0.6	37.7 ± 0.92
Enrollment Age: (Days ± SE)	12.7 ± 1.2	19 ± 1.5	11.2 ± 1.8
Clinical Findings			
Skin Lesions	43 (90)	19 (63)	17 (100)
Brain involvement	35 (73)	30 (100)	0 (0)
Pneumonia	26 (54)	0 (0)	0 (0)
Mortality:			
6 Months	33 (69)	5 (17)	0 (0)
Neurologic Impairment of Survivors:			
Total	9/15 (60)	10/25 (40)	4/16 (25)
Ara-A	8/13 (62)	8/22 (36)	1/8 (12)
Placebo	1/2 (50)	2/3 (67)	3/8[a] (38)

[a]One not included; died—bacterial septicemia. NIAID, National Institute of Allergies and Infectious Diseases, SEM, skin, eyes, mouth.

Infection of the CNS alone or in combination with disseminated disease presents with the classic findings of encephalitis in the newborn. Historically, nearly 70% of babies with neonatal HSV infection have evidence of acute brain infection. Brain infection can occur either as a component of multiorgan-disseminated infection or only as encephalitis with or without SEM involvement. Nealy one-third of all babies with neonatal HSV infection have only the encephalitis component of disease. Likely, the pathogenesis of these two forms of brain infection differ. Babies with disseminated infection probably seed the brain by a bloodborne route, resulting in multiple areas of cortical hemorrhagic necrosis. In contrast, babies who present only with encephalitis likely develop brain disease as a consequence of intraneuronal transmission of virus. Two pieces of data support this contention. First, babies with disseminated disease have documented viremia and present for therapy earlier in life than those with only encephalitis; 9–10 days versus 16–17 days. Second, babies with encephalitis are more likely to receive transplacental antibodies from their mothers, which may foster intraneuronal transmission.

Clinical manifestations of either localized CNS disease or CNS infection in association with disseminated disease include seizures, irritability, poor feeding, temperature instability, bulging fontanelle, and pyramidal tract signs. While babies with disseminated infection often have skin vesicles in association with brain infection, the same is not true for babies with encephalitis alone. In this latter group 60% of the children may have only skin vesicles at any time in the disease course (42,53,54). Cultures of cerebrospinal fluid (CSF) yield virus in 25–40% of all cases. Anticipated findings on CSF examination include pleocytosis and proteinosis (as high as 500–1,000 mg/dl). Although a few babies with CNS infection demonstrated by brain biopsy have been reported to have no alterations in their CSF, this occurs very rarely. Serial CSF assessment provides a useful diagnostic approach, as the infected child with brain disease will demonstrate progressive increases in the CSF protein. The importance of CSF examinations in all infants is underscored by the finding that even subtle changes have been associated with significant developmental abnormalities. Electroencephalography and computed tomography can be very useful in defining the presence of CNS abnormalities. Death occurs in 50% of babies with localized CNS disease who are not treated and is usually related to brainstem involvement. With rare exceptions, survivors are left with neurologic impairment (55).

The long-term prognosis, following either disseminated or localized CNS involvement is particularly poor. As many as 75% of children have some degree of psychomotor retardation, often in association with microcephaly, hydranencephaly, porencephalic cysts, spasticity, blindness, or learning disabilities. It is unclear at this time whether visceral or CNS damage can be progressive after initial clearance of the viral infection, a possibility suggested by long-term assessment of children with SEM disease (29,34,55) and more recently in this group of babies (56).

Several points warrant reiteration. Clinical manifestations in children with localized CNS infection are virtually identical to CNS involvement with disseminated cases, in spite of presumed differences in pathogenesis. For babies with encephalitis, only two of three babies will develop evidence of a vesicular rash characteristic of HSV infection. Thus, a newborn with pleocytosis and proteinosis of the cerebrospinal fluid and without a rash can easily be misdiagnosed as having a bacterial or other viral infection, unless HSV infection is carefully considered. In such circumstances, a history of genital lesions in the mother or her sexual partner may be very important in the incrimination of HSV as a cause of illness.

Infection localized to the SEM is associated with lower mortality, but it is not without significant morbidity. Infections involving the eye may manifest as keratoconjunctivitis, or later as chorioretinitis. When infection is localized to the skin, presence of discrete vesicles remains the hallmark of disease. Clusters of vesicles often appear initially upon the presenting part of the body which was in direct contact with the virus during birth. With time, the rash can progress to involve other areas of the body as well. Vesicles occur in 90% of children with SEM infection. Children with disease localized to the skin, eye, or mouth generally present at about 10–11 days of life. Those babies with skin lesions invariably will suffer from recurrences over the first 6 months of life, regardless of whether or not therapy was administered. Although death is not associated with disease localized to the

SEM, approximately 30% of these children eventually develop evidence of neurologic impairment (29,34,55). Neurologic impairment encountered in these children may be significant and includes spastic quadriplegia, microcephaly, and blindness. Important questions regarding the pathogenesis of delayed onset neurologic impairment are raised by such clinical findings. Despite normal studies in children followed for evidence of early CNS involvement by serial CNS and ophthalmological examinations, several developed severe neurologic impairment, indicating that late involvement of the CNS occurs in a manner similar to that associated with toxoplasmosis or syphilis.

In the absence of skin vesicles, the diagnosis of neonatal HSV infection can be difficult, requiring a high index of suspicion. Histories concerning the possibility of genital or labial herpes obtained from the mother and her sexual partner and, in some situations, health care providers, may be extremely helpful in suggesting and establishing the diagnosis.

DIAGNOSIS

The appropriate utilization of laboratory tools is essential if a diagnosis of HSV infection is to be made. Virus isolation remains the definitive diagnostic method. If skin lesions are present, a scraping of skin vesicles should be made and transferred in appropriate virus transport media to a diagnostic virology laboratory. Clinical specimens should be shipped on ice for inoculation into cell culture systems that are susceptible to the demonstration of the cytopathic effects characteristic of HSV replication. In addition to skin vesicles, other sites from which virus may be isolated include the cerebrospinal fluid, stool, urine, throat, nares, and conjunctivae. It may also be useful in infants with evidence of hepatitis or other gastrointestinal abnormalities to obtain duodenal aspirates for HSV isolation. The virologic results of cultures from these sites, along with clinical findings, should be used in conjunction with clinical findings to establish disease classification.

Typing of an isolate of HSV may be done by one of several techniques that are usually available in only a few diagnostic laboratories. Since outcome with treatment does not appear related to the type of HSV, identification is only of epidemiologic and pathogenetic importance and, therefore, not usually necessary. Commercially available serologic procedures to distinguish between HSV-1 and HVS-2 infections do not appear to be of value.

In the absence of diagnostic virology facilities, cytologic examination of cells from the maternal cervix or the infant's skin, mouth, conjunctivae, or corneal lesions may be useful in making a presumptive diagnosis of HSV infection. Cellular material obtained by scraping the periphery of the base of lesions should be smeared on a glass slide and promptly fixed in cold ethanol. The slide can be stained according to the methods of Papanicolaou, Giemsa, or Wright before examination by a trained cytologist. The presence of intranuclear inclusions and multinucleated giant cells are indicative but not diagnostic of HSV infection. Since the sensitivity of such procedures is only about 50–60%, there is a high prevalence of false-negative results.

In contrast to other neonatal infections, serologic diagnosis of HSV infection is less than optimal. The inability of the commonly available serologic assays to distinguish between antibodies to HSV-1 and HSV-2 as well as to denote the presence of transplacentally acquired maternal IgG, as opposed to endogenously produced antibodies, makes the assessment of the neonate's antibody status difficult during acute infection. Serial antibody assessment may be useful if a mother without a prior history of HSV infection has a primary infection late in gestation and transfers very little or no antibody to the fetus. The most commonly used tests for measurement of HSV antibodies are complement fixation, passive hemagglutination, neutralization, immunofluorescence, and ELISA assay.

Besides HSV infection, other diagnostic considerations in a newborn with a vesicular rash include neonatal melanosis, acrodermatitis enteropathica, congenital varicella, enterovirus, cutaneous candidiasis, congenital syphilis, and *Staphylococcus* skin infection. These diagnoses can be excluded by history and epidemiologic considerations, as well as by proper deployment of laboratory tests (including bacterial cultures and skin biopsies when appropriate).

TREATMENT

Nucleoside analogues have attracted the most attention as therapeutics of neonatal HSV infections. Four have been evaluated: idoxuridine, cytosine arabinoside, vidarabine, and, more recently, acyclovir. Of these compounds, the first three are nonspecific inhibitors of both cellular and viral replication, while the last, acyclovir, is selectively activated by HSV thymidine kinase. Idoxuridine and cystosine arabinoside have no value for systemic antiviral therapy for any viral infection because of toxicity and equivocal efficacy. The first drug demonstrated to be efficacious was vidarabine, as it decreased mortality and improved morbidity in neonatal HSV infection (55). Preliminary analyses of a comparison of vidarabine with acyclovir suggest that these compounds have a similar level of activity against this disease (46).

Vidarabine

In a collaborative study, the use of vidarabine in infants with disseminated or localized CNS disease was associated with a decline in mortality rate from 75–40%, as displayed in Figure 11.1. Significant improvement in morbidity was also achieved when comparing drug and placebo recipients. When outcome was examined according to each of the three disease classifications, as shown in Figure 11.2, the best therapeutic result was achieved in babies with either encephalitis or SEM infection. Mortality was decreased from nearly 90% in babies with disseminated infection to approximately 70% with therapy. This mortality remains unacceptably high, even in the ongoing acyclovir studies. For babies with encephalitis, mortality was decreased from 50–15%, and approximately 30%

of children returned to normal function. Finally, following SEM infection, while there were no deaths, severe neurologic impairment was decreased from 30–10% with therapy (34,55). Notably, there is no enhanced therapeutic benefit if the dosage of vidarabine is increased (34).

Therapy with vidarabine is most efficacious if instituted early. Recognizing that disease is often present in these babies for 4 or 5 days, a window for earlier therapy does exist. This point must be stressed, as earlier therapeutic intervention for any microbial infection will lead to improved outcome, particularly when a vital organ such as the brain is involved. Furthermore, when therapy is instituted early, fewer children will progress from localized skin involvement to more serious forms of infection. In prior studies, progression to more serious forms of infection occurred in 70% of children who received placebo. In the group of infants receiving vidarabine at doses of 15mg/kg/day or 30mg/kg/day, progression occurred in 20% and 5%, respectively (56). Vidarabine can be given intravenously in dosages of 15–30mg/kg/day over a 12-hour period for 10–14 days. At these dosages, there is no evidence of significant toxicity. Although there is no difference in mortality for babies receiving the 15 or 30mg/kg/day dose, a significantly lower percentage of babies receiving 30mg/kg/day progress to more serious forms of illness. Thus, the higher dose appears to be beneficial in preventing progression of the dis-

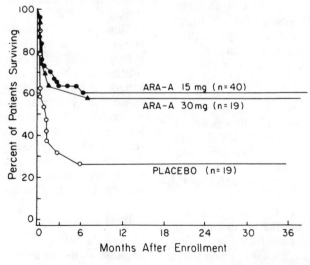

Figure 11.1. Survival of vidarabine-treated and placebo-treated newborns with CNS or disseminated neonatal herpes simplex virus infection. (Reprinted with permission from Whitley RJ, et al: *Pediatrics* 72:779–785, 1983.)

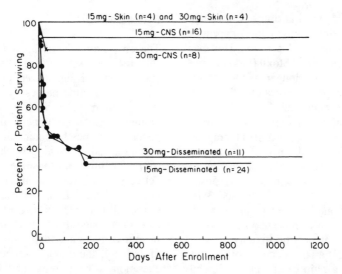

Figure 11.2. Survival of newborns with herpes simplex virus according to disease classification and dose of vidarabine. (Reprinted with permission from Whitley RJ, et al: *Pediatrics* 72:779–785, 1983.)

ease. In some circumstances, longer periods of therapy may be indicated. Approximately 2% of infants treated for 10–14 days appear to have recurrence of infection leading to CNS disease. Whether this clinical event is actually recurrence of disease or simply progression of the original infection remains poorly documented at this time. However, these infants require reinstitution of therapy. Of note, it has been suggested that progressive encephalitic disease can occur (57).

Acyclovir

Acyclovir, a relatively new antiviral compound presently undergoing extensive clinical trials, is a 2nd generation antiviral drug specific for HSV replication. This compound is activated by the thymidine kinase induced by HSV and acts as a competitive inhibitor of HSV DNA polymerase (58). It is a DNA chain terminator. The drug has been administered to numerous infants with neonatal HSV as well as to infants with cytomegalovirus infection for pharmacokinetic and tolerance evaluations. The NIAID Collaborative Antiviral Study Group is currently completing its evaluation of the relative value of vidarabine versus acyclovir for the treatment of neonatal HSV infection. Two aspects of this study are worthy of note. First, as noted above, there does not appear to be a difference in either mortality or morbidity between the two drugs. Furthermore, there are no differences in either adverse effects or laboratory evidence of toxicity. Thus,

the therapeutic index appears to be identical for the two drugs in the treatment of this disease (46). Second, the demographic and clinical information for infants enrolled in the study are worthy of note. Of the babies enrolled, 50% have disease localized to the skin, eye, or mouth (59). This represents a 3-fold increase in babies with SEM involvement from previous studies and historical data. The number of babies with CNS involvement has remained constant at about 30%, while the number of babies with disseminated disease has decreased to 20%. The overall mortality is 19%, and morbidity for this group of infants is significantly reduced from previous studies. This change in the clinical spectrum of neonatal HSV infection and improved outcome may well be related to earlier diagnosis and institution of antiviral therapy, thus preventing progression of disease from SEM to more severe disease. Available data indicate that therapy was begun an average of 3 days earlier for this group of infants. Another factor that may have affected the different spectrum of disease is that a larger number of women have recurrent genital herpes. For infants born to these women, the acquisition of humoral immunity from their mothers through transplacental antibodies may influence the outcome of infection.

Infants with ocular involvement caused by HSV should receive topical antiviral medication in addition to parenteral therapy. Presently, little safety and tolerance data are available for the topical ophthalmic antiviral drugs. In older patients, Viroptic (trifluorothymidine) appears to have the greatest antiviral activity. However, vidarabine ophthalmic and Stoxil (indoxuridine) have been utilized for a longer period of time, and there is more experience regarding their safety in both adults and children.

During the course of therapy, careful monitoring is important in order to assess therapeutic response. Even in the absence of clinical evidence of encephalitis, the CSF should be examined serially for prognostic purposes. Evaluation of certain hepatic (increased SGPT or SGOT) and bone marrow parameters (decreased platelets) may indicate viral involvement of these organs or drug toxicity.

As for all drugs, a consideration of the therapeutic index or a ratio of efficacy to toxicity is important for antiviral compounds. Experience with vidarabine and acyclovir, thus far, has indicated little toxicity when used appropriately. However, the possibility of toxicity should be considered in any child receiving parenteral antiviral therapy and assessed by serially evaluating bone marrow, renal, and hepatic function. Importantly, the potential for long-term harm from these drugs remains to be defined. Since these compounds act at the level of DNA replication, physicians responsible for follow-up of these children should be aware of the possibility of mutagenic or even teratogenic effects that may not appear until decades later. Furthermore, viral resistance may develop; the clinical significance remains to be defined. Caution should be utilized when considering prophylactic therapeutic approaches for children born to women excreting HSV at delivery.

Since the child with neonatal HSV infection, particularly with skin vesicles, will excrete virus in large quantities, isolation of the newborn is important in order to decrease the potential for nosocomial transmission of infection. Many infants with this infection will have life-threatening problems (DIC, shock, respiratory failure) and will require supportive care that is available only at tertiary medical centers.

At present, no other form of therapy is useful for treating neonatal HSV infection. Various experimental modalities, including Bacillus Calmette-Guérin (BCG), interferon, immune modulators, and immunization have been attempted, but none have produced demonstrable effects.

PREVENTION

The only prophylactic approach that has been shown to be useful for prevention of neonatal HSV infection is the delivery of pregnant women with active genital herpes by cesarean section. As a consequence, advisory committees recommend genital cultures of all women with a history of herpes beginning at 34–36 weeks in gestation and continuing weekly until delivery (60). If cultures are positive within a week of delivery or if lesions are present, cesarean section is indicated. Despite these measures, some cases will occur (59,61). Cost-benefit analyses have questioned these screening practices (62). In spite of recommendations for screening prior to delivery, the crucial time to determine viral excretion is at the onset of labor. As recently proven, predelivery cultures are not predictive of those women who will excrete virus when in labor (63). Thus, alternative management approaches will have to be developed.

Furthermore, serious forms of neonatal HSV infections will continue to be associated with significant mortality and morbidity, even with vidarabine therapy. As a consequence, some investigators have suggested that acyclovir may be useful in preventing the occurrence of neonatal HSV infections in infants who are delivered unknowingly through an infected birth canal. The prophylactic use of acyclovir has also been suggested in pregnant women who have a history of genital lesions. No data exist to establish the value of prophylactic therapy for the newborn. Such studies will have to weigh the risk of maternal primary versus recurrent infection for the fetus. Similarly, suppressive therapy of women with a known history of recurrent infection can pose significant risk to the fetus because of nephrotoxicity.

Recent data indicate that the risk of transmission of infection to infants of mothers with primary infections, even if asymptomatic at delivery, is as high as 40%. The risk for infants born to women with recurrent genital herpes is probably no greater than 3% (29,62). In women with primary infection, it is possible that prophylaxis may be of benefit. Unfortunately, substantiating data are not yet available. At present, such an approach would result in treating as many as 200 women to prevent one case of neonatal HSV infection. The potential benefit in such circumstances does not appear to outweigh the risks or costs involved. Similarly, the absence of quantitative pharmacokinetic data for any of the available antiviral drugs in the fetus should temper enthusiasm for such an approach.

Infants delivered vaginally to mothers with active genital herpes should be isolated if possible, and appropriate cultures obtained between 24–48 hours of delivery (Table 11.2). These cultures should be repeated at 2–3 day intervals during the period when infection usually begins—namely the first 2 weeks of life. Sites from which virus should be sought include eye, oro- and nasopharynx, and suspect lesions. These recommendations should serve only as guidelines until formal data are available. Antiviral therapy should be instituted promptly if *any* culture is positive. This latest recommendation is justified since our present information suggests that only a very few infected infants are asymptomatic.

Another issue of frequent concern is whether or not the mother with active genital HSV infection at delivery should be isolated from her child after delivery. Since transmission occurs by direct contact with the virus, appropriate precautions by the mother, including careful handwashing before touching the infant, should prevent the necessity of separation of mother and child. Similarly, breastfeeding is contraindicated only if the mother has vesicular lesions involving the breast. Hospitalization is not prolonged in these children.

At many institutions, a policy which requires transfer or provision of medical leave for nursing or other personnel in nurseries with a labial HSV infection is impractical and causes an excessive burden in those attempting to provide adequate care. Education regarding the risk of transmission of virus and the importance of handwashing when lesions are present should be repeatedly emphasized to health care workers. In addition, hospital personnel should wear masks when active lesions are present.

Finally, the increasing use of day-care for children in this country, including children surviving neonatal HSV infections, has stimulated many questions concerning how these children should receive care. Certainly, there is some risk that children with recurrent skin lesions secondary to a neonatal herpes infection will transmit the virus to other children in this environment. The most reasonable recommendation in this situation appears to be simply to cover the lesions and to attempt to prevent direct contact with the lesions. It is much more likely that HSV-1 will be present in the day care environment in the form of symptomatic or asymptomatic gingivostomatitis. In both cases, virus is present in the mouth and pharynx, so that the frequent exchange of saliva and other respiratory droplets, which probably occurs among children in this setting, makes this route of transmission much more likely. Education of day-care workers and the general public by health care workers concerning herpesvirus infections, their implications, and the frequency with which they occur would do much to calm fears and to correct common misconceptions concerning infections with this virus.

CONCLUSION

Neonatal HSV infection remains a life-threatening infection for the newborn in the United States today. With an increasing incidence of genital herpes and a presumed increase in neonatal HSV infections, it is important that pediatricians, neonatologists, obstetricians, and family practitioners continue to maintain a high index of suspicion in infants whose symptoms may be compatible with HSV infections so that early identification leads to prompt treatment. We hope that over the next decade, the development of safe and efficacious vaccines, as well as a better understanding of factors associated with transmission of virus from mother to baby, will allow ultimate prevention of neonatal HSV infection.

Table 11.2
Contact Isolation Guidelines for Neonatal Herpes Simplex Disease

1. Infant should be placed in a private room, if possible.
2. Gowns should be used if soiling is likely.
3. Gloves should be used for touching infective material.
4. Infants born to infected or colonized mothers should be isolated for the duration of their nursery stay (initial symptoms may occur up to one month after birth).

ACKNOWLEDGMENT

Studies performed by the author and reported in this chapter were supported in part by research grant RR-032 from the Division of Research Resources, National Institutes of Health, grant CA-13148 from the National Cancer Institute, contract NO1-AI-62554 from the Development and Applications Branch from the National Institute of Allergy and Infectious Diseases, and a grant from the State of Alabama.

REFERENCES

1. Mettler C: *History of Medicine* Philadelphia, Blakiston, 1947, pp 356–361.
2. Astruc J: *De Morbis Venereis Libri Sex*, Paris, G. Cavelier, 1736, pp 361–366.
3. Gruter W: Das herpesvirus, seine atiologische und klinische bedeutung. *Munch Med Wschr* 71:1058–1060, 1924.
4. Hass M: Hepatoadrenal necrosis with intranuclear inclusion bodies: report of a case. *Am J Pathol* 11:127–142, 1935.
5. Batignani A: Conjunctivite da virus erpetico in neonato. *Boll Ocul* 13:1217–1221, 1934.
6. Nahmias AJ, Dowdle W: Antigenic and biologic differences in herpesvirus hominis. *Prog Med Virol* 10:110–159, 1968.
7. Nahmias A, Roizman B: Herpes simplex virus. *N Engl J Med* 289:667–672; 719–725; 781–786, 1973.
8. Corey L, Spear P: Infections with herpes simplex viruses. *N Engl J Med* 314:686–691; 749–751, 1986.
9. Roizman B: The organization of the herpes simplex virus genomes. *Annu Rev Genet* 13:25–57, 1979.
10. Spear PG: Glycoproteins specified by herpes simplex virus. In Roizman B (ed): *The Herpesviruses*. New York, Plenum, 1984, vol 3, pp 315–356.
11. Roizman B, Furlong D: The replication of herpesviruses. In Fraenkel-Conrat H, Wagner RR (eds): *Comprehensive Virology* New York, Plenum, 1985, vol 3, pp 229–403.
12. Stevens JG, Cook ML: Latent herpes simplex virus in spinal ganglia of mice. *Science* 173:843–845, 1971.
13. Cabrera CV, Wohlenberg C, Openshaw H: Herpes simplex virus DNA sequences in the CNS of latently infected mice. *Nature* 298: 1068–1070, 1978.
14. Fraser NW, Lawrence WC, Wroblewska Z, Gilden DH, Koprowski H: Herpes simplex virus type 1 DNA in human brain tissue. *Proc Natl Acad Sci USA* 78:6451–6465, 1981.
15. Rock DL, Fraser NW: Detection of HSV-1 genome in central nervous system of latently infected mice. *Nature* 302:523–525, 1983.
16. Baringer JR: Recovery of herpes simplex virus from human trigeminal ganglions. *N Engl J Med* 291:828–830, 1974.
17. Baringer JR, Swoveland P: Recovery of herpes simplex virus from human trigeminal ganglions. *N Engl J Med* 288:648–650, 1973.
18. Warren KG, Brown SM, Wrobelwska Z, Gilden D, Koprowski H, Subak-Sharpe J: Isolation of latent herpes simplex virus from the superior cervical and vagus ganglions of human beings. *N Engl J Med* 298:1068–1070, 1978.
19. Sequiera LW, Jennings LC, Carrasso LH, Lord MA, Curry A, Sutton RN: Detection of herpes simplex virus genome in brain tissue. *Lancet* 2:609–616, 1979.
20. Galloway DA, Fenoglio C, Shevchuk M, McDougall JK: Detection of herpes simplex RNA in human sensory ganglia. *Virology* 95:265–268, 1979.
21. Hill TJ: Herpes simplex virus latency. In Roizman B (ed): *The Herpesviruses*. New York, Plenum, 1985, vol 3, pp 175–240.
22. McClung H, Seth P, Rawls WE: Relative concentrations in human sera of antibodies to cross-reacting and specific antigens of herpes simplex virus types 1 and 2. *Am J Epidemiol* 104:192–201, 1976.
23. Smith IW, Peutherer JF, MacCallum FO: The incidence of herpesvirus hominis antibodies in the population. *J Hyg (Camb)* 65:395–408, 1967.
24. Wentworth BB, Alexander ER: Seroepidemiology of infections due to members of the herpesvirus group. *Am J Epidemiol* 94:496–507, 1971.
25. Nahmias AJ, Josey WE, Naib ZM, Luce CF, Duffey A: Antibodies to herpesvirus hominis types 1 and 2 in humans. *Am J Epidemiol* 91:539–546, 1970.
26. Stavraky KM, Rawls WE, Chiavetta J, Donner AP, Wanklin JM: Sexual and socioeconomic factors affecting the risk of past infections with herpes simplex virus type 2. *Am J Epidemiol* 118:109–121, 1983.
27. Mann SL, Meyers JD, Holmes KL, Corey L: Prevalence and incidence of herpesvirus infections among homosexually active men. *J Infect Dis* 149:1026–1027, 1984.
28. Nahmias AJ, Keyserling H, Bain R, Becker T, Lee F, Coleman M, Dragalin D, Pereira L, Wickliffe C, Wells E, Perry L, Muther J: Prevalence of herpes simplex virus (HSV) type-specific antibodies in a USA prepaid group medical practice population. Abstract, Sixth International Meeting of the International Society for STD Research, London, England, 1985.
29. Nahmias AJ, Keyserling HL, Kerrick CM: Herpes simplex. In Remington JS, Klein JO (eds): *Infectious Diseases of the Fetus and Newborn Infant*. Philadelphia, WB Saunders, 1983, pp 638–677.
30. Hutto C, Arvin A, Jacobs R, Steele R, Stagno S, Lyrene R, Willett L, Powell D, Andersen R, Werthammer J, Ratcliff G, Nahmias A, Christy C, Whitley R: Intrauterine herpes simplex virus infections. *J Pediatr* 110:97–101, 1987.
31. Tejani N, Klein SW, Kaplan M: Subclinical herpes simplex genitalis infections in the perinatal period. *Am J Obstet Gynecol* 135:547, 1978.
32. Vontver LA, Hickok DE, Brown Z, Reid L, Corey L: Recurrent genital herpes simplex virus infection in pregnancy: infant outcome and frequency of asymptomatic recurrences. *Am J Obstet Gynecol* 143:75–84, 1982.
33. Whitley RJ, Nahmias AJ, Visintine AM, Glemin CL, Alford CA and the NIAID Collaborative Antiviral Study Group with special assistance from Yeager A, Arvin A, Haynes R, Hilty M, Luby J: The natural history of herpes simplex virus infection of mother and newborn. *Pediatrics* 66:489–494, 1980.
34. Whitley RJ, Yeager A, Kartus P, Bryson Y, Connor JD, Nahmias AJ, Soong SJ, and the NIAID Collaborative Antiviral Study Group: Neonatal herpes simplex virus infection: followup evaluation of vidarabine therapy. *Pediatrics* 72:778–785, 1983.
35. Corey L, Adams HG, Brown ZA, Holmes KK: Genital herpes simplex virus infections: clinical manifestations, course and complications. *Ann Intern Med* 98:958–972, 1983.
36. Corey L: The diagnosis and treatment of genital herpes. *JAMA* 248:1041–1049, 1982.
37. Sullivan-Bolyai J, Hull HF, Wilson C, Corey L: Neonatal herpes simplex virus infection in King County, Washington: increasing incidence and epidemiologic correlates. *JAMA* 250:3059–3062, 1983.
38. Florman AL, Gershon AA, Blackett PR, Nahmias AJ: Intrauterine infection with herpes simplex virus: resultant congenital malformations. *JAMA* 225:129–132, 1973.
39. South MA, Tompkins WA, Morris CR, Rawls WE: Congenital malformation of the central nervous system associated with genital type (type 2) herpesvirus. *J Pediatr* 75:8–13, 1969.
40. Baldwin S, Whitley RJ: Intrauterine HSV infection. *J Teratol* (in press), 1988.
41. Allen WP, Rapp F: Concept review of genital herpes vaccines. *J Infect Dis* 145:413–421, 1982.
42. Hutto C, Willett L, Yeager A, Whitley RJ: Congenital herpes simplex virus infection—early versus late gestational acquisition. Abstract 1114, Washington, D.C., The Society for Pediatric Research, 1985.
43. Yeager AS, Arvin AM, Urbani LJ, Kemp JA: Relationship of antibody in outcome in neonatal herpes simplex virus infections. *Infect Immunol* 29:532–538, 1980.
44. Prober CG, Sullender WM, Yasukawa LL, Au DS, Yeager AS, Arvin AM: Low risk of herpes simplex virus infections in neonates exposed to the virus at the time of vaginal delivery to mothers with recurrent genital herpes simplex virus infections. *N Engl J Med* 316:240–244, 1987.
45. Nahmias AJ, Josey WE, Naib ZM, Freeman MG, Fernandex RJ, Wheeler JH: Perinatal risk associated with maternal genital herpes simplex virus infection. *Am J Obstet Gynecol* 110:825–837, 1971.
46. Whitley RJ, Arvin A, Corey L, Powell D, Plotkin S, Starr S, Alford C, Connor J, Nahmias AJ, Soong SJ, and the NIAID Collaborative Antiviral Study Group: Vidarabine versus acyclovir therapy of neonatal herpes simplex virus infection. Abstract 987, Washington, D.C., The Society for Pediatric Research, 1986.
47. Francis DP, Herrmann KL, MacMahon JH, Chavigny KH, Sanderlin KC: Maternal and hospital acquired neonatal herpesvirus

hominis infections: a report of four fatal cases. *Am J Dis Child* 129:889–893, 1975.

48. Hammerberg O, Watts J, Chernesky M, Luchsinger I, Rawls W: An outbreak of herpes simplex virus type 1 in an intensive care nursery. *Pediatr Infect Dis* 2:290–294, 1983.

49. Light IJ: Postnatal acquisition of herpes simplex virus by the newborn infant: a review of the literature. *Pediatrics* 63:480–482, 1979.

50. Sullivan-Bolyai JZ, Fife KH, Jacobs RF, Miller Z, Corey L: Disseminated neonatal herpes simplex virus type 1 from a maternal breast lesion. *Pediatrics* 71:455–457, 1983.

51. Hatherley LI, Hayes K, Jack I: Herpesvirus in an obstetric hospital. Asymptomatic virus excretion in staff members. *Med J Aust* 2:273–275, 1980.

52. Schreiner R, Kleinman M, Gresham E: Maternal oral herpes: isolation policy. *Pediatrics* 63:247–249, 1979.

53. Arvin AM, Yeager AS, Bruhn FW, Grossman M: Neonatal herpes simplex infection in the absence of mucocutaneous lesions. *J Pediatr* 100:715–721, 1982.

54. Yeager AS, Arvin AM: Reason for the absence of a history of recurrent genital infections in mothers of neonates infected with herpes simplex virus. *Pediatrics* 73:188–193, 1984.

55. Whitley RJ, Nahmias J, Soong SJ, Galasso CG, Fleming CL, Alford CA: Vidarabine therapy of neonatal herpes simplex virus infection. *Pediatrics* 66:495–501, 1980.

56. Gutman LT, Wilfert CM, Eppes S: Herpes simplex virus encephalitis in children: analysis of cerebrospinal fluid and pro-

gressive neurodevelopmental deterioration. *J Infect Dis* 154:415–421, 1986.

57. Whitley RJ, Hutto C: Neonatal herpes simplex virus infections. *Pediatr in Rev* 7:119–126, 1985.

58. Elion GB, Furman PA, Fyfe JA, deMiranda P, Beauchamp L, Schaeffer HC: Selectivity of action of an antiherpetic agent 9-(2-hydroxyethoxymethyl) guanine. *Proc Natl Acad Sci USA* 74:5716–5720, 1977.

59. Whitley RJ, Hutto C, Corey L, Arvin A, Nahmias AJ, Alford CA, Soong SJ, and the NIAID Collaborative Antiviral Study Group: Changing presentations of neonatal herpes simplex virus (HSV) infections. Abstract 516, Minneapolis, 25th Interscience Conference on Antimicrobial Agents and Chemotherapy, 1985.

60. American Academy of Pediatrics, Committee on Fetus and Newborn and Committee on Infectious Diseases. Perinatal herpes simplex virus infections. *Pediatrics* 66:147–149, 1980.

61. Stone KM, Brooks CA, Guinan ME, Alexander ER: Neonatal herpes—results of one year's surveillance. Abstract 515, Interscience Conference on Antimicrobial Agents and Chemotherapy, 1985.

62. Binkin NJ, Koplan JP, Cates W: Preventing neonatal herpes: the value of weekly viral cultures in pregnant women with recurrent genital herpes. *JAMA* 251:2816–2821, 1984.

63. Arvin AM, Hensleigh PA, Prober CG, Au DS, Yasukawa LL, Wittek AE, Palumbo PE, Paryani SG, Yeager AS: Failure of antepartum maternal cultures to predict the infant's risk of exposure to herpes simplex virus at delivery. *N Engl J Med* 315:796–799, 1986.

12

Cytomegalovirus

Robert F. Pass, M.D. and Sergio Stagno, M.D.

BACKGROUND

The Virus

Cytomegalovirus (CMV) is composed of double-stranded DNA of approximately 240 kilobases, a nucleoprotein core, icosahedral capsid, and envelope (1). The intact virus is approximately 200 nm in diameter and cannot be distinguished from other human herpesviruses by electron microscopic appearance. In tissue culture, CMV produces a focal cytopathic effect characterized by cell swelling, rounding, and appearance of cytoplasmic and nuclear inclusions. Cytopathic effect from clinical isolates is usually not apparent until 10 or more days after inoculation. Only human fibroblasts are permissive for human CMV replication in vitro.

Like other members of the herpesvirus family, CMV persists in host cells indefinitely. Careful in situ cytohybridization studies with a CMV DNA probe containing the gene for immediate early protein have detected CMV-specific RNA in leukocytes from around 70% of normal seropositive adults, none of whom had evidence of CMV gene expression or productive infection (2). Whether the intermittent CMV shedding that has been detected in normal seropositive persons is due to reactivation of virus latent at the site of excretion or by other mechanisms is not known.

Acquired Infection in Adults and Children

In the healthy adult or child, cytomegalovirus rarely produces any signs of illness. Prospective studies in pregnant women have found that only around 5% who have primary CMV infection recall any illness that could be related to CMV during the interval of seroconversion (3–5). Infants who acquire CMV from maternal milk, and children who acquire CMV in day-care centers appear to be even less likely to have any symptoms associated with the onset of CMV excretion (6,7). When primary CMV infection does produce illness in the normal host, it is most likely to be a mononucleosis-like syndrome with fever, malaise, myalgias, rash, and hepatitis lasting from days to weeks (1,8). Adenopathy, hemolytic anemia, pneumonitis, myocarditis, gastrointestinal ulcerations, encephalitis, and Guillain-Barré syndrome have also been reported with CMV infection in normal hosts (1,8). CMV mononucleosis is often accompanied by lymphocytosis and atypical lymphocytes and can be clinically indistinguishable from mononucleosis due to Epstein-Barr virus (EBV). However, the heterophile antibody test is negative with CMV mononucleosis. Specific serologic tests, including detection of IgM antibodies, should be used to distinguish symptomatic CMV infection from that due to EBV, *Toxoplasma gondii*, or other agents that produce similar febrile illnesses.

Blood products (red blood cells, leukocytes, platelets) are an important source of CMV infection that can result in severe illness in immunocompromised hosts, as discussed below. Among CMV seronegative patients free of immunologic impairment, the risk of infection from blood products is clearly associated with receipt of blood from seropositive donors and increases in parallel with increasing number of units transfused. The majority of these infections are asymptomatic, though some have been accompanied by a self-limited mononucleosis-like illness or post-transfusion hepatitis.

The time from initial acquisition of CMV to onset of excretion in normal hosts has not been precisely defined, but is thought to be about 4–6 weeks. In patients who have CMV mononucleosis as well as in those who are asymptomatic, virus is shed from multiple sites (saliva, urine, tears, cervix, semen). Excretion is readily detectable for months to years after primary infection and recurs intermittently thereafter at least in some hosts (1). Around 10% of young seropositive women shed CMV in the genital tract (9,10).

Congenital Infection

Only about 5% of the estimated 35,000 infants (1% of all live births) born annually in the United States with congenital CMV infection are overtly symptomatic at birth with generalized disease, commonly referred to as cytomegalic inclusion disease (CID) (9,11). Another 5% have milder or atypical involvement, and 90% are born with subclinical but chronic infection. Clinically apparent infection is characterized by involvement of multiple organs, in particular the reticuloendothelial system and central nervous system, with or without ocular and auditory damage (12). The abnormalities found most frequently are hepatomegaly, splenomegaly, jaundice, petechiae, and chorioretinitis. In addition, intrauterine growth retardation, prematurity, and microcephaly are commonly seen in symptomatic patients. Intracranial calcifications are less likely to be detected. There are reports suggesting an association between CMV and congenital anomalies involving various organs; most of the studies are retrospective or in the form of single case reports (13). Except for inguinal hernias in males, anomalies of the first branchial arch, and a defect of tooth enamel that becomes apparent when teeth erupt (14), there is little evidence that congenital CMV infection is associated with specific morphologic abnormalities.

From the laboratory standpoint, the following laboratory values are found in decreasing order of frequency: increased cord serum IgM (>20 mg/dl), atypical lymphocytosis, elevated SGOT, thrombocytopenia, conjugated hyperbilirubinemia (indirect serum bilirubin >2 mg/dl), and increased cerebrospinal fluid protein (>120 mg/dl) (12). One or more of these laboratory abnormalities are found in 50–90% of newborns with symptomatic congenital CMV infection.

Among symptomatic infants, mortality may be as high as 30% (12). Most deaths occur in the neonatal period. Mortality during the neonatal period is usually to multiorgan disease with severe hepatic dysfunction, bleeding, dissemi-

nated intravascular coagulation, and secondary bacterial infections. A small number of deaths after the 1st month but during the 1st year have been attributed to progressive liver disease with cirrhosis. Death after the 1st year is usually restricted to severely neurologically handicapped children and is due to malnutrition, aspiration pneumonia, and overwhelming infections. The likelihood of survival with normal intellect and hearing following symptomatic congenital CMV infection is small. Severe intellectual deficits and/or neuromuscular disorders (seizures, paresis, and spasticity) are observed in 50% or more of cases. In addition, sensorineural hearing loss (bilateral or unilateral, severe to profound) and ocular abnormalities have occurred in 60% and 16% respectively of children who were symptomatic as newborns. As the children have aged, it is evident that hearing loss is of a progressive nature in many (15). Psychomotor retardation, delays in expressive language, and learning disabilities have been noted in the majority of these patients who have reached school age. Overall, it can be anticipated that between 90–95% of infants with symptomatic congenital infections who survive will develop handicaps.

As indicated in the previous section, most infants with congenital CMV infections have no early clinical manifestations, and their long-term outcome is much better. Nevertheless, there is now solid evidence derived from controlled prospective studies that at least 5%, and perhaps as many as 15%, are at risk for developmental abnormalities, such as sensorineural hearing loss, which may not be manifest until after the newborn period but usually within the first 2 years and can be progressive (15). Microcephaly with motor defects, such as spastic diplegia or quadriplegia, and various degrees of mental retardation occur in approximately 2–7% of initially asymptomatic patients. Chorioretinitis occurs in approximately 1% of cases, and like the hearing loss, may not be present at the outset. These abnormalities usually become apparent within the first 2 years of life.

Perinatal Infection

Cytomegalovirus can also be transmitted from mother to infant during the birth process and through mother's milk. From 7–28% of pregnant women excrete CMV in the genital tract late in pregnancy (10,16–18). Approximately 50% of infants born to mothers with genital excretion acquire CMV; these infants begin to excrete CMV between 3–10 weeks of age (9,10). Lactating women frequently shed CMV in milk (6). Nearly one-third of seropositive nursing mothers with up to three milk samples tested had virolactia, with most positive samples collected between 2–12 weeks postpartum. Around 30% of infants nursed by seropositive mothers acquire CMV; if milk cultures are positive for CMV, 70% of nursed infants will become infected. Human milk is probably the most common source of CMV infection for infants during their 1st year (19).

The vast majority of infants with maternally derived perinatal CMV infection remain asymptomatic. Most of these infections result from reactivation of maternal virus. Thus, infants are born with variable levels of maternal antibody. Asymptomatic perinatal CMV infection in healthy, term infants has no adverse effect on growth, perceptual functions, or on motor psychosocial development (20). However, CMV has been incriminated as a cause of pneumonitis in infants less than 4 months of age (21). The syndrome is clinically and roentgenographically indistinguishable from other causes of afebrile pneumonia, such as *Chlamydia trachomatis*, respiratory syncytial virus, *Ureaplasma urealyticum*, parainfluenza viruses, influenza viruses, adenoviruses, enteroviruses, and others.

Blood transfusions are a source of CMV infection for premature newborns. Significant morbidity and even death have been noted in premature newborns with transfusion-acquired CMV infection (22–24). From 14–30% of hospitalized premature newborns have been found to be excreting CMV, with virus shedding usually beginning after 4 weeks of age. Some of these patients have had clinical evidence of disseminated CMV infection with a septic appearance, respiratory impairment, hepatosplenomegaly, petechiae, hemolytic anemia, and atypical lymphocytosis (22–24). Epidemiologic studies found a close association between number of transfusions and CMV infection in premature newborns (25,26). Yeager and her coworkers found that greater risk of illness was associated with a seronegative mother, transfusion of more than 50 ml of blood and low birthweight (25). Almost all of the seriously ill newborns reported by Yeager and other investigators had birthweights less than 1200 g (25,26). Prospective randomized clinical trials have shown that use of blood from seronegative donors for seronegative premature recipients will prevent transfusion-acquired CMV infection (25). Use of frozen, deglycerolized red blood cells also reduces the incidence of transfusion-acquired CMV infection in this population (27). Removal of leukocytes from blood by saline washing and serial centrifugation was not effective in preventing transmission of CMV (28).

Premature newborns, like term babies, can acquire CMV from maternal sources, and in sick infants weighing less than 1500 g at birth, some of these maternally derived infections have been associated with a symptom complex similar to that noted with transfusion-acquired infection (29). Though one might expect maternal antibody to be protective, in small, premature newborns passively acquired maternal antibody can decline to undetectable levels within a few weeks. Five of six premature newborns with maternally derived infection reported by Yeager et al. had no detectable serum antibody at the onset of CMV excretion (29). Although perinatal CMV infection in healthy term infants has not been associated with late sequelae, follow-up of premature newborns suggests that some with birthweights less than 2000 g and onset of CMV excretion prior to 8 weeks may have hearing loss, neuromuscular abnormalities, or other central nervous system sequelae (30).

Infants with perinatal as well as congenital CMV infection excrete virus from saliva and urine for years (Fig. 12.1) and may thus be an important source of CMV for other children with whom they have close contact (31,32).

Immunocompromised Hosts

Patients with impaired cell-mediated immunity are at much greater risk for severe disseminated CMV infections. These have been reported frequently in oncology patients on chemotherapy, renal, hepatic, cardiac, and bone marrow transplant recipients, and in patients with acquired immunodeficiency syndrome (AIDS). The principle sources of CMV for these infections have been reactivated latent virus as well as transplanted tissue and blood products. Use of leukocyte transfusions from CMV-seropositive donors for seronegative immunocompromised patients has been shown to carry a high risk for transmission of virus (33,34). Many immunocompromised patients have silent CMV infections accompanied by prolonged viruria.

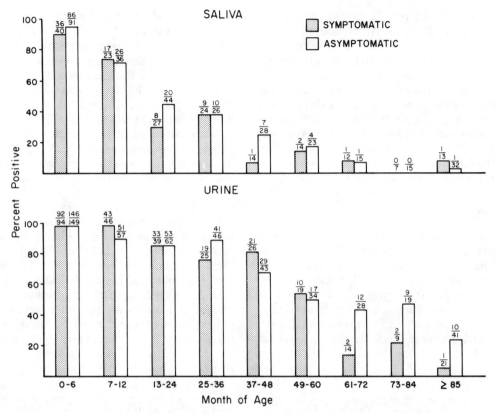

Figure 12.1   Prolonged excretion of virus in children with congenital CMV infection. Children with perinatal CMV infection have similarly persistent CMV shedding. (From Pass RF, Stagno S, Britt WJ, Alford CA: Specific cell mediated immunity and the natural history of congenital infection with cytomegalovirus. *J Infect Dis* 148:953–961, 1983. Reprinted with permission of the publisher.)

Symptomatic infection is more likely when the patient is seronegative prior to transplantation and develops primary CMV infection from blood products or transplanted tissue while immunosuppressed. The frequency of disseminated infection and serious complications from CMV appears to parallel the degree of impairment of cellular immunity. Patients receiving immunosuppressive therapy for rheumatologic disorders and renal transplant patients not treated with antithymocyte globulin (ATG) usually have asymptomatic infection. Renal and cardiac transplant patients treated with ATG, bone marrow recipients, and AIDS patients are more likely to have clinically significant CMV infections (35–37). In each of these categories, it may be difficult to attribute clinical problems clearly to CMV when laboratory evidence of infection is

so common, even in asymptomatic patients, and in patients with immunosuppression, graft rejection, graft versus host disease, or other opportunistic infections that frequently produce similar syndromes. The constellation of findings most consistently associated with CMV infection in renal and cardiac transplant patients is a febrile illness accompanied by malaise, arthralgias, leukopenia, chemical evidence of hepatitis, and a generalized rash (36–39). Although the episodes are usually self-limited, CMV has also been associated with pneumonitis, gastrointestinal ulceration, retinitis, impaired graft function, increased susceptibility to opportunistic infection, and death in these patients. In bone marrow transplant patients, CMV has been associated with graft versus host disease and a persistent diffuse pneumonitis with a high mortality (34,40). Chronic CMV infection has been nearly universal among AIDS patients, who are likely to be infected with other pathogens capable of causing similar syndromes (41,42). Extensive chorioretinitis has been clearly associated with CMV, and may progress to blindness (43). Both chorioretinitis and a chronic CMV-related ulcerating gastroenteritis (44) in AIDS patients have been controlled with the new antiviral drug 9-(1,3-dihydroxy-2-propoxymethyl) guanine (DHPG), though relapse after cessation of treatment was common (45).

POPULATION

Cytomegalovirus infection has been found in every human population that has been studied. Seroepidemiologic surveys have found that the prevalence of antibody to CMV increases with age, with patterns varying widely among populations from different geographic and ethnic backgrounds (Fig. 12.2). In general, CMV is acquired earlier in life in developing countries

and among the lower socioeconomic strata of developed countries (46). Differences between populations can be particularly striking during childhood, with rates of seropositivity of 4–6-year-olds, varying from less than 10% in Great Britain to nearly 100% in Africa and the South Pacific (32). Certain childrearing practices appear to contribute to the spread of CMV among children. Since the virus is often excreted in milk of seropositive women, where rates of maternal seropositivity are high and breastfeeding widely practiced, 80% or more of infants may acquire CMV during the 1st year of life (19). Group care of children as practiced in some developing countries, in kibbutzim in Israel, and in day-care centers in the U.S. and Europe appears to enhance spread of CMV as well (46). Factors that influence incidence of CMV infection after childhood have been less well-characterized. As noted, prevalence of antibody and seroconversion rates are higher for populations of lower socioeconomic status, presumably due to crowding. Sexual contact also contributes to

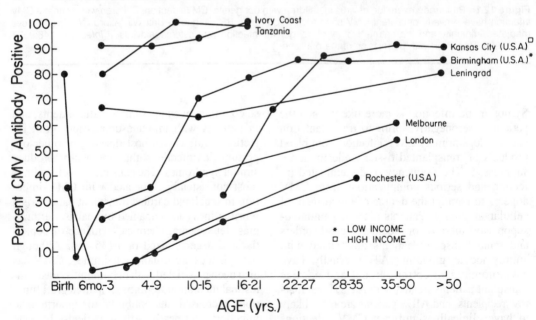

Figure 12.2 Age-related prevalence of antibody to cytomegalovirus in various populations. (From Alford CA, et al: Epidemiology of cytomegalovirus. In Nahmias AJ, Dowdle WR, Schinazi RE (eds): *The Human Herpesviruses*. New York, Elsevier, 1981, p 161. Reprinted with permission of the publisher.)

spread of CMV. High rates of seropositivity have been observed among males and females with multiple sex partners and histories of sexually transmitted diseases (47–49).

It has been frequently stated that CMV is not very contagious. That generalization still appears to be true in spite of evidence for transmission among children in day-care centers and from young children to their parents (50–52). Spread of CMV appears to require direct contact with infected secretions. Every reported case where restriction enzyme analysis of DNA from CMV isolates has been used to confirm person-to-person spread of virus has involved situations where close contact with secretions containing CMV would occur; for example, in nursing infants (53), sex partners (48), and parents of infected toddlers (53,54). Fomites may also play some role here, as CMV has been shown to retain infectivity for hours on plastic surfaces (55), and CMV has been isolated from randomly selected toys and surfaces in a day-care center (56).

DIAGNOSIS

As with most infectious diseases, there are two practical approaches to diagnosis. One is the assessment of the host's immune response; the other, the detection of virus or viral-specific antigen. A variety of methods have been used for each of these approaches (57).

The diagnosis of congenital CMV infection should be entertained in any newborn infant with signs and symptoms compatible with an intrauterine infection, or a maternal history of mononucleosis-like illness or any evidence of a primary maternal infection during pregnancy. The most specific and sensitive method to diagnose congenital CMV infection is tissue culture isolation of virus, which is most commonly accomplished from urine and saliva. In order to distinguish a congenital infection from a perinatally acquired infection, the specimens should be obtained within the first 2 weeks of life. Urine is the preferred specimen, because of larger amounts of virus and greater stability. At refrigerator temperature (4°C), urine without preservative can be stored for up to 1 week without significant loss of infectivity (58). Thus, specimens can be shipped to distant diagnostic laboratories, if necessary. However, under no circumstance should urine be frozen at $-20°C$,

since this results in significant loss of infectivity. A more rapid virologic method combines the use of tissue culture with specific anti-CMV antibodies (monoclonal antibodies or hyperimmune sera) (59,60). This method is based on the fact that CMV infection of fibroblasts induces the production of immediate and early antigens in the nucleus of the cells. The detection of these antigens is possible whether the infection is productive or not and can be reliably demonstrated with antisera or monoclonal antibody as early as 24 hours postinoculation of the monolayers. Centrifugation of monolayers appears to be an important step for this approach. With this method, there is no need to wait for the appearance of typical cytopathic effect, which may take 2 weeks to develop. The major limitation of this method is the need for freshly prepared fibroblast monolayers, but its sensitivity and specificity compare favorably with routine tissue culture methods. These are other alternatives:

1. The detection of viral particles by means of electron microscopy, a rapid test with a sensitivity of 90% and a specificity of 100% for urine specimens obtained during the 1st month of life (61). With electron microscopy, it is impossible to distinguish between CMV and the other members of the herpesvirus family.

2. Detection of CMV antigens in urine by means of solid-phase enzyme-linked immunosorbent assay (ELISA) (62). For this purpose, a monoclonal antibody is used to capture the antigens, and high-titer hyperimmune guinea pig serum is used as detector antibody. When compared with viral isolation, this method had a sensitivity of 65% and a specificity of 100%. These results are still far from being acceptable, and the test cannot be recommended for use as a screening tool for congenital CMV infection.

3. Rapid diagnosis of CMV can also be accomplished by DNA hybridization. Using a radiolabeled CMV-DNA probe, Chou and Merigan were the first to detect CMV DNA in urine specimens by DNA-DNA hybridization (63). Results were available in 24 hours, and if the urine contained 10^3 or more tissue culture infective dose per ml, both specificity and sensitivity were 100%. However, with lower amounts of virus in urine, the sensitivity of this assay has been much lower. Similar results have been reported by Spector et al. with a different DNA probe (64). The major disadvantages of DNA

hybridization are the need to use radiolabeled probes of short shelf life for optimal sensitivity and the relative insensitivity of the current techniques to detect low-titer virus.

Further studies are needed to clearly define the diagnostic value of these new methodologies. Certainly, none of these alternatives to traditional virus culture is yet practical, reliable, and inexpensive enough to be adopted as a routine diagnostic method for congenital CMV infection.

The serologic diagnosis of congenital CMV infection by means of assessments of IgG antibody titers is unfortunately of very little value. A negative result is sufficient evidence to exclude the diagnosis, but a positive result obtained within the first few months of life is generally a reflection of maternal immunity. The approach of demonstrating stable or rising levels of antibody in serial serum specimens over a 6–9-month period does not work in this situation because of the frequent occurrence of perinatal acquisition of CMV. The serologic diagnosis of congenital CMV infection can be more specifically established by demonstrating IgM antibody in cord or early neonatal serum. The indirect immunofluorescent test for IgM antibodies has been used with limited success (58). The test has a sensitivity of only 50–75% in subclinical infections and a poor specificity, with false-positive reactions reported in as many as 20–33% of control sera. Much better results have been obtained with radioimmunoassay (RIA) and ELISA for IgM antibodies (65,66). In our experience with subclinical congenital infection, the RIA-IgM has a sensitivity of 89% and a specificity of 100%, while ELISA-IgM has a sensitivity of 69% and a 5.7% rate of false-positive results. Neither of these tests is currently commercially available for diagnosis of congenital CMV infection. The presence of rheumatoid factors (IgM antibody against IgG antibodies) can cause false-positive reactions and thus must be removed from the serum before testing.

In perinatally acquired infections, isolation of virus in tissue culture is the preferred diagnostic method. Excretion of CMV usually begins between 3–12 weeks after exposure. Differentiation between congenital and perinatal CMV infection is desirable because, except in small premature newborns, risk for acute morbidity

and for long-term sequelae is generally a complication of the former. A negative CMV culture within the first 2 weeks of life or negative maternal serology will rule out congenital infection.

In older subjects (children, adolescents, and adults) the detection of IgG antibodies against CMV indicates that the infection was acquired sometime in the past. Several sensitive and specific diagnostic tests such as complement fixation (CF), indirect immunofluorescence, anticomplement immunofluorescence (ACIF), RIA, ELISA, and indirect hemagglutination, among others, are readily available in diagnostic laboratories. A primary infection is documented by seroconversion (de novo appearance of IgG antibodies), or the simultaneous detection of IgG and IgM antibodies. Greater than 4-fold rises in IgG antibody titer in initially seropositive subjects must be interpreted with caution, as these are occasionally seen years after primary infection. Testing for IgM antibodies should be done in experienced laboratories. The best methods are RIA and ELISA; however, both may give false-positive and false-negative results. It is essential that the laboratory offering tests for IgM antibody to CMV be able to provide data on the sensitivity and specificity of the test in their hands. In immunocompromised patients, primary CMV infection is best proven by demonstration of de novo appearance of IgG antibody. Rising antibody titers and even IgM antibody have been detected in immunocompromised patients with reactivation infections (67). Detection of viremia in immunocompromised patients has correlated with CMV-related disease in some studies, but asymptomatic, viremic patients have also been noted (34,37).

Detection of CMV excretion is best accomplished by virus isolation. Preferred specimens to document excretion are urine, saliva, and genital secretions. The isolation of CMV from other specimens, such as breast milk and leukocytes, may also be valuable. Virus isolation alone, however, cannot distinguish between primary and recurrent or chronic infections. A reactivation of infection or reinfection is defined by the reappearance of viral excretion in a patient known to have been seropositive and not excreting virus in the past. The distinction between reactivation and reinfection is difficult and at this time requires restriction enzyme analysis of viral DNA to demonstrate homology or heterogeneity between viral isolates obtained at different times from the same patient, a problem that is best addressed in research laboratories.

TREATMENT

A small number of systemically administered antiviral agents have been used in therapeutic trials of CMV infection, mostly in immunosuppressed patients, normal adults with mononucleosis syndrome, and infants with symptomatic congenital infection. Trials with idoxuridine, 5-fluor-2' deoxyuridine, cytosine arabinoside, adenine arabinoside, acyclovir, leukocyte interferon, interferon stimulators, transfer factor, or combinations of these agents have proved very disappointing. During therapy, these compounds may cause reductions in the amount of virus excreted, but the effect is short-lived. With the exception of vidarabine and acyclovir, drug-related toxicity is a significant problem. The most recent addition is 9-(1, 3 dihydoxypropoxymethyl) guanine (DHPG), which in preliminary studies has proven partially effective in the treatment of CMV retinochoroiditis, gastroenteritis, and pneumonitis in immunocompromised patients (45,68). However, because of systemic toxicity (bone marrow suppression), DHPG is currently restricted to life-threatening or vision-threatening CMV infections. In summary, there is as yet no safe, effective treatment available for the majority of symptomatic CMV infections.

PREVENTION

Possible strategies for preventing transmission of CMV have not been tested in population-based studies, and an effective vaccine is currently not available. Therefore, recommendations for prevention of spread of CMV are based on a "common sense" approach that recognizes that transmission of this virus appears to require direct contact with infected material.

Hospitalized Patients

Nosocomial CMV infection is a potential risk for recipients of blood products and organ transplants. Although CMV infections in these patients are frequently the result of reactivation of endogenous virus, seronegative patients who receive blood elements or organs from seropositive donors often develop primary CMV infection, which can result in severe multisystem disease,

as noted previously. Prevention of transfusion-acquired CMV infections in nonimmune patients can be accomplished by providing blood products from seronegative donors; use of frozen deglycerolized red blood cells is also effective (27,69). Both of these procedures add expense to the preparation of blood products. Screening of donors also limits the number of donors available for seronegative patients, a problem that will be particularly noted in areas where the majority of the donor population is seropositive. With transplant patients, there are obviously much greater restrictions on organ donor selection.

Because of these problems and the great variability in the course of CMV infections acquired via transfusion or organ transplantation, there has been no consensus on the use of donor selection to prevent these infections. Some hospitals are using only blood from seronegative donors for small seronegative premature newborns. The Committee on Standards of the American Association of Blood Banks has stated, "where transfusion-associated cytomegalovirus (CMV) disease is a problem, components that contain formed elements should be selected or processed to reduce that risk to neonatal recipients weighing less than 1200 g at birth, when either the neonatal recipient or the mother is CMV-antibody-negative or that information is unknown" (70). The wording of this recommendation leaves the local hospital and blood bank with the responsibility for determining whether transfusion-associated CMV disease is a problem. Among immunocompromised patients, the severity of CMV infections seems to parallel the degree of impairment of cellular immunity. In severely compromised patients, such as those undergoing bone marrow transplantation, who are not already CMV-infected, efforts should be made to prevent acquisition of CMV by providing blood products from seronegative donors (71).

Active and passive immunization have been used with success in immunocompromised patients to modify clinical expression of CMV infection-acquired from blood products or transplanted organs. Immunization of susceptible kidney transplant patients with Towne strain live CMV vaccine significantly reduced the morbidity of primary CMV infection, although it did not prevent acquisition of virus (72). There is currently no CMV vaccine licensed for clinical use. Prophylactic treatment with CMV im- munoglobulin (CMV-Ig) has been evaluated in transplant patients. In renal transplant recipi- ents, intravenous CMV-Ig decreased the sever- ity of infection in seronegative patients (73). In bone marrow transplant patients, results of sev- eral trials have shown prevention of CMV in- fection or reduction in disease severity by prophylactic administration of CMV-Ig (74–76). However, Bowden et al. could not confirm the efficacy of CMV-Ig in bone marrow transplant patients, but did demonstrate that use of sero- negative blood products was highly effective in preventing CMV infection (71). Use of passive immunization with intravenous CMV-Ig for ser- onegative transplant patients who will unavoid- ably receive tissue or blood products from seropositive donors appears reasonable at this time. Whether this approach will be effective in preventing transfusion-acquired CMV infection in small premature newborns or others remains to be determined.

Nonparenteral transmission of CMV among patients in a newborn nursery and in a children's hospital was suggested by studies employing restriction endonuclease analysis of viral iso- lates (77,78). However, the very low frequency of CMV infection in neonates who are born to seronegative mothers and are limited to blood products from seronegative donors suggests that acquisition of CMV from fomites or workers' hands is rare. It is likely that handwashing and hygienic practices, which should be a routine part of hospital care, make nonparenteral spread of CMV in the hospital less likely than in the community.

Hospital Workers

Studies of CMV infection risk in nurses and other hospital workers have yielded conflicting results (Table 12.1). Yeager reported a higher seroconversion rate for neonatal (4.1%/yr) and pediatric nurses (7.7%/yr) than for non-nurse hospital employees (0%), but differences were not statistically significant (79). Friedman et al. noted higher seroconversion rates in a pediatric hospital among workers with patient contact, compared with those without such contact (80). Although the difference in rates was not statis- tically significant, when "high-risk" employees (intensive care nurses, blood and i.v. team) were compared with others, a significantly higher rate of CMV infection was found in the former. Dworsky studied nurses in newborn nurseries and other health care workers; no difference was found when their seroconversion rate was com-

Table 12.1
Rates of Primary CMV Infection Among Health Care Workers and Others.[a]

Study (Ref.)	Group	Seroconversions	
		N	%/yr
Yeager 1975 (79)	Non-nurses	27	0
	Neonatal nurses	34	4.1
	Pediatric nurses	31	7.7
Dworsky 1983 (81)	Medical students	89	0.6
	Pediatric residents	25	2.7
	Neonatal nurses	61	3.3
Friedman 1984 (80)	"High risk"-ICU, blood, i.v. team	57	12.3
	"Low risk"-ward nurses, noncontact	151	3.3
Brady 1985 (83)	Pediatric residents	122	3.8
Adler 1986 (84)	Pediatric nurses	31	4.4
	Neonatal nurses	40	1.8
Demmler 1986 (78)	Pediatric nurses	43	0
	Pediatric "therapists"	76	0
Balfour 1986 (82)	Transplant/dialysis nurses	117	1.04
	Neonatal ICU nurses	96	2.28
	Nursing students	139	2.25
	Blood donors	167	1.57
Stagno 1986 (11)	Middle-income pregnant women	4,692	2.5
	Low-income pregnant women	507	6.8

[a]Only Friedman's 1984 study (80) in a children's hospital reported a statistically significant difference in relation to occupational contact.

pared with that of a large group of pregnant women in the community (81). Balfour and Balfour measured incidence of CMV infection among transplant/dialysis nurses, neonatal intensive care nurses, student nurses, and a control group; neither the initial rate of seropositivity nor the annual seroconversion rate differed significantly among any of the groups (82). Their annualized seroconversion rate of 1.84% was very close to rates determined for middle income pregnant women in Birmingham, Alabama (11) and in Sweden (3). Working with hospitalized children will inevitably lead to contact with a child shedding CMV; however, it is important that workers who develop primary infection not assume that their occupational exposure or contact with a specific patient is the source of infection.

Two case reports illustrate this point well. Yow et al. (85) and Wilfert et al. (86) described health care workers who acquired CMV while pregnant and after attending a patient known to be excreting CMV. In each of these reports, restriction endonuclease analysis of DNA from CMV isolates indicated that the source of CMV for the worker and her aborted fetus was not the patient under suspicion. Adler et al. used restriction enzyme methods to study CMV strains from 34 newborns and a nurse who seroconverted; all 35 strains were different, supporting the conclusion that nosocomial spread of CMV to workers or among newborns was not occurring in their nursery (84). Although hospital workers, particularly those who attend children or immunocompromised patients, will likely have occupational exposure to CMV, there is no convincing evidence that their risk of infection is increased. The Centers for Disease Control has

not recommended screening of hospital employees, but has stressed use of simple hygienic practices, such as handwashing (87,88).

Only limited data, some of which is summarized in Table 12.2, is available concerning rates of CMV excretion among various patient groups. Although many, if not most CMV-shedding patients will be asymptomatic and therefore unrecognized, patients who are known to be excreting CMV should be handled with secretion precautions.

Pregnant Women

Questions concerning prevention of CMV during pregnancy often arise in relation to known or suspected occupational exposure to the virus. Although hospital workers do not appear to be at increased risk for CMV infections, women who work in day-care centers almost certainly are. High rates of CMV excretion have been noted in children in this setting (Fig. 12.3), where hygiene is difficult at best. In addition, high rates of seroconversion have been documented in parents of CMV excreting children who attend day-care centers (52) (Fig. 12.4). We recommend that women of childbearing age whose work brings them in contact with CMV-excreting patients or children be provided with the following information as a minimum:

1. They could acquire CMV through their occupational exposure. However, the incidence of CMV infection appears to be no greater for hospital workers than for women in the community; for day-care workers, this rate has not been established.

2. Careful hygiene in the workplace, particularly handwashing and avoiding contact with

Table 12.2
Rates of CMV Excretion Among Various Patient Groups

Group	Site of Excretion	% Shedding CMV	Reference
Newborns			22–24, 81, 82
Well nursery	Urine	1.6	
Neonatal ICU	Not given	1.1	
Premature, > 3 weeks old	Urine	13–30	
Pediatric outpatients			50, 81
9–15 months, low-income	Saliva	9	
9–15 months, middle-income	Saliva	5	
0–5 years	Urine	8	
Renal transplant patients	Not given	5.6	82
Women, delivery/postpartum	Cervix, vagina	7–28	10, 16–18

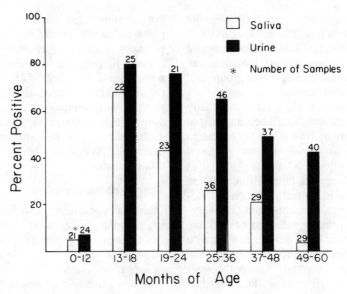

Figure 12.3 Prevalence of CMV shedding by age among children in a single day-care center serving middle-income families.

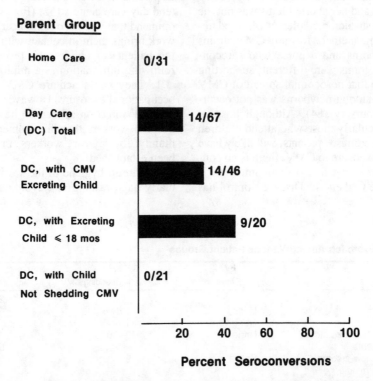

Figure 12.4 Parental seroconversion to CMV in relation to day-care attendance and CMV excretion by the child. (From Pass RF, Hutto C, Ricks R, Cloud GA: Increased rate of cytomegalovirus infection among parents of children attending day-care centers. *N Engl J Med* 314:1414–1418, 1986. Reprinted with permission of the publisher.)

secretions that may contain CMV, should prevent acquisition of CMV, but this has not been proven.

3. The presence of maternal serum antibody to CMV correlates with protection of the fetus from a damaging CMV infection. Congenital CMV infections have been documented when there is preconceptional maternal immunity, but these are thought to be the result of reactivation of endogenous virus. More importantly, damaging fetal infections appear to result principally from primary maternal infection during pregnancy.

Although screening of all women of childbearing age who work in hospitals or day care centers for antibody to CMV has not been recommended (87,88), antibody testing can be helpful in counseling the woman concerned about acquiring CMV during her pregnancy. Those who are seropositive can be strongly reassured. In most day-care centers, exposure to CMV will be less likely if the seronegative worker is limited to care of children 4 years of age or older. Rates of CMV excretion are lower than for children less than 3 years of age, and care of the older children is less likely to require contact with secretions or urine. In providing care for children in hospitals or day-care centers, it is unreasonable to attempt to identify CMV-excreting children so that the concerned worker can avoid contact with them (89). This would necessitate repeated testing of all the children for CMV excretion, since the vast majority of CMV-infected children are asymptomatic. The worker who wished to avoid all possibility of contact with CMV-excreting children during her pregnancy should probably not work with young children in hospitals or day-care centers.

ACKNOWLEDGMENT

This work was supported in part by grants from the National Institutes of Health, NICHD (HD 10699 and HD 17966) and the National Foundation—March of Dimes (No. 15–72).

REFERENCES

1. Alford CA, Britt WJ: Cytomegalovirus. In Fields BN, Knipe DM, Chanock RM, Melnick JL, Roizman B, Shope RE (eds): *Virology*. New York, Raven Press, 1985, pp 629–660.
2. Schrier RD, Nelson JA, Oldstone MBA: Detection of human cytomegalovirus in peripheral blood lymphocytes in a natural infection. *Science* 230:1048–1051, 1985.
3. Ahlfors K, Ivarsson SA, Harris S, Svanberg L, Holmqvist R, Lernmark B, Theander G: Congenital cytomegalovirus infection and disease in Sweden and the relative importance of primary and secondary maternal infections. Preliminary findings from a prospective study. *Scand J Infect Dis* 16:129–137, 1984.
4. Griffiths PD, Baboonian C: A prospective study of primary cytomegalovirus infection during pregnancy: Final report. *Br J Obstet Gynecol* 91:307–315, 1984.
5. Stagno S, Pass RF, Dworsky ME, Henderson RE, Moore EG, Walton PD, Alford CA: Congenital cytomegalovirus infection: The relative importance of primary and recurrent maternal infection. *N Engl J Med* 306:945–949, 1982.
6. Dworsky ME, Yow M, Stagno S, Pass RF, Alford CA: Cytomegalovirus infection of breast milk and transmission in infancy. *Pediatrics* 72:295–299, 1983.
7. Pass RF, Hutto C, Reynolds DW, Polhill RB: Increased frequency of cytomegalovirus in children in group day care. *Pediatrics* 74:121–126, 1984.
8. Cohen JI, Corey GR: Cytomegalovirus infection in the normal host. *Medicine* 64:100–114, 1985.
9. Alford CA, Stagno S, Pass RF: Natural history of perinatal cytomegaloviral infection. In *Perinatal Infections*. Ciba Foundation Symposium. New York, Elsevier, 1980, pp 125–147.
10. Stagno S, Pass RF, Dworsky ME, Alford CA: Maternal cytomegalovirus infection and perinatal transmission. *Clin Obstet Gynecol* 25:563–576, 1982.
11. Stagno S, Pass RF, Cloud G, Britt WJ, Henderson RE, Walton PD, Veren DA, Page F, Alford CA: Primary cytomegalovirus infection in pregnancy: Incidence, transmission to the fetus and clinical outcome in two populations of different socioeconomic backgrounds. *JAMA* 256:1904–1908, 1986.
12. Pass RF, Stagno S, Myers GJ, Alford CA: Outcome of symptomatic congenital cytomegalovirus infection: Results of long-term longitudinal follow-up. *Pediatrics* 66:758–762, 1980.
13. Hanshaw JB: Cytomegalovirus. In Remington JS, Klein JO (eds): *Infectious Diseases of the Fetus and Newborn Infant*, ed 2. Philadelphia, WB Saunders, 1983, pp 126–127.
14. Reynolds DW, Stagno S, Alford CA: Congenital cytomegalovirus infection. In Sever JL, Brent RL (eds): *Teratogen Update: Environmentally Induced Birth Defect Risks*. New York, Alan R Liss, 1986, pp 93–95.
15. Dahle AJ, McCollister FP, Stagno S, Reynolds DW, Hoffman HE: Progressive hearing impairment in children with congenital cytomegalovirus infection. *J Speech Hear Disord* 44:220–229, 1979.
16. Montgomery R, Youngblood L, Medearis DN: Recovery of cytomegalovirus from the cervix in pregnancy. *Pediatrics* 49:524–531, 1972.
17. Numazaki Y, Yano N, Morizuka T, Takai S, Ishida N: Primary infection with human cytomegalovirus: Virus isolation from healthy infants and pregnant women. *Am J Epidemiol* 91:410–417, 1970.
18. Chandler SH, Alexander ER, Holmes KK: Epidemiology of cytomegalovirus infection in a heterogeneous population of pregnant women. *J Infect Dis* 152:249–259, 1985.
19. Pass RF: Transmission of viruses through human milk. In Howell RR, Morriss FH, Pickering LK (eds): *Human Milk in Infant Nutrition and Health*. Springfield, IL, Charles C Thomas, 1986, pp 205–224.
20. Kumar ML, Nankervis GA, Jacobs IB, Ernhart CB, Glasson CE, McMillan PM, Gold E: Congenital and postnatally acquired cytomegalovirus infections: Long term follow up. *J Pediatr* 104:674–679, 1984.
21. Stagno S, Brasfield DM, Brown MC, Cassell GH, Pifer LL, Whitley RJ, Tiller RE: Infant pneumonitis associated with cytomegalovirus, chlamydia, pneumocystis and ureaplasma—a prospective study. *Pediatrics* 68:322–329, 1981.
22. Ballard RA, Drew WL, Hufnagle KG, Riedel PA: Acquired cytomegalovirus infection in preterm infants. *Am J Dis Child* 133:482–485, 1979.
23. Spector SA, Schmidt K, Ticknor W, Grossman M: Cytomegaloviruria in older infants in intensive care nurseries. *J Pediatr* 95:444–446, 1979.
24. Yeager AS: Transfusion-acquired cytomegalovirus infection in newborn infants. *Am J Dis Child* 128:478–483, 1974.
25. Yeager AS, Grumet FC, Hafleigh EB, Arvin AM, Bradley JS, Prober CG: Prevention of transfusion acquired cytomegalovirus infections in newborn infants. *J Pediatr* 98:281–287, 1981.

26. Adler SP, Chandrika T, Lawrence L, Baggett J: Cytomegalovirus infections in neonates acquired by blood transfusions. *Pediatr Infect Dis* 2:114–118, 1983.

27. Brady MT, Milam JD, Anderson DC, Hawkins EP, Speer ME, Seavy D, Bijou H, Yow MD: Use of deglycerolized red blood cells to prevent posttransfusion infection with cytomegalovirus in neonates. *J Infect Dis* 150:334–339, 1984.

28. Demmler GJ, Brady MT, Bijou H, Speer ME, Milam JD, Hawkins EP, Anderson DC, Six H, Yow MD: Posttransfusion cytomegalovirus infection in neonates: Role of saline-washed red blood cells. *J Pediatr* 108:762–765, 1986.

29. Yeager AS, Palumbo PE, Malachowski N, Ariagno RL, Stevenson DK: Sequelae of maternally derived cytomegalovirus infections in premature infants. *J Pediatr* 102:918–922, 1983.

30. Paryani SG, Yeager AS, Hosford-Dunn H, Johnson SJ, Malachowski N, Ariagno RL, Stevenson DK: Sequelae of acquired cytomegalovirus infection in premature and sick term infants. *J Pediatr* 107:451–456, 1985.

31. Pass RF, Stagno S, Britt WJ, Alford CA: Specific cell mediated immunity and the natural history of congenital infection with cytomegalovirus. *J Infect Dis* 148:953–961, 1983.

32. Pass RF, Hutto C: Group day care and cytomegaloviral infections of mothers and children. *Rev Infect Dis* 8:599–605, 1986.

33. Winston DJ, Ho WG, Howell CL, Miller MJ, Mickey R, Martin WJ, Lin CH, Gale RP: Cytomegalovirus infections associated with leukocyte transfusions. *Ann Intern Med* 93:671–675, 1980.

34. Meyers JD, Flournoy N, Thomas ED: Risk factors for cytomegalovirus infection after human marrow transplantation. *J Infect Dis* 153:478–488, 1986.

35. Meyers JD, Spencer HC, Watts JC, Gregg MB, Stewart JA, Troupin RH, Thomas ED: Cytomegalovirus pneumonia after human marrow transplantation. *Ann Intern Med* 82:181–188, 1975.

36. Pollard RB, Rand KH, Arvin AM, Merigan TC: Cell-mediated immunity to cytomegalovirus infection in normal subjects and cardiac transplant patients. *J Infect Dis* 137:541–549, 1978.

37. Pass RF, Whitley RJ, Diethelm AG, Whelchel JD, Reynolds DW, Alford CA: Cytomegalovirus infection in patients with renal transplants: Potentiation by antithymocyte globulin and an incompatible graft. *J Infect Dis* 142:9–17, 1980.

38. Suwansirikul S, Rao N, Dowling JN, Ho M: Primary and secondary cytomegalovirus infection. *Arch Intern Med* 137:1026–1029, 1977.

39. Betts RF, Freeman RB, Douglas RG, Talley TE: Clinical manifestations of renal allograft derived primary cytomegalovirus infection. *Am J Dis Child* 131:759–763, 1977.

40. Lonnqvist B, Ringdén O, Wahren B, Gahrton G, Lundgren G: Cytomegalovirus infection associated with and preceding chronic graft-versus-host disease. *Transplantation* 38:465–468, 1984.

41. Macher AM, Reichert CM, Straus SE, Long DL, Parrillo J, Lane HC, Fauci AS, Rook AH, Manischewitz JS, Quinnan GV: Death in the AIDS patient: Role of cytomegalovirus. *N Engl J Med* 309:1454, 1983.

42. Lerner CW, Tapper ML: Opportunistic infection complicating acquired immune deficiency syndrome: Clinical features of 25 cases. *Medicine* 63:155–164, 1984.

43. Palestine AG, Rodrigues MM, Macher AM, Chan CC, Lane HC, Fauci AS, Masur H, Longo D, Reichert CM, Steis R, Rook AH, Nussenblatt RB: Ophthalmic involvement in acquired immunodeficiency syndrome. *Ophthalmology* 91:1092–1099, 1984.

44. Meiselman MS, Cello JP, Margaretten W: Cytomegalovirus colitis: Report of the clinical, endoscopic, and pathologic findings in two patients with the acquired immune deficiency syndrome. *Gastroenterology* 88:171–175, 1985.

45. Collaborative DHPG Treatment Study Group: Treatment of serious cytomegalovirus infections with 9-(1,3-dihydroxy-2-propoxymethyl) guanine in patients with AIDS and other immunodeficiencies. *N Engl J Med* 314:801–805, 1986.

46. Pass RF: Epidemiology and transmission of cytomegalovirus. *J Infect Dis* 152:243–248, 1985.

47. Drew WL, Mintz L, Miner RC, Sands M, Ketterer B: Prevalence of cytomegalovirus infection in homosexual men. *J Infect Dis* 143:188–192, 1981.

48. Handsfield HH, Chandler SH, Caine VA, Meyers JD, Corey L, Medeiros E, McDougall JK: Cytomegalovirus infection in sex partners: Evidence for sexual transmission. *J Infect Dis* 151:344–348, 1985.

49. Chandler SH, Alexander ER, Holmes KK: Epidemiology of cytomegaloviral infection in a heterogeneous population of pregnant women. *J Infect Dis* 152:249–256, 1985.

50. Hutto C, Ricks R, Garvie M, Pass RF: Epidemiology of cytomegalovirus infections in young children: Day care vs. home care. *Pediatr Infect Dis* 4:149–152, 1985.

51. Yeager AS: Transmission of cytomegalovirus to mothers by infected infants: Another reason to prevent transfusion-acquired infections. *Pediatr Infect Dis* 2:295–297, 1983.

52. Pass RF, Hutto C, Ricks R, Cloud GA: Increased rate of cytomegalovirus infection among parents of children attending day-care centers. *N Engl J Med* 314:1414–1418, 1986.

53. Dworsky M, Lakeman A, Stagno S: Cytomegalovirus transmission within a family. *Pediatr Infect Dis* 3:236–238, 1984.

54. Adler SP: Molecular epidemiology of cytomegalovirus: Evidence for viral transmission to parents from children infected at a day care center. *Pediatr Infect Dis* 5:315–318, 1986.

55. Faix RG: Survival of cytomegalovirus on environmental surfaces. *J Pediatr* 106:649–652, 1985.

56. Hutto C, Little A, Ricks R, Lee JD, Pass RF: Isolation of cytomegalovirus from toys and hands in a day care center. *J Infect Dis* 154:527–530, 1986.

57. Griffiths PD: Diagnostic techniques for cytomegalovirus infection. *Clin Haematol* 13:631–644, 1984.

58. Stagno S, Pass RF, Reynolds DW, Moore MA, Nahmias AJ, Alford CA: Comparative study of diagnostic procedures for congenital cytomegalovirus infection. *Pediatrics* 65:251–257, 1980.

59. Gleaves CA, Smith TF, Shuster EA, Pearson GR: Rapid detection of cytomegalovirus in MRC-5 cells inoculated with urine specimens by using low-speed centrifugation and monoclonal antibody to an early antigen. *J Clin Microbiol* 19:917–919, 1984.

60. Griffiths PD, Stirk PR, Ganczakowski M, Panjwani DD, Ball MG, Blacklock HA: Rapid diagnosis of cytomegalovirus infection in immunocompromised patients by detection of early antigen fluorescent foci. *Lancet* 2:1242–1245, 1984.

61. Lee FK, Nahmias AJ, Stagno S: Rapid diagnosis of cytomegalovirus infection in infants by electron microscopy. *N Engl J Med* 299:1266–1270, 1978.

62. McKeating JA, Stagno S, Stirk PR, Griffiths PD: Detection of cytomegalovirus in urine samples by enzyme-linked immunosorbent assay. *J Med Virol* 16:367–373, 1985.

63. Chou S, Merigan TC: Rapid detection and quantitation of human cytomegalovirus in urine through DNA hybridization. *N Engl J Med* 308:921–925, 1983.

64. Spector SA, Rua JA, Spector DH, McMillan R: Detection of human cytomegalovirus in clinical specimens by DNA-DNA hybridization. *J Infect Dis* 150:121–126, 1984.

65. Griffiths PD, Stagno S, Pass RF, Smith RJ, Alford CA: Congenital cytomegalovirus infection: Diagnostic and prognostic significance of the detection of specific immunoglobulin M antibodies in cord serum. *Pediatrics* 69:544–549, 1982.

66. Stagno S, Tinker MK, Elrod C, Fuccillo DA, Cloud G, O'Beirne AJ: Immunoglobulin M antibodies detected by enzyme-linked immunosorbent assay and radioimmunoassay in the diagnosis of cytomegalovirus infections in pregnant women and newborn infants. *J Clin Microbiol* 21:930–935, 1985.

67. Pass RF, Griffiths PD, August AM: Antibody response to cytomegalovirus after renal transplantation: Comparison of patients with primary and recurrent infections. *J Infect Dis* 147:40–46, 1983.

68. Masur H, Lane HC, Palestine A, Smith PD, Manischewitz J, Stevens G, Fujikawa L, Macher AM, Nussenblatt R, Baird B, Megill M, Wittek A, Quinnan GV, Parrillo JE, Rook AH, Eron LJ, Poretz DM, Goldenberg RI, Fauci AS, Gelmann EP: Effect of 9-(1,3-dihydroxy-2-propoxymethyl)guanine on serious cytomegalovirus disease in eight immunosuppressed homosexual men. *Ann Intern Med* 104:41–44, 1986.

69. Taylor BJ, Jacobs RF, Baker RL, Moses EB, McSwain BE, Shulman G: Frozen deglycerolyzed blood prevents transfusion-acquired cytomegalovirus infections in neonates. *Pediatr Infect Dis* 5:188–191, 1986.

70. Holland PV, Schmitt PJ: *Standards for Blood Banks and Transfusion Services*, ed 12. Arlington, VA, Committee on Standards American Association of Blood Banks, 1987, pp 30–31.

71. Bowden RA, Sayers M, Flournoy N, Newton B, Banaji M, Thomas ED, Meyers JD: Cytomegalovirus immune globulin and seronegative blood products to prevent primary cytomegalovirus infection after marrow transplantation. *N Engl J Med* 314:1006–1010, 1986.

72. Plotkin SA, Friedman HM, Fleisher GR, Dafoe DC, Grossman RA, Smiley ML, Starr SE, Wlodaver C, Friedman AD, Barker CF: Towne vaccine-induced prevention of cytomegalovirus disease after renal transplants. *Lancet* 1:528–530, 1984.

73. Snydman DR, Werner BG, Heinze-Lacey B, Berardi VP, Tilney NL, Kirkman RL, Milford EL, Cho SI, Bush HL Jr, Levey AS, Strom TB, Carpenter CB, Levey RH, Harmon WE, Zimmerman CE II, Shapiro ME, Steinman T, LoGerfo F, Idelson B, Schroter GPJ, Levin MJ, McIver J, Leszczynski J, Grady GF: Use of cytomegalovirus immune globulin to prevent cytomegalovirus disease in renal-transplant recipients. *N Engl J Med* 317:1049–1054, 1987.

74. Condie RM, O'Reilly RJ: Prevention of cytomegalovirus infection by prophylaxis with an intravenous, hyperimmune, native, unmodified cytomegalovirus globulin. Randomized trial in bone marrow transplant recipients. *Am J Med* 76(3A):134–140, 1984.

75. Meyers JD, Leszczynski J, Zaia JA, Flournoy N, Newton B, Snydman DR, Wright GG, Levin MJ, Thomas ED: Prevention of cytomegalovirus infection by cytomegalovirus immune globulin after marrow transplantation. *Ann Intern Med* 98:442–446, 1983.

76. Winston DJ, Ho WG, Lin CH, Bartoni K, Budinger MD, Gale RP, Champlin RE: Intravenous immune globulin for prevention of cytomegalovirus infection and interstitial pneumonia after bone marrow transplantation. *Ann Intern Med* 106:12–18, 1987.

77. Spector SA: Transmission of cytomegalovirus among infants in hospital documented by restriction endonuclease digestion analyses. *Lancet* 1:378–381, 1983.

78. Demmler GJ, Yow MD, Spector SA, Brady MT, Reis SS, Anderson DC, Taber LH: Nosocomial transmission of cytomegalovirus in a children's hospital [Abstract]. *Pediatr Res* 20:308A, 1986.

79. Yeager AS: Longitudinal, serological study of cytomegalovirus infections in nurses and in personnel without patient contact. *J Clin Microbiol* 2:448–452, 1975.

80. Friedman HM, Lewis MR, Nemerofsky DM, Plotkin SA: Acquisition of cytomegalovirus infection among female employees at a pediatric hospital. *Pediatr Infect Dis* 3:233–235, 1984.

81. Dworsky ME, Welch K, Cassady G, Stagno S: Occupational risk for primary cytomegalovirus infection among pediatric health-care workers. *N Engl J Med* 309:950–953, 1983.

82. Balfour CL, Balfour HH: Cytomegalovirus is not an occupational risk for nurses in renal transplant and neonatal units. *JAMA* 256:1909–1914, 1986.

83. Brady MT, Demmler GJ, Anderson DC: Cytomegalovirus infection in pediatric house officers: Susceptibility and risk of primary infection [Abstract]. *Pediatr Res* 19:179A, 1985.

84. Adler SP, Baggett J, Wilson M, Lawrence L, McVoy M: Molecular epidemiology of cytomegalovirus in a nursery: Lack of evidence for nosocomial transmission. *J Pediatr* 108:117–123, 1986.

85. Yow MD, Lakeman AD, Stagno S, Reynolds RB, Plavidal FJ: Use of restriction enzymes to investigate the source of a primary cytomegalovirus infection in a pediatric nurse. *Pediatrics* 70:713–716, 1982.

86. Wilfert CM, Huang ES, Stagno S: Restriction endonuclease analysis of cytomegalovirus deoxyribonucleic acid as an epidemiologic tool. *Pediatrics* 70:717–721, 1982.

87. Prevalence of cytomegalovirus excretion from children in five day care centers—Alabama. *MMWR* 34:49–51, 1985.

88. Onorato IM, Morens DM, Martone WJ, Stansfield SK: Epidemiology of cytomegaloviral infections: Recommendations for prevention and control. *Rev Infect Dis* 7:479–497, 1985.

89. Pass RF, Kinney JS: Child care workers and children with congenital cytomegalovirus infection. *Pediatrics* 75:971–973, 1985.

13

Human Immunodeficiency Viruses

Elliott R. Pearl, M.D.

BACKGROUND

In the three decades since the initial description of agammaglobulinemia, a large body of knowledge has accumulated concerning human immunodeficiency diseases. The cellular defects that underlie many of these disorders have been defined, and internationally recognized clinical and laboratory criteria for their diagnosis and classification have been established (1). In the early 1980s, a syndrome of opportunistic infections, unusual cutaneous malignancies, and laboratory evidence for immunodeficiency was reported in previously healthy individuals (2–4). This new and unique disorder, named the acquired immunodeficiency syndrome (AIDS), had unusual epidemiologic features, suggesting that it was caused by an infectious agent that could be transmitted through sexual contact, by direct inoculation, or from mothers to infants (5–9).

By 1984, two nearly identical RNA-containing retroviruses were isolated from patients in the United States and France (10,11). The American isolate, recovered from a patient with AIDS, belonged to a group of viruses with tropism for human T lymphocytes, and was named human T-lymphotropic virus type III (HTLV-III). The European virus was isolated from a patient who was not immunodeficient but who had generalized lymphadenopathy, and was termed lymphadenopathy-associated virus (LAC). Infection with this virus, commonly referred to as HTLV-III/LAV, was found to elicit a serological response in patients (12,13), and antibody assays soon found widespread clinical application. In 1986, an international panel proposed that the AIDS retroviruses be named human immunodeficiency viruses, or HIV (14). Although it is now clear that there are several viruses responsible for AIDS and disorders related to AIDS, they are all very closely related and, for purposes of clarity, will here be referred to as a single agent.

With the availability of assays for anti-HIV, it has become apparent that the clinical manifestations of HIV disease are diverse, especially in children, but that immunological and neurological disorders predominate (7,8,15–19). The virus attacks the helper/inducer subset of T lymphocytes (T4, CD4), and the loss of this crucial immunoregulatory cell underlies the pathogenesis of AIDS (20,21). Further, autoimmune phenomena, such as immune thrombocytopenia and other immunologic aberrations that can occur with HIV infection in the absence of immunodeficiency disease, may also result from disordered immunoregulatory network function (22–24).

There is substantial evidence that the virus is also tropic for central nervous system (CNS) tissue and may infect the brain independently of the lymphoid system (25,26). Virus has been recovered from cerebrospinal fluid or brain tissue from infected persons, and antiviral antibody synthesis can occur within the blood-brain barrier. Invasion of the CNS by HIV can cause acute or chronic neurological syndromes and eventually results in a serious progressive encephalopathy that commonly accompanies the immunodeficiency disease in both adults and children (27,28).

The number of individuals with HIV disease has steadily increased since 1980, and over 32,000 patients meeting the CDC case definition for AIDS have been reported thus far (29). In addition to those with AIDS, many more infected persons have less severe disorders or have no evidence of disease. The objective of this chapter is to provide information and to allow a rational approach to the hospital care of individuals infected with HIV or who are at risk for infection.

POPULATION AT RISK

The major population groups at increased risk for acquiring HIV (Table 13.1) have not changed since the original descriptions of AIDS (30). At present, HIV infections in pediatric patients occur primarily in adolescents and in infants and preschool children. In adolescents, HIV is transmitted largely by sexual contact with an infected individual or by direct inoculation of contaminated blood or blood products. In this age group, most current patients with AIDS are either homosexual/bisexual males or users of intravenous drugs. Other adolescents at risk include heterosexual partners of infected persons and recipients of blood products contaminated with HIV, including many patients with hemophilia. As with other sexually transmitted diseases, promiscuity, either homosexual or heterosexual, greatly increases the risk of infection. As AIDS begins to appear in heterosexual individuals in the United States, it is clear that virtually all sexually active adolescents are at risk for infection. As with other bloodborne pathogens, such as hepatitis B virus, sharing of needles during intravenous drug use carries a high risk of infection with HIV.

Most children who have AIDS are of preschool age (30,31). The majority acquire the virus from their infected mothers by vertical transmission in utero or during the perinatal period (9). Infants of mothers belonging to a high-risk group constitute the largest number of pediatric patients with HIV disease, including AIDS (7,8,17,19,31). High-risk maternal groups include mothers who are sexually promiscuous, are intravenous drug users, or who have sexual contact with men in high-risk groups. Such women may be asymptomatic and become aware of their infection only after their infants become ill.

A smaller but significant number of infants and young children with HIV infection were recipients of blood or blood products derived from infected donors (30). Many of these patients were premature or sick newborns who received blood transfusions in the course of intensive medical treatment very early in life. This mode of acquisition will, however, become less significant since all blood intended for transfusion is currently being tested for anti-HIV.

Both sexual and parenteral transmission of HIV can occur in victims of child abuse (19). Children who have sexual contact with an infected individual or who are traumatized with contaminated needles can become infected and constitute perhaps the most tragic of all the patients.

Diseases due to HIV are not highly contagious, so there is a notably low risk of HIV infection in health care workers, casual contacts, and nonsexual close household contacts of infected patients (32–38). The paucity of AIDS in the large number of children in the 5–15 year-old age group is one piece of evidence against a significant role for casual social contact as a means of acquiring the virus (30). In hospital workers intensively exposed to patients with AIDS, including those workers suffering accidental needle-stick injuries, the risk of contracting HIV in the workplace is very low, and at least 10 times less likely than contracting hepatitis B virus infection (32–38). Nonetheless, HIV infection has occurred as a result of workers contaminating broken skin with infected secretions (39), thus underscoring the need for infection control practices discussed later in this chapter.

DIAGNOSIS

In pediatric patients, there are few clinical circumstances in which a diagnosis of HIV infection is usually considered. These include the child with proven or suspected immunodeficiency disease; the newborn infant whose mother is infected with HIV or who belongs to a group at increased risk for becoming so; or the adolescent who is a member of a recognized high-

Table 13.1
Risk Groups for HIV Infection

Adolescents/Adults
  Homosexual or bisexual men
  Intravenous drug users
  Hemophiliacs
  Sexual partners of high-risk group members
  Prostitutes
  Transfusion recipients

Infants/Young Children
  Mother in high-risk group
  Father in high-risk group
  Transfusion recipients
  Abused children

risk group. A number of features of symptomatic HIV disease in children are shown in Table 13.2. In contrast to adults, in whom opportunistic infections and Kaposi's sarcoma are major manifestations, the most common presentation of AIDS in children is recurrent bacterial infections and failure to thrive (7,8, 15,19,31). Opportunistic infections do occur, and the agents responsible are similar to those observed in adults (Table 13.3). Many of the manifestations of pediatric AIDS are ones common to primary immunodeficiency syndromes that occur in infants, particularly the severe combined immunodeficiency diseases (SCIDS), including the variant known as Nezelof syndrome (16,40). The epidemiologic, clinical, and laboratory features of childhood AIDS are, however, sufficiently distinct to allow differentiation from the primary immunodeficiency disorders (21).

The diagnosis of pediatric AIDS should be strongly considered in children with recurrent infections who have polyclonal hyperimmunoglobulinemia and evidence of T lymphocyte dysfunction, as this combination of findings is very uncommon in primary immunodeficiency diseases. To confirm a diagnosis of AIDS in an immunodeficient child, one must prove infection with HIV by isolating the virus or by demonstrating an antibody response to it. The great majority of infected children have IgG antibodies to HIV demonstrable in their serum. Screening tests for anti-HIV utilizing enzyme immunoassays and confirming tests employing the Western blot technique are widely available in hospital and reference laboratories. One must

Table 13.2
Features of HIV Infections in Children

Clinical
  Recurrent bacterial infections
  Failure to thrive
  Developmental delay
  Chronic diarrhea
  Opportunistic infections
  Neurological dysfunction
  Chronic pneumonitis
  Hepatosplenomegaly
  Lymphadenopathy

Laboratory
  Polyclonal hyperimmunoglobulinemia
  T helper cell deficiency
  Autoantibodies
  Antibodies to HIV

Table 13.3
Opportunistic Organisms Common in AIDS

Pneumocystis carinii
Mycobacterium avium intracellulare
Herpes simplex
Cytomegalovirus
Candida albicans
Cryptococcus neoformans
Toxoplasma gondii

be aware that children with AIDS may become severely hypoimmunoglobulinemic (16,18), and negative tests for antibody are meaningless under these circumstances. In such cases, viral isolation from blood lymphocytes or other tissues may be necessary to prove HIV infection. Viral isolation techniques are costly, and assays capable of detecting HIV antigen would be very useful where tests for antibody are unreliable or when high-risk individuals are seronegative (41). These assays are under development and should be available shortly.

Infants born to infected mothers may be asymptomatic at birth, but usually develop symptoms of disease early in life (19). As with many other infections that occur in utero, serologic tests for antibody are not helpful in establishing the presence of infection in infants during the newborn period. If the mother is seropositive, antibody present in her circulation will cross the placenta and be detectable in the infant. Demonstrating persistence of antibody or a rising titer through the first 3 or 4 months of life or documenting the presence of virus will establish infection in the newborn with certainty. Infants born to mothers at risk or infected with HIV must be considered infected until proven otherwise.

TREATMENT

At present, there is no satisfactory antiviral agent proven effective against HIV during the incubation or latent periods, so, of course, there is no specific treatment for HIV infection. Early results of experimental therapy of selected symptomatic patients with reverse transcriptase inhibitors, such as 3'-azido 3'-deoxythymidine (AZT) suggest that control of viral replication is possible and may result in clinical improvement (42). Although the drug is clearly toxic to many patients (43), this treatment is a promising strategy and will likely be vigorously pursued. Until specific antiviral therapy is available, treatment of patients is limited to the secondary disorders that result from immunodeficiency or other clinical expressions of HIV infection.

The basic principles of management of infants and children with primary immunodeficiencies have been applied to the treatment of childhood AIDS. These measures include nutritional support, specific immunologic replacement therapy, and early detection and treatment of secondary infections. Chronic malnutrition may develop because of diarrhea, anorexia, or neurological impairment, and may require nutritional resuscitation and intravenous alimentation. As with other serious immunodeficiency diseases, AIDS is associated with secondary infection by opportunistic pathogens (Table 13.3). In addition, in spite of having hyperimmunoglobulinemia, many AIDS patients have defective specific antibody production, which renders them susceptible to a variety of pyogenic infections (24,44,45). For this reason, intravenous immunoglobulin replacement (200–400 mg/kg twice monthly) may be useful in all immunodeficient children and is mandatory in those who become hypoimmunoglobulinemic. Other attempts at immunoreconstitution, such as bone marrow transplantation or treatment with lymphokines, have been unsuccessful. For secondary bacterial, viral, fungal, and protozoal infections, specific antimicrobials can be used, including prophylaxis against *Pneumocystis carinii* infection with trimethoprim-sulfamethoxazole.

While the clinical manifestations of pediatric AIDS are often very severe, there are many children infected with HIV who are not seriously ill. These include asymptomatic infants born to infected mothers, transfused individuals who are seropositive, and patients with less severe clinical disorders associated with HIV. Tragically, many asymptomatic children infected with HIV have suffered social ostracism, educational deprivation, and emotional abuse because of unsubstantiated public fears and misunderstandings about the manner in which AIDS is spread. These children need psychological support and attention to their social and emotional needs. The American Academy of Pediatrics and the Centers for Disease Control have published guidelines regarding school and day-care attendance as well as immunization strategies for children infected with HIV (46–48). In deriving these recommendations, the Academy considered the risks of transmitting HIV as well as the risks of immunodeficient patients acquiring secondary infections in the school, day-care, or foster care environment. These recommendations may be applied to in-hospital education programs as well as to traditional school situations. With few exceptions, school-aged children infected with HIV should be allowed an unrestricted educational setting. Patients who are neurologically impaired or who are unable to adequately control secretions or body fluids should be in a setting that minimizes contact with other children.

Asymptomatic patients require little or no care with respect to HIV, but may have occasion to be hospitalized for other reasons, such as accidents or surgery. Similarly, those with illness associated with HIV other than AIDS may also require inpatient care in community hospitals or secondary centers. For this reason, all hospitals must be prepared to adapt currently used infection isolation precautions for use with patients infected with HIV.

PREVENTION

Prevention of HIV disease in the hospital setting is far simpler than prevention of disease in the general population. Intensive public educational efforts concerning the nature of the virus and its major routes of transmission will be indispensable in achieving effective control over the spread of AIDS. Future development of effective chemotherapy or a useful vaccine will undoubtedly be helpful as well. But for now, the prevention of pediatric AIDS and other HIV illnesses relies on preventing infection in women of childbearing age. All physicians who care for adolescents should assure that they have timely written information concerning AIDS and HIV for distribution to their patients. Matters of venereal disease prevention and the dangers of intravenous drug abuse should be openly discussed. Pediatricians and family physicians must become advocates of intensive AIDS-oriented education in the schools if the heterosexual dissemination of this infection throughout the young adult population is to be stopped. It is worth noting that risk factors for AIDS are really risk behaviors, and all young people must be made aware of the consequences of their behavior.

Acquisition of HIV by casual contact or by close intrafamilial nonsexual contact has not been reported (35). Nonetheless, precautions should be taken when dealing with HIV-infected individuals who are hospitalized in order to reduce the risk to both health care workers and to the patients themselves. Specific guidelines concerning preventing transmission of HIV to hospital and laboratory workers have been published (29) and are applicable to the prevention of many other infections. Such precautions appear to be effective, since their use in hospitals that care for substantial numbers of HIV-infected patients is associated with a negligible risk of nosocomial infection with HIV (32–34,36,38,49).

Since medical history and examination cannot reliably identify all patients with HIV or other bloodborne pathogens, the CDC has recently proposed that the traditional blood secretion precautions be routinely used on *all* hospitalized patients and referred to as "universal precautions" or "universal blood and body fluid precautions," as outlined in Table 13.4 (29). Similar principles have already been successfully introduced into clinical practice (50). This author suggests that all patients with documented HIV infection be placed on the traditional blood and body fluid precautions to maximize technique in the care of the identified case. Patients need not be routinely housed in private rooms, unless demanded by the presence of secondary infection or the need for protective isolation. Sodium hypochlorite 0.5% (1:10 dilution of bleach in water) is an effective disinfectant and should be used for cleaning washable surfaces and for de-

contaminating instruments or sharp items for disposal. To avoid the need for unexpected mouth-to-mouth resuscitation, plastic airways, endotracheal tubes, and ventilation bags should be immediately available. All personnel working in direct contact with a patient's mucous membranes, secretions, drainage fluids, or wounds should be gloved.

Failure to apply the principles of universal or blood and body fluid precautions and to avoid direct skin contact with potentially contaminated secretions or blood is believed to have been responsible for infection of four health care providers, in one case the patient's mother (39,51). It should be emphasized, however, that this latter individual had extremely heavy exposure to contaminated material, and that this is the only instance of transmission of HIV within a family that did not involve sexual contact, needle sharing, or in utero acquisition of the virus.

Other types of isolation may be necessary for HIV-infected children, depending on the presence or absence of immunodeficiency or of secondary infections. The use of strict, respiratory, contact, or enteric isolation precautions should be dictated by the nature of the complicating secondary bacterial, viral, fungal, or protozoal infection and not by the presence of HIV itself. Immunodeficient children are vulnerable to nosocomial infection or infection acquired from visitors. Such patients should be placed in protective isolation, and all their visitors should be screened by the nursing staff prior to being allowed access to the room.

Individuals involved in phlebotomy, care of intravenous lines, or the handling of blood/spinal fluid specimens from all patients, thus assuming all are infected (or potentially infected) with HIV, need to be particularly careful to avoid inadvertent parenteral exposure. Likewise, personnel performing or assisting at invasive procedures, such as bone marrow aspiration, lumbar puncture, or bronchoscopy, need be attentive to the chance for inadvertent exposure. Extreme care should be taken in handling needles or other sharp objects that are potentially contaminated with HIV. Needles should never be bent or recapped, but disposed of promptly at the bedside in a puncture-resistant container of disinfectant. Should an accidental penetrating injury occur, it should be reported to appropriate infection control committees, and individuals involved in

Table 13.4
Universal Blood and Body Fluid Precautions for Containment of HIV Infections

1. Wash hands before and after direct patient contact.
2. Use gloves if handling blood, drainage, secretions, or excretions. Hands should be washed after removing gloves and changed between patients.
3. Masks and protective eyewear should be used during procedures that are likely to generate droplets of blood or other body fluids to prevent exposure of mucous membranes of the mouth, nose, and eyes.
4. Gowns needed if soiling of clothes is likely.
5. All contaminated articles are bagged before removal from room and are clearly labeled for infectious precautions.
6. Surfaces may be disinfected with household bleach 1:10 in water.
7. Needles and disposable sharp instruments should be placed in a puncture-resistant container containing disinfectant.

these exposures should be serologically monitored for an extended period of time. The experience reported from several centers caring for many AIDS patients is that even with needle-stick/sharp injury to health care workers, the risk of acquisition of this infection is extremely low in the absence of other risk factors (33,38,52), but it can occur (53).

As with any potentially bloodborne agent, laboratory specimens from infected patients should be clearly labeled for infectious precautions and carefully transported in sealed plastic bags. In the laboratory, every effort should be made to avoid contact of the specimen with unprotected skin or mucous membranes and, as always, careful handwashing after handling any potentially infectious material is a must.

The occurrence of nosocomial infection with HIV in hospitalized patients is extraordinarily unlikely. There is a risk in the potential for transfusion of contaminated blood products; however, this has been substantially reduced since the introduction of routine screening for anti-HIV by blood banks in 1984. Nonetheless, rare incidences of such transmission may continue to occur (52), since virus has been isolated from the tissues of asymptomatic persons who lacked antibody to HIV (38). Such individuals may transmit infection prior to the appearance of serum antibody and would thus escape current methods of detection. Newly developed assays for viral antigen should prove useful under these circumstances, as they have for hepatitis B.

An undiagnosed but infected patient poses a greater risk than one who is identified and properly managed. As previously mentioned, it has been recommended that all hospitalized patients be treated as potentially infected with HIV (and other blood/secretionborne infectious agents) (29). It is important for all patients to be screened for the presence of personal or family risk factors (Table 13.1). Physician and nursing staff histories should include specific queries about intravenous drug use, homosexual/bisexual contacts, or unprotected sexual contact by household members with anyone who might belong to a group at risk for HIV infection. In this way, suspected at-risk patients can be effectively identified and appropriate studies performed to either diagnose or exclude HIV infection. This is particularly relevant to obstetrical patients who are asymptomatic but who may be infected. These women will give birth to infants who may also

be infected and who may potentially spread the disease.

SUMMARY

Infection with HIV occurs primarily through sexual contact or by direct inoculation, and largely in members of certain high-risk behavior groups or in their newborn infants. Effective means for diagnosing the presence of infection are available and should be utilized if historical information indicates or suggests the presence of recognized risk factors. Patients with proven or suspected HIV infection should be placed on blood/secretion precautions, which are known to be effective in preventing the spread of the disease. Finally, if such identification and management principles are observed and safe needle-handling techniques are utilized, the risk of acquiring HIV disease, including AIDS, in the hospital setting is minimal.

REFERENCES

1. Cooper MD, Faulk WP, Fudenberg HH, Good RA, Hitzig W, Kunkel HG, Roitt IM, Rosen FS, Seligmann M, Soothill JF: Meeting report of the second international workshop on primary immunodeficiency diseases in man. *Clin Immunol Immunopathol* 2:416–445, 1974.
2. Gottlieb MS, Schroff R, Schanker HM, Weisman JD, Fan PT, Wolf RA, Saxon A: *Pneumocystis carinii* pneumonia and mucosal candidiasis in previously healthy homosexual men. *N Engl J Med* 305:1425–1431, 1981.
3. Masur H, Michelis MA, Greene JB, Onorato I, Vande Stouwe RA, Holzman RS, Wormser G, Brettman L, Lange M, Murray HW, Cunningham-Rundles S: An outbreak of community-acquired *Pneumocystis carinii* pneumonia. *N Engl J Med* 305: 1431–1438, 1981.
4. Siegal FP, Lopez C, Hammer GS, Brown AE, Kornfeld SJ, Gold J, Hassett J, Hirschman SZ, Cunningham-Rundles C, Adelsberg BR, Parham DM, Siegal M, Cunningham-Rundles S, Armstrong D: Severe acquired immunodeficiency in male homosexuals manifested by chronic perianal ulcerative herpes simplex lesions. *N Engl J Med* 305:1439–1444, 1981.
5. Harris C, Small CB, Klein RS, Friedland GH, Moll B, Emeson EE, Spigland I, Steigbigel NH: Immunodeficiency in female sexual partners of men with the acquired immunodeficiency syndrome. *N Engl J Med* 308:1181–1184, 1983.
6. Curran JW, Lawrence DN, Jaffe H, Kaplan JE, Zyla LD, Chamberland M, Weinstein R, Lui K-J, Schonberger LB, Spira TJ, Alexander WJ, Swinger G, Ammann A, Solomon S, Auerbach D, Mildvan D, Stoneburner R, Jason JM, Haverkos HW, Evatt BL: Acquired immunodeficiency syndrome (AIDS) associated with transfusions. *N Engl J Med* 310:69–75, 1984.
7. Oleske J, Minnefor A, Cooper R Jr., Thomas K, dela Cruz A, Ahdieh H, Guerrero I, Joshi VV, Desposito F: Immune deficiency syndrome in children. *JAMA* 249:2345–2349, 1983.
8. Rubinstein A, Sicklick M, Gupta A, Bernstein L, Klein N, Rubinstein E, Spigland I, Fruchter L, Litman N, Lee H, Hollander M: Acquired immunodeficiency with reversed T_4/T_8 ratios in infants born to promiscuous and drug-addicted mothers. *JAMA* 249:2350–2356, 1983.
9. Cowan MJ, Hellmann D, Chudwin D, Wara DW, Chang RS, Ammann AJ: Maternal transmission of acquired immune deficiency syndrome. *Pediatrics* 73:382–386, 1984.

10. Barre'-Sinoussi F, Chermann JC, Rey F, Nugeyre MT, Chamaret S, Gruest J, Dauguet C, Axler-Blin C, Vezinet-Brun F, Rouzioux C, Rozenbaum W, Montagnier L: Isolation of a T-lymphotropic retrovirus from a patient at risk for acquired immune deficiency syndrome (AIDS). *Science* 220:868–871, 1983.

11. Gallo RC, Salahuddin SZ, Popovic M, Shearer GM, Kaplan M, Haynes BF, Palker TJ, Redfield R, Oleske J, Safai B, White G, Foster P, Markham PD: Frequent detection and isolation of cytopathic retroviruses (HTLV-III) from patients with AIDS and at risk for AIDS. *Science* 224:500–503, 1984.

12. Brun-Vezinet F, Rouzioux C, Barre-Sinoussi F, Klatzmann D, Saimot AG, Rozenbaum W, Christol D, Gluckmann JC, Montagnier L, Chermann JC: Detection of IgG antibodies to lymphadenopathy-associated virus in patients with AIDS or lymphadenopathy syndrome. *Lancet* 1:1253–1256, 1984.

13. Sarngadharan MG, Popovic M, Bruch L, Schupbach J, Gallo RC: Antibodies reactive with human T-lymphotropic retroviruses (HTLV-III) in the serum of patients with AIDS. *Science* 224:506–508, 1984.

14. Coffin J, Haase A, Levy JA, Montagnier L, Oroszlan S, Teich N, Temin H, Toyoshima K, Varmus H, Vogt P, Weiss R: Human immunodeficiency viruses. *Science* 232:697, 1986.

15. Scott GB, Buck BE, Letterman JG, Bloom FL, Parks WP: Acquired immunodeficiency syndrome in infants. *N Engl J Med* 310:76–81, 1984.

16. Wykoff RF, Pearl ER, Saulsbury FT: Immunologic dysfunction in infants infected through transfusion with HTLV-III. *N Engl J Med* 312:294–296, 1985.

17. Amman AJ: The acquired immunodeficiency syndrome in infants and children. *Ann Int Med* 103:734–737, 1985.

18. Pahwa S, Kaplan M, Fikrig S, Pahwa R, Sarngadharan MG, Popovic M, Gallo RC: Spectrum of human t-cell lymphotropic virus type III infection in children. *JAMA* 255:2299–2305, 1986.

19. Rubinstein A, Bernstein L: The epidemiology of pediatric acquired immunodeficiency syndrome. *Clin Immunol Immunopathol* 40:115–121, 1986.

20. Seligmann M, Chess L, Fahey JL, Fauci AS, Lachmann PJ, L'Age-Stehr J, Ngu J, Pinching AJ, Rosen FS, Spira TJ, Wybran J: AIDS—an immunologic reevaluation. *N Engl J Med* 311:1286–1292, 1984.

21. Amman AJ, Levy J: Laboratory investigation of pediatric acquired immunodeficiency syndrome. *Clin Immunol Immunopathol* 40:122–127, 1986.

22. Walsh C, Krigel R, Lennette E, Karpatkin S: Thrombocytopenia in homosexual patients. *Ann Int Med* 103:542–545, 1985.

23. Saulsbury FT, Boyle RJ, Wykoff RF, Howard TH: Thrombocytopenia as the presenting manifestation of human T-lymphotropic virus type III infection in infants. *J Pediatr* 109:30–34, 1986.

24. Lane HC, Masur H, Edgar LC, Whalen G, Rook AH, Fauci AS: Abnormalities of B-cell activation and immunoregulation in patients with the acquired immunodeficiency syndrome. *N Engl J Med* 309:453–458, 1983.

25. Ho DD, Rota TR, Schooley RT, Kaplan JC, Allan JD, Groopman JE, Resnick L, Felsenstein D, Andrews CA, Hirsch MS: Isolation of HTLV-III from cerebrospinal fluid and neural tissues of patients with neurologic syndromes related to the acquired immunodeficiency syndrome. *N Engl J Med* 313:1493-1497, 1985.

26. Resnick L, diMarzo-Veronese F, Schupback J, Tourtellotte WW, Ho DD, Muller F, Shapshak P, Vogt M, Groopman JE, Markham PD, Gallo RC: Intra-blood-brain-barrier synthesis of HTLV-III-specific IgG in patients with neurologic symptoms associated with AIDS or AIDS-related complex. *N Engl J Med* 313:1498–1504, 1985.

27. Snider WD, Simpson DM, Nielsen S, Gold JWM, Metroka CE, Posner JB: Neurological complications of acquired immune deficiency syndrome: Analysis of 50 patients. *Ann Neurol* 14:403–418, 1983.

28. Epstein LG, Sharer LR, Oleske JM, Connor EM, Goudsmit J, Bagdon L, Robert-Guroff M, Koenigsberger MR: Neurologic manifestations of human immunodeficiency virus infection in children. *Pediatrics* 78:678–687, 1986.

29. Centers for Disease Control: Recommendations for prevention of HIV transmission in health care settings. *MMWR* 36:2s–18s, 1987.

30. Centers for Disease Control: Update: Acquired immunodeficiency syndrome—United States. *MMWR* 35:757–766, 1986.

31. Rogers M: AIDS in children: a review of the clinical, epidemiologic and public health aspects. *Pediatr Infect Dis* 4:230–236, 1985.

32. Hirsch MS, Wormser GP, Schooley RT, Ho DD, Felsenstein D, Hopkins CC, Joline C, Duncanson F, Sarngadharan MG, Saxinger C, Gallo RC: Risk of nosocomial infection with human T-cell lymphotropic virus III (HTLV-III). *N Engl J Med* 312:1–4, 1985.

33. Weiss SH, Saxinger WC, Rechtman D, Grieco MH, Nadler J, Holman S, Ginzburg HM, Groopman JE, Goedert JJ, Markham PD, Gallo RC, Blattner WA, Landesman S: HTLV-III infection among health care workers. *JAMA* 254:2089–2093, 1985.

34. Shanson DC, Evans R, Lai L: Incidence and risk of transmission of HTLV III infections to staff at a London hospital, 1982–85. *J Hosp Infect* 6(suppl C):15–22, 1985.

35. Kaplan JE, Oleske JM, Getchell JP, Kalyanaraman VS, Minnefor AB, Zabala-Ablan M, Joshi V, Denny T, Cabradilla CD, Rogers MF, Sarngadharan MG, Sliski A, Gallo RC, Francis DP: Evidence against transmission of human T-lymphotropic virus/lymphadenopathy-associated virus (HTLV-III/LAV) in families of children with the acquired immunodeficiency syndrome. *Pediatr Infect Dis* 4:468–471, 1986.

36. Henderson DK, Saah AJ, Zak BJ, Kaslow RA, Lane HC, Folks T, Blackwelder WC, Schmitt J, LaCamera DJ, Masur H, Fauci AS: Risk of nosocomial infection with human T-cell lymphotropic virus III/lymphadenopathy-associated virus in a large cohort of intensively exposed health care workers. *Ann Int Med* 104:644–647, 1986.

37. Lifson A, Castro KG, McCray E, Jaffe HW: National surveillance of AIDS in health care workers. *JAMA* 256:3231–3234, 1986.

38. Gerberding JL, Bryant-LeBlanc CE, Nelson K, Moss AR, Osmond D, Chambers HF, Carlson JR, Drew WL, Levy JA, Sande MA: Risk of transmitting the human immunodeficiency virus, cytomegalovirus and hepatitis B virus to health care workers exposed to patients with AIDS and AIDS-related conditions. *J Infect Dis* 156:1–8, 1987.

39. Centers for Disease Control: Update: Human immunodeficiency virus infections in health-care workers exposed to blood of infected patients. *MMWR* 36:285–289, 1987.

40. Amman AJ: Is there an acquired immune deficiency syndrome in infants and children? *Pediatrics* 72:430–432, 1983.

41. Salahuddin SZ, Groopman JE, Markham PD, Sarngadharan MG, Redfield RR, McLane MF, Essex M, Sliski A, Gallo RC: HTLV-III in symptom-free seronegative persons. *Lancet* 2:1418–1420, 1984.

42. Fischl MA, Richman DD, Grieco MH, Gottlieb MS, Volberding PA, Laskin OL, Leedom JM, Groopman JE, Mildvan D, Schooley RT, Jackson GG, Durack DT, King D, and the AZT collaborative group. The efficacy of azidothymidine (AZT) in the treatment of patients with AIDS and AIDS-related complex. A double-blind, placebo-controlled trial. *N Engl J Med* 317:185–191, 1987.

43. Richman DD, Fischl MA, Grieco MH, Gottlieb MS, Volberding PA, Laskin OL, Leedom JM, Durack DT, Nusinoff-Lehrman S, and the AZT collaborative group. The toxicity of azidothymidine (AZT) in the treatment of patients with AIDS and AIDS-related complex. A double-blind, placebo-controlled trial. *N Engl J Med* 317:192–197, 1987.

44. Amman AJ, Schiffman G, Abrams D, Volberding P, Ziegler J, Conant M: B-cell immunodeficiency in acquired immune deficiency syndrome. *JAMA* 251:1447–1449, 1984.

45. Bernstein LJ, Kriger BZ, Novick B, Sicklick MJ, Rubinstein A: Bacterial infection in the acquired immunodeficiency syndrome of children. *Pediatr Infect Dis* 4:472–475, 1985.

46. Centers for Disease Control: Education and foster care of children infected with human T-lymphotropic virus type III/lymphadenopathy-associated virus. *MMWR* 34:517–521, 1985.

47. American Academy of Pediatrics: School attendance of children and adolescents with human T lymphotropic virus III/lymphadenopathy-associated virus infection. *Pediatrics* 77:430–432, 1986.

48. Centers for Disease Control: Immunization of children infected with human T-lymphotropic virus type III/lymphadenopathy-associated virus. *MMWR* 35:595–606, 1986.

49. Gerberding JL: Recommended infection-control policies for patients with human immunodeficiency virus infection. An Update. *N Engl J Med* 315:1562–1564, 1986.

50. Lynch P, Jackson MM, Cummings MJ, Stamm WE. Rethinking the role of isolation practices in the prevention of nosocomial infections. *Ann Int Med* 107:243–246, 1987.

51. Centers for Disease Control: Apparent transmission of human T-lymphotropic virus type III/lymphadenopathy-associated virus from a child to a mother providing health care. *MMWR* 35:76–79, 1986.

52. Centers for Disease Control: Human T-lymphotropic virus type III/lymphadenopathy-associated virus: Agent summary statement. *MMWR* 35:540–548, 1986.

53. Editorial: Needlestick transmission of HTLV-III from a patient infected in Africa. *Lancet* 2:1376–1377, 1984.

54. Centers for Disease Control: Transfusion-associated human T-lymphotropic virus type III/lymphadenopathy-associated virus infection from a seronegative donor—Colorado. *MMWR* 35:389–391, 1986.

14

Hepatitis A Virus, Hepatitis B Virus, and Non-A Non-B Hepatitis

Timothy R. Townsend, M.D.

Hepatitis is an acute or chronic inflammatory process affecting the liver. Numerous bacterial, viral, fungal, chemical, immunological, and physical agents can cause inflammation of the liver. When a clinician is faced with an infant or child with clinical or laboratory evidence of inflammation of the liver, the broad range of etiologic agents should be kept in mind. Suppose, for example, you are presented with a jaundiced one-month-old patient who had been asphyxiated at birth and had been multiply transfused while in a newborn intensive care unit. Could this be a case of shock liver, Epstein-Barr virus, cytomegalovirus, viral hepatitis from blood transfusions, early fungal sepsis, biliary atresia, toxicity from drugs or hyperalimentation, or hepatitis B acquired from the infant's asymptomatic carrier mother? Careful evaluation and testing should help to identify the cause of the hepatitis, but this is likely to be a challenging task.

This chapter will focus only on three of the etiologic agents of liver inflammation—hepatitis A virus (HAV), hepatitis B virus (HBV), and the presumed viral agent or agents of non-A non-B hepatitis (NANB).

HEPATITIS A

Background

HAV is a small 27 nm, nonenveloped, RNA virus belonging to the family Picornaviridae, which also include the rhinoviruses and the enteroviruses. HAV is in the genus enterovirus (enterovirus type 72), but appears to have many unique characteristics compared with other enterovirus, particularly the prototype enterovirus, poliovirus. For example, HAV is more heat stable than poliovirus, so it may persist better in the environment (1). HAV can be grown in tis-

sue culture, but unlike poliovirus, it produces no cytopathic effect. Unlike the situation in the human host where there is no evidence for chronic persistent infection, infection of tissue culture cells results in persistence. This phenomenon has importance for the development of a vaccine against HAV. Although there is some variation in the nucleotide sequences of different specimens of HAV, there appears to be a single antigenic strain of HAV that is consistent worldwide (2).

The pathogenesis of HAV infection is incompletely understood. Although infectious hepatitis has been recognized as a clinical entity for centuries, the etiologic agent was discovered less than 25 years ago. HAV can be transmitted by the fecal-oral route, and rarely by the intravenous route. Irrespective of route of infection, and possibly the size of the infecting inoculum, the incubation period is about 28 days. Despite considerable effort to find an intestinal site of replication of HAV, none has been found, unlike the prototypic enterovirus poliovirus. Pathogenic events from the time of ingestion or injection of HAV to the onset of viral replication in the hepatocytes are largely unknown. Approximately 2 weeks following infection, viral antigen can be detected in hepatocytes, and a brief viremia follows. Approximately 3 weeks after infection, whole virions can be found in the stool, presumably excreted in the bile, since an intestinal site of replication is not thought to exist. Concentration of viral particles in the stool reaches a peak at the time that liver enzyme abnormalities are greatest, just prior to the onset of clinical illness (3). By the time clinical illness is severe enough for patients to seek medical attention or be hospitalized, the concentration of viral particles in their stool is markedly diminished as is their infectivity.

Coincident with the onset of abnormalities of liver enzymes, serum IgM antibodies against HAV are detectable. Serum neutralizing antibodies are found during active viral replication. The finding of little hepatocyte destruction during the early phases of HAV infection and the appearance of hepatocyte destruction coincident with the development of various antibodies to HAV may suggest an immunologic basis for the liver inflammation of HAV infection. IgM antibodies usually persist for only a few months following infection. IgG antibodies can be detected a few weeks after maximal liver enzyme abnormalities and may persist for life, even though they may fall to very low but still protective levels many years following infection (4).

The clinical manifestations of HAV infection are age-dependent. Less than one-fourth of infants and children with HAV infection have symptoms, whereas over three-fourths of infected adults are symptomatic. Diarrhea is a common symptom among children but is uncommon among infected adults. Other manifestations, such as jaundice, dark urine, malaise, and light-colored stools are found in approximately 60–80% of both children and adults with symptomatic infection. Elevated liver enzymes rarely persist for more than few months, and there is no evidence that a chronic or recurrent infectious state exists.

Population

Nosocomial transmission of HAV appears to occur infrequently. Most reported cases are associated with epidemics, and many epidemics have involved pediatric patients (5–8). Epidemics of nosocomial HAV infection generally are of three types. First, foodborne outbreaks affecting patients or hospital staff or both, depending on the food involved in the transmission, have been reported but differ little from outbreaks involving restaurants or other food sources for the general public. Second, transfusion-acquired HAV infection has been reported (5). In several well-documented instances, the donor was bled at a time consistent with the expected brief viremia associated with HAV infection. Such a coincidence is probably rare, but HAV infection must be considered in any patient with a history of transfusion. Third, either direct or indirect (through the environment or hands of hospital personnel) fecal-oral transmission of HAV infection are well-documented (6,7). In most cases, the index case was not suspected of having an HAV infection and was fecally incontinent.

In most reported epidemics, no unusual characteristics of the population at risk of infection were noted. Specifically, no marker of increased susceptibility such as age, sex, race, pregnancy, immunosuppression, etc. were noted. Contact, presumably with infectious material from the index case, seemed to be the most common risk factor in most epidemics. As might be expected, the index cases involved in the epidemics did have unusual characteristics in that they were food handlers, blood donors and recipients, and incontinent patients.

Diagnosis

Since many HAV infections are asymptomatic, particularly in children, and the clinical manifestations of symptomatic cases are often protean, particularly if jaundice is not present, serotesting is the most reliable means to diagnose HAV infection (9). A single serum specimen tested for IgM anti-HAV and IgG anti-HAV can indicate if a person is not clinically or subclinically ill with HAV and if he is either susceptible (negative IgG and IgM), currently or recently infected with HAV (negative IgG, positive IgM), or infected previously and now immune (positive IgG, negative IgM if more than 2–6 months since infection, or positive IgM if less than 2–6 months).

Serotesting should be reserved for confirming the suspected diagnosis of HAV infection. Insufficient data are available to determine if serotesting of patients, blood donors, or food handlers would be cost-effective in preventing nosocomial transmission of HAV infection. There are, however, data to suggest that hospital workers' seroprevalence is no different from the general population's. This finding suggests that there is little endemic HAV transmission from patients to employees and that hospital food services are no more of a problem than public food services (10).

Treatment

Other than supportive symptomatic care, there is no treatment available for HAV infection. Should, in the future, a candidate antiviral compound be considered, it would need to be inexpensive and have minimal side effects since HAV infection, albeit costly in terms of morbidity, is rarely a serious fatal disease.

Prevention

There are three ways to prevent nosocomial HAV transmission: active immunization, passive immunization, and infection control practices. Active immunization is currently not available, but several candidate vaccines are in early human trials. Both inactivated and live attentuated virus vaccine prototypes will undergo testing in the next few years, and at least one should become available within a decade.

Passive immunization using immune serum globulin (ISG) has been used for over a quarter of a century and is 87–98% effective in preventing clinical illness (11). Depending on how long after exposure ISG is administered, it will either prevent infection or infection will occur, but clinical illness will be prevented. The latter situation is called passive-active immunity in that the infection stimulates immunity, but the passively administered antibodies are sufficient to prevent the infection from being severe enough to cause clinical illness. Long-lasting immunity from the subclinical illness ensues. The usual dose of ISG is 0.01 ml per pound of body weight. If ISG is given more than 2 weeks after an exposure, its efficacy is minimal. ISG should be used in the hospital setting for individual patients or personnel with known exposures to infected persons or as an outbreak control measure. Guidelines for who should receive ISG during an outbreak are difficult to formulate because to be effective, it must be given as soon after exposure as possible. The early part of an outbreak is precisely the time when the source or mode of transmission is usually unknown. Since HAV nosocomial outbreaks usually have involved blood, food, or feces (usually incontinent patients), a quick assessment of cases for these common factors may suggest enough of a source or mode of transmission to institute ISG prophylaxis to persons exposed to that source.

Infection control practices are probably effective in preventing nosocomial HAV transmission, although they have never been subjected to the rigors of a randomized clinical trial using HAV as the agent to test the hypothesis. Considering that active immunization is not available, and ISG for all hospital employees every 2–3 months would be expensive, painful, and impractical, infection control practices are obviously a good alternative. In the patient with documented HAV infection, enteric precautions are recommended (12) (Table 14.1). When HAV disease is considered, enteric precautions should be exercised until the diagnosis is eliminated. However, in several of the nosocomial HAV outbreaks, the diagnosis was unsuspected. The patients were incontinent, and their diarrhea was thought to be due to other causes (drugs, feeding changes, etc). To avoid such transmission, infection control practices must be consistently applied to all patients, irrespective of any diseases they may have.

HAV is a hardy virus well-adapted for transmission via the environment. Common sense dictates that if gloves are worn when having contact with any patient's blood, secretions, or excretions, the likelihood of transmitting any contact-transmitted disease is diminished. If handwashing follows the removal of the gloves, the last of any infective material that may have leaked through the gloves or came into contact with the hands during glove removal is eliminated.

HEPATITIS B

Background

Hepatitis B virus (HBV) infection is caused by a 42 nm, incompletely double-stranded DNA virus, belonging to the hepadnavirus group. The complete infectious virion consists of the strand of DNA, a hepatitis B core antigen (HBcAg), a hepatitis B "e" antigen (HBeAg), and a surface protein coat, the hepatitis B surface antigen (HBsAg). When a liver cell, the hepatocyte, is infected with HBV, the virus takes over control of the hepatocyte's function such that the hepatocyte makes thousands of new viruses. In this replication process, the hepatocyte manufactures excess protein coat (HBsAg), which is released along with whole virions into the blood-

Table 14.1.
Enteric Precautions for Hepatitis A

1. Gloves should be worn when in contact with feces or fecally contaminated objects.
2. Gowns should be worn when clothing may be in contact with feces or fecally contaminated objects.
3. Private room is suggested for a patient who is not toilet trained, has diarrhea, or poor personal hygiene.

stream in the form of tubules and 20-nm spherical particles.

Approximately 1000 HBsAg particles are released for every whole virion. The number of whole virions in the blood of an infected individual can be enormous; over 10^9 infectious particles per milliliter is not uncommon. Due to the limits of sensitivity of the radioimmunoassay for detecting HBsAg in blood (10^{-4}–10^{-5}), infectivity titers (10^{-7}–10^{-8} in a chimpanzee animal model) may not correlate with absence of detectable HBsAg in blood (13). This situation requires that to test the efficacy of a sterilization or disinfection process in destroying infectivity rather than simply destroying HBsAg, direct inoculation into primates is necessary (HBV cannot be cultivated in artificial media).

Antibodies directed against each of the viral components noted above have been described. The antibody to HBsAg (anti-HBs) is the protective antibody, appearing in serum after the disappearance of HBsAg following natural infection or in response to the HBV vaccine. The antibody to HBcAg (anti-HBc) indicates previous infection with HBV; the IgM class antibody to HBcAg (IgM anti-HBc) appears in serum 1–2 weeks after HBsAg is detectable and persists for 4–6 months, when it is replaced by the IgG class antibody to HBcAg (IgG anti-HBc). Infectivity correlates with HBeAg, so presence of the antibody to HBeAg (anti-HBe) in serum indicates lesser infectivity, and in the chronic carrier state, indicates lower titer of circulating virus.

Following percutaneous inoculation of the HBV, the virus enters the hepatocyte. In about 7 days, HBsAg can be detected in the serum (14). In contrast, HBsAg appears in serum about 50–60 days following oral ingestion of virus. Within 1–2 weeks, anti-HBc is detectable and persists presumably indefinitely. Fifty–150 days following infection, liver enzymes become elevated. In 10–25% of cases, symptoms of fatigue, jaundice, anorexia, nausea, vomiting, and abdominal pain occur. Increased age correlates directly with symptomatic infection such that fewer than 10% of infected infants and children are symptomatic (15). In infections that resolve, HBsAg disappears from serum, and 1–2 months later, anti-HBs appears in serum and persists indefinitely. HBeAg and anti-HBe generally parallel HBsAg and anti-HBs. In infections that do not resolve, leading to the chronic carrier

state, HBsAg and anti-HBc persist as long as the chronic carrier state persists. Chronic carriers are defined as persons with HBsAg detectable for greater than 6 months; approximately 1% of carriers per year will resolve their infection (16). Young age at the time of infection increases the risk of chronic carriage such that as many as 90% of perinatal infections result in chronic infections.

HBV can be transmitted percutaneously, orally, and perinatally. Perinatal transmission most likely is the result of oral ingestion of maternal blood at the time of delivery, but transplacental transmission, possibly via placental leaks resulting in maternofetal transfusion, can occur (17,18). Sexual transmission or transmission occurring in the hospital or household setting is probably a result of either oral ingestion of virus or contamination of tiny breaks in the skin or mucous membranes with virus. The infectious dose of HBV for humans is unknown, but epidemiologic and laboratory animal data suggest that very small amounts of blood or body fluids containing infectious virus are needed (13,19).

The HBV can persist in an infectious state on inanimate surfaces, yet it is susceptible to heat and many commonly available disinfectants (20,21). Infectivity for chimpanzees of dried infectious blood was destroyed by 10-minute exposure at 20°C of 500 mg/liter-free chlorine from sodium hypochlorite; 10-minute exposure at 20°C of 2% aqueous glutaraldehyde (pH 8.4); 10-minute exposure at 20°C of a 1:16 dilution of a 2% glutaraldehyde - 7% phenate solution (pH 7.9); 10-minute exposure at 20°C of 70% isopropyl alcohol; 10-minute exposure at 20°C of a 1:213 dilution of an iodophor detergent-disinfectant (80 mg available iodine per liter); 5-minute exposure at 24°C of a 1% and a 0.1% aqueous glutaraldehyde (pH 7.2); and 2 minutes of exposure to a temperature of 98°C. Although these data do not satisfy the Environmental Protection Agency requirements for disinfectant label claims of hepatitis B virucidal activity, they can serve as a general guideline for disinfection or sterilization of environmental surfaces that have been thoroughly cleaned so as to reduce the amount of viable virus to a minimum.

Population

The epidemiology of HBV infection varies in different parts of the world partly because of the predominant route of transmission of the virus. In areas of Asia and sub-Saharan Africa, 5–15% of persons are carriers, and virtually the entire population has been infected. Transmission is usually perinatal or in early childhood. In contrast, in this country, the lifetime risk of infection is 5% for the population as a whole, although certain groups are at much higher risk. Transmission is primarily sexual or percutaneous. Groups at higher (10–100%) risk than the population as a whole are intravenous drug abusers, household contacts of HBV carriers, homosexually active males, staff and clients in institutions for the mentally retarded, male prison inmates, and immigrants from parts of the world with high rates of infection. Patients undergoing hemodialysis are at increased risk, although in recent years the risk seems to be decreasing.

Hospital employees who have contact with blood (possibly as little as getting blood on themselves as infrequently as once a week) are at increased risk. For hospital employees, a significant determinant of their risk is the prevalence of actively infected (acute or chronic carriers) persons in the patient population of their particular hospital (22). Since HBV infection is primarily a disease of adults in this country, hospital workers who care for infants and young children probably are at less risk of acquiring infection from their patients than are those who care for adolescents or adults. In the hospital setting, HBV transmission is much more common from patient to hospital worker than from hospital worker to patient, although transmission in each direction has been documented (23–26).

Finally, infants born of HBsAg-positive mothers, particularly those who are also HBeAg-positive are at high risk of infection, and if infection occurs, are at a 90% risk of becoming chronic carriers. Identification of infected pregnant women is the most effective means of identifying which infants are at risk of infection.

Diagnosis

Since HBV infection is usually asymptomatic, particularly among infants and children, a reliable diagnosis is best made serologically. Commercially available, highly sensitive tests for HBsAg, HBeAg, anti-HBs, anti-HBc (IgG and IgM), and anti-HBe are in use in many hospital and reference laboratories. Although the usual interpretation of test results is noted under

"Background" it must be kept in mind that false-positive and false-negative results do occur. The nation's blood supply is routinely tested for evidence of HBV infection in donors, but blood transfusions can still, albeit rarely, transmit HBV.

A positive test for HBsAg is considered a marker for infectivity even though, at least for chimpanzees, direct intravenous inoculation of blood that is below the level of sensitivity of the test for HBsAg can produce infection. A positive test for anti-HBs is considered a marker for immunity to HBV infection, although low levels of anti-HBs may not be protective, depending on the dose and route of a challenging HBV. Despite these caveats, for practical purposes, a patient who has a positive test for HBsAg should be considered infectious, and a person who has a positive test for anti-HBs should be considered noninfectious and immune to future infection.

The routine serotesting of all donors of blood or blood products is recommended. The routine serotesting of patients admitted to the hospital is not recommended unless it is part of a survey to establish policy regarding risk of patient-patient or patient-hospital worker transmission of HBV.

Treatment

Other than symptomatic supportive care, there is no treatment available for HBV infection. To date, no promising antiviral therapy is imminent.

Prevention

HBV infection is indeed preventable. Worldwide, prevention of the acute mortality (about 1%) and mortality from the sequelae of chronic infection, such as cirrhosis and hepatocellular carcinoma (up to a 300-fold increased risk in chronic carriers), demands the highest priority for prevention strategies. The following discussion will focus on prevention of HBV infection in the hospital setting, but the same prevention strategies can be applied to diverse populations (27).

As mentioned earlier, nosocomial transmission of HBV occurs predominantly from patient to hospital worker, occasionally from mother to newborn infant, occasionally from patient to patient, and rarely from hospital worker to patient, and rarely through contaminated blood products.

Serotesting of all blood donors for HBsAg is currently the standard of practice and has markedly reduced HBV transmission via blood and blood products. In addition, most volunteer donor blood banks screen donors for a history of hepatitis and membership in high hepatitis-risk populations. Further reduction in the risk of HBV transmission via blood or blood products seems unlikely in the near future, unless more sensitive serological tests become available.

When a hospital worker is identified as being infectious, either acutely or as a chronic carrier, the preponderance of evidence suggests that reasonable infection control practices are effective against spreading the disease. Such practices include the health care worker's wearing gloves while working with sharp instruments or doing invasive procedures so as to not allow infectious blood to come into contact with the patient (25). Reported instances of health care worker-to-patient transmission frequently document breaks in accepted technique. Fear of loss of livelihood or medicolegal liability has fostered a reluctance on the part of many hospital workers to be tested for the presence of HBsAg (28). It could be argued that if health care workers knew they were infectious, they might make sure to wear gloves when performing procedures that might place their patients at risk. Until the social and medicolegal issues are resolved, little reduction in this relatively infrequent nosocomial HBV transmission can be expected.

Patient-to-patient nosocomial transmission occurs mainly through environmental or inanimate surface contamination. Contamination of the surfaces of hemodialysis machines, then passive transfer on the hands of personnel to shunt connection sites, is an example of this method of HBV transmission. Isolated instances of presumed transmission via contaminated endoscopes or other invasive instruments have been reported, but exclusion of coincidence or other routes of transmission has been lacking (29). Regular serotesting of patients and staff of hemodialysis units, segregation of positive and negative dialysis patients and equipment, use of good infection control techniques, and careful cleaning and disinfection of inanimate surfaces has reduced HBV transmission in hemodialysis units. How great a role the cleaning and disinfection had in contributing to the reduced risk

is unknown. Meticulous cleaning, particularly of the coiled intricate internal parts of endoscopes, is recommended prior to sterilization or high-level disinfection and should reduce any risk of HBV transmission (30).

Maternal-infant transmission of HBV can largely be prevented if the mother is recognized to be HBsAg-positive prior to the time of delivery. It is recommended that women of Asian, Pacific Island, or Alaskan Eskimo descent (immigrant or U.S.-born), women born in Haiti or sub-Saharan Africa, or women with a history of liver disease be serotested for HBsAg prior to delivery (27). In addition, women who have had contact with a hemodialysis unit or an institution for the mentally retarded, or who have been rejected as blood donors, have been multiply transfused, or who have had frequent occupational blood exposure or household contact with an HBV carrier or hemodialysis patient, multiple episodes of venereal diseases, or have used illicit percutaneous drugs should likewise be tested. In a large inner city obstetric population with a 0.5% carrier rate and a 9% rate of current or previous infection with HBV, the sensitivity of a positive response to any one of the preceding recommended questions was no better than 50% (G. McQuillan, T.R. Townsend, unpublished observations). To avoid failure to detect an infectious pregnant woman, routine third trimester serotesting was recently instituted at The Johns Hopkins Hospital based on these observations. Further data testing the sensitivity and specificity of the recommended screening questions in different obstetrical populations may be needed before recommending routine screening. However, considering the large lifetime costs for health care of a single case of perinatal HBV infection and the small costs for routine serotesting of urban obstetrical populations, this may be cost-effective and of significant preventive benefit.

Once a pregnant woman has been identified as being HBsAg-positive, it is recommended that as soon after birth as possible, the infant receive 0.5 ml intramuscularly (clean the injection site thoroughly so as not to carry maternal blood on the needle into the infant's leg) of hepatitis B immune globulin (HBIG), and at a different site, 0.5 ml of hepatitis B vaccine. Repeat doses of vaccine are given at 1 month and 6 months of age. This regimen is about 90% effective in preventing infection and the subsequent chronic carrier state (31). Delays in initiating this regimen reduce its effectiveness. If delays greater than 1 month occur, screen the infant for HBsAg, and if negative, institute HBIG and vaccine (given at 0-, 1-, and 6-month intervals). Following this regimen, the infant should be serotested at 18 months of age for HBsAg (a positive test indicating a failure of prophylaxis) and anti-HBs (a positive test indicating immunity) to provide a basis for prognostication and counseling.

Most nosocomial HBV transmission is from patients to hospital workers who come in contact with infected blood or body fluids. Three prevention strategies are effective in interrupting transmission; preexposure vaccination, postexposure passive immunization and vaccination, and avoidance of infection through infection control techniques.

Hepatitis B vaccine, both the plasma vaccine and the recombinant vaccine are highly effective (32,33). When the vaccine is handled properly and not injected into fatty tissue, such as the buttocks, or subcutaneously, over 90% of normal individuals mount an adequate antibody response and are protected. Certain genetic factors have been linked with poor response (34). The height of the initial antibody response to the vaccine predicts the length of protection. When antibody levels fall to 10 sample ratio units, protection is diminished (35). The need for or timing of booster doses remains unresolved.

HBIG, which is gammaglobulin-derived from preselected donors who have high anti-HBs titers, is effective as postexposure prophylaxis, such as after a needle-stick exposure (36). If given within 7 days of percutaneous exposure and repeated 1 month later, HBIG is 75–95% effective in preventing infection and clinical illness and permits a passive active immunization similar to ISG for HAV infection. After 7 days, its efficacy is questionable.

Infection control techniques are those mentioned previously for HAV infection. Most hospitalized patients who can transmit infection to hospital workers are asymptomatic. On direct questioning for membership in high-risk groups, only 50% of an obstetrical population currently or previously infected with HBV could be identified (G. McQuillan G, T.R. Townsend, unpublished observations). It therefore makes sense for hospital workers to protect themselves against HBV (and other bloodborne diseases, such as

Table 14.2.
Blood/Body Fluid Precautions for Hepatitis-B

1. Gloves should be worn when in contact with blood or body fluids (excretions or secretions), or contaminated objects.
2. Gowns, masks, and protective eyeware should be worn when splashing or spattering of blood or body fluids is anticipated.
3. Infants born to Hb_s Ag-positive mothers should be placed on Blood and Body Fluid Precautions.

syphilis, cytomegalovirus, human immunodeficiency virus, etc.) by wearing gloves when in contact with any patient's blood or body fluids or with objects that have been contaminated with blood or body fluids (Table 14.2).

Infection control techniques should be thought of as the first line of defense in preventing nosocomial transmission of HBV (and other bloodborne infections). As a second line of defense, immunization of all hospital workers who get blood on their hands more than one time per week will provide adequate specific protection. If a particular hospital can document little or no risk of nosocomial transmission to its employees, vaccination may not be necessary. If a hospital decides to initiate a vaccination program for its employees, it should follow recent published guidelines for prevaccination serotesting (27). Finally, postexposure prophylaxis using HBIG and vaccine may be thought of as a failure of the first two lines of defense. Additionally, if an unvaccinated susceptible hospital worker sustains an exposure (needle-stick, blood on hands that have cuts or scratches, etc.), use of HBIG alone without vaccine makes little sense, since that individual has demonstrated that he is at occupational risk of HBV infection, and future overt or covert exposures can be expected.

Through its employee health service, each hospital should develop a protocol for the management of employees who sustain a possible HBV exposure while on the job. The following is a suggested guideline for such a protocol.

1. Educate employees as to what to do should they think they have sustained an exposure. Remind employees that urgency in reporting the exposure is important because delays of even a few days reduces their chances of protection.

2. Designate a limited group of persons who will interview the employee to determine if a significant exposure occurred.

3. Define what constitutes a significant exposure. There must be physical contact with blood or body fluids on skin that has a reasonable probability of cuts, scratches, or other integument breaches (hands, shaved areas, etc.) or mucous membranes (including eyes) or penetrating injury (needle-sticks).

4. Determine if the source of the exposure is known or unknown and, if known, whether the HBsAg status is known (or can be serotested within 24–48 hours) or unknown.

5. Determine the antibody status of the employee, unless the employee has completed the three-dose vaccination series and has been tested within the preceding 12 months and is found to have greater than 10 sample ratio units of antibody.

6. If the employee is unvaccinated or has not completed the three-dose series, and the source of the exposure is known and is HBsAg-positive, give a single 0.06 ml/kg of HBIG, and at a separate site, give the first of the three doses of vaccine (repeat at 1 and 6 months), or if the series has been started, complete the series.

7. If the employee is unvaccinated or has not completed the three-dose series, and the source of the exposure is known but the HBsAg status cannot be determined or is unknown, determine the likelihood that the source is at high risk of being contaminated with HBsAg (e.g., needle poking through a trash bag on a ward where multiply transfused hemophiliac children are treated) or is at low risk of being contaminated with HBsAg (e.g., a needle poking through a trash bag on a general pediatric infant ward). If the source is a high-risk one, give the employee a single 0.06 ml/kg of HBIG, and at a different site, give the first of the three-dose series of vaccine, or if the series has been started, complete the series. If the source is a low-risk one, give the employee the first dose of vaccine or complete the series, if vaccine had been previously started.

8. If the employee is unvaccinated or has not completed the three-dose series and the source of the exposure is unknown, give the employee the first of the three-dose vaccine series or complete an already started series.

9. If the employee has completed the three-dose vaccination series and within the previous 12 months has been documented to have adequate antibody (greater than 10 sample ratio units) and the source of the exposure is known and is

HBsAg positive, no treatment is needed.

10. If the employee has completed the three-dose vaccination series but has not been serotested within the preceding 12 months and the source of exposure is known and is HBsAg-positive, serotest the employee. If adequate antibody is present, no treatment is needed. If inadequate antibody is present, give a 0.06 ml/kg dose of HBIG, and at a separate site, give a booster dose of vaccine.

11. If the employee has completed the three-dose vaccination series and within the preceding 12 months has been documented to have adequate antibody, and the source of the exposure is known but the HBsAg status cannot be determined or if the source is unknown, no treatment is needed.

12. If the employee has completed the three-dose vaccination series and within the preceding 12 months has not been serotested and the source of the exposure is known, but the HBsAg status cannot be determined, or if the exposure is unknown, no treatment is needed. Serotesting is optional if the employee has a history of multiple exposures.

NON-A NON-B HEPATITIS
Background

Non-A non-B hepatitis (NANB) is an illness that clinically resembles HAV or HBV infection, and the evidence to date suggests that it is caused by a filterable, transmissible agent or agents that are probably one or more viruses. With the availability for more than a decade of tests to diagnose HAV, HBV, Epstein-Barr virus, and cytomegalovirus infections, which can produce the clinical picture of NANB hepatitis, recognition of this entity has been possible. It is a diagnosis of exclusion.

There appear to be two epidemiologically distinct forms of NANB. One is similar to HBV and is the form almost exclusively seen in the U.S. The other resembles HAV in that it seems to be transmitted by the fecal-oral route. It has been described in outbreaks in Asia, has not been as extensively studied, and does not appear to be a problem in the U.S. (37,38). The remainder of this discussion will focus on the form seen in the U.S.

Prior to the routine screening of all donated blood, post-transfusion hepatitis was thought to be "serum hepatitis" or HBV infection. In retrospect, however, there were two distinct incubation periods, one longer (12–14 weeks) and one shorter (6–9 weeks). The longer one is now known to be HBV and the shorter is NANB. Today 85–95% of all post-transfusion hepatitis is NANB. Symptomatic or asymptomatic NANB occurs following transfusion in 7–10% of transfused patients (38).

There are some data to suggest there may be two or more separate agents producing NANB. The most convincing data come from cross-challenge studies of chimpanzees using well-characterized infectious sera from humans who have transmitted NANB.

Following injection of infectious blood, clinical illness indistinguishable from HAV or HBV infection occurs in 20% of infected persons. The mean incubation is 7 weeks, and 90% of cases will have incubation periods of 5–12 weeks. Liver enzymes rise but usually not as high as with HAV or HBV infection. In 40–60% of cases, the elevated liver enzymes persist, often in a waxing-and-waning pattern and often for month or years. A chronic carrier state often ensues, in which infectiousness can persist for at least 6 years (39). Ten percent of blood donors have been shown to transmit NANB to their recipients (40). Chronic active hepatitis leading to cirrhosis may occur in 10–20% of chronic carriers.

As with HBV infection, there are other modes of transmission besides blood transfusion. Percutaneous and sexual transmission are well-described. Among sporadic cases of NANB hepatitis, a history of drug abuse, employment as a health care worker in contact with blood, and personal contact with a person who had had hepatitis were significantly more common than among controls, suggesting routes of transmission similar to HBV infection (41).

Population

Blood or blood products are the primary source of NANB hepatitis, so contact with these substances define the population at risk. In some populations of patients with coagulopathies (e.g., hemophilia) that require repeated transfusions and factor concentrates, virtually 100% have NANB hepatitis. Patients undergoing hemodialysis, renal transplantation, platelet support, or cardiac surgery requiring multiple transfusions, are frequently infected. Injection of illicit

drugs is also a significant risk factor. Although not as well-described as with HBV infection, maternal-fetal transmission has been documented.

There are no data to suggest that there is any age predilection for NANB hepatitis. Any differences in age distribution would be reflective of the presence of risk factors: transfusion and blood products in all ages and percutaneous drug use and sexually acquired infection in adolescents and young adults.

Diagnosis

NANB hepatitis is a diagnosis of exclusion once HAV, HBV, Epstein-Barr virus, and cytomegalovirus infections and drug or toxin exposure have been ruled out. There are no reliable tests for NANB in spite of a plethora of reported antigen-antibody systems, indirect markers, and the like published recently (42). The typical clinical picture of hepatitis with negative tests for the other agents and no drug or toxin exposure and chronic waxing and waning of liver enzymes is sufficient to make the diagnosis.

Treatment

No treatment of proven efficacy is currently available. Recombinant human alpha interferon may suppress abnormal liver enzymes temporarily, but the long-term benefit is unknown (43).

Prevention

The situation with NANB is reminiscent of that of AIDS in the early 1980s: no infectious agent identified, the epidemiology reasonably well-understood as far as risk factors are concerned, and no treatment or vaccine in sight. NANB is not uniformly fatal, but along with alcohol, may be one of the major causes of liver disease in hospitalized populations.

Since the major route of transmission is blood and blood products, several means of making these substances safer are under study. Screening blood donors for elevated alanine aminotransferase may reduce the risk of NANB by 25%, but the predictive value of that screen is only about 60%, meaning that approximately one-half of the discarded units of blood using this screening method would be thrown away needlessly (42). Screening blood donors for anti-HBc has been proposed, but there are conflicting opinions as to whether this would be better than alanine aminotransferase screening. Various treatments, such as heating factor concentrates

**Table 14.3.
Blood/Body Fluid Precautions for
Non-A Non-B Hepatitis**

1. Gloves should be worn when in contact with blood
or body fluids (excretions or secretions) or
contaminated objects.
2. Gowns, masks, and protective eyewear should be
worn when splashing or spattering of blood or
body fluids is anticipated.

to 60°C for 10 hours, appear to destroy infectivity.

Most patients with NANB are not symptomatic, may be chronic carriers capable of transmitting NANB for years, and may not be obvious
members of a high-risk group (e.g., the mother
forgets to tell the nurse or doctor her son had a
transfusion in the neonatal period 3 years ago).
Gloves, handwashing after removing the gloves,
and the common sense to use gloves and make
it a habit when the possibility of contact with
blood or body fluids exists, are the only preventive measures currently available for the health
care worker (Table 14.3).

REFERENCES

1. Siegl G: The biochemistry of hepatitis A virus. In Gerety RH
(ed): *The Hepatitis A Virus.* New York, Academic Press, 1984,
pp 81–100.
2. Weitz M, Siegl G: Comparison of HAV strains isolated in far
apart geographical regions. In Gerety RH (ed): *The Hepatitis A
Virus.* New York, Academic Press, 1984, p 704.
3. Rakela J, Mosley JW: Fecal excretion of hepatitis A virus in
humans. *J Infect Dis* 135:933–938, 1977.
4. Villarejos VM, Serra CJ, Anderson-Visona K, Mosely JW:
Hepatitis A virus infection in households. *Am J Epidemiol*
115:557–586, 1982.
5. Azimi PH, Roberto RR, Guralnik J, Livermore T, Hoag S,
Hagens S, Lugo N: Transfusion-acquired hepatitis A in a premature infant with secondary nosocomial spread in an intensive
care nursery. *Am J Dis Child* 140:23–27, 1986.
6. Krober MS, Bass JW, Brown JD, Lemon SM, Rupert KJ: Hospital outbreak of hepatitis A: risk factors for spread. *Pediatr
Infect Dis* 3:296–299, 1984.
7. Reed CM, Gustafson TL, Seigel J, Duer P: Nosocomial transmission of hepatitis A from a hospital-acquired case. *Pediatr
Infect Dis* 3:300–303, 1984.
8. Meyers JD, Romm FJ, Tihen WS, Bryan JA: Food-borne hepatitis A in a general hospital. *JAMA* 231:1049–1053, 1975.
9. Mathiesen LR, Feinstone SM, Wong DC, Skinhoej P, Purcell
RH: Enzyme-linked immunosorbant assay for detection of hepatitis A antigen in stool and antibody to hepatitis A antigen in
sera: comparison with solid-phase radioimmunoassay, immune
election microscopy, and immune adherence hemagglutination
assay. *J Clin Microbiol* 7:184–193, 1978.
10. Maynard JE: Viral hepatitis as an occupational hazard in the
health care profession. In Vyas GN, Cohen SN, Schmid R (eds):
*Viral Hepatitis: A Contemporary Assessment of Epidemiology,
Pathogenesis and Prevention.* Philadelphia, Franklin Institute
Press, 1978, p 321.
11. Landrigan PJ, Huber DH, Murphy GD, Creech WB, Bryan JA:
The protective efficacy of immune serum globulin in hepatitis
A. *JAMA* 223:74–75, 1973.
12. Garner JS, Simmons BP: CDC guideline for isolation precautions in hospitals. *Infect Control* 4:245–325, 1983.
13. Tabor E, Purcell RH, London WT, Gerety RJ: Use of and
interpretation of results using inocula of hepatitis B virus with
known infectivity titers. *J Infect Dis* 147:531–534, 1983.
14. Krugman S, Overby LR, Mushahwar IK, Ling C, Frosner GG,
Deinhardt F: Viral hepatitis, type B. *N Engl J Med* 300:101–
106, 1979.
15. McMahon BJ, Alward WLM, Hall DB, Heyward WL, Bener
TR, Francis DP, Maynard JE: Acute hepatitis B virus infection:
Relation of age to the clinical expression of disease and subsequent development of the carrier state. *J Infect Dis* 151:599–
603, 1985.
16. Alward WLM, McMahon BJ, Hall DB, Heyward WL, Francis
DP, Bender TR: The long-term serological course of asymptomatic hepatitis B virus carriers and the development of primary
hepatocellular carcinoma. *J Infect Dis* 151:604–609, 1985.
17. Lee AKY, Ip HMH, Wong VCW: Mechanisms of maternal-
fetal transmission of hepatitis B virus. *J Infect Dis* 138:668–
671, 1978.
18. Goudeau A, Yvonnet B, Lesage G, Barin F, Denis F, Coursaget
P, Chiron JP, Mar ID: Lack of anti-HBc IgM in neonates with
HBsAg carrier mothers argues against transplacental transmission of hepatitis B virus infection. *Lancet* 2:1103–1104, 1983.
19. Pattison CP, Boyer KM, Maynard JE, Kelly PC: Epidemic
hepatitis in a clinical laboratory: Possible association with computer card handling. *JAMA* 230:854–857, 1974.
20. Bond WW, Favero MS, Petersen NJ, Ebert JW: Inactivation of
hepatitis B virus by intermediate-to-high-level disinfectant
chemicals. *J Clin Microbiol* 18:535–538, 1983.
21. Kobayashi H, Tsuzuki M, Koshimizu K, Toyama H, Yoshihara
N, Shikata T, Abe K, Mizuno K, Otomo N, Oda T: Susceptibility of hepatitis B virus to disinfectants or heat. *J Clin Microbiol* 20:214–216, 1984.
22. Storch GA, Perrillo RP, Miller JP, Benz B, Kahn RA: Prevalence of hepatitis B antibodies in personnel at a children's hospital. *Pediatrics* 76:29 -35, 1985.
23. Snydman DR, Hindman SH, Wineland MD, Bryan JA, Maynard JE: Nosocomial viral hepatitis B. *Ann Intern Med* 85:573–
577, 1976.
24. Gerber MA, Lewin EB, Gerety RJ, Le CT: The lack of nurse-
infant transmission of type B hepatitis in a special care nursery.
J Pediatr 91:120–122, 1977.
25. LaBrecque DR, Muhs JM, Lutwick LI, Woolson RF, Hierholzer
WR: The risk of hepatitis B transmission from health care workers to patients in a hospital setting—a prospective study. *He-
patology* 6:205–208, 1986.
26. Grob PJ, Bischof B, Naeff F: Cluster of hepatitis B transmitted
by a physician. *Lancet* 2:1218–1220, 1981.
27. Anonymous: Recommendations of the immunization practices
advisory committee: Recommendations for protection against
viral hepatitis. *MMWR* 34:313–324, 329–335, 1985.
28. Mosley JW: The HBV carrier—A new kind of leper? *N Engl
J Med* 292:477–478, 1975.
29. Birnie GG, Quigley EM, Clements GB, Follet EAC, Watkinson
G: Endoscopic transmission of hepatitis B virus. *Gut* 24:171–
174, 1983.
30. Bond WW, Moncada RE: Viral hepatitis B infection risk in
flexible fiberoptic endoscopy. *Gastrointest Endoscopy* 24:225–
230, 1978.
31. Beasley RP, Hwang L, Lee GC, Lan L, Roan C, Huang F,
Chen C: Prevention of perinatally transmitted hepatitis B virus
infections with hepatitis B immune globulin and hepatitis B
vaccine. *Lancet* 2:1099–1102, 1983.
32. Szmuness W, Stevens CE, Harley EJ, Zang EA, Oleszko WR,
William DC, Sadovsky R, Morrison JM, Kellner A: Hepatitis
B vaccine. *N Engl J Med* 303:833–841, 1980.
33. Jilg W, Lorbeer B, Schmidt M, Wilski B, Zoulek G, Deinhardt
F: Clinical evaluation of a recombinant hepatitis B vaccine.
Lancet 2:1174–1175, 1984.

34. Nowicki MJ, Tong MJ, Bohman RE: Alterations in the immune response of nonresponders to the hepatitis B vaccine. *J Infect Dis* 152:1245–1248, 1985.

35. Hadler SC, Francis DP, Maynard JE, Thompson SE, Judson FN, Echenberg DF, Ostrow DG, O'Malley PM, Penley KA, Altman NL, Braff E, Shipman GF, Coleman PJ, Mandel EJ: Long-term immunogenicity and efficacy of hepatitis B vaccine in homosexual men. *N Engl J Med* 315:209–214, 1986.

36. Seef LB, Wright EL, Zimmerman HJ, Alter HJ, Dietz AA, Felsher BF, Finklestein JD, Garcia-Pont P, Gerin JL, Greenlee HB, Hamilton J, Holland PV, Kaplan PM, Kiernan T, Koff RS, Leevy CM, McAuliffe VJ, Nath N, Purcell RH, Schiff ER, Schwartz CC, Tamburro CH, Vlahcevic Z, Zemel R, Zimmon DS: Type B hepatitis after needlestick exposure: Prevention with hepatitis B immune globulin. *Ann Intern Med* 88:285–293, 1978.

37. Khuroo MS: Study of an epidemic of non-A, non-B hepatitis. *Am J Med* 68:818–824, 1980.

38. Dienstag JL: Non-A, non-B hepatitis. I. Recognition, epide-

miology, and clinical features. *Gastroenterology* 85:439–462, 1985.

39. Tabor E, Seef LB, Gerety RJ: Chronic non-A, non-B hepatitis carrier state. *N Engl J Med* 303:140–143, 1980.

40. Aach RD, Szmuness W, Mosley JW, Hollinger FB, Kahn RA, Stevens CE, Edwards VM, Werch J: Serum alanine aminotransferase of donors in relation to the risk of non-A, non-B hepatitis in recipients. *N Engl J Med* 304:989–994, 1981.

41. Alter MJ, Gerety RJ, Smallwood LA, Sampliner RE, Tabor E, Deinhardt F, Frosner G, Matanoski GM: Sporadic non-A, non-B hepatitis: Frequency and epidemiology in an urban U.S. population. *J Infect Dis* 145:886–893, 1982.

42. Dienstag JL: Non-A, non-B hepatitis. II. Experimental transmission, putative virus agents and markers, and prevention. *Gastroenterology* 85:743–768, 1985.

43. Hoofnagle JH, Mullen KD, Jones DB, Rustgi V, Bisceglie AD, Peters M, Waggoner JG, Park Y, Jones EA: Treatment of chronic non-A, non-B hepatitis with recombinant human alpha interferon. *N Engl J Med* 315:1575–1578, 1986.

15

Respiratory Syncytial Virus

M. Dianne Murphy, M.D.

BACKGROUND

Introduction

Despite its enormous impact on the health of children and infants as the most frequent cause of lower respiratory disease in young infants, respiratory syncytial virus has acquired little of the household familiarity that has been accorded the influenza virus. Respiratory syncytial virus (RSV) is not only unknown to much of the lay public but, because of the adult orientation of medicine, many physicians are unfamiliar with this etiologic agent which annually causes epidemics of respiratory illness in thousands of children. The increased understanding of the spectrum of disease caused by this virus and the growth of a susceptible population at high risk for severe consequences when exposed to this virus make RSV of great significance. Even more important, RSV has become one of the few viral diseases for which there is now an effective and approved antiviral agent.

RSV is an RNA virus that was shown, in 1956, to cause coryza in chimpanzees (1) and was therefore originally called the chimpanzee coryza agent. A year later, this virus was isolated from humans with bronchopneumonia and laryngotracheobronchitis (2). In keeping with both its clinical presentation in humans and its ability to form syncytia in tissue culture, it was renamed respiratory syncytial virus. In 1961, Kapikian clearly demonstrated that RSV was a major cause of respiratory tract infections in the early years of life (3), and in 1962, Chanock described RSV as the most important single cause of severe respiratory disease in early life (4). Both the severity of this disease (5–7) and its ubiquitous nature make it an extremely important pathogen in the young infant.

Pathogenesis

Depending on the site of maximal involvement, the clinical presentation of RSV extends from the asymptomatic or mildly ill individual with rhinorrhea to the gasping cyanotic infant with pneumonia or the wheezing, dyspneic child with bronchiolitis. The common mediators of the clinical presentation are the chemical substances causing edema, mucus production, and airway obstruction. The most common site of involvement is the small bronchiolar airway, which, because of the tiny lumen in infants, is easily obstructed. Minimal edema and production of inflammatory products within the lumen may have marked effects on airflow. The discussion concerning the role of smooth muscle in the young infant's airway will be only tangentially addressed. If there is a response to a bronchodilator drug, then certainly the use of these therapeutic agents, which affect smooth muscle and enlarge the airway, is indicated. The main pathology, however, should be recognized as one of inflammation and edema. As defined by W. Aherne, "In acute bronchiolitis the main lesion is epithelial necrosis when a dense plug is formed in the bronchiolar lumen leading to trapping air and other mechanical interference with ventilation. The interstitial pneumonia there is widespread inflammation and necrosis of lung parenchyma and severe lesions of the bronchial and bronchiolar mucosa as well" (8). Because of this mechanical obstruction, the main thrust of therapy is aimed at enhancing oxygenation and ventilation by removal of mucus and decreasing edema by stopping or inhibiting viral replication.

Epidemiology

It is now well-appreciated that RSV not only causes winter epidemics of bronchiolitis and

207

pneumonia, but also presents as apnea and sudden death (7,9). As many of these infants are afflicted at home, and some die before reaching medical care, it would be best to first review the intrafamilial spread of RSV. In a study of 36 families and a total of 178 family members, greater than 40% of the members become infected with RSV (10). The highest infectivity occurred in the young infants (Table 15.1). Secondary attack rates within a family were 27% overall, but 45% for infants. Severity of disease was higher in the younger age group. This phenomena, and the fact that 80% of RSV disease occurs in children less than 6 months of age, appears to be related to maternal antibody. Glezen et al. found that neutralizing antibody titers to RSV in the cord sera of 68 infants with culture-proven RSV were significantly lower than those of 575 randomly selected cord serum samples from infants born at the same time (11).

The peak age of attack is under 6 months of age, and greater than half of the children living through their first RSV epidemic will have been infected with the virus. By 2 years of age, 50% of all children will have neutralizing antibody, and 75% by 3 years of age. Although the first infection is nearly always a symptomatic one, the older child will experience less respiratory impairment and will probably be more responsive to bronchodilators. The risk of severe disease appears to be additionally increased in urban and lower socioeconomic groups (12,13).

The unfailing predictability of RSV epidemics is one of the puzzles surrounding this organism. There is no antigenic change to account for milder epidemics. Despite this lack of variation, there is usually little difference in the number of children affected each year. Seasonality is another interesting facet of RSV epidemics (13). In Washington, D.C., over an interval of 13 years, RSV was most active during the period from January–April and virtually absent from the community during August and September (14). It has been suggested that pharyngeal carriage is an important mechanism for maintenance and dissemination of the virus in the population (14).

POPULATION

The symptomatic expression of this disease occurs most frequently in young infants. Adults, however, do acquire and transmit this virus. Approximately 17% of exposed adults will develop symptoms, although these symptoms will almost always be limited to upper airway congestion or bronchitis (Table 15.1) (15). Nasal congestion and cough are more common presentations in older individuals, while bronchiolitis and pneumonia are more common in infants (16). Fever also occurs more commonly in children less than 2 years of age. Adult nursing personnel have been shown to acquire and spread RSV with minimal symptomatology (17,18). RSV infection is not always a benign process in the adult. Clinical studies have demonstrated high absenteeism and prolonged abnormalities in pulmonary function determinations (15).

It is becoming increasingly evident that certain types of patients will suffer disproportionately higher morbidity and mortality from RSV infection. One of the highest mortalities occurs

Table 15.1.
Attack Rate of Respiratory Syncytial Virus in Families According to Age[a]

Age	Crude Rate		Attack Rate[b] Rate in RSV-Positive Families		Secondary Rate[d]	
(yr)	N[c]	%	N[c]	%	N[c]	%
<1	10/34	29.4	10/16	62.5	5/11	45.4
1–<2	2/7	28.6	2/5	40.0	0/3	0.0
2–<5	9/34	26.4	9/19	47.0	2/12	16.6
5–<17	9/48	18.7	9/24	38.0	4/19	21.0
17–45	9/55	16.8	9/21	43.0	6/18	33.3
Total	39/178	21.9	39/85	45.9	17/63	27.0

[a]Reproduced with permission from Hall et al: Respiratory syncytial virus infections within families. *N Engl J Med* 1976; 294(8):414–419.
[b]Crude attack rate according to age is shown for all family members studied and for members of RSV-positive families. The secondary attack rate is also shown for members of RSV-positive families, excluding all primary and co-primary cases.
[c]Number of persons infected with RSV.
[d]Total number of persons exposed.

in infants with congenital heart disease whose death rate from nosocomial RSV infection is 44% in contrast to 5% mortality for other hospitalized infants who become infected. The RSV-related mortality is increased to 73% in the infant with associated pulmonary hypertension (19). Patients with cystic fibrosis (20) and children with compromised immune function (21,22) experience more frequent RSV infections with hospitalizations, higher mortality, and more severe disease.

In neonates, illness with RSV may be overlooked because of its atypical presentation where its only manifestation may be apnea or sudden death (6), and occasionally may present as a "sepsis-like" syndrome (23). Infants with prior pulmonary compromise or hospitalized intubated infants also experience a higher mortality from RSV infection (24).

Besides causing severe acute respiratory symptoms in children, RSV may produce abnormalities of the respiratory tract which appear to be associated with long-term (years) pulmonary dysfunction (22,25). Besides causing more severe wheezing in children who may already have a propensity to reactive airway disease, RSV will also produce pulmonary abnormalities that may predispose to wheezing in children without reactive airway disease (26).

DIAGNOSIS

Clinical

Dr. Holt's (27) description of a child with "bronchitis of the smaller tubes" remains without improvement:

The severe form . . . . differs from the preceding variety mainly in the greater severity of all its symptoms. The onset may be like that just described, the severe symptoms not appearing until the patient has been sick two or three days, or they may be severe from the outset. If the latter, it is indistinguishable from that of broncho-pneumonia. There are cough, dyspnoea, accelerated breathing, fever, and moderate, sometimes severe, prostration. The cough is tighter, and more frequently of a short, teasing character than severe and paroxysmal. There is difficulty in nursing. Dyspnoea may be quite marked and is shown by the active dilation of the alae nasi and the recession of all the soft parts of the chest on inspiration. The respirations as a rule are from 50–80 a minute. The temperature for the first day or two is usually 101°

or 102°, but it may be 103° or 104° F. So high a temperature does not continue unless pneumonia develops. The prostration is in most cases more closely related to the dyspnoea and the rapidity of respiration than to the temperature. Often there is slight cyanosis.

In the beginning, the chest is filled with sibilant and sonorous rales, many of them of a musical character. In 12 or 24 hours these are replaced by moist rales—coarse or fine, according as they are produced in the large or medium-sized tubes. There are often loud, wheezing rales on expiration. The respiratory murmur is feeble; the resonance on percussion is normal or slightly exaggerated. As the case progressed toward recovery, the finer rales are the first to disappear. The rales are always best heard behind, but they are present all over the chest.

Wheezing is the most prominent clinical finding. In a 13-year surveillance of respiratory infections at the Children's Hospital in Washington, D.C., greater than 40% of children admitted to the hospital with the diagnosis of bronchiolitis were culture positive for RSV, and 25% of those with pneumonia had RSV isolated from their respiratory secretions (13).

By combining the data obtained from the clinical presentation (wheezing, cough, pneumonia) with the season (winter) and the age of the infant (the majority of patients are under 12 months of age), we can accurately say that a clinical diagnosis of RSV lower respiratory disease can often be made before the rapid viral diagnostic test results are available.

Major considerations in the differential diagnosis are asthma (unlikely in this age group), other viral agents such as influenza or adenovirus (not as common), and bacterial infections, although these usually have a more abrupt onset and lobar infiltration on chest radiographs. Definitive etiologic diagnosis is extremely useful in the rapid treatment and isolation of these patients.

All patients with suspected RSV bronchiolitis should receive a trial administration of a bronchodilator to evaluate responsiveness. If a child responds to bronchodilator therapy, it does not mean that he has "asthma," but that he has a component of reactive airway as part of the disease process. Only the development of recurrent episodes of wheezing in the future will define if the child has "asthma" without a viral precipitating cause. The child with asthma frequently requires long-term therapeutic interventions, while the child with RSV bronchiolitis usually recovers without requiring long-term administration of bronchodilators. The child with influenza may benefit from other antiviral agents, and the child with a bacterial pneumonia infection will need antibacterial drugs.

It has been known for years that it is important to identify patients who have RSV infections for isolation and infection control purposes. It is now even more imperative to make a specific etiologic diagnosis so that ribavirin may be used early in the course of disease for those patients who are at high risk of suffering severe morbidity and even death from an RSV infection.

Radiologic and laboratory tests are useful in confirming a viral diagnosis that is not complicated by a secondary bacterial infection. The chest radiograph of a child presenting with classical RSV bronchiolitis or pneumonia will demonstrate flattened diaphragms with hyperaeration, peribronchial thickening, or diffuse "patchy" infiltrates, although it must be emphasized that the radiograph in bronchiolitis in infants may be nonspecific (28). An isolated lobar process is either a secondary bacterial complication or evidence of atelectasis and mucus plugging. As with most viral illnesses, the hematologic picture of an uncomplicated case of RSV will usually demonstrate a lymphocytosis.

Laboratory

The key to RSV diagnosis is rapidity. Serologic diagnosis no longer has a place in the routine diagnostic approach to the patient with suspected RSV infection. The three most commonly used techniques for viral identification are fluorescent antibody stains of infected nasal epithelial cells, enzyme-linked immunosorbent assays (ELISA) on nasal/pharyngeal secretions, and viral culture of the respiratory secretions. Infants will usually shed virus for approximately 7 days with a range of 1-21 days (29). It has been demonstrated that a nasal washing, as compared with a pharyngeal or nasal swab, will increase the yield of collected virus and the percentage of positive results (30). Swabbing a patient's throat is easier but much more likely to give a poor sample, and often does not provide adequate cells for rapid testing with fluorescent antibody stain.

Collection of the proper specimen cannot be overemphasized. A nasal wash in infants or a nasal "snort" from adults will yield more virus and cells. Transporting the specimen on ice (*not* freezing) and inoculating cells within 2 hours of collection will also increase the yield of positive results. Sending a viral culture for RSV via an overnight mail service is wasting your patient's mucus and money. Specimens should be placed onto cells within 2 hours of collection (31).

A nasal wash is easily performed using material available on any pediatric hospital service (Fig. 15.1). Either a mucus trap or a syringe attached to a "butterfly" with the needle and tubing cut off about 2 inches from the hub can be used. One-5 ml, of saline is delivered with a syringe into a nares and then immediately aspirated. Only mucoid material should be kept for processing. If clear water is aspirated, repeat the wash. The specimen can be sent in the syringe on ice, or some can be ejected into viral "holding" media and the rest into a sterile urine cup and sent immediately on ice to the laboratory. Specimens should be ordered for collection, before pulmonary toilet, in an effort to maximize mucus yield and to avoid excess time from collection to placement on the proper cell line.

A nasal snort requires that the individual obstruct one nostril, sniff saline into the other nostril, and then blow his nose into a beaker or sterile urine cup. Adults prefer performing this in private, but the adequacy of the specimen should be evaluated before accepting it for transport to the virology laboratory.

Fluorescent staining of cells obtained in the aforementioned manner will correlate 95-100% with culture results (32). The attractiveness of this test is the availability of the results within 1-2 hours from the time of collection. The next most rapid approach uses ELISA technology. It has been demonstrated that this technique is 83-97% sensitive (33,34). Because this is an antigen detection test, the ELISA is useful for specimens that may have been mishandled (frozen, delayed in transport, etc.). It does, however, take more time (2-8 hours), requires additional technical support, and does not provide information about other viruses that may be present. However, for laboratories without individuals with fluorescent microscopy expertise, this may be the "rapid" test of choice.

In addition to the rapid tests, it is still important to simultaneously perform a viral cul-

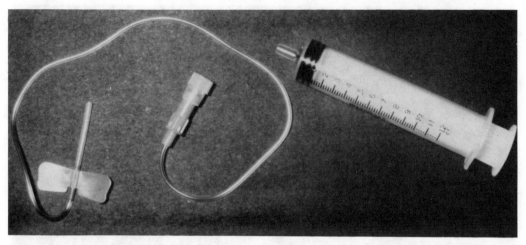

Figure 15.1. Materials needed to perform a nasal wash: mucous trap (syringe attached to a "butterfly" with the needle and tubing cut off about 2 inches from the hub).

ture. RSV may not be the pathogen and other antiviral drugs may be useful, i.e., acyclovir for herpes or amantadine for influenza. Additionally, some process should be in place to intermittently, routinely verify the rapid test results. By use of centrifugation techniques, our virology laboratory has been able to reduce the time for a positive culture to less than 72 hours (35).

In summary, by utilizing collection of optimal specimen samples early in the course of disease, an accurate specific diagnosis for RSV is possible within 1–72 hours. This is important for both infection control and therapeutic endeavors (36).

TREATMENT

In 1985, ribavirin (1-B-D-ribofuranosyl-1,2,4-triazole-3-carboxamide) was released for use in the treatment of RSV. Until this time, the only therapeutic interventions available for treatment of RSV infections were supportive in nature and not a direct assault on the causative viral agent. Ribavirin is a quanosine analogue that is thought to function as an antiviral agent by inhibiting viral RNA polymerase (37). This agent is known to have antiviral properties against many RNA and DNA viruses, including influenza A and B (38–40). Many of the original studies of this agent were performed in adults with influenza using an oral formulation of ribavirin. In these early studies, the therapeutic effects of the drug

were not particularly impressive, and it was not until the drug was utilized as an aerosol that a significant beneficial effect was demonstrated (41). By aerosolizing ribavirin, the drug is delivered directly onto the infected surface instead of depending on diffusion or transport from the vascular system into the outer mucosal cellular layers of the airway. The aerosol provides a much higher concentration of the drug in the immediate infective milieu while decreasing potential systemic adverse effects. The systemic adverse effects of aerosolized ribavirin are limited to bone marrow suppression, which is usually a reversible anemia. One adverse effect that may occur with the aerosol mode of delivery is bronchospasm. In a few infants, the small particles reaching the lower airway have acted as an irritant and have actually caused deterioration of pulmonary functions. This is not the usual effect, but it must be considered when delivering ribavirin as an aerosol.

The water particles upon which the drug is nebulized must be 3 µm or smaller, or they will precipitate in the larger airway. This can be accomplished only with a special nebulization apparatus called a "small-particle aerosol generator" or SPAG (Fig. 15.2). At present, this unit is provided with the drug by the drug manufacturer. As the most severely infected infants are under 1 year of age, the aerosol is usually delivered into a croup tent, oxygen hood, or, rarely, a mask. The aerosolization of this drug

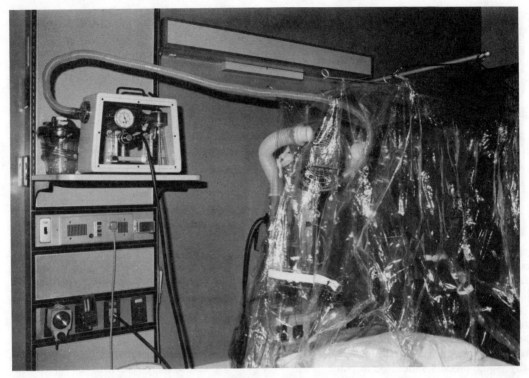

Figure 15.2. Small-particle aerosol generator (SPAG)—an effective nebulization apparatus.

is most successful when delivered into a tent because the mask is usually not tolerated by an infant or small child for the required 18-24 hours per day. The drug tends to precipitate in the small airspace inside the oxygen hood. Ribavirin can be used with a ventilator, but there are major delivery problems due to particle precipitation in the lines and filters. The patient's tidal volume also affects the amount of drug delivered from a solution that is approximately 20 mg/ml of ribavirin.

The goal of ribavirin therapy should be to prevent the need for mechanical ventilation in the high-risk patient. These patients, as defined earlier in this chapter, should have aerosolized ribavirin instituted early in the course of hospitalization. It is the high-risk infant who is in greatest danger and has the highest morbidity and mortality from RSV infections. Efforts at early diagnosis and use of ribavirin aerosol are necessary if mortality is to be decreased and ventilatory support is to be avoided. Premature infants who have had severe pulmonary disease

often have adverse residual damage to their cilia, mucosa, and small airways. These affected areas will have great difficulty in containing and clearing the viral infection. The child whose cardiac disease involves high pulmonary artery flow and/or pulmonary hypertension will have increased difficulties in responding to the increased metabolic and pulmonary flow requirements associated with fever and viral illness, and will frequently suffer from a more severe degree of hypoxemia.

The normal infant would be one who had been born at term (38-40 weeks gestational age) and has no pulmonary or cardiac abnormalities that would affect the child's ability to effectively respond to the viral infection. The normal infant without risk factors, who is in minimal respiratory distress, can be observed and initially treated only with supportive measures. Therapy with ribavirin should be instituted if the child's pulmonary status deteriorates, as manifested by increasing respiratory effort, and/or increasing hypoxemia, and hypercarbia. It should be kept in mind that the earlier antiviral therapy is instituted, the greater the beneficial effect.

Despite the excitement surrounding the use of a new therapeutic agent, it is essential to remember that this agent will only slow viral replication. The initial injury from the RSV infection and the resultant complications of that injury must be addressed and pursued aggressively if simple mechanical obstruction of the airways is to be prevented. Supportive therapy includes administration of oxygen, bronchodilators, hydration, and nutrition with vigorous pulmonary toilet, and close monitoring for apnea.

Because almost all children with RSV have some element of hypoxia, oxygen should be administered to all hospitalized patients. Arterial blood gas determinations will be necessary to follow the changes in a severely affected infant, but the infant who is not cyanotic will benefit from low levels (30-40%) of inspired oxygen and use of capillary blood gases to follow venous pH and PCO_2 (42).

Because these infants are febrile, tachypneic, and expending extra energy in efforts to breathe, they will require additional fluids. Using a 12% increase in caloric requirements for each degree centigrade above 37.8 °C and 10–30% increase in caloric requirements for increased activity, fluid requirements will be increased by 125 ml for every extra 100 calories expended (43). Once well-hydrated, fluid therapy should be carefully monitored, as the inflammation and edema that are associated with the infectious process may enhance fluid collection in the lung and may actually intensify the arterial venous block. The child who is in congestive heart failure or whose pulmonary status deteriorates with extra vascular volume will necessitate modification of fluid therapy.

Because the pathology involved in an RSV infection causes an increase in mucus plugging of small airways, efforts aimed at removal of this mucus is desired. Coughing should not be suppressed. Gentle vibratory percussion and suctioning of secretions should be instituted.

Infants with moderate to severe respiratory distress will frequently be unable to take adequate fluids or calories by mouth and will require intravenous fluid therapy. Prolonged efforts in starting intravenous lines and/or collecting blood specimens may push the tiring, barely compensated infant into worsening respiratory distress or respiratory failure. Therefore, common sense, as always, should be employed in deciding the technical instrumentation required. If vascular access is particularly difficult, it may be prudent to first apply oxygen, pulmonary toilet, and careful monitoring of capillary gases or pulse oximetry.

The use of bronchodilators remains controversial, and much has been written concerning the differences between reactive airway disease and bronchiolitis. Not withstanding etiologic and pathologic differences, a trial of aerosolized bronchodilators is warranted. This inflammatory process may cause or exacerbate irritation of airway smooth muscle when it is present, particularly in the older infant. If bronchodilator drugs appear to be clinically beneficial and/or improve gaseous exchange, they should be continued. The potential for such adverse effects as tachycardia and irritability indicate a need to discontinue use of these agents if no improvement is noted (44).

Steroids have not been demonstrated to make any difference in outcome except when combined with albuterol (45).

PREVENTION

Prevention of nosocomial RSV disease is based on knowing the modes of transmission of the virus, identifying the population at high risk for serious complications, and being able to reliably and rapidly identify the etiologic agent. This latter point is particularly important if proper use of ribavirin is to be instituted and isolation procedures are to be effected, and so that laxity of handwashing habits does not occur. As nicely delineated by Drew (46), viral diagnosis of RSV is rapid, useful, and economically warranted. To effectively prevent nosocomial RSV infection, the medical and infection control staff must be familiar with and utilize rapid diagnostic procedures and then judiciously and vigorously apply infection control policies to the at-risk population. These efforts should emphasize handwashing, identification, early isolation, and, where appropriate, early treatment.

Education of nurses, resident physicians, ancillary personnel, and medical staff is an important part of this process. Even though peak RSV season does not usually occur until January or later, it is useful to begin your information and inservice programs in October or November. This is the time of year public health officials institute efforts to vaccinate individuals for the upcoming influenza season.

By using an education program based on diagnosis and control of RSV infections coordinated through infection control, the virology laboratory, pediatric nursing and medical staffs, the pediatric unit of the University of Tennessee Medical Center at Knoxville, weathered the 1986 RSV epidemic with only one documented nosocomial RSV infection (Table 15.2). From December 1985 to March 1986, 41 of 127 submitted respiratory specimens were proven to be RSV, but only one was found, using Centers for Disease Control criteria, to have been nosocomially acquired. This type of program requires a commitment from your head nurse, virology supervisor, infection control nurse, infectious disease physicians, and medical staff (Murphy et al., presented at the American Academy of Pediatrics Meeting, Washington, D.C., October 1986). The emphasis of the program is to identify all respiratory illnesses that are clinically consistent with RSV, implement immediate handwashing-isolation procedures on admission, obtain adequate and proper specimens for rapid viral diagnosis, such as FA and ELISA (47,48), and administer ribavirin to all high-risk infants or infants in severe respiratory distress. This approach should prevent unnecessary isolation of other illnesses, decrease unwarranted use of antibiotics, decrease viral shedding by infected infants, and enhance recovery from the disease process. The latter two effects of the program will facilitate earlier discharge of the

infected patient from the hospital, thus decreasing the "viral load" available for spread to other patients.

The type of isolation necessary for the infant infected with RSV is based on information that has evolved from the 1970s (Table 15.3). Many of the physicians caring for infants in the 1970s commented on the severity of RSV nosocomial infections (5,17,49) as well as on the lack of effectiveness of the usual isolation procedures and the role of adult carriage (17,49–51). A classic study by Hall et al. in 1981 clearly defined the contribution of large particles (or droplets), fomites and small-particle aerosols to acquisition of RSV infections (52). Their study

Table 15.3
Contact Isolation Policies for Respiratory Syncytial Virus Disease

1. Rapid identification of RSV in suspected patients.
2. Contact isolation—may be instituted by nursing personnel.
3. Strict handwashing—additional signs on door or bed.
4. Gown use for contact care.
5. If available, eye-nose goggles for personnel providing direct patient care, such as suctioning and pulmonary toilet.
6. Cohort nursing if possible; emphasis on preventing simultaneous care of uninfected high-risk patient and RSV-infected patient.
7. Cohort-documented RSV infected cases if necessary for space and nursing.
8. Avoid elective admissions of high-risk patients (pulmonary, cardiac, immunocompromised patients) during peak RSV seasons.
9. Therapy of high-risk patients with proven infection with aerosolized ribavirin.

Table 15.2.
Laboratory Verification of Respiratory Syncytial Virus

Month	Inpatient No. RSV Specimens	No. Positive[a] for RSV	RSV Nosocomial Cases	Admissions, General Pediatrics, and PICU
Oct. 1985	1	0	0	159
Nov. 1985	3	1	0	152
Dec. 1985	23	7	0	115
Jan. 1986	47	16	1	165
Feb. 1986	41	14	0	139
Mar. 1986	16	4	0	121
Apr. 1986	7	1	0	154
May 1986	4	0	0	142
Total	142	43	1	1147

[a]Culture and/or FA positive.

suggested that spread of RSV in a hospital occurs by close contact with large droplets of infected material (coughing into the face, secretions contaminating hands) or by self-inoculation after touching contaminated surfaces. An average of over two surfaces, from the four to eight which were cultured in each of the study infants' rooms, were positive for RSV. Further evidence for the role of medical care personnel and for fomites in the spread of RSV to both personnel and patients was presented recently when Hall et al. demonstrated a significant decrease in acquisition of disease by both personnel and patients when personnel used eye-nose goggles when caring for patients (53). Previous studies (18,54,55) that demonstrate no impact on ac-

quisition of disease by either personnel or patients with the use of gown and mask or gown alone have indicated that self-inoculation of the eye and/or nose may be an important mode of RSV transmission with the hospital. It would appear that personnel contaminate their hands, fail to wash them, and then touch their eyes and nose. Personnel then become infected, secrete virus, contaminate surfaces, and probably transmit disease to infants in close-care situations. A subsequent study by LeClair et al. concluded that glove and gown precautions can significantly reduce nosocomial transmission of RSV (56).

Because good handwashing habits are difficult to maintain (57), a special effort needs to

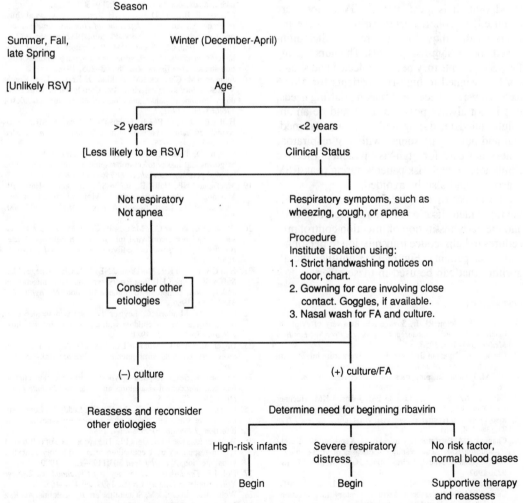

Figure 15.3.   Algorithm for approach to diagnosis and treatment of infant with possible RSV.

be made to identify the RSV-infected patients so that extra reminders can be attached to their doors and charts. These reminders are in addition to the usual contact isolation card with instructions, which is placed on the door of the room of RSV-infected patients. Some programs have used large "Teddy Bear cards" that state "Handwashing Makes a Difference", and others have instructed parents of hospitalized high-risk infants to become advocates for their children and request personnel to wash their hands before touching their infant.

The use of a single room is helpful (49), although this approach by itself has not been shown to significantly decrease nosocomial RSV infection rates. Cohorting of multiple documented cases of RSV has been helpful from a nursing standpoint. It is ideal, if the RSV patients are cohorted, to cohort nurses caring for these patients so that they do not care for other uninfected and/or high-risk patients. The nurse caring for RSV patients may become infected and should not be assigned to high-risk patients for 4 or 5 days. However, because of nursing staffing needs, this is not always possible. It should be an absolute mandate, during RSV season, that medical and nursing personnel with any respiratory illness not care for high-risk patients. Elective admissions of high-risk patients during peak RSV season should also be avoided.

The objective of infection control efforts is the rapid identification of infants excreting RSV and the early institution of infection control procedures to help reduce transmission to personnel and other patients. Figure 15.3 outlines the algorithm that can be used in these efforts.

REFERENCES

1. Morris JA, Blount RE Jr, Savage RE: Recovery of cytopathogenic agent from chimpanzees with coryza. *Proc Soc Exp Biol Med* 92:544–549, 1956.
2. Chanock R, Roizman B, Myers R: Recovery from infants with respiratory illness of a virus related to chimpanzee coryza agent (CCA). I. Isolation, properties and characterization. *Am J Hyg* 66:281–290, 1957.
3. Kapikian AZ, Bell JA, Mastrota FM, Johnson KM, Huebner RJ, Chanock RM: An outbreak of febrile illness and pneumonia associated with respiratory syncytial virus infection. *Am J Hyg* 74:234–248, 1961.
4. Chanock RM, Parrott RH, Vargosko AJ, Kapikian AZ, Knight V, Johnson KM: Acute respiratory diseases of viral etiology. IV. Respiratory syncytial virus. *Am J Public Health* 52:918–925, 1962.
5. Gardner PS, Turk DC, Aherne WA, Bird T, Holdaway MD, Court SDM: Deaths associated with respiratory tract infections in childhood. *Br Med J* 4:316–320, 1967.
6. Hall CB, Kopelman AE, Douglas RG Jr, Geiman JM, Meagher MP: Neonatal respiratory syncytial virus infection. *N Engl J Med* 300:393–396, 1979.

7. Downham MAPS, Gardner PS, McQuillin J, Ferris JAJ: Role of respiratory viruses in childhood mortality. *Br Med J* 1:235–239, 1975.
8. Aherne W, Bird T, Court SDM, Gardner PS, McQuillin J: Pathological changes in virus infections of the lower respiratory tract in children. *J Clin Pathol* 23:7–18, 1970.
9. Adams JM: Primary virus pneumonitis with cytoplasmic inclusion bodies: a study of an epidemic involving 32 infants, with 9 deaths. *JAMA* 116:925–933, 1941.
10. Hall CB, Geiman JM, Biggar R, Kotok DI, Hogan PM, Douglas RG Jr: Respiratory syncytial virus infections within families. *N Engl J Med* 294:414–419, 1976.
11. Glezen WP, Paredes A, Allison JE, Taber LH, Frank AL: Risk of respiratory syncytial virus infection of infants from low-income families in relationship to age, sex, ethnic group, and maternal antibody level. *J Pediatr* 98:708–715, 1981.
12. Parrott RH, Kim HW, Brandt CD, Chanock RM: Respiratory syncytial virus in infants and children. *Prev Med* 3:473–480, 1974.
13. Parrott RH, Kim HW, Arrobio JO, Hodes DS, Murphy BR, Brandt CD, Camargo E, Chanock RM: Epidemiology of respiratory syncytial virus infection in Washington, D.C. II. Infection and disease with respect to age, immunologic status, race and sex. *Am J Epidemiol* 98:289–300, 1973.
14. Chanock R, Brandt CD, Parrott RH: Respiratory syncytial virus. In Evans AS (ed): *Viral Infections of Humans*: *Epidemiology and Control*, ed 2. New York, Plenum, 1982, pp 365–382.
15. Hall WJ, Hall CB, Speers DM: Respiratory syncytial virus infection in adults: clinical, virologic and serial pulmonary function studies. *Ann Intern Med* 88:203–205, 1978.
16. Johnson KM, Chanock RM, Rifkind D, Kravetz HM, Knight V: Respiratory syncytial virus. IV. Correlation of virus shedding, serologic response, and illness in adult volunteers. *JAMA* 176:663–667, 1961.
17. Hall CB, Douglas RG Jr, Geiman JM, Messner MK: Nosocomial respiratory syncytial virus infections. *N Engl J Med* 293:1343–1346, 1975.
18. Murphy D, Todd JK, Chao RK, Orr I, McIntosh K: The use of gowns and masks to control respiratory illness in pediatric hospital personnel. *J Pediatr* 99:746–750, 1981.
19. MacDonald NE, Hall CB, Suffin SC, Alexson C, Harris PJ, Manning JA: Respiratory syncytial virus infection in infants with congenital heart disease. *N Engl J Med* 307:397–400, 1982.
20. Wang EEL, Prober CG, Manson B, Corey M, Levison H: Association of respiratory viral infections with pulmonary deterioration in patients with cystic fibrosis. *N Engl J Med* 311:1653–1658, 1984.
21. Hall CB, Powell KR, MacDonald NE, Gala CL, Menegus ME, Suffin SC, Cohen HJ: Respiratory syncytial virus infection in children with compromised immune function. *N Engl J Med* 315:77–81, 1986.
22. Gurwitz D, Mindorff C, Levison H: Increased incidence of bronchial reactivity in children with a history of bronchiolitis. *J Pediatr* 98:551–555, 1981.
23. Unger A, Tapia L, Minnich LL, Ray CG: Atypical neonatal respiratory syncytial virus infection. *J Pediatr* 100:762–764, 1982.
24. Krasinski K: Severe respiratory syncytial virus infection: clinical features, nosocomial acquisition and outcome. *Pediatr Infect Dis* 4:250–257, 1985.
25. Hall CB, Hall WG, Gala CL, MaGill FB, Leddy JP: Long-term prospective study in children after respiratory syncytial virus infection. *J Pediatr* 105:358–364, 1984.
26. Welliver RC, Kaul TN, Ogra PL: The appearance of cell-bound IgE in respiratory-tract epithelium after respiratory syncytial virus infection. *N Engl J Med* 303:1198–1202, 1980.
27. Holt LE: *The Diseases of Infancy and Childhood*, ed 2. New York, Appleton-Century-Crofts, 1899, pp 464–465.
28. Wohl MEB, Chernick V: State of the art: bronchiolitis. *Am Rev Respir Dis* 118:759–781, 1978.
29. Hall CB, Douglas RG Jr, Geiman JM: Respiratory syncytial virus infections in infants: quantitation and duration of shedding. *J Pediatr* 89:11–15, 1976.

30. Treuhaft MW, Soukup JM, Sullivan BJ: Practical recommendations for the detection of pediatric respiratory syncytial virus infections. *J Clin Microbiol* 22:270–273, 1985.

31. Bromberg K, Daidone B, Clarke L, Sierra MF: Comparison of immediate and delayed inoculation of HEp-2 cells for isolation of respiratory syncytial virus. *J Clin Microbiol* 20:123–124, 1984.

32. Waner JL: Isolation and identification of viruses from respiratory specimens. *Pan American Group for Rapid Diagnosis* 12(1), February 1986.

33. Swensen PA, Kaplan MH: Rapid detection of respiratory syncytial virus in nasal pharyngeal aspirates by a commerical enzyme immunoassay. *J Clin Microbiol* 23:485–488, 1986.

34. Hornsleth A, Frilis B, Krasilnikof PA: Detection of respiratory syncytial virus in nasopharyngeal secretions by a biotin-avidin ELISA more sensitive than the fluorescent antibody technique. *J Med Virol* 18:113–117, 1986.

35. Stout C, Roberts R, Murphy M, Kattine A: Comparison of shell vial centrifugation, standard culture and fluorescent antibody (FA) techniques for diagnosis of respiratory syncytial virus (RSV). Presented at the Second Annual Clinical Virology Symposium, April 1986, University of South Florida, Clearwater, Florida.

36. Eriksson M, Forsgren M, Sjoberg O, Van Sydow M, Wolontis S: Respiratory syncytial virus infection in young hospitalized children. Identification of risk patients and prevention of nosocomial spread of rapid disgnosis. *Acta Paediatr Scand* 72:47–51, 1983.

37. Oberg B, Johannsson NG: The relative merits and drawbacks of new nucleoside analogues with clinical potential. *J Antimicrob Chemother* 14 (Suppl A):5–26, 1984.

38. Knight V, McClung HW, Wilson SZ, Waters BK, Quarles JM, Cameron RW, Greggs SE, Zerwas JM, Couch RB: Ribavirin small-particle aerosol treatment of influenza. *Lancet* 2:945–949, 1981.

39. Taber LH, Knight V, Gilbert BE, McClung WH, Wilson SZ, Norton HJ, Thurson JM, Gordon WH, Atmar RL, Schlaudt WR: Ribavirin aerosol treatment of bronchiolitis associated with respiratory syncytial virus infection in infants. *Pediatrics* 72:613–618, 1983.

40. Hall CB, McBride JT, Gala CL, Hildreth SW, Schnabel KC: Ribavirin treatment of respiratory syncytial viral infection in infants with underlying cardiopulmonary disease. *JAMA* 254:3047–3051, 1985.

41. Hall CB, McBride JT, Walsh EE, Bell DM, Gala CL, Hildreth S, Ten Eyck LG, Hall WJ: Aerosolized ribavirin treatment of infants with respiratory syncytial viral infection: a randomized double-blind study. *N Engl J Med* 308:1443–1447, 1983.

42. Mellins RB: Bronchiolitis: comments on pathogenesis and treatment. *Pediatr Res* 11:268–269, 1977.

43. Biller JA, Yeager AM: *The Harriet Lane Handbook*, ed 9. Chicago, Year Book, 1981, pp 201–204.

44. Ellis EF: Therapy of acute bronchiolitis. *Pediatr Res* 11:263–264, 1977.

45. Nahata MC, Johnson JA, Powell DA: Management of bronchiolitis. *Clin Pharmacol* 4:297–303, 1985.

46. Drew WL: Controversies in viral diagnosis. *Rev Infect Dis* 8:814–827, 1986.

47. Gardner PS, Court SDM, Brocklebank JT, Downham MAPS, Weightman D: Virus cross-infection in paediatric wards. *Br Med J* 2:571–574, 1973.

48. Mintz L, Ballard RA, Sniderman SH, Roth RS, Drew WL: Nosocomial rspiratory syncytial virus infections in an intensive care nursery: rapid diagnosis by direct immunofluorescence. *Pediatrics* 64:149–153, 1979.

49. Ditchburn RK, McQuillin J, Gardner PS, Court SDM: Respiratory syncytial virus in hospital cross-infection. *Br Med J* 3:671–673, 1971.

50. Sims DG, Downham MAPS, Webb JKG, Gardner PS, Weightman D: Hospital cross-infection on children's wards with respiratory syncytial virus and the role of adult carriage. *Acta Paediatr Scand* 64:541–545, 1975.

51. Sterner G: Respiratory syncytial virus in hospital cross-infection. *Br Med J* 1:51–52, 1972.

52. Hall CB, Douglas RG Jr: Modes of transmission of respiratory syncytial virus. *J Pediatr* 99:100–103, 1981.

53. Gala CL, Hall CB, Schnabel KC, Pincus PH, Blossom P, Hildreth SW, Betts RF, Douglas RG Jr: The use of eye-nose goggles, to control nosocomial respiratory syncytial virus infection. *JAMA* 256:2706–2708, 1986.

54. Donowitz LG: Failure of the overgown to prevent nosocomial infection in a pediatric intensive care unit. *Pediatrics* 77:35–38, 1986.

55. Hall CB, Geiman JM, Douglas RG Jr, Meagher MP: Control of nosocomial respiratory syncytial virus infections. *Pediatrics* 62:728–732, 1978.

56. LeClair JM, Freeman J, Sullivan BF, Crowley CM, Goldmann DA: Prevention of nosocomial respiratory syncytial virus infections through compliance with glove and gown isolation precautions. *N Engl J Med* 317:329–334, 1987.

57. Albert RK, Condie F: Handwashing patterns in medical intensive care units. *N Engl J Med* 304: 1465–1466, 1981.

16

Measles and Rubella Viruses

Gregory F. Hayden, M.D. and Walter A. Orenstein, M.D.

MEASLES

Background

Measles (rubeola) is a highly contagious disease that is caused by a paramyxovirus and has been recognized for centuries. In a typical case, symptoms begin 8–12 days after exposure, and consist initially of fever and one or more of the three C's: cough, coryza, and conjunctivitis (and/or photophobia). The pathognomonic enanthem (Koplik's spots) appears a few days later on the buccal and labial mucosa as pinpoint, bluish-white specks on an erythematous base. A few days later, when the enanthem is fading or gone (approximately 2–4 days after onset of the prodrome and an average of 14 days after exposure), the generalized rash appears as a maculopapular eruption around the face and neck, which then spreads centrifugally. The rash often becomes confluent, and after a few days begins to fade in the order of appearance, sometimes leaving in its wake a fine, brawny desquamation. The overall duration of illness is about 10 days, prompting the lay term "10-day measles." Complications of measles may include otitis media, encephalitis, bronchitis, pneumonia, diarrhea, and hemorrhagic measles. Measles may exacerbate underlying conditions, such as malnutrition, thereby increasing mortality. A single attack confers solid, lifelong immunity.

Two uncommon forms of measles have been described. *Atypical measles* is a syndrome of fever, hypersensitivity pneumonia, and a pleomorphic, peripheral rash which can occur following exposure to wild measles virus in persons who received inactivated measles vaccine available in the United States between 1963–1967 (1). This clinical syndrome is thought to represent an abnormal immune response in a previously sensitized host. Laboratory findings classically include eosinophilia and a sharply elevated titer of measles antibodies. Affected patients are probably not contagious. *Modified measles* is simply a mild clinical case of measles due to the mitigating effect of measles antibodies (2). This syndrome has been described among children who became ill after receiving immune globulin (IG) for known measles exposures and among infants whose transplacentally acquired passive immunity has waned partially. The incubation period may be prolonged up to 20 days in such instances; the illness is short, mild, and rarely followed by complications. Respiratory shedding of virus may occur, however, so these patients must be considered potentially infectious.

Measles is highly contagious. Spread is usually via direct contact with infectious droplets, but airborne spread has also been documented (3,4). Patients generally become infectious at the onset of the prodrome up to 3–5 days before rash onset, and remain infectious up to 4 days after rash onset.

Population

Measles remains a very important cause of morbidity and mortality in the developing world. The introduction and widespread use of measles vaccine in the United States, however, have resulted in an over 98% reduction in reported measles compared with the prevaccine era (5). Fewer than 6,300 cases of measles were reported in the United States in 1986. Unvaccinated preschool children have had the highest risk in recent years, but many cases have been reported among children who had been vaccinated unsuccessfully and among high school and college students (6).

Most measles transmission in recent years has been school- or home-based, but up to 3–5%

of cases involved transmission in medical settings (7). In one recent outbreak alone, more than 20 patients probably acquired their infection in medical facilities (8). Approximately 75% of such cases have occurred among patients or visitors, with the remainder among medical personnel, including physicians, nurses, laboratory technicians, clerks, and members of other employee categories (7). Transmission is most commonly from an infected patient to a susceptible patient, staff member, or visitor. In some instances, transmission has occurred when the infected patients were in the prodrome of their illness before rash onset, but in other instances, transmission resulted from inadequate isolation of patients with rash illness. Measles transmission has been reported in a broad variety of medical settings, including hospital, physician's office, nonhospital outpatient clinic, pharmacy, nonhospital emergency center, drug rehabilitation center, and medical laboratory (7). Unfortunately, the age groups that appear most likely to acquire measles in medical settings are infants and young adults, the same age groups at highest risk for measles complications (9).

Most children in the United States are immune to measles. Vigorous enforcement of school immunization laws in recent years has resulted in marked increases in immunization rates among young school-age children. Immunization levels are somewhat lower, however, among preschool children. A small proportion (up to 5%) of vaccinees may fail to respond to vaccine and will remain susceptible (10).

The great majority of hospital employees are immune to measles on the basis of previous disease or vaccination. In one recent study, only one of 266 employees tested with sensitive serologic assays was found to be serosusceptible (11). Levels of susceptibility may increase, however, as cohorts of current high school and college students enter the hospital workforce. The accumulation of susceptibles in this young adult population has resulted from lack of vaccination, inadequate vaccination, and occasional failures of appropriate vaccination, all in the setting of minimal exposure to measles disease.

Diagnosis

Early recognition of measles cases requires a strong index of suspicion because the early signs of illness are nonspecific, and the disease is now encountered only infrequently in this country. Careful attention must therefore be paid to obtaining a history of exposure to rash illness at the time of presentation to the medical facility. Once the exanthem has developed, the clinical diagnosis of measles is much easier, but transmission may already have occurred by this time.

A clinical diagnosis of measles can be confirmed in the medical laboratory. Measles virus can be isolated in cell culture from blood, urine, or nasopharyngeal secretions, but this procedure is expensive, slow, and technically difficult. The usual means of confirmation is therefore serologic with demonstration of a significant increase in titer of measles antibodies between acute and convalescent serum specimens. Alternatively, detection of IgM antibodies against measles virus in an appropriately timed single specimen is considered diagnostic of primary measles infection.

Treatment

There is no specific antiviral treatment for uncomplicated measles, so that only supportive measures are available. Antimicrobial therapy may be useful, however, for unusual instances of bacterial superinfection.

Prevention

Once the presumptive diagnosis of measles has been made, several steps need to be taken to prevent or limit the transmission of the illness to staff and other patients at the medical facility. Respiratory isolation (Table 16.1) should be instituted as soon as the diagnosis is suspected, rather than waiting for serologic or virologic confirmation. At the same time, efforts should be undertaken to protect potentially exposed patients and staff. For epidemiologic purposes, a probable case has been defined as occurring in a patient with fever ($\geq$101°F); generalized rash of 3 or more days duration; and one or more of cough, coryza, and conjunctivitis. A confirmed case meets the same clinical definition but requires either supportive laboratory evidence (culture or serology) or epidemiologic connection to another probable or confirmed case. These suggested case definitions may have retrospective epidemiologic value in describing a measles outbreak, but are not meant to impede swift and decisive measures to control the spread of disease. Action should ideally be taken as soon as

Table 16.1.
Respiratory Isolation for Measles Infection

1. Isolation should be instituted as soon as the diagnosis is considered, rather than waiting for serologic or virologic confirmation.
2. Confirm diagnosis with culture or serology.
3. Susceptible persons should not enter the patient's room.
4. Immune persons may enter room without mask.
5. Isolation should continue for at least 4 days after onset of the rash.
6. Exposed susceptible staff should be given live attenuated measles vaccine or immunoglobulin and furloughed from days 6–21 following exposure, or if they become ill, until 4 days after the onset of rash.
7. Exposed susceptible patients should be isolated from the 6th–21st day after exposure, or discharged if at all possible.

the diagnosis of measles is suspected, preferably before rash has been present for 3 or more days. An inpatient with suspected measles should remain in respiratory isolation until at least 4 days after rash onset (12). Susceptible persons should, if possible, stay out of the room, whereas immune persons need not wear a mask. An immunocompromised patient who develops measles may shed virus for a more prolonged interval than usual and should be isolated for the duration of the illness.

Outpatients with suspected measles should be isolated from other patients as completely as possible. Some contacts of such patients with the medical facility can be averted by means of judicious home visits by members of the medical staff. If such patients must be seen at the facility, and the visit is planned in advance, scheduling at the end of the day may help to reduce the number of possible exposures. Patients who present for urgent care without an appointment should be identified at the time of registration and, to the extent possible, should be kept in separate waiting and examining rooms to minimize their contacts with other children, especially those likely to be susceptible to measles (e.g., those under age 15 months). Masks placed on the suspected patient upon entry into the medical facility may also help to reduce possible exposures.

The next step is to determine which patients and hospital employees have been exposed to measles. Those persons having close, direct

contact with the patient in the few days preceding rash onset are at greatest risk. Since airborne transmission in medical facilities has been described, however, it is prudent to assume that all persons on the affected ward or clinic area during the patient's contagious period have been exposed and are therefore at risk. The exposed employee population will likely include physicians, nurses, clerical staff, dietary personnel, and perhaps others, such as students, volunteers, therapists, and laboratory personnel.

The next step is to determine which of the exposed patients and staff are susceptible to measles. Determination of susceptibility often requires some understanding of the two types of measles vaccine used in the United States. In 1963, two different measles vaccines were licensed, a live attenuated vaccine (Edmonston B strain) and an inactivated or killed vaccine (KMV). The KMV proved ineffective, was soon associated with the hypersensitivity syndrome of atypical measles, and was withdrawn from the market in 1967. During this brief interval between 1963–1967, only approximately 600,000–900,000 persons were vaccinated with KMV; the majority of vaccinees received a live measles vaccine. The live, attenuated vaccine was frequently administered with immune globulin (IG) to reduce the frequency and severity of side effects, principally rash and fever. Live, further attenuated strains that induced fewer and milder reactions were licensed in 1965 and 1968, and were not intended to be administered with IG. After 1975, only these live, further attenuated vaccines were available in the United States. All strains of live measles vaccine induce immunity in ≥95% of recipients at ≥15 months of age.

The following criteria suggest immunity to measles among exposed children:

1. Physician-documented measles;
2. Documented history (with date) of live measles vaccination on or after the first birthday; or
3. Laboratory evidence of serologic immunity to measles.

Presence of any one of the three previously mentioned criteria is good evidence of immunity among hospital staff, but one additional criterion for immunity is often applied to adults. Persons born before 1957 are very likely to be immune to measles since they lived several years in the prevaccine era, when measles transmission was widespread and few susceptibles escaped infection during early childhood. Presumably, the earlier the birthdate before 1957, the greater the likelihood of measles immunity. Confirmation of immunity among such older employees by means of serologic testing may sometimes be desirable.

One issue of concern in some settings is age at vaccination. As mentioned earlier, ≥95% of children vaccinated when 15 months of age or older develop antibodies and are presumably protected against measles. However, efficacy in persons vaccinated at 12 months of age appears to be somewhat lower, ranging from 80%–95% (13). Because efficacy is still relatively high, even with vaccination at age 12 months, it has not been recommended to routinely revaccinate persons initially vaccinated between 12–14 months of age. However, revaccination of such persons might be considered in hospital outbreaks if persons vaccinated between 12–14 months of age appear to be playing an important role in transmission.

Another issue of potential concern is the degree of protection provided to employees by measles vaccination many years previously. Live measles vaccination at or after 15 months of age induces long-lasting immunity in about 95% or more of vaccinees. Although vaccination of persons between 12–14 months of age may induce slightly lower rates of seroconversion, those persons who do respond appear to have long-term, probably lifelong, protection from disease. Some vaccinees who seroconvert may lose measurable serologic evidence of immunity after many years, but such persons typically demonstrate a booster-type immune response when revaccinated, suggesting that they had remained functionally immune to measles (14). During the early vaccine era, however, some persons were vaccinated with an ineffective vaccine or in a suboptimal manner and may be susceptible as follows:

1. Received live measles vaccine before 1 year of age;
2. Received live, further attenuated measles vaccine with concurrent IG;
3. Received only killed (or inactivated) measles vaccine or killed vaccine followed by live measles vaccine within 3 months;

4. Received measles vaccine of unknown type between 1963–1967 when the inactivated vaccine was still being distributed.

Once those patients and personnel who are potentially susceptible to measles have been identified, the next step is to decide what preventive measures should be undertaken. When given within 72 hours of exposure, live, further attenuated measles vaccine may be helpful. Further, if the exposure did not result in infection, the vaccine should protect the recipient against subsequent measles exposures. Contraindications to vaccination include acute febrile illness, altered immunity, pregnancy, and anaphylactic hypersensitivity to neomycin. Protocols have been developed for cautious vaccination of persons hypersensitive to egg protein (15). Another option is to give IG, which will prevent or modify measles infection if given within 6 days of exposure. The recommended intramuscular dose is 0.25 ml/kg (or 0.5 ml/kg for an immunocompromised host) with a maximum dose of 15 ml. Since IG imparts only short-lived protection, it should be followed by live measles vaccination 3 months later in persons older than age 15 months to provide long-lasting protection. IG is particularly useful for the protection of children under 1 year of age who have had close contact with a person with measles, and for persons for whom measles vaccine is contraindicated.

All exposed inpatients should be isolated from the 6th–21st day after exposure or until they are discharged. Only immune hospital staff should care for these exposed patients. Exposed, susceptible patients should be discharged from the hospital as soon as possible so as to reduce the likelihood of additional measles exposures in the hospital.

The best means of preventing staff from transmitting measles is to ensure that they are immune before any potential exposures to measles. At present, the vast majority of hospital personnel appear to be immune, but younger employees, particularly recent high school and college students, can be expected to have higher rates of susceptibility. Assuring that all persons born after 1956 have adequate evidence of immunity to measles is one means of protecting both staff and patients from disease. Such a program can be implemented in conjunction with rubella immunization efforts. Use of combined vaccines containing both measles and rubella antigens offers the potential of inducing immunity against both diseases at only a small extra cost for the second vaccine. There is no known harm in vaccinating someone already immune.

RUBELLA

Background

Rubella (German measles) is a usually mild clinical illness caused by an RNA-containing member of the togavirus family. The infection is commonly inapparent and unrecognized. Symptomatic illness is usually manifested by rash and lymphadenopathy commonly involving the posterior auricular and suboccipital nodes. The rash begins as discrete, pink maculopapules on the face, which spread to the trunk and then progress centrifugally. The usual duration of rash is 2–5 days, prompting the lay term ''3-day measles.'' Arthralgia and arthritis may be seen, especially in adult women, but serious complications are rare. Some adults experience a prodrome consisting of low-grade fever, malaise, anorexia, headache, sore throat, and in severe cases, cough, coryza, and conjunctivitis, as seen in measles. In general, however, patients with rubella appear much less ill than patients with measles, and these two illnesses can usually be differentiated clinically. It is more commonly difficult to distinguish rubella from other nonspecific viral illnesses than from measles.

Rubella attains major public health significance because of its potentially devastating effects on the developing fetus. Both clinically apparent and inapparent primary infections can cause fetal damage. Defects of virtually every organ system have been described in children with congenital rubella infection, with the clinical expression of infection closely related to the gestational timing of rubella. Infection in the 1st trimester may result in major anomalies such as cataract or glaucoma, heart disease (e.g., patent ductus arteriosus and pulmonary stenosis), sensorineural deafness, and psychomotor retardation in 25% or more of infants.

Rubella spreads primarily via respiratory droplets or direct contact. The period of maximum communicability extends from the few days before rash onset until 5–7 days after rash onset. Infants with congenital rubella may continue to shed large amounts of virus in nasopharyngeal secretions and urine for prolonged periods; in some cases, 1 year or more. The incubation period averages 16–18 days (range 14–21 days).

Population

Before the licensure of rubella vaccine in 1969, rubella occurred in epidemic form in the United States in an approximate 6–9-year cycle. A major epidemic in 1964 resulted in the birth of approximately 20,000 infants with congenital rubella (16). Following widespread vaccination, another major outbreak has not occurred, and reported rubella has dropped to all-time low levels (16). Fewer than 550 cases were reported in the United States in 1986.

The population at greatest risk of infection during the prevaccine era was young school-aged children. In the early years of the vaccine era, primary emphasis was placed on the vaccination of young children, and the reported incidence of rubella among this age group dropped sharply. Disease activity did not decrease as dramatically among adolescents and young adults, with numerous outbreaks reported among high school and college students (16,17). As cohorts of vaccinated children entered adolescence and adulthood, and with increased attention in the 1980s to the identification and vaccination of susceptible adolescents and adults, especially women, reported rubella among these age groups has dropped substantially as well.

Several outbreaks of rubella have been reported in medical settings (18–24). Exposures have occurred in both inpatient and outpatient settings, and cases have been reported both among patients and among medical, nursing, and ancillary staff. Illnesses among obstetrical staff members, both male and female, and exposures in prenatal clinics have caused particular concern (21–24). Although no known cases of congenital rubella have resulted among infected pregnant staff, several infected women have elected to terminate their pregnancies (19).

Diagnosis

Since clinical manifestations may be absent or minimal, the clinical diagnosis of postnatal rubella is difficult or impossible in the nonepidemic setting. A clinical suspicion of rubella should therefore be confirmed in the medical laboratory, especially when infection is suspected in a pregnant female or a newborn infant. Viral isolation from nose, throat, blood, or urine specimens is feasible but expensive, slow, and technically difficult. Demonstration of a significant rise in titer of antirubella antibodies between acute and convalescent serum specimens is therefore preferred in most instances. Detection of rubella-specific IgM antibodies in a single appropriately timed serum specimen strongly suggests recent primary infection and may allow more rapid diagnostic confirmation.

The clinical diagnosis of congenital rubella infection depends on the constellation of signs and symptoms with a history compatible with maternal gestational rubella. Since the clinical presentation may sometimes be confused with congenital infection with other agents (including toxoplasmosis, cytomegalovirus, and syphilis), laboratory confirmation is desirable via viral isolation; presence of rubella-specific IgM antibodies, which unlike IgG antibodies, cannot cross the placenta; or persistence of a significant titer of rubella antibodies between 6–11 months of age, by which time passively acquired maternal antibodies should have dropped to negligible levels.

Treatment

There is no specific antiviral therapy for rubella. Patients with fever, malaise, or arthritis may benefit from symptomatic therapy.

Prevention

The first step in managing a possible rubella exposure in the inpatient setting is to place the patient under contact isolation for 7 days after onset of the rash (Table 16.2). Infants with known or suspected congenital rubella should be con-

Table 16.2.
Contact Isolation for Rubella Infection

1. Contact isolation should be instituted as soon as the diagnosis is considered, rather than waiting for serologic or virologic confirmation.
2. Children with congenital rubella should be considered contagious until 1 year of age and placed in contact isolation.
3. Confirm diagnosis with culture or serology.
4. Isolation should continue for at least 7 days after onset of rash.
5. Exposed susceptible staff should be furloughed from day 7 to 21 days after exposure, or if they become ill, until 1 week after the onset of rash.
6. Exposed susceptible patients should be isolated from 7–21 days after exposure, or discharged if at all possible.

sidered potentially contagious until 1 year of age (unless negative nasopharyngeal and urine cultures have been obtained after 3 months of age), and likewise placed in contact isolation (12).

The second step is to determine which patients and employees have been exposed. Patients with rubella differ markedly in their ability to spread infection, perhaps related to the presence of respiratory symptoms, such as sneezing and coughing. It is therefore prudent to assume the worst case of high communicability from approximately 7 days before until 5 days after rash onset. Persons with subclinical rubella can also transmit infection, as can infants with congenital rubella.

The third step is to determine whether the exposed persons are susceptible to rubella. A history of clinically diagnosed rubella without serologic documentation is unreliable and should not be accepted as proof of immunity. Acceptable evidence of rubella immunity would include documented (with date) history of rubella vaccination on or after the 1st birthday or serologic evidence of rubella immunity. With the conventional serologic methods (e.g., hemagglutination inhibition), the presence of any level of rubella-specific antibody has been considered to indicate previous infection and presumed immunity from primary infection and viremia. Conversely, the absence of such antibody has been assumed to indicate probable susceptibility. Many newer serologic techniques for rubella have been introduced in recent years, however, the significance of absent or low titers using these methods needs to be defined more clearly (25,26). Assessment of rubella immunity based on a single serologic specimen may therefore require familiarity with the test method used and its levels of diagnostic sensitivity and specificity. In general, however, even persons with low titers are immunologically primed and demonstrate a secondary immune response if challenged with rubella vaccine. Viremia appears rare under these circumstances. Therefore, if the test is truly measuring rubella antibodies, even in very low titer, the patient with a positive test can be considered immune (27,28).

The final step is to counsel the exposed susceptibles. Standard IG given after exposure may suppress or modify symptoms but will not prevent infection or viremia. Limited experimental experience with high-titer human rubella immunoglobulin has been favorable, but this material is not generally available (29,30). The use of rubella vaccine after exposure is not known to be harmful, but is of uncertain value. If the recent exposure has not resulted in incubating infection, vaccine should provide protection against subsequent exposures.

What should be done in the special case of an exposed pregnant patient or employee? Since many women have had a rubella serology performed for purposes of entrance into college or the military or as part of routine prenatal care, a quick history or chart review will often reveal evidence of immunity and provide rapid reassurance. If not obtained previously, a rubella antibody titer should be performed immediately. If the interval since exposure has been less than 7 days, any positive titer by conventional tests such as hemagglutination inhibition and complement fixation likely indicates previous infection (or vaccination) with resultant immunity. If no rubella antibodies are detected, it will be necessary to repeat the testing in 2 weeks. If rubella antibodies are present in this second specimen, rubella infection can be assumed to have occurred. If this second specimen is again negative, the test should be repeated a third time, 1 month later. A negative test at this time, 6 weeks after exposure, indicates that infection has not occurred. If a period longer than 1 week has elapsed between the rubella exposure and the time of an initial serology that is positive, the interpretation becomes more difficult (31). The presence of rubella-specific IgM antibodies, however, suggests recent primary infection. IG following exposures in early pregnancy is not of proven benefit, and should be contemplated only for a woman who would not undergo therapeutic abortion. Pregnant women should not be given rubella vaccine.

The traditional concern with rubella within the hospital setting has been that a pregnant employee might contract rubella from an infected patient. For this reason, female employees who might become pregnant should be required to prove rubella immunity for their own protection. Rubella transmission is a two-way street, however, and in several recent outbreaks, infected employees have exposed pregnant patients. In several instances, the infected employee was a male physician. To protect the patients, it is advisable that all hospital employees, male and female, in contact with pregnant patients have documented rubella immunity.

Careful, advance attention to the verification of rubella immunity among hospital staff can help to reduce or avoid the panic that can otherwise accompany a rubella exposure in the hospital setting.

Many questions need to be addressed when planning a program to improve levels of rubella immunity among hospital staff. First, there should be concern about the safety of rubella vaccines in susceptible postpubertal populations. Ample evidence indicates that the risk of side effects is higher in such populations compared with comparable populations of children. However, the reactions are generally mild, primarily involving transient arthralgia, and do not cause significant absenteeism (32). An additional safety issue relates to the unintentional vaccination of women who are either pregnant or become pregnant within 3 months of vaccination. The Centers for Disease Control has collected information on 155 infants born to 153 susceptible women vaccinated with RA27/3 rubella vaccine between 3 months before and 3 months after the estimated date of conception (33). No babies had defects compatible with congenital rubella syndrome. Since no cases of congenital rubella syndrome have been observed, the risk appears to be so small as to be negligible. While women who are known to be pregnant should not be vaccinated, vaccination of a woman later found to be pregnant should not ordinarily be a reason to consider interruption of pregnancy. Reasonable precautions for a rubella vaccination program of adult women include asking the women whether they are pregnant; excluding those who claim to be pregnant or uncertain; explaining the theoretical risks to the others; and offering vaccine to the others, explaining that they should avoid pregnancy for 3 months.

In addition to questions about safety, there are questions about how to implement the most effective program. Will employee participation in the program be voluntary or mandatory? Will the employees be screened via serologic testing before vaccination? If so, how and where will the vaccination of susceptibles be accomplished? These and other questions have caused much debate among medical and nursing staff, public health officials, hospital administrators, and others (34,35). Cited obstacles to establishing programs to screen and vaccinate employees have included cost, liability issues, and high employee turnover (36). Compliance with voluntary programs has generally been poor, especially among physicians and male employees (20,32,37). A low rate of compliance with voluntary vaccination after mandatory serologic screening has also been reported (38). Many hospitals have therefore instituted mandatory programs under which rubella immunity is a prerequisite to employment. At some hospitals, the employee health service has proven a suitable site for the necessary serologic testing and vaccination (39). Enforcement of such programs to identify and vaccinate susceptible personnel provides the opportunity for preventing rubella outbreaks with their accompanying disruption of hospital services and risk of fetal rubella infection.

REFERENCES

1. Annunziato D, Kaplan MH, Hall WW, Ichinose H, Lin JH, Balsam D, Paladino VS: Atypical measles syndrome: Pathologic and serologic findings. *Pediatrics* 70:203–209, 1982.
2. Krugman S, Katz SL, Gershon AA, Wilfert CM: *Infectious Diseases of Children*, ed 8. St Louis, CV Mosby, 1985, p 157.
3. Bloch AB, Orenstein WA, Ewing WM, Spain WH, Mallison GF, Herrmann KL, Hinman AR: Measles outbreak in a pediatric practice: Airborne transmission in an office setting. *Pediatrics* 75:676–683, 1985.
4. Remington PL, Hall WW, Davis IH, Herald A, Gunn RA: Airborne transmission of measles in a physician's office. *JAMA* 253:1574–1577, 1985.
5. Bloch AB, Orenstein WA, Stetler HC, Wassilak SG, Amler RW, Bart KJ, Kirby CD, Hinman AR: Health impact of measles vaccination in the United States. *Pediatrics* 76:524–532, 1985.
6. Amler RW, Orenstein WA: Measles in young adults: The case for vigorous pursuit of immunization. *Postgrad Med* 77(1):251–161, 1985.
7. Davis RM, Orenstein WA, Frank JA Jr, Sacks JJ, Dales LG, Preblud SR, Bart KJ, Williams NM, Hinman AR: Transmission of measles in medical settings, 1980 through 1984. *JAMA* 255:1295–1298, 1986.
8. Dales LG, Kizer KW: Measles transmission in medical facilities. *West J Med* 142:415–416, 1985.
9. Foulon G, Cottin JF, Matheron S, Perronne C, Bouvet E: Transmission and severity of measles acquired in medical settings. *JAMA* 256:1135–1136, 1986.
10. Hayden GF: Measles vaccine failure: A survey of causes and means of prevention. *Clin Pediatr* 18:155–167, 1979.
11. Chou T, Weil D, Arnow PM: Prevalence of measles antibodies in hospital personnel. *Infect Control* 7:309–311, 1986.
12. Garner JS, Simmons BP: Guidelines for isolation precautions in hospitals. *Infect Control* 4:245–325, 1983.
13. Orenstein WA, Markowitz L, Preblud SR, Hinman AR, Tomasi A, Bart KJ: Appropriate age for measles vaccination in the United States. *Devel Biol Standard* (in press).
14. Krugman S: Further attenuated measles vaccine: Characteristics and use. *Rev Infect Dis* 5:477–481, 1983.
15. Herman JJ, Radin R, Schneiderman R: Allergic reactions to measles (rubeola) vaccine in patients hypersensitive to egg protein. *J Pediatr* 102:196–199, 1983.
16. Orenstein WA, Bart KJ, Hinman AR, Preblud SR, Greaves WL, Doster SW, Stetler HC, Sirotkin B: The opportunity and obligation to eliminate rubella from the United States. *JAMA* 251:1988–1994, 1984.
17. Hinman AR: Measles and rubella in adolescents and young adults. *Hosp Practice* 17:137–146, 1982.
18. Greaves WL, Orenstein WA, Stetler HC, Preblud SR, Hinman AR, Bart KJ: Prevention of rubella transmission in medical facilities. *JAMA* 248:861–864, 1982.
19. Heseltine PNR, Ripper M, Wohlford P: Nosocomial rubella—consequences of an outbreak and efficacy of a mandatory immunization program. *Infect Control* 6:371–374, 1985.
20. Polk BF, White JA, DeGirolami PC, Modlin JF: An outbreak of rubella among hospital personnel. *N Engl J Med* 303:541–545, 1980.
21. Strassburg MA, Imagawa DT, Fannin SL, Turner JA, Chow AW, Murray RA, Cherry JD: Rubella outbreak among hospital employees. *Obstet Gynecol* 57:283–288, 1981.
22. Fliegel PE, Weinstein WM: Rubella outbreak in a prenatal clinic: Management and prevention. *Am J Infect Control* 10:29–33, 1982.
23. Gladstone JL, Millian SJ: Rubella exposure in an obstetric clinic. *Obstet Gynecol* 57:182–186, 1981.
24. McLaughlin MC, Gold LH: The New York rubella incident: A case for changing hospital policy regarding rubella testing and immunization. *Am J Public Health* 69:287–289, 1979.
25. Sever JL, Cleghorn C: Rubella diagnostic tests: What is a significant result? *Postgrad Med* 71(3):73–77, 1982.
26. Vejtorp M: Serodiagnosis of postnatal rubella: A survey of methods with special reference to the enzyme-linked immunosorbent assay. *Danish Med Bull* 30:53–66, 1983.
27. Orenstein WA, Herrmann KL, Holmgreen P, Bernier R, Bart KJ, Eddins DL, Fiumara NJ: Prevalence of rubella antibodies in Massachusetts schoolchildren. *Am J Epidemiol* 124:290–298, 1986.
28. Preblud SR: Some current issues relating to rubella vaccine. *JAMA* 254:253–256, 1985.
29. Urquhard GED, Crawford RJ, Wallace J: Trial of high-titer human rubella immunoglobulin. *Br Med J* 2:1331–1332, 1978.
30. Schiff GM: Titered lots of immune globulin (Ig): Efficacy in the prevention of rubella. *Am J Dis Child* 118:322–329, 1969.
31. Mann JM, Preblud SR, Hoffman RE, Bradling-Bennett AD, Hinman AR, Herrmann KL: Assessing risks of rubella infection during pregnancy: A standardized approach. *JAMA* 245:1647–1652, 1981.
32. Orenstein WA, Heseltine PNR, LaGagnoux SJ, Portnoy B: Rubella vaccine and susceptible hospital employees: Poor physician participation. *JAMA* 245:711–713, 1981.
33. Centers for Disease Control: Rubella vaccination during pregnancy—United States, 1971–1985. *MMWR* 35:275–276, 281–284, 1986.
34. Evans ME, Schaffner W: Rubella immunization of hospital personnel: A debate. *Infect Control* 2:387–390, 1981.
35. Schoenbaum SC: Rubella policies for hospitals and health workers. *Infect Control* 2:366–417, 1981.
36. Sacks JJ, Olson B, Soter J, Clark C: Employee rubella screening programs in Arizona hospitals. *JAMA* 249:2675–2678, 1983.
37. Hartstein AI, Quan MA, Williams ML, Osterud HT, Foster LR: Rubella screening and immunization of health care personnel: Critical appraisal of a voluntary program. *Am J Infect Control* 11:1–9, 1983.
38. Kohl HW III: Rubella screening and vaccination follow-up by a hospital employee health office. *Am J Infect Control* 13:124–127, 1985.
39. Weiss KE, Falvo CE, Buimovici-Klein E, Magill JW, Cooper LZ: Evaluation of an employee health service as a setting for a rubella screening and immunization program. *Am J Public Health* 69:281–283, 1979.

17

Hemophilus influenzae

Trudy V. Murphy, M.D.

BACKGROUND

Hemophilus influenzae are small, pleomorphic Gram-negative rods. Some *H. influenzae* strains elaborate a serologically distinct polysaccharide capsule. These strains can be separated into six serotypes designated a–f (1). In previously healthy children, 97% of systemic infection caused by *H. influenzae* are caused by serotype b strains. The most common infections are meningitis, cellulitis, pneumonia, epiglottitis, and arthritis (2). Other serotypes of *H. influenzae* are rarely isolated from children with systemic infection (3–5).

H. influenzae, which do not elaborate capsule, nontypeable, or nonencapsulated strains, differ from encapsulated strains in their antigenic and genetic characteristics, and in the spectrum of infections (6). Nontypeable *H. influenzae* frequently are isolated from aspirates of the middle ear in children with acute otitis media (7). They are also commonly found in sputum, sinus, and occasionally in blood cultures from patients with acute bronchitis, sinusitis, or pneumonia (8,9). Nontypeable *H. influenzae* are pathogens of invasive disease, primarily in adults (6). They are isolated occasionally from neonates with systemic infection (10–12), from immunocompromised patients (13,14), and rarely from previously healthy children (2,15).

The usual habitat of *H. influenzae* in humans is the oronasopharynx. In the absence of exposure to a patient with systemic type b infection, fewer than 5% of preschool children and fewer than 1% of adults are colonized with type b strains (16–18). By contrast, 15–90% of well preschool children and adults are colonized in the nasopharynx by nontypeable strains of *H. influenzae* (19,20).

At least 80% of patients with systemic *H. influenzae* type b infection are pharyngeal carriers of the organism (21,22). Persistence of colonization after 12–24 hours of intravenous therapy occurs uncommonly (22,23). Nevertheless, resurgence of pharyngeal colonization after completion of antibiotic therapy has been demonstrated in 3–80% of patients (23,24).

Transmission of *H. influenzae* is reported to occur by direct contact or by inhalation of droplets of infected respiratory secretions (25). It is unknown whether fomites contaminated with secretions play a role in the transmission of *H. influenzae* type b. *H. influenzae* die rapidly with drying or heating (20). However, when the concentration of organisms in respiratory secretions is high, as in infected nasal mucus, organisms can be recovered from contaminated fomites for 2–18 hours (26,27).

POPULATION

Outbreaks of *H. influenzae* Type b Disease in Acute and Chronic Care Hospitals

Based on anecdotal experience, invasive *H. influenzae* type b disease resulting from transmission of *H. influenzae* type b in acute care hospitals is exceedingly rare. The most likely explanation for this observation is the low rate of positive pharyngeal cultures in patients during parenteral antibiotic therapy, the few opportunities for patients to share secretions, and an emphasis on prompt release from the hospital after treatment (22,23).

Transmission of type b *Hemophilus* from patients to personnel also would seem unlikely, except during the first 12–24 hours after initiation of antibiotic therapy. A preliminary investigation, to detect transmission of *H. influenzae* type b to 40 pediatric house officers who provided care to 97 patients, did not demonstrate acquisition of colonization (28).

A single case report suggests the possibility of transmission of *H. influenzae* type b in an acute care hospital (29). A child developed type b *H. influenzae* meningitis after being placed in the same room as an infant who was recovering from *H. influenzae* meningitis. *Hemophilus* isolated from both patients had the same rare strain markers. The index patient may have had persistence of nasopharyngeal colonization or reacquisition of the strain from a visiting family member. Although the two patients had no direct contact, the authors suggest that the organism could have been transmitted in secretions or on the hands of personnel (29).

Outbreaks of systemic *H. influenzae* type b infection are reported in chronic care hospitals for children (30–32). In one outbreak, the prevalence of colonization in "healthy" patients was 24%, and in staff members it was 11%. The authors hypothesized that intimate and frequent contact with patients' secretions may have accounted for the relatively high rate of colonization among staff members (30).

In another outbreak of type b *Hemophilus* infection, the prevalence of colonization in chronically ill patients was also high (20%). However, no members of the staff were colonized. Two of five cases in this outbreak were in patients with conditions that might increase their risk of systemic type b *Hemophilus* infection: hydrocephalus and asplenia (32).

Hospital-Acquired Infection with Endogenous *H. influenzae*

Infection with *H. influenzae* may ensue when access to normally sterile tissues is provided either by procedures or by changes in the normal host barriers and defenses. Such infections are more often caused by *H. influenzae* that are nontypeable and serotypes other than type b, these being the more prevalent *H. influenzae* colonizing the respiratory tract.

A retrospective review of 134 cases of hospital-acquired meningitis at Boston City Hospital identified five cases caused by *H. influenzae* (33,34). Patients had been hospitalized from 5–21 days when meningitis was diagnosed. Most patients had head injuries or were recovering from neurosurgical or otorhinological proce-

dures. It is not possible to determine from this report whether any of the hospital-acquired cases were in children, and serotyping was not performed on the isolates. At our own institution, we have observed *H. influenzae* meningitis in children complicating skull fracture, persistent cerebrospinal fluid leak, and cranial surgery. Both nontypeable and encapsulated strains of *H. influenzae* have been recovered.

It is well known that prolonged endotracheal intubation or tracheostomy are occasionally complicated by pneumonia (35,36). Changes in the mucosa, reduced mucociliary clearance, and aspiration of secretions may increase the susceptibility to local tissue invasion by colonizing bacteria, such as *H. influenzae*. Repeated aspiration of oral secretions in the neurologically compromised patient may also result in pneumonia caused by this organism.

Prolonged nasotracheal or nasogastric intubation are known to obstruct the sinus ostia. *H. influenzae* must be considered in the differential diagnosis of ipsilateral sinusitis that develops in such patients (37).

A rare complication observed twice at our institution was the development of local cellulitis at the site of traumatic procedures in patients bacteremic with type b *H. influenzae* disease. In one such patient, cellulitis developed in the neck following repeated attempts at intubation for epiglottitis. In the other patient, cellulitis developed at the site of a venepuncture.

H. influenzae is an uncommon cause of pneumonia and bacteremia in the neutropenic or otherwise immunocompromised patient. Patients who are asplenic may be at particular risk (38–40).

Neonatal sepsis or conjunctivitis are thought to be acquired through exposure to the colonized genital tract of the mother (12,41). The majority of these patients have onset of the infection in the first 48 hours after birth (11).

DIAGNOSIS

Hospital-acquired *H. influenzae* infection should be suspected in three groups of patients whose clinical status deteriorates: infants and immunocompromised patients with sepsis; patients with compromise of the physical barriers to the central nervous system (e.g., skull fracture, surgical procedures); and patients with aspiration of oral and respiratory secretions.

In the first two groups of patients, diagnosis is made after careful physical examination and a complete septic evaluation. Cultures of blood, cerebrospinal and pleural fluids, and radiographs of the chest should be obtained. In patients with aspiration or tracheal intubation, cultures of sputum or tracheal aspirates should also be obtained.

Gram stain of body fluids, including cerebrospinal fluid, may be helpful. Gram stain of tracheal secretions that contain neutrophils and a predominance of small, pleomorphic Gram-negative rods suggests infection with a *Hemophilus* species. Initial therapy should include appropriate antibiotics for *H. influenzae* pending confirmation by cultures and susceptibility testing.

TREATMENT

A wide spectrum of antibiotics is currently available for treatment of systemic *H. influenzae* infections. The principles of treating hospital-acquired infection do not differ from those of treating community-acquired infection.

An increasing proportion of *H. influenzae* isolated from patients are β-lactamase-producing (42,43) or resistant to ampicillin by mechanisms other than β-lactamase production (44). Thus, until susceptibility test results are available, therapy should include a second or third generation cephalosporin (e.g., cefuroxime, cefotaxime, ceftriaxone), or chloramphenicol (45–47). Confirmation that the organism isolated from the patient is suceptible to the antibiotic of choice is essential (44,48–50).

Most serious invasive infections caused by *H. influenzae* respond to 10 days (7–14 days) of parenteral therapy. Areas of loculated pus, e.g., pleural empyema, usually require drainage to hasten improvement and to prevent relapse. Sinusitis may require a more prolonged course of therapy (up to 3 weeks) but can be treated with an oral antibiotic such as amoxicillin or cefaclor (51). Removal of any tubes that obstruct the sinus ostia is desirable.

PREVENTION

H. influenzae Type b Infection

During the first 12–24 hours of hospitalization, it is currently recommended that patients with meningitis, pneumonia, and epiglottitis suspected to be caused by type b *H. influenzae* should be on respiratory isolation, and individuals having close contact with them should wear masks (Table 17.1) (52). Patients with other invasive type b *Hemophilus* infections are also thought to have nasopharyngeal colonization at the time of diagnosis and are therefore managed with the same initial precautions. Staff and visiting family members should be made aware of the potential transmission of this organism in respiratory secretions and be encouraged to use good technique and frequent handwashing.

At the end of therapy, patients with proven *H. influenzae* type b disease should be treated prophylactically with rifampin (20 mg/kg/day to a maximum 600 mg/dose, in a single daily dose, for 4 days) according to the recommendations of the Committee on Infectious Diseases of the American Academy of Pediatrics (25). There are little data to support the necessity of treating patients with rifampin simply because they remain in the hospital after discontinuation of parenteral antibiotics. However, if contact with other infants is anticipated, rifampin could be considered to reduce any small chance of transmission of persisting type b *H. influenzae* to staff or to other patients.

Nontypeable and Nonserotype b *H. influenzae* Infections

Because nontypeable strains and nontype b serotypes of *H. influenzae* are considered to be part of the normal oral flora, no special precautions are necessary for patients found to be infected. However, staff and visitors should be encouraged to use good technique and handwashing after contact with either their own or the patient's respiratory secretions. Rifampin prophylaxis is not indicated after *H. influenzae* infections other than type b.

Table 17.1.
Respiratory Isolation for *Hemophilus influenzae* Type b Infections

1. Private room for the first 12–24 hours of therapy.
2. Masks for close patient contact in the first 12–24 hours.
3. Careful handling of respiratory secretions.
4. Rifampin for eradication of nasopharyngeal colonization suggested for patients of any age who continue to be hospitalized after therapy, *and* according to the recommendations of the American Academy of Pediatrics Committee on Infectious Diseases (25).

Acknowledgment

Preparation of this chapter was funded in part by the National Institutes of Health grant no. AI21842.

REFERENCES

1. Kilian M: *Haemophilus*. In Lennett EH, Balows A, Hausler WJ Jr, Shadomy HJ (eds): *Manual of Clinical Microbiology*, ed 4. Washington, D.C., American Society for Microbiology, 1985, pp 387–393.
2. Murphy TV, Osterholm MT, Pierson LM, White KE, Breedlove JA, Seibert GB, Kuritsky JN, Granoff DM: Prospective surveillance of *Haemophilus influenzae* type b disease in Dallas County, Texas and Minnesota. *Pediatrics* 79:173–180, 1987.
3. Controni G, Rodriguez WJ, Chang MJ: Meningitis caused by *Haemophilus influenzae* type e, biotype IV. *Southern Med J* 75:78, 1982.
4. Sundwall DA, Bergeson ME, Ortiz A: Reye's sydrome associated with *Haemophilus influenzae* infection. *Clin Pediatr* 19:357–360, 1980.
5. Gray BM: Meningitis due to *Hemophilus influenzae* type f. *J Pediatr* 90:1031, 1977.
6. Murphy TF, Apicella MA: Nontypable *Haemophilus influenzae*: A review of clinical aspects, surface antigens, and the human immune response to infection. *Rev Infect Dis* 9:1–15, 1987.
7. Harding AL, Anderson P, Howie VM, Ploussard JH, Smith DH: *Haemophilus influenzae* isolated from children with otitis media. In Sell SH, Karzon DT (eds): *Hemophilus influenzae*. Nashville, TN, Vanderbilt Univ Press, 1983, pp 21–28.
8. Musher DM: *Haemophilus influenzae* infections. *Hosp Pract* 18:158–170, 1983.
9. Wald ER, Milmoe GJ, Bowen A, Ledesma-Medina J, Salamon N, Bluestone CD: Acute maxillary sinusitis in children. *N Engl J Med* 304:749–754, 1981.
10. Friesen CA, Cho CT: Characteristic features of neonatal sepsis due to *Haemophilus influenzae*. *Rev Infect Dis* 8:777–780, 1986.
11. Campognone P, Singer DB: Neonatal sepsis due to nontypable *Haemophilus influenzae*. *Am J Dis Child* 140:117–121, 1986.
12. Finkelstein E, Weinberger S, Kandall S: Neonatal *Hemophilus influenzae* sepsis. *N York State J Med* 86:106–107, 1986.
13. Chilcote RR, Baehner RL: Septicemia in association with acute lymphoblastic leukemia. *J Pediatr* 94:715–718, 1979.
14. Howard MW, Strauss RG, Johnston RB: Infections in patients with neutropenia. *Am J Dis Child* 131:788–790, 1977.
15. Gilsdorf JA: *Haemophilus influenzae* non-type b infections in children. *Am J Dis Child* 141:1063–1065, 1987.
16. Hampton CM, Barenkamp SJ, Granoff DM: Comparison of outer membrane protein subtypes of *Haemophilus influenzae* type b isolates from healthy children in the general population and from diseased patients. *J Clin Microbiol* 18:596–600, 1983.
17. Turk DC: Distribution of *Haemophilus influenzae* in healthy human communities. In Turk DC and May JR (eds): *Haemophilus influenzae: Its Clinical Importance*. London, English University Press, pp 13–23.
18. Michaels RH, Poziviak CS, Stonebraker FE, Norden CW: Factors affecting pharyngeal *Haemophilus influenzae* type b colonization rates in children. *J Clin Microbiol* 4:413–417, 1976.
19. Sell SH, Turner DJ, Federspiel CF: Natural infections in children: I. types identified. In Sell SH and Karzon DT (eds): *Haemophilus influenzae*. Nashville, TN, Vanderbilt Univ Press, 1973, pp 3–12.
20. Smith DH: *Haemophilus influenzae*. In Mandell GL, Douglas RG Jr, Bennett JE (eds): *Principles and Practice of Infectious Diseases*. New York, John Wiley & Sons, 1979, vol 2, pp 1759–1767.
21. Gilsdorf JR: Dynamics of nasopharyngeal colonization with *Haemophilus influenzae* b during antibiotic therapy. *Pediatrics* 77:242–245, 1986.
22. Murphy TV, Del Rio M, Chrane D: Persistent pharyngeal colonization during therapy in patients with *Haemophilus influenzae* type b meningitis. *J Infect Dis* 152:489, 1985.
23. Alpert G, Campos JM, Smith DM, Barenkamp SJ, Fleisher GR: Incidence and persistence of *Haemophilus influenzae* type b upper airway colonization in patients with meningitis. *J Pediatr* 107:555–557, 1985.
24. Michaels RH, Norden CW: Pharyngeal colonization with *Haemophilus influenzae* type b: A longitudinal study of families with meningitis or epiglottitis due to *H. influenzae* type b. *J Infect Dis* 136:222–228, 1977.
25. Committee on Infectious Diseases. *Haemophilus influenzae Infections*, ed 20. Evanston, IL, American Academy of Pediatrics, 1986, pp 169–174.
26. Gilsdorf JR, Herring G: Recovery of *Haemophilus influenzae* b from hospital and environmental surfaces. *Am J Infect Control* 15:33–35, 1987.
27. Murphy TV, Clements JF: Survival of *Haemophilus influenzae* type b on surfaces in day care. Presented at the 25th Interscience Conference on Antimicrobial Agents and Chemotherapy. Setember 29–October 2, 1985, Minneapolis, MN, p 213.
28. Jenkins MB, Barrett FF, Gigliotti, Jones DP: *Haemophilus influenzae* type b colonization among pediatric house officers. *Clin Res* 34:249A, 1986.
29. Barton LL, Granoff DM, Barenkamp SJ: Nosocomial spread of *Haemophilus influenzae* type b infection documented by outer membrane protein subtype analysis. *J Pediatr* 102:820–824, 1983.
30. Shapiro ED, Wald ER: Efficacy in eliminating pharyngeal carriage of *Haemophilus influenzae* type b. *Pediatrics* 66:5–8, 1980.
31. Yogev R, Lander HB, Davis AT: Effect of TMP-SMX on nasopharyngeal carriage of ampicillin-sensitive and ampicillin-resistant *Hemophilus influenzae* type b. *J Pediatr* 93:394–397, 1978.
32. Glode MP, Schiffer MS, Robbins JB, Khan W, Battle CU, Armenta E: An outbreak of *Hemophilus influenzae* type b meningitis in an enclosed hospital population. *J Pediatr* 88:36–40, 1976.
33. Finland M, Barnes MW: Acute bacterial meningitis at Boston City Hospital during 12 selected years, 1935–1972. *J Infect Dis* 136:400–415, 1977.
34. Finland M, Barnes MW: Duration of hospitalization for acute bacterial meningitis at Boston City Hospital during 12 selected years, 1935–1972. *Am J Med Sci* 274:4–12, 1977.
35. Blanc VF, Tremblay NAG: The complications of tracheal intubation: A new classification with a review of the literature. *Anesth Analg* 53:202–213, 1974.
36. Miller EH Jr, Caplan ES: Nosocomial *Hemophilus* pneumonia in patients with severe trauma. *Surg Gyn Obstet* 159:153–156, 1984.
37. Caplan ES, Hoyt NJ: Nosocomial sinusitis. *JAMA* 247:639–641, 1982.
38. Chilcote RR, Baehner RL, Hammond D: Septicemia and meningitis in children splenectomized for Hodgkin's disease. *N Engl J Med* 295:798–800, 1976.
39. Siber GR: Bacteremias due to *Haemophilus influenzae* and *Streptococcus pneumoniae*. Their occurrence and course in children with cancer. *Am J Dis Child* 134:668–672, 1980.
40. Lerman SJ: Systemic *Hemophilus influenzae* infection: a study of risk factors. *Clin Pediatr* 21:360–364, 1982.
41. Albritten WL, Brunton JL, Meier M, Bowman MN, Slaney LA: *Haemophilus influenzae*: Comparison of respiratory tract isolates with genitourinary tract isolates. *J Clin Microbiol* 16:826–831, 1982.
42. Nelson JD: The increasing frequency of β-lactamase-producing *Haemophilus influenzae* b. *JAMA* 244:239, 1980.
43. Mason EO Jr, Kaplan SL, Lamberth LB, Hinds DB, Kvernland SJ, Louiselle EM, Feigin RD: Serotype and ampicillin susceptibility of *Haemophilus influenzae* causing systemic infections in children: 3 years of experience. *J Clin Microbiol* 15:543–546, 1982.

44. Rubin LG, Medeiros AA, Yolken RH, Moxon ER: Ampicillin treatment failure of apparently β-lactamase-negative *Haemophilus influenzae* type b meningitis due to novel β-lactamase. *Lancet* II:1008–1010, 1981.
45. Marks WA, Stutman HR, Marks MI, Abramson JS, Ayoub EM, Chartrand SA, Cox FE, Geffen WA, Harrison CJ, Harrison D, Paryani S, Tolpin MD: Cefuroxime versus ampicillin plus chloramphenicol in childhood bacterial meningitis: a multicenter randomized controlled trial. *J Pediatr* 109:123–130, 1986.
46. Odio CM, Faingezicht I, Salas JL, Guevara J, Mohs E, McCracken GH Jr: Cefotaxime vs. conventional therapy for the treatment of bacterial meningitis of infants and children. *Pediatr Infect Dis* 5:402–407, 1986.
47. Del Rio MA, Chrane D, Shelton S, McCracken GH Jr, Nelson JD: Ceftriaxone versus ampicillin and chloramphenicol for treatment of bacterial meningitis in children. *Lancet* I:1241–1244, 1983.
48. Mendelman PM, Doroshow CA, Gandy SL, Syriopoulou V, Weigen CP, Smith AL: Plasmid mediated resistence in multiply resistant *Haemophilus influenzae* type b causing meningitis: Molecular characterization of one strain and review of the literature. *J Infect Dis* 150:30–39, 1984.
49. Campos J, Garcia-Torrel S, Gairí JM, Fábregues I: Multiply resistant *Haemophilus influenzae* type b causing meningitis: Comparative clinical and laboratory study. *J Pediatr* 108:897–902, 1986.
50. Mendelman PM, Chaffin DO, Clausen C, Stull TL, Williams JD, Smith AL: Failure to detect ampicillin-resistant, non-β-lactamase-producing *Haemophilus influenzae* by standard disk susceptibility testing. *Antimicrob Agents Chemother* 30:274–280, 1986.
51. Wald ER, Reilly JS, Casselbrant M, Ledesma-Medina J, Milmoe GJ, Bluestone CD, Chiponis D: Treatment of acute maxillary sinusitis in childhood: a comparative study of amoxicillin and cefaclor. *J Pediatr* 104:297–302, 1984.
52. Garner JS, Simmons BP: Guideline for isolation precautions in hospitals. *Infect Control* 4(Suppl):245–325, 1983.

18

Meningococcus

Eugene D. Shapiro, M.D.

BACKGROUND

Neisseria meningitidis is a Gram-negative diplococcus that can be subclassified into serogroups A,B,C,D,X,Y,Z,W-135, and 29-E on the basis of the chemical structure of its polysaccharide capsule (1,2). These serogroups can also be subdivided into antigenically distinct serotypes based on their outer membrane proteins. The organism causes a variety of infections in humans that include meningitis, overwhelming sepsis (purpura fulminans), arthritis, pericarditis, pneumonia, conjunctivitis and urethritis (1). There is a less common subacute form of invasive disease, that is termed "chronic meningococcemia" (3). The organism has also been implicated as a cause of occult bacteremia in children (4).

N. meningitidis is the second most common cause of bacterial meningitis (after *Haemophilus influenzae* type b) in the United States (5). In 1984, there were 2,746 cases of meningococcal infection reported to the Centers for Disease Control (1.2 cases/100,000 people), of which nearly 50% occurred in children under 5 years of age (6). The highest age-specific annual incidence of meningococcal meningitis occurred among 3–5-month-old infants (11.5 cases/100,000) (7). This incidence gradually diminished to 3.8 cases/100,000 among children 1–2 years of age and 0.7 cases/100,000 among children 5 years of age and older (7). Meningococcal disease is an endemic disease in the United States, although the occurrence of epidemics in the military, schools, and day-care centers as well as widespread outbreaks in cities and countries in underdeveloped nations is well recognized (8–15). In the United States, endemic meningococcal disease is caused most

commonly by serogroup B, followed in frequency by serogroups W-135, C, and Y (16).

Humans are the only known reservoir of *N. meningitidis*. The organism colonizes the posterior nasopharynx and is transmitted by respiratory droplets or oral secretions. Because droplets are usually transmitted only a short distance, close contact with infected individuals is important in the transmission of the organism. High rates of colonization with *N. meningitidis* among close contacts of colonized individuals (whether or not they developed invasive disease), such as among members of the same family, household, or military barracks, support this assumption (8,17–24). *N. meningitidis* may also infect the genital tract and the anal canal of both men and women, thus making possible transmission of the organism via sexual contact (25–27).

The prevalence of carriage of *N. meningitidis* varies in different populations, but it is estimated to be approximately 2–10% during non-epidemic periods (17,19,24,28–30). By contrast, 17–50% of household contacts of people with either invasive meningococcal infection or pharyngeal colonization with meningococci are themselves colonized with the organism (17,19,21,23,24). In military populations, the prevalence of colonization is even higher, ranging up to 80% (17,24,31).

Invasive disease may develop in susceptible individuals after colonization with *N. meningitidis*, presumably via bacteremic spread after invasion of the bloodstream from the pharynx. The factors that determine susceptibility to invasive meningococcal disease are imperfectly understood, although certain factors have been shown to be important. Bactericidal serum antibodies are clearly a major factor in immunity to meningococci (32). A prime reason for the

231

attack rate of meningococcal disease being greatest among infants is the delay in the development of humoral antibodies against T-cell-dependent antigens, such as the polysaccharide capsular antigens of *N. meningitidis* and *H. influenzae* type b, until the 2nd year of life. Serum antibodies develop in response not only to pharyngeal colonization with *N. meningitidis*, but also from pharyngeal or intestinal colonization with bacteria that are antigenically cross-reactive with *N. meningitidis*, as well as from colonization with unencapsulated (nongroupable) meningococci (29,33). Defects in the complement system have been clearly associated with the development of invasive meningococcal disease (34). Some studies have suggested that antecedent viral infections may potentiate invasive disease (23,35). Other factors associated with the development of disease include deficiencies of specific subclasses of IgG, the presence of circulating IgA antibodies that block bactericidal antibodies, and strains of meningococci that produce a protease that is specific for human IgA (36–38). Data about the role of crowding and shared sleeping quarters in promoting the transmission of meningococci have been conflicting; some studies suggest that these factors promote transmission (9,28,39), whereas other studies conducted in the military found that the degree of crowding seemed to be unrelated to an enhanced risk of either the transmission of meningococci or the development of invasive disease (12,40,41).

POPULATION

There is little information about the risks of nosocomial meningococcal disease in pediatric patients. By contrast, there are substantial data about "secondary" meningococcal disease in households and in the military, information that may illuminate the problem of nosocomial disease (42–45). Secondary cases of meningococcal disease have been defined arbitrarily as cases in contacts of the index case that occur between 1–30 days later. The risk of secondary disease among members of the household of the index case has been estimated to be up to 1,000 times greater than the risk of invasive meningococcal disease in the general population (42,46–48). The rate of colonization with meningococci of household contacts of index cases far exceeds that of the general population, ranging up to 50% (8,18,21,39). Because of this high rate of

colonization and the relatively intimate and frequent contact among household members, the likelihood is great that uncolonized individuals will encounter and eventually become colonized with the organism. In susceptible individuals, invasive disease may follow colonization. Although there is often fear among close contacts of a patient with meningococcal disease that the patient might have spread the infection to one of the contacts, it is more probable that the patient acquired the bacteria from a colonized close contact, rather than vice versa (49). This is because invasive disease usually occurs relatively shortly after acquisition of a virulent organism in a susceptible host.

Genetic factors have been shown to be associated with susceptibility to infection with encapsulated bacteria in children, and similar factors are also likely to be associated with susceptibility to invasive meningococcal infections (49,50). Family members of a patient with invasive disease are also more likely than others to share genetic susceptibility to meningococcal disease.

Although anecdotes about nosocomial meningococcal disease are common, documented nosocomial disease is very rare (51–56). Most of the documented cases of nosocomial infection have occurred in association with patients who had proven or suspected pneumonia due to *N. meningitidis* (51–55). In addition, there has been at least one instance in which meningococcal disease was suspected of being acquired in a microbiology laboratory (57).

For nosocomial infection to occur as a result of the hospitalization of a patient with an invasive meningococcal infection, the organism must be transmitted from the affected patient to a susceptible individual, either directly or via another colonized person. Studies have been done to try to assess the risk of transmission of meningococci from patients with invasive disease to their contacts in the hospital. Artenstein and associates found that the rate of carriage of meningococci in hospital contacts of cases was nearly identical to that of a control group of persons with no contact with these cases (58). Omer and associates also found that the rate of carriage of meningococci among other patients on wards with patients with meningococcal meningitis was not higher than would have been expected in the general population (59).

Maki and associates prospectively assessed the risk of nosocomial acquisition of *N. men-*

ingitidis among 287 hospital personnel who were exposed to 10 patients with invasive meningococcal disease that was not initially recognized (60). Consequently, no isolation precautions were in effect for these patients for from 1–5 days (median, 2 days). Although none of the 77 personnel who were exposed to the 7 patients with meningococcemia or meningococcal meningitis became colonized, 9% of the 210 personnel who had been exposed to the 3 patients with meningococcal pneumonia were colonized with the same serogroup of meningococcus as that of the index patient. By comparison, in a control group of 94 personnel who had no exposure to the index patients with pneumonia during the same time period, only 1% were colonized with meningococci of the same serogroup ($P < 0.01$). None of the contacts developed invasive meningococcal infection. Maki concluded that the risk of nosocomial transmission of meningococci is substantially increased among contacts of patients with unrecognized meningococcal pneumonia. The results are consistent with other reports of nosocomial colonization and invasive disease in association with patients with meningococcal pneumonia (51–56,61).

Nosocomial transmission of meningococci is most likely to occur among the contacts in the hospital who have the closest contact with the patient's oral secretions and aerosolized respiratory particles. Thus, personnel who have had close contact with the patient's secretions, such as during mouth-to-mouth resuscitation or intubation, would be at especially high risk of acquisition of the organism. However, any person who may have had contact with oral or respiratory secretions of the patient is at risk of acquiring the organism. Nevertheless, it must be emphasized that nosocomial transmission of *N. meningitidis* is rare, and invasive disease as a result of nosocomial transmission of the organism is extraordinarily rare because most contacts in the hospital have protective serum antibodies and are immune.

DIAGNOSIS

The most important factor in the early detection of nosocomial meningococcal infection is to maintain an awareness of the possibility that such infections, though rare, may occur. By maintaining a reasonable index of suspicion, prompt evaluation of symptomatic hospital contacts of patients with meningococcal infections should lead to early treatment and isolation of affected individuals.

Because asymptomatic colonization with *N. meningitidis* is so common, it is not reasonable to do nasopharyngeal cultures of contacts or of the hospital staff in general for surveillance. Prolonged high rates of carriage of meningococci among hospital personnel without the development of invasive disease have been documented (17,41). In addition, a single positive culture provides no information about how long that individual has been colonized. Because colonization often persists for many months, it is quite possible that the colonized person has developed immunity to the organism. Indeed, the individual whose culture is negative for *N. meningitidis* may be at greater risk.

Because a large proportion of other members of the household of a patient with infection with *N. meningitidis* are also colonized, a high index of suspicion must also be maintained for such individuals. If a close contact of the index patient has meningococcal pneumonia that is untreated, then that person may pose a risk to other patients and hospital personnel during visits to the hospital (56). Consequently, any such persons who develop petechiae or symptoms of either a systemic illness or lower respiratory disease should be evaluated promptly for the possibility of meningococcal infection. Likewise, personnel who have cared for a patient with meningococcal disease should be evaluated promptly if they develop such signs or symptoms.

TREATMENT AND PROPHYLAXIS

Chemoprophylaxis for hospital personnel is indicated only for the rare instances in which someone has unusually intimate contact with the respiratory secretions of a patient with meningococcal disease (except pneumonia), such as someone who either performed mouth-to-mouth resuscitation or suctioned or intubated the patient. In addition, chemoprophylaxis is indicated for both personnel and other patients who have had contact with a person with meningococcal pneumonia (caused by an encapsulated strain) before respiratory isolation of that person was effected. Because the majority of personnel who care for patients with meningococcal infections do not have this kind of contact with the patient, chemoprophylaxis is usually not indicated (62,63). If chemoprophylaxis is indicated, sulfadiazine should be used if the strain of *N. meningitidis* is known to be susceptible to this drug. If the strain of bacteria is resistant to sulfadiazine, or if its susceptibility to specific antimicrobials is unknown, then rifampin should be used. The dosages of both rifampin and sulfadiazine are shown in Table 18.1. If chemoprophylaxis is indicated, it should be administered promptly. Chemoprophylaxis is not 100% effective, and it may be taken too late to have an effect. Consequently, the possibility of meningococcal infection in a contact should not be dismissed because chemoprophylaxis had been taken. In the unlikely event that nosocomial meningococcal infection should occur, the affected person should be treated as anybody would be treated, with penicillin administered parenterally in high dosages.

Finally, there is a licensed polysaccharide vaccine against serogroups A,C,Y and W-135 that is recommended for prophylactic use for household contacts of a patient with meningococcal disease and to halt epidemics in a community. There are no official recommendations for its use in hospital personnel. While the vaccine is not indicated in most situations in hospitals, its availability should be kept in mind if an ongoing epidemic should occur in a hospital.

PREVENTION

The most important measures to take to prevent nosocomial transmission of *N. meningitidis* are to recognize (or suspect) the diagnosis promptly and to institute respiratory isolation immediately (64). Recommendations for isolation of patients with meningococcal disease are outlined in Table 18.2. Infected patients should have a private room. All persons who enter the room or who have close contact with the patient should wear masks. Gowns and gloves are unnecessary. However, hands of both personnel and visitors must be washed after either the pa-

Table 18.2.
Respiratory Isolation of Patients with Proven or Suspected Meningococcal Disease

1. Respiratory isolation for 24 hours.
2. Private room.
3. Masks for all who enter the room (Gowns and gloves are unnecessary).
4. Strict handwashing after contact with the patient.

tient or articles that may have been contaminated by the patient are touched. Respiratory isolation should be maintained for 24 hours after the institution of effective antimicrobial therapy. If this policy is strictly followed, chemoprophylaxis of contacts of the patient should not be necessary.

There have been no studies that have assessed the persistence of pharyngeal colonization with *N. meningitidis* in patients with invasive disease after the institution of parenteral antimicrobial therapy. This question is of importance because penicillin, standard therapy for invasive disease, is not effective in eradicating pharyngeal colonization in the usual doses that are administered orally (65). This issue has been studied in patients with disease caused by *H. influenzae* type b, a bacteria that is not always eradicated from the pharynx by standard parenteral therapy (45). However, although the organism may persist in the pharynx after parenteral therapy is completed, during parenteral therapy its concentration (and presumably its transmissibility) is markedly reduced (66). By inference, it is likely that the same thing occurs with patients with meningococcal disease. Consequently, although the patient with meningococcal disease should receive either sulfadiazine or rifampin after parenteral therapy is completed (if chemoprophylaxis was administered to the household, daycare center, or other close contacts), the risk of nosocomial transmission of the organism more than 24 hours after parenteral treatment has begun seems to be negligible.

Table 18.1.
Dosages for Prophylaxis of Meningococcal Disease

Drug	Age of Contact	Dosage
Rifampin	Adults	600 mg every 12 hours for 2 days
	1 month–12 years	10 mg per kg of body weight every 12 hours for 2 days
Sulfadiazine	Adults	1 g every 12 hours for 2 days
	1–12 years	500 mg every 12 hours for 2 days
	<1 year	500 mg every 24 hours for 2 days

REFERENCES

1. Glode MP, Smith AL: Meningococcal disease. In Feigen RD, Cherry JD, (eds): *Textbook of Pediatric Infectious Diseases.* Philadelphia, WB Saunders, 1981, pp 916–928.
2. Feldman HA: Meningococcal infections. In Evans AS, Feldman HA (eds): *Bacterial Infections of Humans: Epidemiology and Control.* New York, Plenum, 1982, pp 327–344.
3. Benoit FL: Chronic meningococcemia. *Medicine* 35:103–112, 1963.
4. Dashefsky B, Teele DW, Klein JO: Unsuspected meningococcemia. *J Pediatr* 99:231–233, 1981.
5. Schlech WF III, Ward JI, Band JD, Hightower A, Fraser DW, Broome CV: Bacterial meningitis in the United States, 1978 through 1981: The national bacterial meningitis surveillance study. *JAMA* 253:1749–1754, 1985.
6. Centers for Disease Control: Annual summary 1984: Reported morbidity and mortality in the United States. *MMWR* 33 (No. 54):38, 1986.
7. Klein JO, Feigin RD, McCracken GH Jr: Report of the task force on diagnosis and management of meningitis. *Pediatrics* 78(Suppl):959–982, 1986.
8. Gauld JR, Nitz RE, Hunter DH, Rust JH, Gauld RL: Epidemiology of meningococcal meningitis at Ford Ord. *Am J Epidemiol* 82:56–72, 1965.
9. Feigen RD, Baker CJ, Herwaldt LA, Lampe RM, Mason EO, Whitney SE: Epidemic meningococcal disease in an elementary-school classroom. *N Engl J Med* 307:1255–1257, 1982.
10. Hudson PJ, Vogt RL, Heun EM, Brondum J, Coffin RR, Plikaytis BD, Bolan G: Evidence for school transmission of *Neisseria meningitidis* during a Vermont outbreak. *Pediatr Infect Dis* 5:213–217, 1986.
11. Jacobson JA, Felice GA, Holloway JT: Meningococcal disease in day care centers. *Pediatrics* 59:299–300, 1977.
12. Artenstein MS, Rust JH, Hunter DH, Buescher EL: Acute respiratory disease and meningococcal infection in army recruits. *JAMA* 201:1004–1008, 1967.
13. Greenwood BM, Hassan-Kind M, Whittle HC: Prevention of secondary cases of meningococcal disease in household contacts by vaccination. *Br Med J* 1:1317–1319, 1978.
14. Munford RS, Sussaurana de Vasconcelos Z, Phillips CJ, Gelli DS, Gorman GW, Risi JB, Feldman RA: Eradication of carriage of *Neisseria meningitidis* in families: A study in Brazil. *J Infect Dis* 129:644–649, 1974.
15. Binkin N, Band J: Epidemic of meningococcal meningitis in Bamako, Mali: Epidemiological features and analysis of vaccine efficacy. *Lancet* 2:315–317, 1982.
16. Band JD, Chamberland ME, Platt T, Weaver RE, Thornsberry C, Fraser DW: Trends in meningococcal disease in the United States, 1975–1980. *J Infect Dis* 148:754–758, 1983.
17. Aycock WL, Mueller JH: Meningococcus carrier rates and meningitis incidence. *Bacteriol Rev* 14:115–160, 1950.
18. Greenfield S, Feldman HA: Familial carriers and meningococcal meningitis. *N Engl J Med* 277:497–502, 1967.
19. Marks ML, Frasch CE, Shapera RM: Meningococcal colonization and infection in children and their household contacts. *Am J Epidemiol* 109:563–571, 1979.
20. Nicolle LE, Postl B, Kotelewetz E, Remillard F, Bourgault AM, Albritton W, Harding GKM, Ronald A: Chemoprophylaxis for *Neisseria meningitidis* is an isolated arctic community. *J Infect Dis* 145:103–109, 1982.
21. Munford RS, Taunay A de E, de Morais JS, Fraser DW, Feldman RA: Spread of meningococcal infection within households. *Lancet* 1:1276–1278, 1974.
22. Saez-Nieto JA, Campos J, Latore C, Juncosa T, Sierra M, Garcia-Tornell T, Garcia-Barreno B, Lopez-Galindez C, Casel J: Prevalence of *Neisseria meningitidis* in family members of patients with meningococcal infection. *J Hyg (Cambridge)* 89:139–148, 1982.
23. Olcen P, Kjellander J, Danielsson D, Lindquist BL: Epidemiology of *Neisseria meningitidis*: Prevalence and symptoms from the upper respiratory tract in family members to patients

with meningococcal disease. *Scand J Infect Dis* 13:105–109, 1981.
24. Broome CV: The carrier state: *Neisseria meningitidis*. *J Antimicrob Chemother* 18(Suppl A):25–34, 1986.
25. Givan KF, Thomas BW, Johnston AG: Isolation of *Neisseria meningitidis* from the urethra, cervix, and anal canal: Further observations. *Br J Vener Dis* 53:109–112, 1977.
26. Blackwell C, Young H, Bain SSR: Isolation of *Neisseria meningitidis* and *Neisseria catarrhalis* from the genitourinary tract and anal canal. *Br J Vener Dis* 54:41–44, 1978.
27. Talbot MD, Collins BN: Presumed sexual transmission of meningococci. *J Infect* 3:273–276, 1981.
28. DeWals P, Gilquin C, De Maeyer S, Bouckaert A, Noel A, Lechat MF, Lafontaine A: Longitudinal study of asymptomatic meningococcal carriage in two Belgian populations of schoolchildren. *J Infect* 6:147–156, 1983.
29. Gold R, Goldschneider I, Lepow ML, Draper TF, Randolph M: Carriage of *Neisseria meningitidis* and *Neisseria lactamica* in infants and children. *J Infect Dis* 137:112–121, 1978.
30. Greenfield S, Sheehe PR, Feldman HA: Meningococcal carriage in a population of "normal" families. *J Infect Dis* 123:67–73, 1971.
31. Fraser PK, Bailey GK, Abbott JD, Gill JB, Walker DJC: The meningococcal carrier rate. *Lancet* 1:1235–1237, 1973.
32. Goldschneider I, Gotschlich EC, Artenstein MS: Human immunity to the meningococcus: I. The role of humoral antibodies. *J Exp Med* 129:1307–1326, 1969.
33. Goldschneider I, Gotschlich EC, Artenstein MS: Human immunity to the meningococcus: II. Development of natural immunity. *J Exp Med* 129:1327–1348, 1969.
34. Ellison RT III, Kohler PF, Curd JG, Judson FN, Reller LB: Prevalence of congenital or acquired complement deficiency in patients with sporadic meningococcal disease. *N Engl J Med* 308:913–916, 1983.
35. Young LS, LaForce FM, Head JJ, Feeley JC, Bennett JV: A simultaneous outbreak of meningococcal and influenza infections. *N Engl J Med* 287:5–9, 1972.
36. Bass JL, Nuss R, Mehta KA, Morganelli P, Bennett L: Recurrent meningococcemia associated with IgG₂-subclass deficiency (letter). *N Engl J Med* 309:430, 1983.
37. Griffiss JM, Bertram MA: Immunoepidemiology of meningococcal disease in military recruits. II. Blocking of serum bactericidal activity by circulating IgA early in the course of invasive disease. *J Infect Dis* 136:733–739, 1977.
38. Mulks MH, Plant AG: IgA protease production as a characteristic distinguishing pathogenic from harmless Neisseriaciae. *N Engl J Med* 299:973–975, 1978.
39. Kaiser AB, Hennekens CH, Saslaw MS, Hayes PS, Bennett JV: Seroepidemiology and chemoprophylaxis of disease due to sulfonamide-resistant *Neisseria meningitidis* in a civilian population. *J Infect Dis* 130:217–224, 1974.
40. Artenstein MS: Prophylaxis for meningococcal disease. *JAMA* 231:1035–1037, 1975.
41. Dudley SF, Brennan JR: High and persistent carrier rates of *N. meningitidis* unaccompanied by cases of meningitis. *J Hyg (Cambridge)* 34:525–541, 1934.
42. The Meningococcal Disease Surveillance Group: Meningococcal disease: Secondary attack rate and chemoprophylaxis in the United States, 1974. *JAMA* 235:261–265, 1976.
43. The Meningococcal Disease Surveillance Group: Analysis of endemic meningococcal disease by serogroup and evaluation of chemoprophylaxis. *J Infect Dis* 134:201–204, 1976.
44. McCormick JB, Bennett JV: Public health considerations in the management of meningococcal disease. *Ann Intern Med* 83:883–886, 1975.
45. Shapiro ED: Prophylaxis for bacterial meningitis. *Med Clin N Amer* 69:269–280, 1985.
46. Norton JF, Gordon JE: Meningococcus meningitis in Detroit in 1928–1929. *J Prev Med* 4:207–214, 1930.
47. Lee WW: Epidemic meningitis in Indianapolis, 1929–1930. *J Prev Med* 5:203–209, 1931.
48. Juels C, Morrison FR, Overturf GD, Roberto RR, Chin J: Men-

ingococcal disease in California: Epidemiology and management. *West J Med* 128:195–202, 1978.

49. Wenzel P, Davies JA, Mitzel JR, Beam WE Jr: Non-usefulness of meningococcal carriage-rates (letter). *Lancet* 2:205, 1973.

50. Ambrosino DM, Schiffman G, Gotschlich EC, Schur PH, Rosenburg GA, DeLange GG, vanLoghem E, Siber GR: Correlation between G2m(n) immunoglobulin allotype and human antibody response and susceptibility to polysaccharide encapsulated bacteria. *J Clin Invest* 75:1935–1942, 1985.

51. Granoff DM, Shackleford PG, Suarez BK, Nahm MH, Cates KL, Murphy TV, Karasic R, Osterholm MT, Pandey JP, Daum RS, and the Collaborative Group: *Haemophilus influenzae* type b disease in children vaccinated with type b polysaccharide vaccine. *N Engl J Med* 315:1584–1590, 1986.

52. Barnes RV, Dopp AC, Celberg HJ, Silva J Jr: *Neisseria meningitidis*: A cause of nosocomial pneumonia. *Am Rev Resp Dis* 111:229–231, 1975.

53. Rose HD, Lenz IE, Sheth NK: Meningococcal pneumonia: A source of nosocomial infection. *Arch Intern Med* 141:575–577, 1981.

54. Bureau of Biologics: Nosocomial meningococcemia—Wisconsin. *MMWR* 27:358–363, 1978.

55. Cohen MS, Davies JA, Baltimore R, von Graevenitz A, Pantelick E, Camp B, Root RK: Possible nosocomial transmission of group Y *Neisseria meningitidis* among oncology patients. *Ann Intern Med* 91:7–12, 1979.

56. Trapana Y, Holzman B, Neill M: Nosocomial meningococcemia. *Am J Infect Control* 11:152, 1983, (abstract).

57. Bhatti AR, DiNinno VL, Ashton FE, White LA: A laboratory-acquired infection with *Neisseria meningitidis*. *J Infect* 4:247–252, 1982.

58. Artenstein MS, Ellis RE: The risk of exposure to a patient with meningococcal meningitis. *Milit Med* 133:474–477, 1968.

59. Omer EE, Williams RF: Epidemiology of contact and non-contact meningococcal carrier rate in hospital patients. *E Afr Med J* 56:339–341, 1979.

60. Maki DG, McCormick R, Zilz M, Hassemer C, Alvarado C: Prospective study of the risk of transmission of *N. meningitidis* to hospital personnel (abstract). *Clin Res* 33:887A, 1985.

61. Reich RM, Maki DG: Transmission of *Neisseria meningitidis* in a critical care unit (abstract). Presented at the 21st Interscience Conference on Antimicrobial Agents and Chemotherapy, Washington, D.C., American Society for Microbiology, 1981.

62. Reingold AL, Broome CV: Nosocomial central nervous system infections. In Bennett JV, Brachman PS (eds): *Hospital Infections*, ed 2. Boston, Little, Brown, 1986, pp 521–529.

63. Williams WW: CDC guideline for infection control in hospital personnel. *Infect Control* 4:339, 1983.

64. Garner JS, Simmons BP: CDC guideline for isolation precautions in hospitals. *Infect Control* 4:259, 1984.

65. Hoeprich PD: Prediction of antimeningococcic chemoprophylactic efficacy. *J Infect Dis* 123:125–133, 1971.

66. Ogle JW, Rabalais GP, Glode MP: Duration of pharyngeal carriage of *Haemophilus influenzae* type b in children hospitalized with systemic infections. *Pediatr Infect Dis* 5:509–511, 1986.

19

Pertussis

James W. Bass, M.D., M.P.H.

BACKGROUND

Pertussis (whooping cough) is a communicable infection of the respiratory tract characterized by severe paroxysms of cough, terminating in a gasping stridulous inspiratory effort. This characteristic musical whooping-like sound is responsible for the term "whooping" cough. Pertussis, which means intensive cough, is a more appropriate term than whooping cough since not all patients with pertussis whoop. The term "pertussis" is usually reserved for the clinical illness produced by infection with *Bordetella pertussis*; however, pertussis-like syndromes are occasionally noted in association with infection due to *B. parapertussis, B. bronchiseptica, Chlamydia trachomatis*, adenovirus, respiratory syncytial virus, and combinations of these organisms. When pertussis-like illnesses are associated with agents other than *B. pertussis*, the disease is usually milder and of shorter duration.

Clinical Manifestations

Clinical manifestations of pertussis evolve in three stages (1–5): the catarrhal, prodromal, or preparoxysmal stage; the paroxysmal or spasmodic cough stage; and the convalescent stage. *The catarrhal stage* develops after an incubation period of 7–10 days (range 5–21 days) and is manifested by a period of 1 to several days of clear mucoid rhinorrhea, nasal congestion, and cough. This stage is indistinguishable from the common cold. As the disease progresses, the cough grows more persistent and severe, particularly at night, and the nasopharyngeal secretions become more profuse, thick, and tenacious. There is heavy shedding of *B. pertussis* organisms in these secretions. It is at this stage that the organism is most easily cultured and the patient is most contagious.

The paroxysmal stage of the disease begins when protracted bouts of cough occur in distinct paroxysms lasting up to several minutes. These paroxysms may number from only 2–3 or up to 50 or more episodes daily. In older infants and young children, the characteristic inspiratory whooping is often heard as the child gasps for breath during cough paroxysms. The paroxysms are frequently terminated by vomiting of previously swallowed thick ropy secretions. Severe cough paroxysms may be associated with florid venous engorgement of the head and neck with secondary petechiae, periorbital edema, and subconjunctival and scleral hemorrhages. In older children and young adults with relatively larger airways, the characteristic whoop is often absent and the disease may present only as a severe persistent cough, lasting up to 2–3 months (6–8). Also, in young, weaker infants less than 6 months of age, cough paroxysms may not be associated with the characteristic whoop but are more often terminated in exhaustion, vomiting, aspiration, cyanosis, apnea, and loss of consciousness (9–11). Without resuscitation, these episodes may result in anoxic brain damage or death. The paroxysmal stage averages about 2 weeks in duration, but it may last only a few days or persist for up to 3–4 weeks. Coughing gradually decreases in frequency and severity until paroxysms no longer occur.

The convalescent stage begins when chronic cough replaces paroxysms. This stage usually lasts 3–4 weeks, but rarely it may persist for months. Figure 19.1 shows the wide variation between the duration of these three clinical stages of pertussis among different individuals and the relationship to the shedding of pertussis organisms during these stages in untreated individuals. Although low-grade fever may be seen in patients in the late catarrhal and early parox-

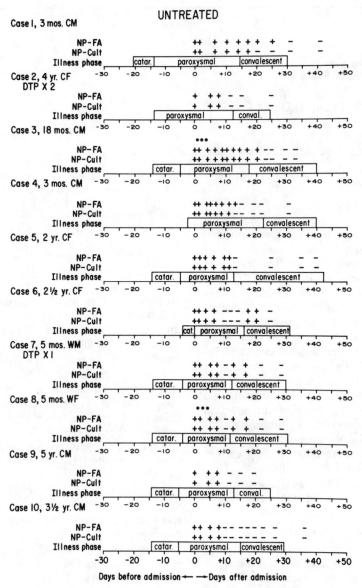

Figure 19.1. Clinical course of pertussis in 10 hospitalized patients who received no antimicrobial therapy. NP-FA indicates nasopharyngeal fluorescein-conjugated antibody test and NP-Cult indicates nasopharyngeal culture for *Bordetella pertussis* organisms. Variations in duration of positive NP-FA, NP-Cult, and catarrhal, paroxysmal, and convalescent stages of illness are shown. (From Bass JW, et al.: Antimicrobial treatment of pertussis. *J Pediatr* 75:768, 1969.)

ysmal stages of pertussis, significant fever is not a feature of the disease (2–4). Its presence suggests the development of a suppurative complication.

Epidemiology and Pathogenesis

The epidemiology and pathogenesis of pertussis have been studied extensively. It is spread by the airborne route directly from droplet and droplet nuclei from aerosols generated by the intense cough of infected individuals. It is one of the most highly communicable human diseases. Attack rates in families and in some community outbreaks approach 100% of susceptible contacts (12). Infection begins when aerosol particles containing viable pertussis organisms settle onto the mucus film overlying the respiratory passages of susceptible individuals. Here they adhere to the cilia of the epithelial cells that line the mucosal surface of the respiratory passages from the nasopharynx to the respiratory bronchioles in the lung. Only here do they replicate, and they do not invade further. Their presence in large numbers on these surfaces is associated with elaboration of profuse tenacious mucus and ciliastasis, resulting in stagnation of mucus flow and inspissation of air passages. Patchy atelectasis and bronchitis are constant, and secondary bronchopneumonia is common. As the disease progresses, specific secretory antibodies are elaborated in increasing quantities into the respiratory secretions. The organism is gradually eliminated from the respiratory passages, ciliary movement is restored, thick mucous secretions are diminished, mucous inspissations are resolved, and the airway returns to normal. No anatomic or functional residua remain. Gross and microscopic (including scanning and transmission electron-microscopy) examination of tissues of patients and experimental animals infected with *B. pertussis* organisms have led to this present understanding of the pathogenesis and the pathophysiology of pertussis (2,4). However, the mechanisms causing cough paroxysms that characterize the disease, the encephalopathy that sometimes complicates the illness, and the principles of immunity against pertussis are less clearly understood.

Complications

Complications from pertussis can be grouped into three categories (2–4): suppurative secondary infections; tissue and organ injury from increased pressure effects due to severe cough paroxysms and vomiting; and central nervous system manifestations due to anoxia caused by cough paroxysms or direct effect from pertussis toxin or toxins. Suppurative complications include pneumonia, which occurred in 16% of hospitalized patients with pertussis in a recent report (13); acute otitis media; and sinusitis. Although *B. pertussis* organisms may be directly involved in these infections, treatment should also be directed toward the usual bacterial pathogens that cause these infections in children relative to age. Suppurative complications should be suspected when patients develop significant fever or elevation of the erythrocyte sedimentation rate since neither of these findings are characteristic of uncomplicated pertussis. Complications due to increased tissue and organ pressure from severe persistent coughing include petechial hemorrhages of the face, neck, conjunctiva, and sclera as well as subarachnoid hemorrhages and subdural hematoma; interstitial, mediastinal, and subcutaneous emphysema; pneumothorax, rectal prolapse, rupture of the diaphragm and umbilical and inguinal hernia. Persistent vomiting may lead to dehydration, metabolic alkalosis with tetany and inanition. Central nervous system complications include convulsions, which occurred in 1.9%, and encephalopathy, which occurred in 0.3% of hospitalized patients in a recent report (13), coma, paralysis, deafness, blindness, mental retardation, and epilepsy.

POPULATION

The World Health Organization estimates that there are 60 million cases of pertussis annually worldwide and that the disease is responsible for ½–1 million deaths each year (5). However, these estimates are probably very low, since reliable statistics on the incidence rates are not available. In developing countries, the great majority of cases are not likely to be reported either because of deficiencies in the reporting system or because the patient does not come in contact with health services. Even in developed countries, it has been estimated that only 10–20% of cases are reported. The incidence of pertussis in developed countries is still significant where pertussis vaccines are not used or where ineffective vaccines are used.

In the United States, where an effective pertussis vaccine has been used with good compliance for many years, the incidence of the disease has declined greater than 99.6% from a high of 265,269 cases with 7,000 deaths reported in 1934 to a low of 1,010 cases with seven deaths reported in 1976 (14). Most authorities credit this remarkable public health achievement to the use of pertussis vaccine. The pertussis vaccines used in the United States and most other countries today are whole cell vaccines that are essentially the same as the original pertussis vaccines that were developed in the United States in the 1930s, field tested in the late 1930s and in the 1940s, and widely accepted for general use since the 1950s. Early vaccine trials showed 85–94% protection (15–17), and recent studies reassessing current efficacy confirm 91% (18) to 94% (13) protection for children in the United States and 95% protection for children in England (19).

As with smallpox, humans are the only reservoir of pertussis, and an asymptomatic carrier state does not exist (20). For these reasons, it has been proposed that with better pertussis vaccine compliance, herd immunity could be attained and, like smallpox, eradication of pertussis could be achieved (21). Although pertussis vaccine compliance has reached greater than 90% in the United States during the past several years (13,22) careful analysis of the epidemiology of pertussis reveals ominous trends (14). Before 1950, most individuals contracted pertussis in childhood and developed lifelong immunity. Since 1950, most preschool children have received pertussis vaccine, so for the past 3 decades, most preschool and school-aged children and most adults have not been susceptible to the disease. The only pertussis-susceptible age group that existed during this period were newborn and very young infants, since passive immunization against pertussis does not occur even from mothers who have had the disease and are themselves immune. These young infants cannot be considered immunized until they have received at least the first three pertussis vaccine injections, which in the United States are routinely given at 2, 4, and 6 months of age. Accordingly, during the 1950s, 1960s, and 1970s this pertussis-susceptible population persisted but had little chance for exposure to the disease since most preschool and school-aged children were immune because of prior immunization. Adults were also immune because they had had the disease when they were children.

These circumstances are now changing. Unlike the natural disease, which confers permanent immunity, pertussis vaccine confers only partial and transient immunity. Eighty–95% protection persist for 3 years, decreasing thereafter to 12 years, after which no protection is evident (12). Because pertussis vaccine is the most reactigenic of all vaccines routinely given to children, and reactions appear to increase with age, primary immunization or even booster vaccine administration are not advised beyond 7 years of age (23). For these reasons, the epidemiology of pertussis in the United States is changing. As children born since 1950 grow into adulthood, their vaccine-induced immunity has waned, and they are rapidly emerging as a steadily enlarging new group of pertussis susceptible adults. Meanwhile, the older group of adults born before 1950 with pertussis-induced lifelong immunity grows older and smaller. This changing epidemiology of pertussis infection among different age groups resulting from widespread use of pertussis vaccine was documented at one medical center when the epidemiology of pertussis cases seen during the 1960s was compared with that of cases seen during the 1970s (8). A recent analysis of the evolving populations of pertussis-immune and pertussis-susceptible individuals on a national scale reveals that these trends should become increasingly more dramatic in the 1980s and coming years (14).

These changes are further complicated by other epidemiological factors. Since pertussis in adults and infants younger than 6 months of age is usually atypical and often lacks the whoop that leads to suspicion of the diagnosis, there is usually a significant delay before the diagnosis is made. This leads to further spread of the disease, since control measures including isolation and the use of antibiotics are also delayed. Adults with atypical symptoms often unknowingly infect young infants whose severe life-threatening apneic and cyanotic episodes usually prompt their hospitalization for observation and intensive care management. The diagnosis of pertussis often remains unsuspected in the infants, who may then infect young medical personnel whose vaccine immunity has waned, including pediatric house officers, nurses, and other personnel, as well as other susceptible infants in the intensive care area. Two such large hospital outbreaks have been reported (24,25) and other nosocomial pertussis epidemics appear to be occurring with increasing frequency across the United States (26,27).

This problem will grow worse in coming years unless a better pertussis vaccine is developed. In order to reverse these trends, a vaccine is needed, one that will produce lasting immunity or is sufficiently safe and well-tolerated to allow booster administration at appropriate intervals to maintain immunity throughout life, as has been achieved with diphtheria and tetanus toxoids.

Recently, two substances that appear to induce specific protective antibodies against pertussis have been identified. These substances are produced by *B. pertussis* organisms. Filamentous hemagglutinin (FHA) allows adherence of pertussis organisms to the cilia of respiratory tract epithelial cells, which is essential for the organism to replicate and initiate infection. Here, replicating organisms produce lymphocytosis-promoting-factor hemagglutinin (LPF), called pertussis toxin by some investigators, which, upon absorption, binds to specific receptors of certain tissue cells. This process allows entrance of the toxin into the cell, thereby altering the function of the cell. These actions appear to be responsible for the symptoms of the disease. In limited studies, acellular vaccines containing purified FHA and LPF antigens have been shown to protect experimental animals against pertussis. These acellular vaccines have been used exclusively in Japan since 1981 (28) and are presently undergoing early clinical trials in the United States (29,30). With over 20 million doses given to children in Japan and in the limited studies conducted to date in the United States, protective efficacy has been established to be equal to whole cell vaccines, with vaccinees showing higher anti-FHA and anti-LPF antibody titers to that seen in individuals who had received whole cell vaccine and similar titers to that seen after natural pertussis infection. These vaccines have been associated with less local and systemic reactions than whole cell vaccines. Most importantly, they have been associated with less severe life-threatening reactions, including collapse, shock, and encephalopathic reactions.

These acellular vaccines could lead to improved pertussis vaccine acceptance and compliance, better and more lasting pertussis vaccine protection (including acceptance of booster vaccine administration throughout life, if needed) and the possibility of eradication of the disease. However, at this time, the exact risk of severe life-threatening reactions associated with the use of these vaccines, duration of immunity, safety, and effectiveness of booster administration are unknown. Even if these developments are validated and refined, it would be several years before such a new pertussis vaccine program could be implemented. Meanwhile, the problems outlined related to the continued use of present-day whole-cell vaccine will probably grow worse, and pertussis infections will remain a significant nosocomial problem.

Until a better pertussis vaccine program is perfected and implemented, it is essential that use of present-day whole-cell pertussis vaccine be continued if suppression of the disease, which has been achieved with these vaccines, is to be maintained. Recent experiences in England and Japan should reinforce the validity of this recommendation. In England, where unfavorable publicity on the risk-benefit of pertussis vaccine appeared in the medical literature (31–33) and in the lay press in the mid-1970s, pertussis immunization rates decreased from 79% in 1973 to 13% in 1978. From 1977–1980, a major pertussis epidemic ensued, and 102,500 individuals contracted whooping cough, 5,000 were hospitalized with the disease, 200 developed secondary pneumonia, 83 experienced seizures, and 28 died. A comparable experience occurred in Japan in the mid-1970s (28,34). In that country, 152,072 cases of pertussis, with 17,001 deaths, were reported in 1947. Similar data were recorded for the next few years until 1951 when a whole-cell pertussis vaccine similar to that used in the United States and England was used on a nationwide scale. The incidence of pertussis declined in ensuing years. Fewer than 1,000 cases, with only 2–5 deaths, were reported annually from 1970–1974. In late 1974, two deaths were reported due to pertussis vaccine–associated shock and encephalopathy. Pertussis vaccine use was halted, and immunization rates declined from 78% in 1974 to less than 14% in 1976. During the period from 1975–1979, a major epidemic of pertussis occurred, with 31,730 cases and 113 deaths.

DIAGNOSIS

The clinical diagnosis of pertussis is clearly evident when the disease presents in its classical form. However, many cases are probably reported without laboratory confirmation (13,22), and most atypical cases, where the diagnosis is unsuspected, go unreported. A history of contact with a person known to have pertussis is helpful, but this will generally be negative in a highly immunized population.

The laboratory diagnosis is confirmed by isolation and identification of *B. pertussis* organisms in respiratory tract secretions. This is best performed by culture of posterior nasopharyngeal swabs directly onto fresh (bright cherry-red and moist) Bordet-Gengou (BG) medium containing 15–20% rabbit blood. Cough plates are no longer recommended. An additional plate containing 2.5 µg/ml of methicillin should also be inoculated. This modification will help to inhibit growth of normal nasopharyngeal bacterial flora and to prevent overgrowth of *B. pertussis*. The BG plate without methicillin should be included because some strains of the organism may be inhibited by methicillin at this concentration. The plates should be streaked and sealed with masking tape to prevent drying during the relatively long incubation period required for growth of *B. pertussis*. Incubation should be at 35°C, and the plates should be inspected daily. Growth of pertussis organisms is seldom evident before 72 hours, so colonies resembling *B. pertussis* appearing before this time should be suspect. However, *B. parapertussis*, which has similar colony morphology, often exhibits appreciable growth as early as 48 hours. Growth of *B. pertussis* is usually first seen at the end of the 3rd day of incubation as small pinpoint-like colonies with a metallic luster resembling droplets of mercury when examined with a hand lens under reflected light. When growth is heavy and confluent, it may appear as a silvery sheen resembling aluminum foil. Maximal growth usually occurs after 5 days, but plates should not be discarded until after 7 days. Suspected colonies can be confirmed as *B. pertussis* by Gram staining, agglutination with specific antiserum, and staining with specific fluorescein-conjugated antiserum with examination under fluorescent microscopy. Presumptive diagnosis can be made within minutes by direct examination of the nasopharyngeal smear on glass slides stained with fluorescein-conjugated *B. pertussis* and *B. parapertussis* antiserum.

Serological tests, including agglutination and complement fixation, are not helpful in early diagnosis. Even when paired acute and convalescent sera are available for testing for 4-fold rises in *B. pertussis* agglutination and complement fixation antibodies, the sensitivity and specificity of these tests are lacking. Some individuals with culture-proven pertussis fail to develop agglutinins to pertussis, whereas some who have not had the disease or prior immunization can be shown to have agglutinins. Laboratory tests that detect specific *B. pertussis* antigens in respiratory tract secretions or antibodies to these antigens in respiratory tract secretions or serum early in the course of the disease are under development (28,35).

Absolute lymphocytosis is a valuable presumptive diagnostic aid. It is usually present in the typical disease in the late catarrhal and early paroxysmal stages. The degree of lymphocytosis usually parallels the severity of the patient's disease. However, lymphocytosis may be absent, especially in infants under 6 months of age, partially immunized individuals, and those with atypical illness.

TREATMENT

Supportive Treatment

Supportive treatment is most important. Severe disease and a high incidence of complications occur most often in young infants. Most infants who die are only 2, 3, or 4 months old, so it is wise to hospitalize very young infants with pertussis, particularly those who have severe cough paroxysms with cyanotic and apnea episodes. Gentle suctioning and supplemental oxygen administration are indicated during severe bouts of paroxysmal cough. Fluid depletion from suctioning of secretions, vomiting, and inadequate oral fluid intake may necessitate parenteral fluid and electrolyte administration. Parenteral hyperalimentation may be necessary in patients with protracted disease to prevent malnutrition. Intensive care management of these patients with experienced and efficient nursing care is probably the most important factor in survival.

Cough suppressants, expectorants, antispasmodics, sedatives, and mucolytic agents have not been shown to be of benefit. Mist therapy is not helpful, but continuous well-humidified oxygen is indicated for patients who show sustained evidence of hypoxemia. Blood gas determinations should be performed in patients with labored respirations, unstable vital signs, or alterations in mental status. Such patients usually have significant complications such as atelectasis, bronchopneumonia, or encephalopathy.

Specific Treatment

Specific treatment modes of proven benefit are few. Pertussis hyperimmune globulin was marketed for many years for treatment of pertussis and for prevention of pertussis in exposed susceptible contacts. More recent, well-controlled clinical trials evaluating the effectiveness of this product for these purposes have failed to show any benefit (36,37). It is no longer recommended and it is no longer available in the United

States. Specific modes of treatment that may be of benefit include the use of antimicrobial agents, corticosteroids, and β_2-adrenergic stimulants, specifically albuterol, which is marketed outside the United States as salbutamol.

Antimicrobial Agents

Antimicrobial agents have limited usefulness in the treatment of pertussis. Pertussis organisms are eradicated from patients with the disease if they are treated with agents that are active against *B. pertussis* organisms, provided that the drug diffuses in significant concentrations into respiratory tract secretions (38–42). As illustrated in Figure 19.2, erythromycin, the tetracyclines, and chloramphenicol have been shown to be effective in achieving early bacteriologic cures. However, no antimicrobial agent alters the subsequent course of the illness when given in the

paroxysmal stage of the disease, when the diagnosis is most often first suspected. There is evidence that these drugs may be effective in preventing the disease when administered in the incubation period (culture-positive asymptomatic susceptibles) and in attenuating the disease when given in the catarrhal or preparoxysmal stage of the disease. Their administration to patients at any stage of pertussis may render them noninfectious. These reasons constitute the rationale for the use of antimicrobials in pertussis. For these purposes, erythromycin appears to be the most effective and least toxic drug studied to date. Ampicillin is not effective (38,39).

Some studies have shown a failure of erythromycin to eradicate pertussis organisms from patients with pertussis or bacteriologic relapse after treatment is discontinued (26,27). Since erythromycin resistance of *B. pertussis* organ-

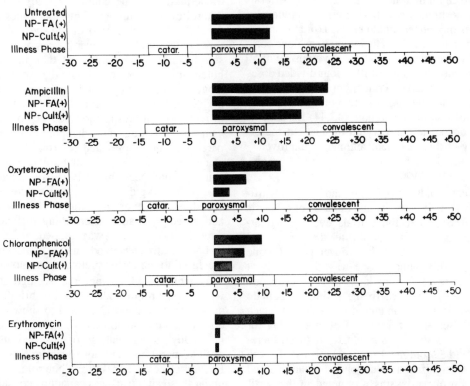

Figure 19.2. Clinical course of pertussis in 10 patients who received no antimicrobial therapy compared with 10 each who received ampicillin, oxytetracycline, chloramphenicol, or erythromycin. NP-FA, nasopharyngeal fluorescein-conjugated antibody test; NP-Cult, culture for *Bordetella pertussis* organisms. Group means are shown for duration of therapy, persistence of positive NP-FA and NP-Cult, and duration of catarrhal, paroxysmal, and convalescent stages of illness. (From Bass JW, et al.: Antimicrobial treatment of pertussis. *J Pediatr* 75:768, 1969.)

isms has not been reported, other reasons for these differences in treatment response have been sought. A recent critical review of these studies (42) concluded that the reports showing failure compared with reports where good results were achieved revealed two differences between the two groups. These differences were in the preparation of erythromycin that was used and in duration of treatment. The erythromycin used in the studies that showed good results was the estolate ester, while those used in the studies that showed failures were other esters that are known to produce lower serum and respiratory tract secretion levels when both are given at the same recommended dosage. Another reason for the difference observed between the groups was duration of treatment. All erythromycin preparations were associated with bacteriologic relapse if treatment was for less than 14 days. It is concluded that erythromycin remains the drug of choice for treatment of patients with pertussis with the limited benefits described previously. The estolate ester should be used (or a treatment regimen that can be relied upon to achieve comparable serum concentrations) in a dosage of 50 mg/kg/day (maximum 1 g) in four divided doses daily for 14 days. Trimethoprim-sulfamethoxazole 8–40 mg/kg/day in two oral doses for 14 days is a possible alternate (43,44) for patients who do not tolerate erythromycin, but the efficacy of this treatment regimen is unproven.

Corticosteroids

Corticosteroids have been shown to significantly alter the severity and duration of pertussis in two controlled clinical trials, even when treatment was not begun until after the paroxysmal stage of the disease had developed. In one study (45), betamethasone was given orally at a dose of 0.075 mg/kg/day. In the second study (46), hydrocortisone sodium succinate (Solu-Cortef, Upjohn Pharmaceuticals) was given intramuscularly at a dose of 30 mg/kg/day for 2 days; the dose was gradually reduced thereafter and discontinued after several days. In both studies, significant reduction in the number and duration of paroxysms was noted in the corticosteriod-treated groups compared with untreated controls. Other anecdotal observations attesting to the effectiveness of corticosteroids in the treatment of pertussis have been reported (47). Additional controlled studies are needed, but it appears that corticosteroids may be beneficial in the treatment of pertussis, particularly in very young infants with life-threatening paroxysms. One of these regimens may be used or other corticosteriod preparations at comparable dosages, should be equally effective.

Albuterol

Albuterol (salbutamol) has been shown to be effective in the treatment of pertussis in a number of studies reported over the past several years. Earlier studies suggested that β-adrenergic blockade occurs in individuals with pertussis and that β_2-blockade may be responsible for some of the cough, cough paroxysms, and the whoop, which are the major clinical features of the disease (48). These observations have led investigators to evaluate the use of albuterol, a potent β_2-adrenergic stimulant in the treatment of pertussis. In one controlled study (49), albuterol-treated children (1 mg four times daily for children below 2 years of age and 2 mg four times daily for children over 2 years of age) had significantly fewer paroxysms than in non-albuterol-treated controls. In another study (50), albuterol in a dosage of 0.5 mg/kg/day in three divided doses was associated with a better rate of recovery with respect to frequency of paroxysms of coughing and whooping when compared with placebo-treated controls. In a study evaluating the effect of albuterol in pertussis using sound spectrum analysis (51), albuterol (0.3–0.5 mg/kg/day in three divided doses) reduced the frequency and duration of the whoops and eased the patient's breathing difficulties. After 3 days, the drug was stopped, and within 24 hours the frequency and duration of the whoops increased to the earlier pretreatment maximum, and apneic episodes reappeared. A single study, which was randomized, double-blind, and crossover in design (52), failed to show a benefit of albuterol treatment. This study involved nine study patients; only six of these had culture-positive pertussis, and none were critically ill. Failure to show a benefit for albuterol treatment under these circumstances cannot be considered conclusive. A recently reported study of similar design (53) involving only one patient with pertussis who had severe paroxysmal coughing with cyanosis requiring ventilatory support showed a dramatic effect due to albuterol (0.5 mg/kg/day in three doses) treatment.

Although the safety and effectiveness of albuterol has not been established in children less than 2 years of age, its use may be indicated for treatment of pertussis in small infants with severe life-threatening paroxysms. A dosage of 0.3–0.5 mg/kg/day in three divided doses has been shown to be effective and well-tolerated.

PREVENTION AND CONTROL OF OUTBREAKS

There are only three effective measures in the prevention of pertussis: vaccination; isolation of infected individuals; and possibly antimicrobial prophylaxis in selected circumstances. Passive protection of exposed susceptible contacts with pertussis hyperimmune globulin has been proven to be ineffective and is no longer recommended (32). The effectiveness of pertussis vaccine in the prevention of pertussis before exposure has been discussed. Attempts to active immunization after exposure affords no benefit (54). Pending the development of a better pertussis vaccine, the only means available for control of pertussis outbreaks are early indentification and isolation of infected individuals (23,41); booster pertussis vaccine administration for selected partially immunized individuals under 7 years of age (23); and attempts at antimicrobial prophylaxis (23,25,38,40–42).

Individuals suspected of having pertussis should be placed in respiratory isolation, pending laboratory confirmation of the diagnosis (Table 19.1). Attempts at antimicrobial prophylaxis should be initiated in the patient, and all significant contacts using erythromycin in the dosage given and for the duration outlined under treatment. Isolation should be continued for at least 5 days after starting erythromycin (3 weeks after onset of paroxysms, if antimicrobials are not given) in those individuals whose naso-

pharyngeal smears are shown to be positive for *B. pertussis* organisms by fluorescent microscopy or culture. Children less than 7 years old who have had at least four doses of pertussis vaccine should receive a booster dose, usually DTP, unless the fourth dose had been given within the past 3 years or after the 4th birthday. Children less than 7 years old who have received their third dose 6 months or more before exposure should be given their fourth dose at this time. Children who have had culture-proven pertussis need not receive further pertussis immunization, and individuals older than 7 years of age should not receive pertussis vaccine.

REFERENCES

1. Gordon JE, Hood RI: Whooping cough and its epidemiological anomalies. *Am J Med Sci* 222:333–469, 1951.
2. Olson L: Pertussis. *Medicine* 54:427–469, 1975.
3. Cherry JD: The epidemiology of pertussis and pertussis immunization in the United Kingdom and the United States. *Current Prob in Pediatr* 19:7–77, 1984.
4. Pittman M: The concept of pertussis as a toxin-mediated disease. *Pediatr Infect Dis* 3:467–486, 1984.
5. Muller AS, Leeuwenburg J, Pratt DS: Pertussis: epidemiology and control. *Bull WHO* 62:899–908, 1986.
6. Morse SI: Pertussis in adults. *Ann Intern Med* 68:953–954, 1968.
7. Linnemann CC, Hasenbeny J: Pertussis in adults. *Annu Rev Med* 28:179–195, 1977.
8. Nelson JD: The changing epidemiology of pertussis in young infants. *Am J Dis Child* 132:371–373, 1978.
9. Strangert K: Clinical course and prognosis of whooping-cough in Swedish children during the first six months of life. *Scand J Infect Dis* 2:45–48, 1978.
10. Congeni BL, Orenstein DM, Nankervis GA: Three infants with neonatal pertussis. *Clin Pediatr* 17:113–118, 1978.
11. McGregor J, Ogle JW, Curry-Kane G: Perinatal pertussis. *Obstet Gynecol* 68:582–586, 1986.
12. Lambert HJ: Epidemiology of a small pertussis outbreak in Kent County, Michigan. *Public Health Rep* 89:365–369, 1965.
13. Centers for Disease Control: Pertussis: United States, 1982 and 1983. *MMWR* 33:573–575, 1984.
14. Bass JW, Stephenson SR: The return of pertussis. *Pediatr Infect Dis* 6:141–144, 1987.
15. Kendrick PL, Eldering G: Progress report on pertussis immunization. *Am J Public Health* 26:8–11, 1936.
16. Kendric PL: Use of alum-treated pertussis vaccine and of alum-precipitated combined vaccine and diphtheria toxoid for active immunization. *Am J Public Health* 32:615–626, 1942.
17. Kendrick PL: A field study of alum-precipitated combined pertussis vaccine and diphtheria toxoid for active immunization. *Am J Hyg* 38:193–202, 1943.
18. Broome CE, Fraser DW: Pertussis in the United States, 1979: a new look at vaccine efficacy. *J Infect Dis* 144:187–190, 1981.
19. Preston NW: Protection by pertussis vaccine, little cause of concern. *Lancet* 1:1065–1067, 1976.
20. Bass JW: Is there a carrier state in pertussis? *Lancet* 1:96, 1987.
21. Kendrick PL: Can whooping cough be eradicated? *J Infect Dis* 132:707–712, 1975.
22. Centers for Disease Control: Pertussis, Maryland. *MMWR* 32:297–305, 1983.
23. Report of the Committee on Infectious Diseases (Red Book), ed 20. Elk Grove Village IL, American Academy of Pediatrics, 1986, pp 266–275.
24. Kurt TL, Yeager AS, Guenette S, Dunlop S: Spread of pertussis by hospital staff. *JAMA* 221:264–267, 1972.

Table 19.1.
Respiratory Isolation Guidelines for Pertussis Infection

1. Isolate all suspected or proven cases for minimum of 5 days in treated patients or 3 weeks after onset of paroxysms in untreated patients.
2. Private room required.
3. Mask required for close patient contact.
4. Booster pertussis vaccine administration for partially immunized individuals under 7 years of age.
5. Erythromycin therapy for index patient.
6. Erythromycin prophylaxis for significant contacts.

25. Linemann CC, Perlstein PH, Ramundo N, Minton SD, Englender GS: Use of pertussis vaccine in an epidemic involving hospital staff. *Lancet* 2:540–543, 1975.
26. Valenti WM, Pincus PH, Messner MK: Nosocomial pertussis: possible spread by a hospital visitor. *Am J Dis Child* 134:520–521, 1980.
27. Halsey NA, Welling MA, Lehman RM: Nosocomial pertussis: a failure of erythromycin treatment and prophylaxis. *Am J Dis Child* 134:521–522, 1980.
28. Sato Y, Fukumi H, Kimura M: Development of a pertussis component vaccine in Japan. *Lancet* 1:122–126, 1984.
29. Edwards KM, Lawrence E, Wright PF: Diphtheria, tetanus and pertussis vaccine: a comparison of the immune response and adverse reactions to conventional and acellular pertussis components. *Am J Dis Child* 140:867–871, 1986.
30. Lewis K, Cherry JD, Holroyd HJ, Baker LR, Dudenhoefler FE, Robinson RG: A double-blind study comparing an acellular pertussis-component DTP vaccine with a whole-cell pertussis-component DTP vaccine in 18-month-old children. *Am J Dis Child* 140:872–876, 1986.
31. Miller DL, Alderslade R, Ross EM: Whooping cough and whooping cough vaccine: the risks and benefit debate. *Epidemiol Rev* 4:1–24, 1982.
32. Griffith AH: Medicine and the media: vaccination against whooping cough. *J Biol Stand* 9:475–482, 1981.
33. Joint Committee on Vaccination and Immunization: *The Whooping Cough Epidemic 1977–1979.* London, Her Majesty's Stationers, 1981.
34. Kanai K: Japan's experience in pertussis epidemiology and vaccination in the past thirty years. *Jpn J Sci Biol* 33:107–143, 1980.
35. Mertsola J, Ruuskanen O, Eerola E, Viljanen MK: Intrafamilial spread of pertussis. *J Pediatr* 103:359–363, 1983.
36. Morris D, McDonald JC: Failure of hyperimmune globulin to prevent whooping cough. *Arch Dis Child* 32:236–239, 1957.
37. Balagtas RC, Nelson KE, Levin S: Treatment of pertussis with pertussis immune globulin. *J Pediatr* 79:203–208, 1971.
38. Bass JW, Klenk ET, Kotheimer JB, Linnemann CC, Smith MHD: Antimicrobial treatment of pertussis. *J Pediatr* 75:768–781, 1969.
39. Islur J, Anglin CS, Middleton PJ: The whooping cough syndrome: a continuing problem. *Clin Pediatr* 14:171–176, 1975.
40. Baraff LJ, Wilkins J, Wehrle PF: The role of antibiotics, immunizations and adenoviruses in pertussis. *Pediatrics* 61:224–230, 1978.
41. Bass JW: Pertussis: current status of prevention and treatment. *Pediatr Infect Dis* 4:614–619, 1985.
42. Bass JW: Erythromycin for treatment of pertussis. *Pediatr Infec Dis* 5:154–157, 1986.
43. Adcock KJ, Reddy S, Okubadejo QA, Montefiore D: Trimethoprim-sulphamethoxazole in pertussis; comparison with tetracycline. *Arch Dis Child* 47:311–313, 1972.
44. Henry RL, Dorman DC, Skinner JA: Antimicrobial therapy of in whooping cough. *Med J Aust* 2:27–28, 1981.
45. Chandra H, Rao CS, Karan S, Mathur YC: Evaluation of betamethasone and isoniazid along with chloramphenicol in managment of whooping cough. *Indian Pediatr* 9:70–73, 1972.
46. Zoumboulakis D, Anagnostakis D, Albanis V, Matsaniotis N: Steroids in treatment of pertussis: a controlled clinical trial. *Arch Dis Child* 48:51–54, 1973.
47. Barrie H: Treatment of whooping cough. *Lancet* 2:830–831, 1982.
48. Badr-El-Din MK, Aref GH, Mazloum H, El-Towesy YS, Kassem AS, Addel-Moneim MA, Abbassy AA: The beta-adrenergic receptors in pertussis. *J Trop Med Hyg* 79:213–217, 1976.
49. Badr-El-Din MK, Aref GH, Kassem HS, Addel-Moneim MA, Abbassy AA: The beta-adrenergic stimulant, salbutamol, in the treatment of pertussis. *J Trop Med Hyg* 79:218–219, 1976.
50. Pavesio D, Ponzone A: Salbutamol and pertussis. *Lancet* 1:150–151, 1977.
51. Peltola H, Michelsson K: Efficacy of salbutamol in the treatment of infant pertussis demonstrated by sound spectrum analysis. *Lancet* 1:310–312, 1982.
52. Krantz I, Norrby SR, Trollfors B: Salbutamol vs. placebo for treatment of pertussis. *Pediatr Infect Dis* 4:638–640, 1985.
53. Brunskill A, Langdon D: Salbutamol and pertussis. *Lancet* 2:282–283, 1986.
54. Cohn P, Weichsel M, Lapin JH: A comparative study of therapeutic agents in the treatment of pertussis. *J Pediatr* 16:30–35, 1940.

20

Tuberculosis

Jane D. Siegel, M.D.

INTRODUCTION

The continued occurrence of tuberculosis in children is indicative of the ongoing transmission of tuberculous infection in our society. It is of particular concern that the overall rate of decline of tuberculosis in the United States slowed in association with the large influx of Southeast Asian refugees in 1978–1981 and with the increase in human immunodeficiency virus (HIV) infections in 1984–1985 [Figure 20.1 (1)]. In 1986, a provisional total of 22,575 (9.4/100,000 population) cases were reported to the Centers for Disease Control (CDC). This represents a 1.7% increase over the 1985 final total of 22,201 cases and is the first year since 1953 that a substantial increase has been observed [Fig. 20.2 (2)]. The 1986 increase is accounted for by HIV-infected patients, minorities, the homeless, and persons born in foreign countries. The incidence in children has also failed to decline (3). Of the 1,261 cases in children less than 15 years of age, 789 (62.6%) occurred in children younger than 5 years of age (4). Thus, physicians caring for children who are at high risk for the development of tuberculous infection as well as the more severe forms of disease should be familiar with the potential for nosocomial spread from patients and their visitors to employees and other patients as well as from hospital employees to patients. Recommendations for prevention and treatment will be discussed in this chapter.

BACKGROUND

Pathogenesis

It is important to first distinguish between the terms *tuberculous infection* and *tuberculosis*. When tuberculous infection occurs, the tubercle bacillus becomes established in the body, but the patient is asymptomatic and has negative bacteriologic and roentgenographic studies; diagnosis is made by a positive tuberculin skin test. "Tuberculosis" implies the presence of an active disease process in one or more organs. The presence of disease is confirmed by appropriate bacteriologic and other studies. Development of disease is dependent upon multiple host, environmental, and bacterial virulence factors. Only 5–15% of patients with tuberculous infection become ill with tuberculosis. Active disease is most likely to occur within the first 2 years following infection. Although the likelihood that disease will develop decreases over time, the untreated, infected patient has a lifetime risk for active tuberculosis.

Tuberculous infection is spread primarily by airborne droplet nuclei, as demonstrated in two early observations. In their classic studies, Riley and coworkers (5) demonstrated airborne transmission of infection from patients with active tuberculosis to guinea pigs whose only air supply was air exhausted from these patients' ward. Variable patient infectivity was recognized when 35 of the 48 guinea pig infections were associated with exposure to only 3 of the 77 patients with active disease. These studies estimated one infectious particle per 11,000 cubic feet of air for most patients with pulmonary tuberculosis, but as much as one infectious particle per 200 cubic feet of air for the highly infectious patient with laryngeal tuberculosis (6). These concepts were supported by the report of an outbreak of tuberculosis aboard a naval vessel whose air supply was entirely recirculated (7). Nearly 50% of the 308 men aboard ship at the same time as a subject with undiagnosed tuberculosis became infected. Many of the infected men had no direct contact with the index case, but shared a com-

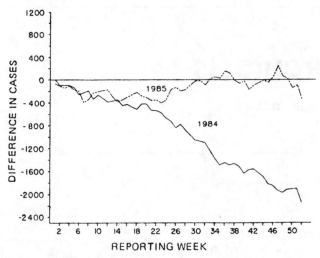

Figure 20.1. Difference in cumulative tuberculosis cases between 1984 and 1983 and between 1985 and 1984, by *MMWR* reporting week—United States

mon air supply only; six of seven who developed active disease had intense contact in common sleeping quarters and work assignments. Similar examples of airborne spread have been documented in general hospital outbreaks of tuberculosis (8; C.E. Haley, unpublished observations).

Once one or more tubercle bacilli come in contact with an alveolus of a susceptible person, a nonspecific, asymptomatic bronchopneumonia develops, and bacilli drain to regional lymph nodes. Then there is the potential for lympho-hematogenous dissemination throughout the body. Most infected persons are able to maintain localized pulmonary infection with healing, granuloma formation, and calcification. Disease develops in newly infected individuals when healing does not occur, and the inflammatory process progresses in the lung or in other organs. In patients who have been remotely infected and untreated, a granuloma may at any time break down, tubercle bacilli multiply, and symptomatic disease develops. Exogenous reinfection may occur in the elderly after the skin test has reverted to negative, indicating loss of immunity (9).

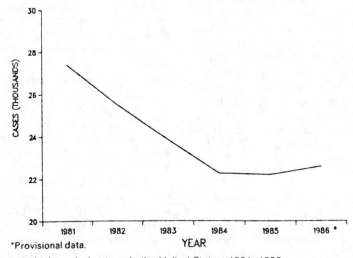

*Provisional data.

Figure 20.2. Reported tuberculosis cases in the United States, 1981–1986

Risk of Transmission

Ninety-five percent of persons with tuberculosis rarely transmit infection to others. Four–5% of patients with tuberculosis infect family members and other close contacts. Only 1% of patients are considered "dangerous disseminators" and transmit infection to their remote contacts. Years of observations and scientific investigations have identified the risk factors that are most highly associated with the transmission of infection. Relative concentration of viable tubercle bacilli in sputum and intimacy of exposure (duration, proximity) are the two most important determinants of transmission (10). The concentration of bacilli present in sputum is directly correlated with the extent of pulmonary disease and the presence of cavitation. Smear-negative, culture-positive sputum contains 5000–9000 bacilli/ml. A cavity with central necrosis may contain 10^3- to *more* than 10^6-fold more bacilli than a nodule of equivalent size (11). Although 10,000 bacilli/ml is the critical concentration required for infectivity, in most circumstances (10), patients with a negative sputum smear and scant organisms on culture have the potential for being infectious. Patient behavior substantially affects infectivity. Frequency of cough, failure to cover mouth and nose when coughing and sneezing, aerosolization of infected sputum during procedures such as endotracheal intubation and bronchoscopy, and ventilation of the patient's room will influence the density of droplet nuclei and therefore the degree of infectivity. Since infants and young children with pulmonary tuberculosis generally do not have cavitary lesions and are unable to generate a forceful cough, they are not considered infective. Chemotherapy renders patients noninfective by decreasing both the frequency of cough and concentration of viable bacilli in sputum and in the droplet nuclei generated (12). Although sputum may not become smear-negative for several weeks after the initiation of chemotherapy, most patients are virtually noninfective after only a few days of effective treatment.

POPULATIONS

Age is an important determinant of the development of active tuberculosis. Complications occur most often in infants and children younger than 5 years of age because of their reduced ability to limit lymphohematogenous dissemination. Progressive pulmonary disease with cavitary lesions is unusual in this age group. Risk for active disease is again increased during adolescence, especially in females, since puberty has a depressant effect on calcium and nitrogen retention, resulting in poor healing of the primary focus of tuberculous infection. The adult type of pulmonary disease with cavitation is a common manifestation of active disease in this age group. Finally, waning immunity in the elderly who have been infected years previously accounts for their characteristic pattern of slowly progressive disease with chronic cavities and bronchogenic spread.

A variety of conditions that compromise host defenses are associated with an increased risk for tuberculosis: congenital or acquired immunodeficiency syndromes, hemophilia, hematologic or reticuloendothelial malignancies and associated chemotherapeutic regimens, nutritional deficiency, weight loss, poorly controlled diabetes mellitus, chronic renal failure, silicosis, and intravenous drug abuse. Of particular importance is the recent recognition of the association between human immunodeficiency virus (HIV) infection and tuberculosis (1,13). It is likely that the increased risk observed in hemophiliacs and intravenous drug abusers is related to the presence of HIV infection. Tuberculosis in immunocompromised patients may be especially difficult to identify because of the frequency of falsely negative skin tests. In the United States, certain ethnic groups have high rates of endemic tuberculosis, the most notable of which are Southeast Asians, Hispanics, Haitians, Indians, and Alaskan Eskimos. Rates of INH resistance of tubercle bacilli recovered from Southeast Asian, Hispanic, and Haitian patients may vary from 13–60% as compared with only 7% in the U.S. population overall (14).

Health care workers comprise another high-risk group for acquisition and transmission of tuberculous infection (15–17). Since 1950, there has been a significant decline in the rate of infection acquired by physicians. Yet, age-specific infection rates among physicians were at least twice the U.S. average in a questionnaire survey of graduates of seven California medical schools reported in 1979 (15). Annual conversion rates during medical school were 1–2%. Infection rates after medical school were largest in internal medicine (14.0%), pediatrics (9.6%), and surgery (9.1%). Annual skin test conversion rates as high as 2.0–8.0% amongst hospital employees have been reported during the modern chemotherapeutic era (16). Not all skin test conversions in hospital workers can, however, be attributed to nosocomial acquisition due to the booster effect of serial tuberculin testing (18) and the high rates of disease to which some groups of employees may be exposed outside of the workplace. In fact, Ruben et al. (19) found no difference in hospital employee conversion rates between the groups with large and small degrees of exposure to patients with tuberculosis.

Exposure to patients with known tuberculosis is rarely associated with transmission of infection unless there is gross contamination of an inadequately ventilated environment (C.E. Haley, unpublished observations). It is generally the patient with undiagnosed tuberculosis who transmits infection to caregivers (8,20–22). In one urban teaching hospital, 35% of 60 tuberculin-negative hospital personnel were infected after 57 hours of exposure to a patient with undiagnosed pulmonary tuberculosis (8). In pediatric hospitals where infants and young children with tuberculosis are considered noninfectious, it is actually the visiting family member with unsuspected cavitary disease who is likely to infect both employees and other patients (22). George and coworkers reported transmission of infection to 30 of 137 (21.9%) exposed children by the mother of a child with tuberculosis of the spine. The mother's cavitary disease was not diagnosed until the child's 29th hospital day. Active disease developed in 23 of these infected children, all of whom were immunocompromised. Most other children beyond the neonatal period reported to have acquired tuberculosis nosocomially had underlying disorders that increased their susceptibility (22–24). Microbiology laboratory workers and postmortem attendants may also be at increased risk of infection due to the aerosolization of tubercle bacilli from unsuspected specimens of infected sputum, pus, and urine or from infected tissue at autopsy of undiagnosed patients (25,26). Thus, prompt diagnosis and contact evaluation are critical for the prevention of nosocomial transmission of tuberculosis.

Transmission of infection from unidentified personnel to susceptible patients has been of particular concern in the neonatal nursery. There are five reports of exposure of large numbers of infants in the newborn nursery to a nurse or nurse's aide with undiagnosed pulmonary tuberculosis [Table 20.1 (27–31)]. Two exposed infants developed miliary tuberculosis in each of two nurseries (27,30), but there was no evidence of nosocomial infection in the more than 700 infants skin tested in the other three reports (28,29,31). Of interest, the source case in one nursery (30) was identified only in retrospect when it was noted that two infants born within 4 days of each other developed miliary tuberculosis at ages 2.5 and 5.5 months of age, and no household sources could be identified. These authors recommend that any infant with tuberculosis who is less than 6 months of age without an identified source be reported to the hospital nursery that cared for that infant. Although the overall infection rate is low, the increased morbidity and mortality in the neonate demands meticulous ongoing surveillance of all nursery personnel.

DIAGNOSIS

A diagnosis of tuberculous infection or tuberculosis is confirmed by the presence of a positive skin test and/or isolation of *Mycobacterium tuberculosis* from infected body fluids or tissues. Chest roentgenograms are not helpful for routine screening and should be reserved for evaluation of symptomatic patients, recent contacts of infectious patients, or patients with special risk factors (32,33).

Skin Testing

Tuberculin skin testing is the method of choice for diagnosis of tuberculous infection (34). Skin hypersensitivity develops within 2–10 weeks following infection. There may, however, be a delay of several months in infected neonates. Both multiple puncture devices and intracutaneous (Mantoux) tests are available. The Mantoux technique is preferred for testing high-risk populations because of the poor control of the exact dose of antigen injected by the multiple puncture devices and the associated high false-positive and false-negative rates. Two preparations of tuberculin are currently available in the United States: old tuberculin (OT) and purified protein derivative (PPD). OT is a filtrate prepared from heat-sterilized concentrated broth cultures of tubercle bacilli. PPD is a more highly

Table 20.1.
Nosocomial Transmission of Tuberculosis in the Newborn Nursery

Study (Ref.)	Index Case	No. Exposed Infants Tested (%)	No. Infants Infected (%)	No. Infants Pos. CXR (%)	Comments
Pope, 1942 Boston (27)	Nurse SX: Cough × 6 months PPD: unknown CXR: RUL infiltrate Sputum: Pos. smear/culture	426/506 (84.2)	26/426 (6.1)	7/26 (26.9)	2/7 (28.6%) fatal miliary disease
Light, 1974 Cincinnati (28)	Aide SX: Cough × 1 month PPD: 60 mm CXR: RUL infiltrate, cavity Sputum: Pos. smear/culture	392/437 (89.7)	0	0	Index case diagnosed by routine CXR
Keim, 1974 Iowa (29)	Aide SX: None PPD: 22 mm CXR: RUL infiltrate, cavity Sputum: Neg. smear Pos. culture	91/97 (93.8)	0	0	Index case diagnosed by routine CXR
Steiner, 1976 New York (30)	Aide, 30 yr SX: None PPD: 25 mm CXR: LUL infiltrate, cavity Sputum: Neg. smear/culture 5 mos after exposure	1,647/1,666 (98.9)	2 (0.1)	2/2 (100)	Retrospective testing after diagnosis of miliary disease in 2 infants born 4 days apart; uneventful recovery in both
Burk, 1978 Alabama (31)	Nurse, 49 yr SX: Fever, cough × 2 months PPD: 15 mm CXR: RUL infiltrate, cavity Sputum: Pos. smear/culture	514/528 (97.3)	0	0	Ultraviolet light in all rooms. No excessive deaths

CXR, chest x-ray; SX, symptoms; PPD, purified protein derivative; RUL, right upper lobe; LUL, left upper lobe.

purified protein precipate obtained from filtrates of OT. The standard tuberculin test contains 5 tuberculin units (5 TU or "intermediate strength") per 0.1 ml of standard purified protein derivative (PPD). One TU per 0.1 ml is used only if there is a suspected tuberculous eye lesion, phlyctenular conjunctivitis, which would be associated with excessive hypersensitivity reactions. "Second strength" or 250 TU per 0.1 ml is used in very rare circumstances because a positive reaction may occur in patients with either tuberculous or atypical mycobacterial infection. Old tuberculin (OT) is available only on multiple puncture devices and should not be used when *M. tuberculosis* infection is suspected, due to the greater cross-reactivity with the atypical mycobacteria.

Reactions occurring within the first 24 hours are mediated by IgG antibodies to cross-reacting antigens of environmental mycobacteria and may not correlate with a true cell-mediated response. A skin test is considered positive if there are 10 or more ml of induration at 48–72 hours. A skin test reaction of 5 or more ml of induration in close contacts of infectious patients should, however, be considered positive. The distinction between true tuberculous infection and exposure to atypical mycobacteria or immunization with BCG in skin test-positive subjects is often questioned. Reactions of 10 ml or greater in persons who have been immunized with BCG are indicative of tuberculous infection due to the usually small reaction associated with BCG and the waning of tuberculin sensitivity over time (34). Epidemiologic history and chest roentgenogram aid in the differentiation of typical from atypical mycobacterial infection with reactions between 10–15 ml. When repeated in 8–12 weeks, the skin test reaction increases with tuberculous infection but decreases or remains the same with atypical mycobacterial infection (35).

Occasionally, falsely negative skin tests may occur. Recently infected patients who have not yet converted their skin tests but have a highly suggestive exposure history or physical examination should be evaluated with a chest roentgenogram and a repeated Mantoux test in 4–12 weeks. Similarly, patients with overwhelming miliary disease, meningitis, or peritonitis may be anergic at the time of initial presentation, but will convert their skin test within 4 weeks of effective therapy. Complete evaluation, including appropriate specimens for bacteriologic

studies, presumptive therapy, and repeat skin testing are indicated in such cases. Anergy in states of malnutrition or chronic disease should be confirmed by skin testing with an appropriate control antigen; DT 1:100 has proved to be useful in immunized patients.

The incidence of tuberculosis in most areas of the United States is too low to warrant screening of all hospital admissions. However, patients with pneumonia, fever of unknown origin, or extrapulmonary infectious processes of uncertain etiology, as well as patients in the high-risk groups previously described should be skin tested. Persistent lymphadenitis, chronic draining ears with mastoiditis, meningitis, and osteomyelitis of the spine are the most frequently encountered extrapulmonary manifestations of tuberculosis in children. Since tubercle bacilli are slow-growing and may not be isolated for 3–6 weeks, the skin test provides a rapid diagnosis in such children. Immunocompromised patients who may be anergic should be screened with a chest roentgenogram as well.

A controversial aspect of skin testing hospital employees is the routine use of the "two-step" method. According to this method, a second Mantoux test is applied 1–3 weeks following the first test in any employee who has an insignificant or negative reaction. An increase of greater than 6 ml from a baseline of less than 10 ml to a final value of greater than 10 is considered a positive "booster" response. Such booster responses are caused by remote tuberculous infection that occurred many years previously, sensitization by atypical mycobacteria, or immunization with BCG vaccine rather than new infection. The median age for employees with booster responses is 45 years, with a continued increase as age advances (18). Identification of employees with such responses at initial testing would avoid the mistaken conclusion that conversion at the annual testing is due to recent infection rather than primary infection many years previously. Since not all hospitals have a significant number of employees with booster responses, it is currently recommended that a pilot study be done to determine the applicability of the two-step method to a specific hospital population (36).

Bacteriologic Studies

All infected body fluids or tissues collected for bacteriologic studies from patients with suspected tuberculosis should have acid-fast smears and cultures performed. Susceptibility testing is recommended for all organisms isolated. When no organism can be recovered from pediatric patients, it can be assumed that the susceptibility pattern is the same as that of the adult source case (37). For special epidemiologic studies of community or institutional outbreaks, mycobacteriophage typing of the outbreak isolates may be requested from the Centers for Disease Control (38).

Adults with pulmonary tuberculosis and older children with adult-type pulmonary disease should submit three to five sputum specimens for acid-fast smear and culture. Sputum specimens may be obtained either by spontaneous expectoration or may be induced by inhaled aerosols. Since young infants and children are unable to produce sputum, the fasting gastric aspirate is a useful alternative. The gastric aspirate contains swallowed sputum and will have a positive acid-fast smear and/or culture in 50% of children with parenchymal disease. Although mycobacteria other than *M. tuberculosis* may be present in the gastric aspirate and account for a falsely positive smear, a strongly positive smear in the appropriate clinical setting supports the presumptive diagnosis of tuberculosis. Best results are obtained when early morning specimens are collected on 3 consecutive days. The patient should be fasted for 8 hours, and 50–75 ml of sterile water (not saline) is utilized for lavage. The gastric acidity should be neutralized with 10% sodium bicarbonate to a pH of 7.0 if there will be a delay of several hours before concentration and culture of the specimen can be performed. This attempt to obtain the organism for identification and susceptibility testing is particularly important in the young child whose index case is unidentified.

Tubercle bacilli may also be identified in bone marrow, urine, or liver biopsy in miliary disease. Liver biopsy is especially helpful in diagnosing congenital infection. Acid-fast smears of cerebrospinal fluid are positive in 85% of patients with tuberculous meningitis if 10–20 ml are submitted and centrifuged before staining. Repeated specimens may be necessary in some patients.

TREATMENT

Active Disease

Since the discovery of streptomycin in 1944, many chemotherapy regimens for tuberculosis have been studied in animals as well as in large clinical trials in humans conducted worldwide. The introduction of isoniazid (INH) in 1952 and of rifampin in the 1960s allowed the development of short-course, intermittent chemotherapeutic regimens. Both 6- and 9-month regimens are now recommended by the American Thoracic Society and the CDC for the treatment of adults (39). The 9-month regimen is preferred for treatment of children because of the paucity of data supporting efficacy of the shorter course in this age group.

The success of these short, intermittent regimens is based on sound bacteriologic principles (40). There are four populations of tubercle bacilli that exist in an infected host:

1. Large, active extracellular multiplication in cavitary lesions;
2. Slow or intermittent multiplication in closed caseous lesions;
3. Slow intracellular multiplication within macrophages;
4. Completely dormant bacilli.

The first-line drugs, isoniazid, rifampin, pyrazinamide, streptomycin, and ethambutol, act on different populations of organisms. Streptomycin is active only against the tubercle bacilli in cavitary lesions, and pyrazinamide is active only against the intracellular macrophage population. Although INH and rifampin have some activity against all populations except the completely dormant bacilli, rifampin is particularly active against the very slowly multiplying organisms that remain dormant most of the time with only intermittent bursts of activity (41). Rifampin and pyrazinamide have greater sterilizing activity, and INH and rifampin have the most effective penetration into cavities, abscesses, and cerebrospinal fluid (42). Ethambutol has only bacteriostatic activity and is less effective than the other first-line drugs. This drug is not used in children less than 13 years of age because of the inability to perform reliable visual field testing for detection of optic neuritis, which is occasionally associated with it. There are no drugs that are active against the population of completely dormant bacilli which are therefore dependent upon host defenses for clearance. The slow multiplication rate (14–22 hours) of even the most active organisms allow once-a-day dosing. Much longer multiplication rates for the intermittently multiplying population which persists after the first 4–8 weeks of treatment are conducive to biweekly dosing for the remaining 4–8 months. The dose of INH is, however, increased during the biweekly phase.

Currently recommended treatment regimens are summarized in Tables 20.2 and 20.3. Important principles are as follows:

1. INH and rifampin are essential components of short-course regimens;
2. Regimens less than 6 months are associated with unacceptably high relapse rates (5% or more);
3. There is no advantage to continuing streptomycin or pyrazinamide beyond 2 months;
4. Pyrazinamide is now the preferred third drug to be added to INH and rifampin, when indicated;
5. Most cases of extrapulmonary tuberculosis may be managed according to the same protocols used for pulmonary tuberculosis;
6. Successful treatment requires at least two bactericidal agents to which the tubercle bacilli are susceptible; therefore, a four-drug regimen is recommended when resistance is suspected. Once the drug susceptibility pattern is known, therapy should be completed with either two or three active drugs, depending on the degree of INH resistance.

Tubercle bacilli are more commonly resistant to INH or streptomycin (10%) than to rifampin, pyrazinamide, or ethambutol (≤1%). The rate of INH resistance varies widely among different racial and ethnic populations. For the overall United States population, the rate of INH resistance is 7.1%. Rates as high as 30–40% have been observed among Hispanic and Asian populations who have recently arrived in the United States, whereas the incidence of INH resistance of isolates from Hispanics, Haitians, and Asians who have been living in the United States is 12–13% (14). It is disturbing that while the rates of resistance to INH, streptomycin, and ethambutol have remained relatively constant during the 1961–1984 period, there has been a significant increase in the resistance rate to rifampin from 1.0% in the 1969–1980 period to 15.8% in the 1981–1984 period in strains isolated from children at the Kings County Medical Center in Brooklyn (43).

The use of corticosteroids as an adjunct to chemotherapy is controversial. Efficacy has been demonstrated in a well-controlled trial for endobronchial disease only (44). Because dramatic clinical improvement has been observed in several other clinical conditions, many authorities advise the use of steroids for treatment of the following conditions: meningitis, acute pericardial effusion with tamponade, pleural effusion with mediastinal shift and severe respiratory compromise, miliary disease with severe alveolocapillary block, endobronchial disease with severe respiratory compromise and collapse/consolidation, and Pott's disease with neurologic compromise (39). The recommended dose is 1 mg/kg/day of prednisone for 6–8 weeks with gradual tapering over the last few weeks. Corticosteroids should never be administered in the absence of two active antituberculous drugs, and the course should not be extended beyond 8 weeks.

Active tuberculosis during pregnancy requires treatment with INH and rifampin (39). Ethambutol is added as a third drug if INH resistance is suspected. Streptomycin should not be used during pregnancy because it interferes with development of the ear and may cause congenital deafness. Pyrazinamide is also contraindicated in pregnancy because of its potential

Table 20.2.
Summary of Recommended First Line Drug Dosages for Treatment of Tuberculosis[a]

Drug	Route	Daily Dose Children[b]	Daily Dose Adults	Twice Weekly Dose Children	Twice Weekly Dose Adults	Maximum Daily Dose
Isoniazid (INH)	P.O.	10–20 mg/kg	5 mg/kg	20–40 mg/kg	15 mg/kg	300 mg[c]
Rifampin (RIF)	P.O.	10–20 mg/kg	10 mg/kg	10–20 mg/kg	10 mg/kg	600 mg
Pyrazinamide (PZA)	P.O.	15–30 mg/kg	15–30 mg/kg	50–70 mg/kg	50–70 mg/kg	2 g
Streptomycin[d] (STREP)	I.M.	20–40 mg/kg	15 mg/kg	25–30 mg/kg	25–30 mg/kg	1 g
Ethambutol (ETHMB)	P.O.	15–25 mg/kg	15–25 mg/kg	50 mg/kg	50 mg/kg	2.5 g

[a]Adapted from Bass JB, et al. (39).
[b]Children whose weight is more than 40 kg should receive the adult dosage regimens.
[c]Maximum daily dose of INH may be increased to 900 mg for twice weekly regimen.
[d]10 mg/kg, maximum 750 mg in persons older than 60 years of age.

Table 20.3.
Summary of Recommended Regimens for Treatment of Tuberculosis[a]

Clinical Manifestations	Drug	Duration
Asymptomatic converter	INH	9–12 months, daily
Household contact, PPD[b]—neg.	INH	3 months daily, repeat skin test, complete 9–12 months if positive
Pulmonary		
INH-susceptible	INH, RIF	9 months or at least 6 months beyond time of sputum conversion: 1–2 months daily, followed by twice weekly for remainder of course.
	INH, RIF, PZA	6 months:[c] 2 months daily followed by INH, RIF twice weekly for 4 months
INH-resistant	INH, RIF, PZA, STREP	9 months: 2 months daily followed by RIF, STREP, PZA twice weekly for 7 months
Extrapulmonary[d]		
uncomplicated[e]	INH, RIF	9 months
extensive	INH, RIF, PZA	9–12 months
meningitis	INH, RIF, PZA	9–12 months

[a]Adapted from Bass JB, et al. (39).
[b]PPD, purified protein derivative; INH, isoniazid; RIF, rifampin; PZA, pyrazinamide; STREP, streptomycin.
[c]Recommended for adults only.
[d]Twice weekly regimens recommended after the first 4–8 weeks or later if clinical improvement has been delayed.
[e]Lymphadenitis.

teratogenicity. INH preventive therapy during pregnancy is recommended only if the woman has been recently infected; it should be initiated after the first trimester. Pyridoxine is administered to all pregnant women receiving INH. INH is secreted in breast milk, but the levels are subtherapeutic and have no harmful effect on the nursing infant.

Management of the neonate born to a tuberculous mother has been well-defined by the Academy of Pediatrics [Table 20.4 (45)]. It is most important to determine the infectivity of the mother and other household contacts and to separate the infant from infective contacts. Repeated skin testing and chest roentgenograms are indicated in order to determine if the infant has become infected. INH should be administered for 3 months while contact investigation and observation are being conducted. Immunization with BCG should be considered if ongoing exposure and poor compliance is anticipated.

Toxicity

INH-induced liver injury is clinically, biochemically, and histologically indistinguishable from viral hepatitis. It occurs most commonly in patients with severe tuberculous disease and increases with advancing age. The incidence of clinical hepatitis in children is less than 0.5%, but biochemical abnormalities may be demonstrated in 10% of patients. Beyond age 35, the incidence of clinical hepatitis steadily increases and may be as great as 5% in those patients older than 50–55 years with biochemical abnormalities in 20% of such patients (46). Hepatitis occurs most frequently within 30–60 days of the initiation of therapy, but may be seen at any time during therapy. Most studies suggest that toxic metabolites of INH produce hepatocellular necrosis. With severe tuberculous disease, INH-associated hepatitis is a result of hepatotoxic products liberated by the tubercle bacilli in the liver after destruction by antituberculous drugs. The risk of hepatitis is increased with doses of more than 20 mg/kg/day, daily alcohol intake, the concomitant administration of other hepatotoxic drugs, or coinfection with a hepatitis virus (47). Genetically controlled rapid acetylation of INH is not predictive of hepatotoxicity (48).

Patients must be followed by a physician at monthly intervals to detect treatment failure, progressive disease, drug toxicity, and to assure compliance. Pretreatment liver function studies should be obtained from patients with extensive tuberculous disease or underlying liver disease, from those receiving multiple hepatotoxic agents,

Table 20.4.
Summary of Management of Newborn Whose Mother Has Tuberculosis at Delivery[a]

Recommended Intervention	Stage of Disease in Mother			
	I Pos. PPD,[b] no active disease	II Minimal disease, noncontagious at delivery	III Active disease, contagious at delivery	IV Disseminated tuberculosis
1. Extensive investigation, skin tests of contacts	Yes	Yes	Yes	Yes
2. Skin test infant[c] (5 TU PPD)	Yes	Yes	Yes	Yes[e]
3. Chest roentgenogram (CXR)[d] of infant	No	Yes	Yes	Yes[e]
4. INH	Until investigation of contacts completed	D/C after 6 months if PPD-neg.	D/C after 6 months if PPD-neg. and mother noncontagious	D/C after 6 months if PPD-neg. and mother noncontagious
5. Rifampin	No	Yes, if CXR-pos.	Yes, if CXR-pos.	Yes, if congenital tuberculosis suspected
6. Separate infant from mother	No	No	Yes	Yes
7. Breast feeding	Yes	Yes	No	No
8. BCG: Consider for all infants expected to have continued contact with noncompliant infective persons.				

[a]Adapted from the Report of the Committee on Infectious Diseases (45).
[b]PPD, purified protein derivative; CXR, chest x-ray; D/C, discontinue; INH, isoniazid; BCG, Bacillus of Calmette and Guérin.
[c]Skin test at 4–6 weeks; if negative, repeat at 3, 6, 12 months.
[d]Check at 4–6 weeks, 3–4 months, 6 months.
[e]Obtain promptly after birth if congenital tuberculosis suspected.

or from all others older than 35 years of age. Liver function studies are repeated in patients younger than 35 years only at the time patients develop symptoms suggestive of hepatitis: unexplained fever for more than 3 days, anorexia, nausea, vomiting, fatigue, or weakness. Hepatic enzymes should, however, be measured periodically in persons older than 35 years of age because of the increased risk of hepatitis. Liver enzymes will return to normal in most persons under 35 years of age while they are continuing to receive INH. If any of the enzyme tests exceed 3–5 times the upper limit of normal, INH should be discontinued. Once the enzymes return to normal, INH may be cautiously restarted.

A chest roentgenogram should be repeated at 2–3 months after the initiation of therapy to document the maximum progression of disease and then upon completion of therapy. Complete resolution of the chest roentgenogram may not occur within the 6- or 9-month course of therapy. This is not an indication to prolong therapy in the patient who has had prompt clinical and bacteriologic response. Chest roentgenograms in such patients should be repeated at 6-month intervals until completely resolved.

Sputum samples should be obtained from adults for acid-fast smear and culture at 2–4 week intervals until sterile. Once effective chemotherapy is initiated, smear positivity does not correlate with infectivity. Sputum may contain large numbers of nonviable organisms for a prolonged period of time, or there may be a substantial decrease in the number of organisms visualized with a persistently positive culture. After 3 months of treatment with regimens containing INH and rifampin, more than 90% of patients have negative sputum smears and cultures (39). Therefore, positive sputum culture at 3 months should prompt a careful evaluation of compliance, drug susceptibility, absorption, and dosage of drugs.

Considering patients infected with resistant organisms, a 6-month goal of 95% sputum conversion is more realistic (49).

PREVENTION

Isolation

Current CDC guidelines (50) for AFB (acid-fast bacilli) isolation are designed for patients with pulmonary tuberculosis who have a positive sputum smear or a chest roentgenogram strongly suggestive of active disease, especially if a cavitary lesion is present. Since young children rarely have this type of transmissible disease, isolation is not recommended. However, it is prudent to place such patients in AFB isolation until the tuberculin status of the visiting family members can be determined. This practice will limit exposure of other patients and employees to visitors with previously unidentified cavitary disease. Patients with draining wounds that contain tubercle bacilli should be isolated until the wound is no longer draining.

The requirements for AFB isolation are outlined in Table 20.5 and are as follows:

1. Private room with negative pressure ventilation and door closed. The type of ventilation, negative or positive, can be readily determined by completely closing the door and placing a tissue at the bottom of the door. Negative pressure ventilation causes the tissue to be blown into the room, whereas positive pressure ventilation causes the tissue to be blown out of the room into the hallway (51). Ultraviolet irradiation of air is a useful adjunct when use of high efficiency filters and negative pressure ventilation cannot be assured (6,21,52).

Table 20.5.
Acid-Fast Bacilli Isolation for Tuberculosis

1. Private room with negative pressure isolation should be provided and door should be kept closed.
2. Masks should be worn if patient is coughing.
3. Gowns should be worn if contamination of clothing with infected body fluids is likely.
4. Gloves should be worn if contamination of hands is likely.
5. Hands should be washed after touching patient or contaminated articles and before caring for another patient.
6. Contaminated articles or instruments should be thoroughly cleaned, sterilized, or discarded.

---

2. Masks should be worn if patient is coughing. Molded, conical masks provide better protection than the looser fitting masks that are used in the operating room (53).
3. Gowns should be worn if contamination of clothing with infected body fluids is likely.
4. Gloves are not required but are beneficial if contamination of hands is likely.
5. Hands must be washed after touching the patient or contaminated articles and before caring for another patient.
6. Contaminated articles or instruments should be thoroughly cleaned, sterilized, or discarded. Fiberoptic bronchoscopes in particular have been implicated in the transmission of disease and should therefore be sterilized by exposure to ethylene oxide for 5 hours or disinfected by immersion in 2% glutaraldehyde for 10–30 minutes, as outlined by Leers (54).

Patients who require AFB isolation should be transported outside the room only for procedures or studies that cannot be performed within the room. Elective procedures are best deferred until infectivity has been substantially reduced by effective chemotherapy. The patient with adult-type pulmonary tuberculosis must wear a mask and have draining wounds well-dressed while being moved through the hallways and in the elevators. Personnel in the area to which the patient is going must be informed in advance so that appropriate precautions can be taken. Most surgical and radiology suites have 80% recirculation of their air supply. Therefore, it is prudent to schedule patients requiring AFB isolation at the end of the day when there will be few, if any, patients in the area who are exposed to the potentially contaminated air. Efforts must be made to be certain that immunocompromised patients will not be exposed to infective patients with tuberculosis during surgical, endoscopic, or radiologic procedures.

Duration of infectivity of patients with positive sputum on treatment is uncertain (55). Most authorities consider patients to be noninfective after 2 weeks of effective chemotherapy; by this time, there is a substantial decrease in both frequency of cough as well as in the number of viable tubercle bacilli. Once appropriate chemotherapy is initiated, infectivity does not always correlate with smear positivity, and recommendations for isolation or return to work must be individualized. Outpatients are not considered to be a significant risk to their household contacts once coughing has decreased and they have been on treatment for 1 week. Such contacts have usually received maximal exposure prior to the time of diagnosis. Separation from neonates or immunocompromised persons should be continued for a minimum of 2 weeks or until the sputum smear becomes negative. Inpatients or infected visiting family members should remain in AFB isolation for a minimum of 2 weeks, unless three consecutive sputum smears obtained on separate days show a substantial reduction in the number of organisms visualized before that time (50).

Employee Health Program

A tuberculosis screening and prevention program is a vital component of all hospital employee health services. Such a program must be formulated with an understanding of the local epidemiology of this disease. Skin testing with the 5 TU PPD by the Mantoux technique is recommended for all personnel at the time of initial employment. In some areas, those persons with a negative response should be retested in 1–3 weeks in order to detect a booster response as described above. A chest roentgenogram should be obtained from all health care workers who have a positive PPD response, a recent exposure to tuberculosis, or pulmonary symptoms suggestive of active disease. After the initial tuberculin screening test, policies for repeat testing should be individualized. The prevalence of tuberculosis in the hospital, community, and employee's ethnic group, personal host susceptibility factors, and degree of exposure to high-risk patients will determine the frequency of screening. Annual screening with skin tests is appropriate for most institutions. There is no benefit to obtaining annual chest roentgenograms as part of a tuberculosis control program (32,33).

Hospital employees with human immunodeficiency virus (HIV) infection and anergy will require routine chest roentgenograms every 3–12 months, depending on their clinical condition (56). Tuberculosis cannot be readily distinguished from other pulmonary infections in these patients on the basis of clinical and radiographic findings; infiltrates may be present in any lung zone, and cavitation is uncommon (57). Therefore, sputum examination or bronchoscopy with

lavage may be required for definitive diagnosis. Tuberculosis surveillance in these employees is best managed by the personal physicians who maintain close communication with the infection control officer.

Personnel who are exposed to an infective patient or family member prior to diagnosis and implementation of appropriate AFB isolation techniques should be skin-tested at 10 weeks following the exposure (58). When there has been gross contamination of the environment from highly infective patients requiring intubation, those personnel in close contact should be tested even if appropriate isolation precautions were taken. If the closest contacts demonstrate conversion, testing should be extended to more remote contacts, including those who may have had only airborne exposure. A baseline skin test should be placed as soon as possible on an exposed employee who has not had a recent skin test to determine if a positive test at 10 weeks will represent a recent conversion. Only those personnel with close, direct contact should be tested if the source patient had a negative sputum smear.

Once an employee with active disease has been identified and chemotherapy is initiated, duration of infectivity must be individualized. The guidelines for hospital personnel returning to work are more conservative than those for patients returning to their own homes, because of the greater risk to new contacts who have not previously been exposed to tuberculosis. Employees should not be allowed to return to work until they are no longer coughing and the sputum is free of bacilli on three consecutive smears obtained on separate days (58). Demonstration of sputum negativity before returning to work is crucial for employees known or suspected of infection with resistant organisms.

Chemoprophylaxis

Chemoprophylaxis, the administration of INH to persons who have asymptomatic tuberculous infection to prevent the development of overt clinical disease, is a critical strategy for the prevention of tuberculosis. Less commonly, INH may be given to prevent the development of new infection when there is a high risk of infection for a limited duration of time. Several large randomized, double-blinded, placebo-controlled studies conducted by the U.S. Public Health Service have demonstrated 70–80% efficacy of a 1-year course of INH in decreasing the incidence of active tuberculosis during the year of treatment (59,60). Efficacy approaches 100% when compliance is assured by administration of medication under direct supervision (60,61). Duration of protection has been established for 20 years following therapy and is likely to last throughout life (62,63). The lack of development of active disease in patients treated before the age of 4 years and the absence of adolescent reactivation in children experiencing subclinical infection between ages 4–15 years further support the likelihood of permanent cure resulting from INH prophylaxis (63).

With the introduction of short courses of chemotherapy for active disease, public health officials have given much consideration to reducing the duration of the course for chemoprophylaxis. It is clear that the efficacy of a 3-month regimen is inferior to regimens of longer duration (60). Efficacy for a 6-month INH regimen has been demonstrated in a study of 28,000 persons in seven Eastern European countries (64). Some patients with fibrotic lesions larger than 2 cm^2 on chest roentgenogram did, however, benefit from an additional 6 months of therapy. A cost-effectiveness analysis recently performed by the CDC has demonstrated the superiority of the 6-month regimen over a 3- or 12-month regimen (65). Although additional data must be gathered in the United States to justify a change in our public health policy, it is likely that shorter courses, 6 or 9 months, will be adopted in the future.

In addition to compliance, the risk of INH-induced hepatitis has been an important limitation to the use of chemoprophylaxis. Current chemotherapy policies are based on information obtained from large numbers of patients enrolled in carefully designed studies. Chemoprophylaxis is recommended for groups of infected persons for whom the risk of developing active tuberculosis is larger than the risk of developing adverse reactions to INH. Both personal and public health aspects must be considered in prescribing prophylactic INH to each individual with subclinical infection. The public health implications are especially important when making policies for hospital personnel. Having considered the various conflicting points of view on this controversial issue, the American Thoracic Society and CDC (39) recommend preventive therapy for the following groups:

1. Household members and other close associates of potentially infectious tuberculosis cases. Such persons have been recently infected and are therefore at greatest risk of developing disease. A PPD reaction of 5 ml or more without a history of past reaction is an indication for preventive therapy. High-risk contacts, such as children or immunocompromised patients who have negative PPD responses initially, are best protected by a 3-month course of INH followed by a repeat skin test. If the 3-month PPD is negative, therapy may be discontinued; if the reaction is positive, the usual chemoprophylactic course should be completed;
2. Newly infected persons: Skin test conversion within the past 2 years and all reactors under 5 years of age;
3. Persons with past tuberculosis that has not been previously treated with adequate chemotherapy;
4. Persons with significant tuberculin reactions and radiographic findings consistent with nonprogressive or previous tuberculosis disease. The risk of developing progressive tuberculosis in such patients is 0.5–5% per year if untreated. The risk is less for those with the smallest lesions and the longest radiographic stability.
5. Persons with significant tuberculin reactions who have any of the high-risk host susceptibility factors previously described (immunodeficiency diseases, immunosuppressive therapy, diabetes mellitus, chronic malnutrition, etc.);
6. Tuberculin skin test reactors under 35 years of age without any of the above risk factors.

The management of close contacts of cases of tuberculosis associated with INH-resistant organisms remains uncertain. Three alternative courses of action have been suggested (39): (*a*) Administer INH alone assuming that there may still be some in vivo efficacy. (*b*) Prescribe another drug in addition to INH or another single or double drug regimen likely to be effective. (*c*) Observe only and do not treat unless active disease develops. The vulnerability of the individual candidate for chemoprophylaxis and the likely susceptibility patterns will determine the course of action in each case. The Academy of Pediatrics (45) currently recommends the addition of rifampin (10 mg/kg/day, maximum 600 mg) to INH until susceptibility testing results are available. If the organisms are completely resistant to INH, INH is discontinued and rifampin continued for the complete course. If the organism is only partially resistant to INH, both INH and rifampin should be continued. Ethambutol may be considered as a second drug with rifampin for preventive therapy in adults infected with INH-resistant organisms.

Bacillus of Calmette and Guérin (BCG)

Calmette and Guérin bacillus (BCG) vaccines are derived from a strain of *Mycobacterium bovis* attenuated through years of serial passage in culture by Calmette and Guérin at the Pasteur Institute in France. When administered to tuberculin-negative individuals, BCG vaccine produces an attenuated infection that should confer immunity to infection with *M. tuberculosis*. The tuberculin skin test will become positive within 2–3 months following immunization, but the reaction is not larger than 10 ml and decreases in size over time.

Although the many BCG vaccines available throughout the world are derived from the original strain, there is considerable variation in immunogenicity, efficacy, and reactogenicity. This variation results from genetic changes in the bacterial strains, differences in production techniques, and in methods of vaccine administration. Protection rates demonstrated in controlled trials in both children and adults varied from 0–80% (66). Since the larger efficacy rates were demonstrated in the methodologically superior trials, it is generally accepted that currently available BCG vaccines will provide protection against progressive or disseminated disease in most populations (67). Protection is less likely in areas where nonspecific tuberculin sensitivity has been induced by exposure to the nontuberculous mycobacteria and where most disease is of the reinfection type (68).

BCG vaccine is considered to be one of the safest vaccines in use. There has never been noted a transformation from attenuation back to virulence. The rare but dramatic complications have received much attention in the literature. The death of 72 children in Germany in 1930 was the result of accidental contamination of the vaccine with a virulent strain (66). Disseminated infection with fatal outcome has been reported in less than one case per 1,000,000 immunizations in individuals with underlying immune deficiency (69). Up to 10% of children immunized before 2 years of age have developed localized ulceration and lymphadenitis, but such reactions are usually caused by too-deep injections. Osteoarticular lesions have been described in the neonate and may be strain related. The incidence of this complication in Sweden decreased from 29 cases per 100,000 neonates immunized to zero when the associated BCG strain was replaced by another strain in 1979 (70).

BCG is routinely used for prevention of tuberculosis in areas of the world where disease rates are excessive and continued surveillance and treatment of infected individuals is not possible. Within a single country, there may be high-risk population groups who would benefit from immunization when too few cases may occur in the population overall to justify general BCG immunization of newborns (70). In the United States, disease rates are relatively low and public health programs for case-finding and treatment have been quite successful. Therefore, BCG is recommended for only two special situations in this country: Young infants who are tuberculin-negative but have repeated exposure to persistently untreated or noncompliant patients with sputum-positive pulmonary tuberculosis, and population groups in which the annual tuberculin conversion rates are 1% or more and the usual surveillance and treatment programs have failed or are not feasible (71). Hospital employee health services in the United States prefer routine surveillance and chemotherapy over BCG administration for the prevention of tuberculosis, even in urban centers where the endemic rates of tuberculosis are relatively high. Those employees who have received BCG in the past are considered infected with *M. tuberculosis* if the tuberculin reaction is larger than 10 ml, as recommended by the CDC (58).

REFERENCES

1. Tuberculosis—United States, 1985—and the possible impact of human T-lymphotropic virus type III/lymphadenopathy-associated virus infection. *MMWR* 35:74–76, 1985.
2. Tuberculosis provisional data—United States, 1986. *MMWR* 36:254–255, 1987.
3. Tuberculosis in minorities—United States. *MMWR* 36:77–80, 1987.
4. Powell KE, Meador MP, Farer LS: Recent trends in tuberculosis in children. *JAMA* 251:1289–1292, 1984.
5. Riley RL, Mills CC, Nyks W, Weinstock N, Storey PB, Sultan LU, Riley MC, Wells WF: Aerial dissemination of pulmonary tuberculosis. *Am J Hyg* 70:185–196, 1959.
6. Riley RL, Mills CC, O'Grady F, Sultan LU, Wittstadt F, Shivpuri DN: Infectiousness of air from a tuberculosis ward: Ultraviolet irradiation of infected air. *Am Rev Resp Dis* 85:511–525, 1962.

7. Houk VN, Kent DC, Baker JH, Sorenson K: The epidemiology of tuberculosis infection in a closed environment. *Arch Environ Health* 16:26–35, 1968.

8. Ehrenkranz NJ, Kicklighter JL: Tuberculosis outbreak in a general hospital: Evidence for airborne spread of infection. *Ann Int Med* 77:377–382, 1972.

9. Nardell E, McInnis B, Thomas B, Weidhaas S: Exogenous reinfection with tuberculosis in a shelter for the homeless. *N Engl J Med* 315:1570–1575, 1986.

10. Rose CE, Zerbe GO, Lantz SO, Bailey WC: Establishing priority during investigation of tuberculosis contacts. *Am Rev Resp Dis* 119:603–609, 1979.

11. Rouillon A, Perdrizet S, Parrot R: Transmission of tubercle bacilli: the effects of chemotherapy. *Tubercle* 57:275–299, 1976.

12. Gunnels JJ, Bates JH, Swindoll H: Infectivity of sputum-positive tuberculous patients on chemotherapy. *Am Rev Resp Dis* 209:323–330, 1974.

13. Sunderam G, McDonald RJ, Maniatis T, Oleske J, Kapila R, Reichman LB: Tuberculosis as a manifestation of the acquired immunodeficiency syndrome (AIDS). *JAMA* 256:357–361, 1986.

14. Pitchenik AE, Russell BW, Cleary T, Pejovic I, Cole C, Snider DE: The prevalence of tuberculosis and drug resistance among Haitians. *N Engl J Med* 307:162–165, 1982.

15. Barrett-Connor E: The epidemiology of tuberculosis in physicians. *JAMA* 241:33–38, 1979.

16. Berman J, Levin ML, Tangerose S, Desi L: Tuberculosis risk for hospital employees: Analysis of a five-year tuberculin skin testing program. *Am J Pub Health* 71:1217–1222, 1981.

17. Geiseler PJ, Nelson KE, Crispen RG, Moses VK: Tuberculosis in physicians: A continuing problem. *Am Rev Resp Dis* 133:773–778, 1986.

18. Thompson NJ, Glassroth JL, Snider DE, Farer LS: The booster phenomenon in serial tuberculin testing. *Am Rev Resp Dis* 119:587–597, 1979.

19. Ruben FL, Norden CW, Schuster N: Analysis of a community hospital employee tuberculosis screening program 31 months after its inception. *Am Rev Resp Dis* 115:23–28, 1977.

20. Craven RB, Wenzel RP, Atuk NO: Minimizing tuberculosis risk to hospital personnel and students exposed to unsuspected disease. *Ann Int Med* 82:628–632, 1975.

21. Catanzaro A: Nosocomial tuberculosis. *Am Rev Resp Dis* 125:559–562, 1982.

22. George RH, Gully PR, Gill ON, Innes JA, Bakhshi SS, Connolly M: An outbreak of tuberculosis in a children's hospital. *J Hosp Infect* 8:129–142, 1986.

23. Stewart CJ: Tuberculosis infection in a paediatric department. *Br Med J* 1:30–32, 1976.

24. Beddall AC, Hill FGH, George RH, Williams MD, Al-Rubei K: Unusually high incidence of tuberculosis among boys with haemophilia during an outbreak of the disease in hospital. *J Clin Pathol* 38:1163–1165, 1985.

25. Allen BW, Darrell JH: Extrapulmonary tuberculosis: A potential source of laboratory-acquired infection. *J Clin Pathol* 34:404–407, 1981.

26. Grist NR: Infections in British clinical laboratories 1980–81. *J Clin Pathol* 36:121–126, 1983.

27. Pope AS: An outbreak of tuberculosis in infants due to hospital infection. *J Pediatr* 20:297–300, 1942.

28. Light IJ, Saidleman M, Sutherland JM: Management of newborns after nursery exposure to tuberculosis. *Am Rev Resp Dis* 109:415–419, 1974.

29. Keim LW: Management of newborns after nursery exposure to tuberculosis. *Am Rev Resp Dis* 110:522–523, 1974.

30. Steiner P, Rao M, Victoria MS, Rudolph N, Buynoski G: Miliary tuberculosis in two infants after nursery exposure: Epidemiologic, clinical, and laboratory findings. *Am Rev Resp Dis* 113:267–271, 1976.

31. Burk JR, Bahar D, Wolf FS, Greene J, Bailey WC: Nursery exposure of 528 newborns to a nurse with pulmonary tuberculosis. *South Med J* 71:7–10, 1978.

32. Reeves SA, Noble RC: Ineffectiveness of annual chest roentgenograms in tuberculin skin test positive hospital employees. *Am J Infect Control* 11:212–216, 1983.

33. Cope R, Hartstein AI: The annual chest roentgenogram for the control of tuberculosis in hospital employees: Recent changes and their implications. *Am Rev Resp Dis* 125:106–107, 1982.

34. Snider DE: The tuberculin skin test. *Am Rev Resp Dis* 125:108–118, 1982.

35. Schuit KE, Powell DA: Mycobacterial lymphadenitis in childhood. *AJDC* 132:675–677, 1978.

36. Valenti WM: Prevention and control of tuberculosis. *Infection Control* 6:169–171, 1985.

37. Steiner P, Rao M, Mitchell M, Steiner M: Primary drug-resistant tuberculosis in children: Correlation of drug-susceptibility patterns of matched patient and source case strains of *mycobacterium tuberculosis. AJDC* 139:780–782, 1985.

38. Snider DE, Jones WD, Good RC: The usefulness of phage typing *Mycobacterium tuberculosis* isolates. *Am Rev Resp Dis* 130:1095–1099, 1984.

39. Bass JB, Farer LS, Hopewell PC, Jacobs RF: Treatment of tuberculosis and tuberculosis infection in adults and children. *Am Rev Resp Dis* 134:355–363, 1986.

40. Dutt AK, Stead WW: Present chemotherapy for tuberculosis. *J Infect Dis* 146:698–704, 1982.

41. Dickinson JM, Mitchison DA: Experimental models to explain the high sterilizing activity of rifampin in the chemotherapy of tuberculosis. *Am Rev Resp Dis* 123:367–371, 1981.

42. Smith MD: What about short course and intermittent chemotherapy for tuberculosis in children. *PID* 1:298–303, 1982.

43. Steiner P, Rao M, Mitchell M, Steiner M: Primary drug-resistant tuberculosis in children: Emergence of primary drug-resistant strains of *M. tuberculosis* to rifampin. *Am Rev Resp Dis* 134:446–448, 1986.

44. Nemir RL, Cardona J, Vaziri F, Toledo R: Prednisone as an adjunct in the chemotherapy of lymph node-bronchial tuberculosis in childhood: A double-blind study. *Am Rev Resp Dis* 95:402–410, 1967.

45. *Report of the Committee on Infectious Diseases*, ed 20. American Academy of Pediatrics, Elk Grove Village, IL, 1986, pp 374–390.

46. Mitchell JR, Zimmerman HJ, Ishak KG, Thorgeirsson UP, Timbrell JA, Snodgrass WR, Nelson SD: Isoniazid liver injury: Clinical spectrum, pathology, and pathogenesis. *Am Int Med* 84:181–192, 1981.

47. O'Brien RJ, Long MW, Cross FS, Lyle MA, Snider DE: Hepatoxicity from INH and rifampin among children treated for tuberculosis. *Pediatrics* 72:491–499, 1983.

48. Martinez-Roig A, Cami J, Llorens-Terol J, de la Torre R, Perich F: Acetylation phenotype and hepatotoxicity in the treatment of tuberculosis in children. *Pediatrics* 77:912–915, 1986.

49. Bacteriologic conversion of sputum among tuberculosis patients—United States. *MMWR* 34:747–750, 1985.

50. Garner JS, Simmon BP: CDC guideline for isolation precautions in hospitals. *Infect Control* 4:259, 280–281, 1983.

51. Rutala WA, Sarubbi FA: Comparative evaluation of a traditional and a "tissue technique" method for determining air pressure differentials in hospital isolation rooms. *Am J Infect Control* 12:96–99, 1984.

52. Riley RL: Ultraviolet air disinfection for control of respiratory contagion. In Kundsin RB (ed): *Building Design and Indoor Microbial Pollution*. New York, Oxford University Press (in press).

53. Guyton HG, Decker HM: Respiratory protection provided by five new contagion masks. *Appl Microbiol* 11:66–68, 1963.

54. Leers WD: Disinfecting endoscopes: How not to transmit *Mycobacterium tuberculosis* by bronchoscopy. *Can Med Assoc J* 123:275–280, 1980.

55. Noble RC: Infectiousness of pulmonary tuberculosis after starting chemotherapy. *Am J Infect Cont* 9:6–10, 1981.

56. Diagnosis and management of mycobacterial infection and disease in persons with human immunodeficiency virus infection, Centers for Disease Control. *Ann Int Med* 106:254–256, 1987.

57. Pitchenik AE, Rubinson HA: The radiographic appearance of tuberculosis in patients with the acquired immune deficiency syndrome (AIDS) and pre-AIDS. *Ann Rev Resp Dis* 131:393–396, 1985.

58. Williams WW: CDC guidelines for infection control in hospital personnel. *Infect Control* 4:344–345, 1983.
59. Ferebee SH: Controlled chemoprophylaxis trials in tuberculosis: A general review. *Adv Tuberc Res* 17:28–106, 1970.
60. Farer LS: Chemoprophylaxis. *Am Rev Resp Dis* 125:102–107, 1982.
61. Grzybowski S, Halbraith JD, Dorken E: Chemoprophylaxis trial in Canadian Eskimos. *Tubercle* 57:263–269, 1976.
62. Comstock GW, Baum C, Snider DE: Isoniazid prophylaxis among Alaskan Eskimos: A final report of the Bethel isoniazid studies. *Am Rev Resp Dis* 119:827–830, 1979.
63. Hsu KHK: Thirty years after isoniazid: Its impact on tuberculosis in children and adolescents. *JAMA* 251:1283–1285, 1984.
64. Thompson NJ: Efficacy of various durations of isoniazid preventive therapy for tuberculosis: Five years of followup in the IUAT trial. *Bull WHO* 60:555–564, 1982.
65. Snider DE, Caras GJ, Kaplan JP: Preventive therapy with isoniazid: Cost-effectiveness of different durations of therapy. *JAMA* 255:1579–1583, 1986.
66. Luelmo F: BCG vaccination. *Am Rev Resp Dis* 125:70–72, 1982.
67. Clemens JD, Chuong JJH, Feinstein AR: The BCG controversy: A methodological and statistical reappraisal. *JAMA* 249:2362–2369, 1983.
68. ten Dam HG, Pio A: Pathogenesis of tuberculosis and effectiveness of BCG vaccination. *Tubercle* 63:225–233, 1982.
69. Lotte A, Wasz-Hockert O, Poisson N, Dumitrescu N, Verron M, Couvet E: BCG complications. *Adv Tuberc Res* 21:107–193, 1984.
70. Romanus V: Tuberculosis in Bacillus Calmette-Guerin-immunized and unimmunized children in Sweden. *PID* 6:272–280, 1987.
71. Springett VH: The value of BCG vaccination. *Tubercle* 46:76–84, 1965.

21

Coagulase-Negative Staphylococci

Michael A. Pfaller, M.D. and Richard P. Wenzel, M.D., M.Sc.

BACKGROUND

In recent years, it has become obvious that Gram-positive cocci and, particularly, the coagulase-negative staphylococci have emerged as very important hospital pathogens (1–8). Among the coagulase-negative bacteria, *S. epidermidis* is the most frequently isolated species, occurring in the majority of nosocomial bloodstream infections (9–11). The postulated reasons for the current prevalence and clinical importance of these organisms include their great numbers on the skin, their selection as a result of widespread usage of broad spectrum antibiotics in the hospital, their ability to attach to vascular catheters and other medical devices by virtue of an extracellar glycocalyx of "slime," and the species' meager nutritional requirements (12–18). In the pediatric population, the groups at the highest risk are those babies in the newborn intensive care unit and those whose therapy includes long-term use of vascular catheters or implantation of medical devices (9,19,20).

Epidemiology

In a 7-year study of nosocomial bacteremia caused by *S. epidermidis*, Ponce de Leon and Wenzel studied 100 cases, 20 (20%) of whom were premature infants under age 1 year (9). The mortality in premature babies with a gestational age less than 36 weeks was 30%, whereas those prematures with a gestational age over 36 months and normal-term babies had a mortality of 19% and 22%, respectively. In another study at the same hospital, Haley and colleagues showed that in 1976–1978, 30% of nosocomial bloodstream infections in the newborn intensive care unit were caused by Gram-positive bacteria, whereas

between 1979–1981, the proportion had increased to 60% (21). Moreover, during the latter period, 28% of the bloodstream infections were due to *S. epidermidis*. The changes in the newborn ICU were mirrored by changes in etiologic agents, causing nosocomial bloodstream infection throughout the hospital: between 1975–1978, the rate of infection for Gram-positive organisms was 29/10,000 admissions, but it increased to 43/10,000 in the period 1979–1982 (21). During the same period, rates for coagulase-negative staphylococci increased from 5.2 to 12.4/10,000, and coagulase-negative staphylococci accounted for 17% of all nosocomial bloodstream infections. From these and other studies, it is clear that the causes of bloodstream infection in the hospital have changed in recent years, that the Gram-positive cocci have emerged as the most prevalent pathogens, that *S. epidermidis* species comprise most of the latter and are a significant problem for newborns up to age 1 year (9, 21–25).

Risk factors for bloodstream infection with coagulase-negative staphylococci have been critically examined in only a few studies. Haley and colleagues identified three important risk factors: use of Broviac central venous catheters, prior surgery, and prior intravenous hyperalimentation (21). Risk factors varied with birthweight category, and in the population under 1500 g, only the prior use of Broviac catheters was independently associated with a high risk of subsequent bloodstream infection.

Recently, Simpson and her colleagues in England have examined the colonization of babies in a special care unit with gentamicin-resistant *S. epidermidis* (26). The proportion of clinically significant isolates had increased from 7% in 1976–1977 to 33% in 1980. All babies investigated during the 3-month study period became colonized at some time. The median time for colonization of the nose, umbilicus, or skin of the chest wall were 5, 8, and 8 days, respectively. Twenty-two of the 25 babies received gentamicin (26). Thirty–60% of staff personnel were also carrying the epidemic strain. Although none of the babies sampled suffered an infection, two babies who were not sampled developed a significant infection with the antibiotic-resistant strain. Thus, the colonization of this strain was widespread, occurred within a week of the babies' hospitalization, and was accompanied by a high proportion of carriage by staff members.

It is possible that the high prevalence of gentamicin use selected for resistant staphylococcal organisms, as it has been shown recently for Gram-negative rods in the hospital (27). In this respect, the study by Sprunt is relevant. She examined pharyngeal bacterial flora of newborns who had or had not received antibiotics during colonization (28). Only 14% of those given antibiotics versus 91% not given antibiotics had "normal" pharyngeal flora, predominating with α-hemolytic streptococci. Moreover, 15% of those abnormally colonized, and only 0.2% of those colonized with normal flora, developed an infection during the study period, 1978–1979. Of interest is that infection rates in those abnormally colonized fell to 6% and 3%, respectively, in 1980 and 1981 during the period when pharyngeal colonization changed predominately from Gram-negative rods to *S. epidermidis* (29). This European study is important because it confirms the change in flora of organisms causing infection in newborn units and suggests that antibiotics may have selected for resistant organisms likely to cause infection. Furthermore, it suggests that invasion may be less likely after colonization with *S. epidermidis* than the situation expected after colonization with Gram-negative rods.

Until recently, it has been assumed that all *S. epidermidis* infections were caused by the patients' organisms, perhaps influenced by the hospital's plasmids coding for antibiotic resistance. Knowledge of the extent to which this is true has been hampered by the lack of simple epidemiologic markers for bacterial typing. Nevertheless, Maki and colleagues have shown that, in some circumstances, infection can be spread from a hospital carrier to patients (29).

Although his patients were postoperative adults, and the carrier was a surgeon, the study is important in stimulating a further examination of transmission in other hospital areas, including the newborn intensive care unit.

From the point of view of the host, Fleer and colleagues have emphasized the immature bacterial defense mechanisms of the neonate (30). In their experience, over 90% of pediatric cases occur in the neonatal ICU in patients of low birthweight (less than 2500 g). They showed a positive correlation between opsonic activity against *S. epidermidis* in sera from premature neonates and gestational age. Additionally, opsonic IgG antibodies to *S. epidermidis* were found to be completely lacking from premature newborns. This was true even if the mothers had such antibodies. Thus, either the IgG opsonic antibodies are inactivated in transplacental transfer, or they fail to cross the placenta (30).

Furthermore, it has been postulated that the *S. epidermidis* slime may interfere with normal white cell function. In one study, however, when slime-positive or slime-negative organisms were incubated with neutrophils, no differences in phagocytosis or killing were observed over a 3-hour period (17). However, when organisms were allowed to grow on the surface of a plastic plate for longer periods in a surface phagocytosis assay, these organisms, which could produce slime over an 18-hour period, were not phagocytosed as readily as organisms grown for only 2 hours (31). In addition, incubation of neutrophils with 50 μg or more of slime inhibited subsequent chemotaxis (31).

In summary, it would appear that a number of existing circumstances have led to the emergence of coagulase-negative staphylococci as major neonatal pathogens. The organisms are present in large numbers on the skin and are readily cultured after hospitalization. They may have been selected by current antibiotic preference and use in the hospital, and they possess the ability to attach to catheters and become enmeshed in a protective layer of slime. In addition, host defenses in the neonate may be defective for coagulase-negative staphylococci. Current evidence suggests that the reservoirs of these organisms are usually the patients themselves and that transmission occurs via medical devices to the bloodstream. All these concepts, however, need to be evaluated more fully.

MICROBIOLOGY

Staphylococci are members of the family micrococcaceae. There are 20 recognized species of staphylococci, and 12 of them are found as part of the normal flora of humans (32–37). They are nonmotile, Gram-positive, facultatively anaerobic-clustering cocci that produce catalase. The biochemical diversity among species is great and has been discussed extensively in several recent reviews (32,35,38,39).

Originally, of all the staphylococci, only *Staphylococcus aureus* was considered pathogenic and was delineated from the other species on the basis of coagulase production, mannitol fermentation, and the presence of protein A on the cell wall surface. All other species were grouped under the species designation *S. albus*, which was subsequently changed to *S. epidermidis* and were considered nonpathogens (37,40). The work of Kloos, Kloos and Schleifer, and Kloos and Wolfshohl (36–39) redefined the coagulase-negative staphylococci (CNS) so that 15 species are now recognized (Table 21.1). Presently, it is clear that, in addition to *S. aureus*, those staphylococci of documented clinical importance are *S. epidermidis* and *S. saprophyticus*. In studies that have attempted to correlate species identification with clinical significance, *S. epidermidis* has accounted for the majority (75%) of the CNS isolates (33–35). This is most likely due to the overwhelming preponderance of *S. epidermidis* on the skin (33–35); however, *S. epidermidis* may also possess virulence factors absent in other CNS isolates (33,34,36). *S. saprophyticus* appears to be a significant cause of urinary tract infections in young women, but has rarely been implicated in other types of infections (33–37). Previous recognition of this group of organisms as significant pathogens may have been obscured due to inaccurate laboratory identification. Other species of CNS, including *S. hominis*, *S. haemolyticus*, and *S. simulans*, have each been isolated from 5–20% of the total human infections attributed to the CNS (33,35). Occasionally, *S. warneri*, *S. saccharolyticus*, and *S. cohnii* have been isolated from infection. Thus, in most clinical situations, it is important to identify *S. epidermidis* and *S. saprophyticus* with a high degree of accuracy. This can be accomplished on the basis of colony morphology, coagulase and phosphatase activities, acid production from D-mannitol, D-trehalose, maltose, sucrose, and D-xylose, and novobiocin susceptibility (32–35,38,39). The identification of other species of CNS can be accomplished using these tests plus the determination of acid production from certain additional carbohydrates and certain enzyme activities (33–35,38,39).

These observations have increased the demand for a more exact identification of CNS in the clinical microbiology laboratory. Unfortunately, because the conventional methods of Kloos and Schleifer (38) are considered too slow and cumbersome for use in the routine clinical microbiology laboratory, and because *S. epidermidis* is the predominant pathogen among the CNS, many clinical laboratories routinely report all such isolates as *S. epidermidis*. However, with the recent recognition of CNS as important nosocomial pathogens, it has become apparent that this practice may not be acceptable in every clinical situation. In addition to the value of having an exact etiological diagnosis, identification increases the knowledge of the pathogenicity of the various species of CNS, provides useful epidemiologic information, and contributes to the predictive value of an isolate's being of clinical significance versus a contaminant (17). Further delineation of individual strains, as well as species of CNS, may be extremely useful as an epidemiologic tool for investigating infections (14,40,41).

The commercial availability of rapid and miniaturized identification systems provides virtually every clinical laboratory with the capability of identifying CNS to the species level. Several manufacturers of commercial kit identification systems or automated instruments have recently released products that are relatively simple and rapid and allow the identification of CNS species with an accuracy of 70–90% when combined with coagulase testing and novobiocin susceptibility (35,39). The systems that are currently available include the API Staph-Ident System® (Analytab), the API Staph-Trac System® (Analytab), Pos Combo Panel® (American Micro Scan), Minitek Gram-Positive System® (BBL), and the Vitek Gram-Positive Identification Card® (Vitek). Although some authors have questioned the need for routine species identification of all CNS isolated from clinical specimens (40), the availability of these commercial test kits should facilitate additional research efforts in this area.

Table 1.
Species of Coagulase-Negative Staphylococci[a]

Common Pathogens
    S. epidermidis
    S. saprophyticus

Uncommon Pathogens
    S. haemolyticus
    S. hominis
    S. warneri
    S. saccharolyticus
    S. cohnii
    S. simulans

Rare Pathogens
    S. auricularis
    S. xylosus
    S. carnosus
    S. sciuri
    S. lentus
    S. caseolyticus
    S. capitis

[a]Data from references 37 and 40.

Recently, Christensen and coworkers (14) have shown that biotype determination using the API Staph-Ident System® in conjunction with antibiotic susceptibility patterns (antibiogram) can be used to enhance the reliability of strain differentiation among multiple isolates of CNS. In general, repeated isolation of CNS, with similar biotypes and antibiograms, from one or more sites suggests an ongoing infectious process (40,41). The finding of isolates of a different species or strain indicates contamination. Additional methods for the characterization of distinct strains of CNS include phage typing and plasmid profiling (14,40–42). Of the two, plasmid profiling may have the greater potential for routine use (14,40–42).

Antimicrobial Susceptibility Testing

The susceptibility of CNS to antimicrobial agents is extremely variable. Although environmental or community-acquired isolates are frequently susceptible to a wide variety of agents, strains isolated from hospitalized patients have been noted to be increasingly resistant to a number of antibiotics (5,43–46). A marked increase in the resistance of *S. epidermidis* to gentamicin, erythromycin chloramphenicol, and methicillin has recently been reported (5,43,44,46). Karchmer et al. reported that 83% of *S. epidermidis* isolates from their patients with prosthetic valve endocarditis were methicillin-resistant (43), and

Archer found that 67% of clinical isolates obtained from blood, CSF, or heart valve tissue were resistant to six or more antibiotics (44).

There are several pitfalls in the performance of antimicrobial susceptibility testing of CNS which should be recognized and avoided. Resistance to penicillin is very common, particularly among hospital strains of CNS, and is frequently mediated by a β-lactamase-producing plasmid (44,47).

β-lactamase-mediated resistance to penicillin is frequently not detected by routine microdilution methods, and all isolates that appear susceptible to penicillin or ampicillin should be tested for β-lactamase production (47). Because the β-lactamase enzyme in staphylococci is inducible, it may not be fully expressed in all isolates and therefore must be induced prior to β-lactamase testing by exposure of the isolate to an appropriate inducing agent, such as oxacillin, in order to avoid a false-negative β-lactamase test (47,48). Recently, Selepak and Witebsky (48) demonstrated that up to 60% of clinical isolates of CNS would be misclassified as β-lactamase-negative if β-lactamase testing were performed without prior induction. They recommended that the β-lactamase tests be performed using induced organisms taken from the edge of the zone around a 1 μg oxacillin disc (47,48).

In contrast to penicillin resistance, resistance of staphylococci to methicillin and other penicillinase-resistant penicillins (PRP), such as oxacillin and nafcillin, is not mediated by β-lactamase production, but rather is thought to be due to an altered penicillin-binding protein (49). The accurate detection of CNS that are resistant to the PRPs is a major problem because PRP-resistant isolates are phenotypically heteroresistant to methicillin and the other PRPs (43,44,50,51). This means that each culture contains both resistant and susceptible subpopulations. The resistant subpopulation generally constitutes only a small fraction (10^{-6}–10^{-4}) of the entire population and thus may easily be missed when in vitro testing is performed (43,44,50–54). The PRP-resistant subpopulation, in general, grows more slowly than the susceptible subpopulation. However, the resistant cells grow faster at incubation temperatures of 30–35°C and in the presence of 2–5% salt added to the medium (51). Thus, the expression of resistance as detected by in vitro testing methods is influenced by several factors, including inoculum size and preparation, time and temperature of incubation, and medium composition and osmolality (51,54). It is important to realize that routine susceptibility testing with methicillin, oxacillin, or nafcillin discs, automated turbidimetric systems, and microdilution systems may all yield false-susceptible results.

There are several recommended modifications of the standard disc diffusion and broth dilution susceptibility methods that will provide improved detection of PRP-resistant strains of staphylococci (52). The current recommendations for optimal detection of PRP resistance are as follows:

1. The inoculum should be prepared by suspending organisms taken directly from an overnight (18–24/hour) growth on an agar plate to the turbidity of a 0.5 McFarland Standard. These conditions favor the growth of the resistant subpopulation.
2. The inoculum size should be 1×10^8 CFU/ml for disc diffusion testing and 5×10^5 CFU/ml for broth dilution testing. Lower inocula may result in false-susceptible results.
3. The medium used for broth dilution testing should be cation-supplemented Mueller-Hinton broth (CSMH) that has been further supplemented with NaCl (2% final concentration) in the PRP-containing wells only.
4. All tests should be incubated at 35°C for a full 24 hours. Higher temperatures and/or shorter incubation times may result in the failure to detect PRP resistance.
5. When performing disc diffusion testing, one should use either oxacillin or methicillin, rather than nafcillin-, cloxacillin-, or dicloxacillin-containing discs.
6. Examine the zone of inhibition surrounding the oxacillin or methicillin disc, using transmitted light, for the presence of small colonies or a haze of growth, indicating the presence of a resistant subpopulation.

Additional clues to the presence of a PRP-resistant staphylococcus include resistance to multiple antibiotics, including erythromycin, clindamycin, tetracycline, chloramphenicol, and gentamicin, an intermediate result to methicillin or oxacillin, and resistance to one but not all PRPs. The use of a larger inoculum and/or prolonged incubation time (greater than 24 hours) is not generally recommended and may result

in false-resistant or intermediate results in some strains (51,53).

An additional confusing issue is the question of cross-resistance between cephalosporins and the PRPs. Routine susceptibility testing will frequently show PRP-resistant *S. epidermidis* to be susceptible to 1st- and 2nd-generation cephalosporins when, in fact, cross-resistance is extensive (43,44,50–54).

For clinical purposes, all PRP-resistant staphylococci should be reported as resistant to all β-lactam agents, regardless of their in vitro susceptibility (52).

To date, there have been no confirmed reports of vancomycin-resistant CNS (8,32,43). Vancomycin susceptibility testing of CNS is reliable and generally is predictive of in vivo response. In vitro studies done with combinations of vancomycin and other antistaphylococcal agents, such as gentamicin or rifampin, have demonstrated synergy against clinical isolates of CNS (43).

DIAGNOSES AND THERAPY

There are no simple guidelines by which one can rely to differentiate infection from colonization with *S. epidermidis*. Nevertheless, when this organism is isolated from the bloodstream of a patient in a critical care unit or a patient who has a medical device in place or who is immunocompromised, it must be viewed seriously as a potential pathogen. The positive predictive value (for a significant blood isolate) increases in the newborn ICU setting compared with a routine ward setting. Additionally, one cannot rely on culturing the organism in two or more sets to distinguish an important isolate from a contaminant (9). Furthermore, it has been reported that the positive predictive value increases if one knows that the species of coagulase-negative staphylococcus is *S. epidermidis*, and is better still if one knows that it is both *S. epidermidis* and a slime-producing organism (17).

In terms of therapy, the treating physician needs to know if the organism is sensitive to methicillin. In large centers, the proportion of methicillin-resistant organisms is as high as 40–60%, and the drug of choice is vancomycin. By analogy with *S. aureus*, some authors suggest that methicillin-resistant strains are resistant—clinically—to all β-lactam antibiotics, regardless of the in vitro results. The authors are not aware of any comparative studies, however, for the pediatric population.

The question of the need to remove a central catheter is frequently asked and has been addressed in a study of pediatric oncology patients by Johnson et al. (55). In their study of Broviac catheter–related infections, the authors found an infection rate (exit site, vascular, and combined) of 2.8/1000 catheter-days. Overall, 70% of their patients were "cured" without removal of the catheter, including 83% of bloodstream infections. However, the subsequent infection-free period was reduced in such patients compared with those whose catheters were not infected. Johnson and his colleagues concluded that the insertion of a new catheter may be necessary in patients who need prolonged intravenous access.

PREVENTION

Frequent handwashing by all health care personnel is of primary importance in limiting staff-to-patient and patient-to-patient spread of CNS. The use of patient isolation, barrier precautions, and disposable gloves may also be indicated when caring for patients infected with CNS in order to minimize the risk of transmission of the infecting organism to other high-risk patients (8,32,56–60). Limiting the amount of intraoperative bacterial contamination by meticulous surgical technique, proper preoperative skin preparation, and proper draping of the operative site are all important in minimizing the risk of surgical infections (57,59,61). Strict attention to protocols for the insertion and management of intravenous and arterial catheters are clearly important in minimizing the risk of catheter-related infections (56). Subsequently, daily surveillance of all intravascular lines and limiting the duration of placement of peripheral venous catheters to no more than 72 hours can greatly reduce the risk of catheter-related infections (56).

The role of antimicrobial agent prophylaxis in preventing infections due to CNS is presently unclear and may, in fact, have significant adverse consequences (8,32,59–62). The findings of Wade et al. (6) in granulocytopenic cancer patients suggests that the addition of vancomycin to their prophylactic oral nonabsorbable antibiotic regimen reduced the alimentary tract colonization with CNS and resulted in a decline in both bacteremic and nonbacteremic infections due to *S. epidermidis*. While this is encourag-

ing, there are little, if any, additional data to support the routine use of prophylactic vancomycin in these patients.

Although the benefits of antistaphylococcal prophylaxis in cardiac and orthopaedic surgery remain uncertain, it has become standard practice to use such prophylaxis (60,62). The value of antimicrobial prophylaxis in cardiac surgery has never been tested in a placebo-controlled trial, and there is very little information available on infection rates in patients not receiving antibiotics. A study by Archer and Tenenbaum (63) demonstrated that widespread use of antibiotics for prophylaxis in cardiac surgery patients led to an increased prevalence of methicillin resistance in *S. epidermidis* isolates obtained from these patients. Furthermore, these investigators found that a high percentage of the methicillin-resistant postoperative isolates were also resistant to multiple antibiotics: penicillin, nafcillin, cephalosporins, and aminoglycosides (63). Subsequently, Archer and Armstrong (45) found that cardiac surgery patients receiving a combination of rifampin and nafcillin prophylaxis became colonized with strains of *S. epidermidis* resistant not only to rifampin and nafcillin, but also to gentamicin. The antibiotic resistance patterns shown by *S. epidermidis* isolates in these studies were similar to those found in isolates from cases of *S. epidermidis* prosthetic valve endocarditis in other studies (44). The studies demonstrate that antibiotic prophylaxis changed the coagulase-negative flora of surgery patients by selecting for multiply resistant strains capable of causing serious postoperative infections (44). In addition, the organisms can possibly serve as a reservoir of resistant strains that can be transferred from patient to staff, staff to patient, and among patients within the hospital (42–45,62). Thus, despite the increasing importance of CNS as agents of nosocomial infection, it is not at all clear that additional antimicrobial prophylaxis is indicated or desirable. Certainly, further clinical and experimental studies are needed. Ideally, the prevention of CNS infections should be based on a better understanding of neonatal host defenses against these microorganisms, particularly those associated with foreign devices.

REFERENCES

1. Wenzel RP: The evolving art and science of hospital epidemiology. *J Infect Dis* 153:462–470, 1986.
2. Morrison AJ, Freer CV, Searcy MA, Landry SM, Wenzel RP: Nosocomial bloodstream infections: secular trends in a statewide

surveillance program in Virginia. *Infect Control* 7:550–553, 1986.

3. Centers for Disease Control: *MMWR* 32:12AA and 33:18SS, 1984.

4. Stillman RI, Donowitz LG, Wenzel RP: The emergence of coagulase-negative staphylococci as major nosocomial bloodstream pathogens. *Infect Control* 8:108–112, 1987.

5. Christensen GD, Bisno AL, Parisi JT, McLaughlin B, Hester MG, Luther RW: Nosocomial septicemia due to multiply antibiotic-resistant *Staphylococcus epidermidis*. *Ann Intern Med* 96:1–10, 1982.

6. Wade JC, Schimpff SC, Newman KA: *Staphylococcus epidermidis*: an increasing cause of infection in patients with granulocytopenia. *Ann Int Med* 97:503–508, 1982.

7. Senell CM, Clarridge JE, Young EJ, Guthrie RK: Clinical significance of coagulase-negative staphylococci. *J Clin Microbiol* 16:236–239, 1982.

8. Lowy FD, Hammer SM: *Staphylococcus epidermidis* infections. *Ann Int Med* 99:834–839, 1983.

9. Ponce de Leon S, Wenzel RP: Hospital-acquired bloodstream infections with *Staphylococcus epidermidis*: review of 100 cases. *Am J Med* 77:639–644, 1984.

10. Ponce de Leon S, Guenthner SH, Wenzel RP: Microbiologic studies of coagulase-negative staphylococci isolated from patients with nosocomial bacteremias. *J Hosp Infect* 7(2):121–129, 1986.

11. Eng RH, Wang C, Person A, Keihn TE, Armstrong D: Species identification of coagulase-negative staphylococcal isolates from blood cultures. *J Clin Microbiol* 15:439–442, 1982.

12. Wenzel RP: The reemergence of gram positive cocci as major nosocomial pathogens. *Infect Control* 7:118–119, 1986.

13. Bayston R, Penny SR: Excessive production of mucoid substance in staphylococcus S II A: a possible factor in colonization of Holter shunts. *Dev Med Child Neurol* 14 (Suppl 27):25–28, 1972.

14. Christensen GD, Parisi JT, Bisno AL, Simpson WA, Beachey EH: Characterization of clinically significant strains of coagulase-negative staphylococci. *J Clin Microbiol* 18:258–269, 1983.

15. Christensen GD, Simpson WA, Bisno AL, Beachey EH: Experimental foreign body infections in mice challenged with slime-producing *Staphylococcus epidermidis*. *Infect Immun* 40:407–410, 1983.

16. Peters G, Locci R, Pulverer G: Adherence and growth of coagulase-negative staphylococci on surfaces of intravenous catheters. *J Infect Dis* 146:479–483, 1982.

17. Ishak MA, Groschel DH, Mandell GL, Wenzel RP: Association of slime with pathogenicity of coagulase-negative staphylococci causing nosocomial septicemia. *J Clin Microbiol* 22:1025–1029, 1985.

18. Davenport DS, Massanari RM, Pfaller MA, Bale MJ, Streed SA, Hierholzer WJ Jr: Usefulness of a test for slime production as a marker for clinically significant infections with coagulase-negative staphylococci. *J Infect Dis* 153:332–339, 1986.

19. Shurtleff DB, Foltz EL, Weeks RD, Loeser J: Therapy of *Staphylococcus epidermidis* infections associated with cerebrospinal shunts. *Pediatrics* 53:55–62, 1974.

20. Okadr DM, Chow AW, Bruce VT: Neonatal scalp abscess and fetal monitoring: factors associated with infection. *Am J Obstet Gynecol* 129:185–189, 1977.

21. Donowitz LG, Haley CE, Gregory WW, Wenzel RP: Neonatal intensive care unit bloodstream infections: emergence of gram positive bacteria as major pathogens. *Am J Infect Control* 15:141–147, 1987.

22. Goldmann DA: Bacterial colonizations and infection in the neonate. *Am J Med* 70:417–422, 1978.

23. Battisti O, Mitchison R, Davies PA: Changing blood culture isolates in a referral neonatal intensive care unit. *Arch In Child* 56:775–778, 1981.

24. Oto A: Major bacterial infection in a referral neonatal intensive care unit. *J Infect* 5:117–126, 1982.

25. Baumgart S, Hall SE, Campos JM, Polin RA: Sepsis with coagulase-negative staphylococci in critically ill newborns. *Am J Dis Child* 137:461–463, 1983.

26. Simpson RA, Spencer AF, Speller DCE, Marples RR: Colonization by gentamicin-resistant *Staphylococcus epidermidis* in a special care baby unit. *J Hosp Infect* 7:108–120, 1986.

27. Goosens H, Ghysels G, Van Laethem N, De Wit S, Levy J, De Mol P, Clumeck N, Butzler JP, Wenzel RP: Predicting gentamicin resistance from annual usage in hospital. *Lancet* 2:804–805, 1986.

28. Sprunt K: Practical use of surveillance for prevention of nosocomial infections (review). *Semin Perinatal* 9:47–50, 1985.

29. Maki DG, Zilz M, Alvarado C, Robbins J, Parisi JT: Multiple-resistant *Staphylococcus epidermidis* surgical wound infections linked to a chronic carrier (meeting). *Clin Res* 30(2):A 373, 1982.

30. Fleer A, Verhoef J, Hernandez AP: Coagulase-negative staphylococci as nosocomial pathogens in neonates. *Am J Med* 80 (Suppl 68):161–165, 1986.

31. Johnson GM, Lee DA, Regelmann WE, Gray ED, Peters G, Quie PG: Interference with granulocytic function by *Staphylococcus epidermidis* slime. *Infect Immun* 54:13-20, 1986.

32. Dunne WM Jr, Franson TF: Coagulase-negative staphylococci: the Rodney Dangerfield of pathogens. *Clin Microbiol Newslett* 8:37–42, 1986.

33. Oeding P: Taxonomy and identification. In Easmon CSF, Adlam C (eds): *Staphylococci and Staphylococcal Infections*. New York, Academic Press, 1983, vol 1, pp 1–31.

34. Schleifer KH: Taxonomy of coagulase-negative staphylococci. In Mardh PA, Schleifer KH (eds): *Coagulase-Negative Staphylococci*. Stockholm, Almqvist and Wiksell International, 1986, pp 11–26.

35. Kloos WE, Jorgensen JH: Staphylococci. In Lennette EH, Balows A, Hausler WJ Jr, Shadomy HJ (eds): *Manual of Clinical Microbiology*, Washington, DC, American Society for Microbiology, 1985, pp 143–153.

36. Kloos WE: Natural populations of the genus staphylococcus. *Annu Rev Microbiol* 34:559–592, 1980.

37. Kloos WE: Coagulase-negative staphylococci. *Clin Microbiol Newslett* 4:75–79, 1982.

38. Kloos WE, Schleifer KH: Simplified scheme for routine identification of human *Staphylococcus* species. *J Clin Microbiol* 1:82–88, 1975.

39. Kloos WE, Wolfshohl J: Identification of *Staphylococcus* species with the API STAPH-IDENT system. *J Clin Microbiol* 16:509–516, 1982.

40. Parisi JT: Coagulase-negative staphylococci and the epidemiologic typing of *Staphylococcus epidermidis*. *Microbiol Rev* 49:126–139, 1985.

41. Archer GL, Karchmer AW, Vishniavsky N: Plasmid-pattern analysis for the differentiation of infecting from noninfecting *Staphylococcus epidermidis*. *J Infect Dis* 149:913–920, 1984.

42. Parisi JT, Hecht DW: Plasmid profiles in epidemiologic studies of infections by *Staphylococcus epidermidis*. *J Infect Dis* 141:637–643, 1980.

43. Karchmer AW, Archer GL, Dismukes WE: *Staphylococcus epidermidis* causing prosthetic valve endocarditis: microbiologic and clinical observations as guide to therapy. *Ann Intern Med* 98:447–455, 1983.

44. Archer G: Antimicrobial susceptibility and selection of resistance among *Staphylococcus epidermidis* isolates recovered from patients with infections of indwelling foreign devices. *Antimicrob Agents Chemother* 14:353–359, 1978.

45. Archer GL, Armstrong BC: Alterations of staphylococcal flora in cardiac surgery patients receiving antibiotic prophylaxis. *J Infect Dis* 147:642–649, 1983.

46. Hamilton-Miller JMT, Iliffe A: Antimicrobial resistance in coagulase-negative staphylococci. *J Med Microbiol* 19:217–226, 1985.

47. Gill VJ, Manning CB, Ingalls CM: Correlation of penicillin minimum inhibitory concentrations and penicillin zone edge appearance with staphylococcal beta-lactamase production. *J Clin Microbiol* 14:437–440, 1981.

48. Selepak ST, Witebsky FG: Beta-lactamase detection in nine staphylococcal species. *J Clin Microbiol* 20:1200–1201, 1984.

49. Ubukata K, Yamashita N, Konno M: Occurrence of a beta-lactam-inducible penicillin-binding protein in methicillin-resis-

tant staphylococci. *Antimicrob Agents Chemother* 27:851–857, 1985.

50. Hansen BG: Population analysis of susceptibility to methicillin, vancomycin, and three cephalosporins in two methicillin-resistant strains of *Staphylococcus epidermidis*. *Acta Pathol Microbiol Immunol Scand B* 91:279–284, 1983.
51. Thornsberry C: Methicillin-resistant (heteroresistant) staphylococci. *Antimicrob Newslett* 1:43–47, 1984.
52. McDougal LK, Thornsberry C: New recommendations for disk diffusion antimicrobial susceptibility tests for methicillin-resistant (heteroresistant) staphylococci. *J Clin Microbiol* 19:482–488, 1984.
53. McDougal LK, Thornsberry C: The role of beta-lactamase in staphylococcal resistance to penicillinase-resistant penicillins and cephalosporins. *J Clin Microbiol* 23:832–839, 1986.
54. Thornsberry C, McDougal LK: Successful use of broth microdilution in susceptibility tests for methicillin-resistant (heteroresistant) staphylococci. *J Clin Microbiol* 18:1084–1091, 1983.
55. Johnson PR, Decker MD, Edwards KM, Schaffner W, Wright PF: Frequency of Broviac catheter infections in pediatric oncology patients. *J Infect Dis* 154:570–578, 1986.
56. Maki DG: Infections associated with intravascular lines. In Remington JS, Swartz MN (eds): *Current Clinical Topics in Infectious Diseases*. New York, McGraw-Hill, 1982, vol 3, pp 309–363.
57. Hovany ET, Marples RR, Weir I, Mourant AJ, DeSaxe J, Singleton B: Problems in the investigation of an apparent outbreak of coagulase-negative staphylococcal systicaemia following cardiac surgery. *J Hosp Infect* 8:224–232, 1986.
58. Reybrouck G: Handwashing and hand disinfection. *J Hosp Infect* 8:5–23, 1986.
59. Cruse P: Surgical infection: incisional wounds. In Bennett JV, Brachman PS (eds): *Hospital Infections*, Boston, Little, Brown & Co., 1986, pp 423–436.
60. Burke JP: Infections of cardiac and vascular prostheses. In Bennett JV, Brachman PS (eds): *Hospital Infections*. Boston, Little, Brown & Co., 1986, pp 437–451.
61. Mayhall CG: Surgical infections including burns. In Wenzel RP (ed): *Prevention and Control of Nosocomial Infections*. Baltimore, Williams & Wilkins, 1987, pp 344–384.
62. Hirschmann JV, Inui TS: Antimicrobial prophylaxis: a critique of recent trials. *Rev Infect Dis* 2:1–23, 1980.
63. Archer GL, Tenenbaum: Antibiotic-resistant *Staphylococcus epidermidis* in patients undergoing cardiac surgery. *Antimicrob Agents Chemother* 17:269–272, 1980.

3
HIGH-RISK PATIENTS

22

The Neonate

John D. Nelson, M.D.

BACKGROUND

Infections in newborn infants can result from transplacental intrauterine seeding of the fetus, from ascending infection after rupture of the amniotic membranes, from contamination during delivery, and from environmental sources in the nursery. As a result, it is often difficult to ascertain whether or not an infection has been nosocomially acquired. For example, group B streptococcal infection in a neonate can have its genesis in any of the routes mentioned above. Even the time of onset of disease does not help differentiate among congenital, perinatal, or nosocomial sources because there can be a lag of many days between infection and clinical expression of that infection. For example, a group B streptococcal osteomyelitis first recognized at 3 weeks of age could be the end result of a transient bacteremia during the perinatal period. Similarly, congenital syphilis commonly does not manifest itself until after the neonatal period.

Because it is often difficult to ascertain whether neonatal infection has a nosocomial source, the National Nosocomial Infections Study (NNIS), conducted by the Centers for Disease Control, designates all infections in the first 28 days of life as nosocomial, regardless of the actual source of those diseases. This decision by the NNIS has created confusion and renders their data virtually uninterpretable. Infection control measures clearly have no impact on vertical transmission from mother to child. In this chapter, the word ''nosocomial'' is used in the narrower sense of ''hospital-acquired.''

Incidence and Types of Infection

The hospitals participating in the NNIS reported a mean nosocomial infection rate in newborn nurseries of 1.4%, with a range from 0.9% in community hospitals to 1.7% in large university hospitals (1). For reasons mentioned earlier, it is uncertain how many of the reported infections were truly nosocomial in origin.

Rates of infection vary, depending on the population served by a particular nursery and the prevalence of certain risk factors discussed below. Rates as high as 25% have been reported in neonatal intensive care units (NNICU) (2–4). In the most comprehensive study of nosocomial infections in a children's hospital, the nosocomial infection rate of 22.2 per 100 hospital discharges in the NNICU was the highest rate of any service in the hospital (2). (The overall rate for the entire hospital was 4.1 per 100 hospital discharges.) That hospital is a tertiary care center, and its newborn population included many high-risk infants. By contrast, primary care community hospital nurseries populated mainly by healthy, term infants had a nosocomial infection rate of only 0.86% (1). In the Children's Hospital Medical Center of Cincinnati, the infection rate during a 24-month period was 0.6% in the normal newborn nursery and 16.9% in the NNICU (5).

Skin infections, diarrhea, respiratory infections, and septicemia are the most common nosocomial infections encountered in a nursery. The etiologic agents are varied, and outbreaks are common. Epidemic situations are particularly characteristic of organisms that colonize skin and mucous membranes with a high colonization-to-disease ratio. In this manner, the organism is able to perpetuate itself in the environment over a prolonged time while causing invasive disease in a small proportion of infants periodically.

Major, often inexplicable shifts in etiologic agents occur about once each decade. Nationwide in the United States, a severe problem with invasive strains of *Staphylococcus aureus* emerged in the 1950s and disappeared in the 1960s largely unrelated to the many attempts that were made to control the problem. Since then, the strains of *S. aureus* causing periodic outbreaks of skin lesions have not been invasive, virulent organisms. In the 1960s, *Pseudomonas aeruginosa* was a serious nosocomial pathogen in many nurseries and a particularly nasty one because of high case fatality rates. Contaminated water in incubators and respiratory therapy equipment was the source of *Pseudomonas*. The 1970s were the decade of group B streptococcal infections, while in the 1980s, methicillin-resistant strains of *S. aureus* and *Staphylococcus epidermidis* have emerged as difficult nosocomial problems in NNICUs. Group B streptococci remain important as pathogens in vertical transmission from mother to baby, but their role as nosocomial agents, which was common in many nurseries (6–8), is largely a thing of the past. Occasionally, clusters of cases suggesting nosocomial transmission turn out to be unrelated coincidences if strain markers are investigated. An outbreak of seven cases of late onset group B streptococcal disease in an NNICU during a brief period was shown to be spurious because the bacteriophage types for the individual strains were different (9). Restriction endonuclease digestion analysis has been helpful in evaluating putative cases of nosocomial herpes simplex virus and cytomegalovirus infection. Differing antimicrobial susceptibility patterns ("antibiograms") of common bacterial infections is another method of disproving identity of strains.

It is common for different types of microorganisms to cause similar clinical pictures in neonates, but certain generalizations can be made. Viruses cause respiratory, cardiac, gastrointestinal, and central nervous system infections. Gram-positive cocci cause skin lesions, sepsis, and pneumonia. Aerobic Gram-negative enteric bacilli cause sepsis, meningitis, and urinary tract infections. Anaerobic Gram-negative enteric bacilli are associated with intraabdominal sepsis and occasionally with abscesses elsewhere. *Pseudomonas aeruginosa* causes conjunctivitis, necrotizing pneumonia, and ecthymatous skin lesions. *Citrobacter diversus* has a great proclivity to cause brain abscesses. *Candida* species cause skin and mucous membrane lesions and occasionally fungemia or endocarditis. Regardless of these generalizations, the phy-

sician evaluating a neonate for infection should assume that virtually any type of microorganism can cause virtually any clinical syndrome and proceed accordingly with the laboratory investigation.

Neonatal nosocomial infections are significant determinants of mortality, especially in low birthweight infants (10,11). Their prevention, recognition and appropriate management should be a goal of all physicians who take care of neonates.

Risk Factors

Immunologic Factors. All newborn infants are immunologically deficient. The degree of immunologic deficiency relates principally to immature gestational age, but it is further compromised by intensive care measures. Invasive procedures violate mechanical barriers to infection, and humoral factors and phagocytic cells are depleted by blood-drawing.

The skin and mucous membranes are the first lines of defense against microbial invasion. By 37 weeks gestation, the skin is an effective barrier, but in premature infants with scant stratum corneum, the skin is quite permeable (12). This not only leads to the problem of excessive water loss through the skin; it also allows easy entry of bacteria, especially in the preterm baby of less than 32 weeks gestation who typically has translucent skin. After approximately 2 weeks of age, the stratum corneum is quite well-developed, regardless of the gestational age.

The normal microflora of the skin and mucous membrane present in older individuals plays a major role in defense against pathogens (13). These tissues are sterile at the moment of birth, unless there has been intrauterine infection; hence this important barrier to pathogens is lacking in most newborns.

Once a pathogen gains entry to blood or other body fluids and tissues, humoral and phagocytic factors are of paramount importance in defense. Polymorphonuclear leukocytes (PMNs) and monocytes exhibit sluggish migration toward exogenous antigens with chemotactic activity being only ½–¼ that of adult PMNs (14–16). Neonatal PMNs have essentially normal phagocytic activity when they are suspended in adult serum, but phagocytosis is decreased in neonatal serum, suggesting the presence of an inhibitory factor (17,18). Contrary to the defects in chemotaxis and phagocytosis, intracellular bactericidal activity of neonatal PMNs is normal (19–21).

Reticuloendothelial activity is decreased in the term neonate, and in the preterm baby, it is essentially absent (22). Both the classic and the alternate pathways of the complement system have decreased activity (23,24), and fibronectin is deficient (25).

Maternal IgG begins passing transplacentally to the fetus at about 15 weeks of gestation, and the fetus begins synthesizing IgM at about 30 weeks of gestation. The major portion of maternal antibody is delivered to the fetus during the last trimester by an active mechanism that allows neonatal IgG concentrations in excess of maternal concentrations at term (26). However, the preterm infant at 32 weeks gestation has a serum IgG concentration that is less than half that of a term infant. Preterm infants commonly have a large portion of their blood volume withdrawn for diagnostic laboratory tests. This further depletes humoral factors. The situation is aggravated by the usual practice of replenishing the infant with packed red blood cells rather than with whole blood. As a consequence, many sick preterm babies have severely depleted immunoglobulin stores (27).

Sources of Infection and Modes of Transmission.   The opportunities for a neonate to acquire infection and for infection to be transmitted from baby to baby are abundant. Routine and invasive procedures all carry a risk.

Intrapartum fetal scalp electrodes have been associated with infections caused by several aerobic Gram-positive and Gram-negative bacteria, by anaerobes, and by herpes simplex virus (28–30). At Johns Hopkins hospital, nine infections (0.9%) occurred in 1030 infants in whom spiral scalp electrodes were used (29). The severed umbilical cord stump is at risk of colonization with invasive pathogens (31). Endotracheal suctioning has resulted in transmission of herpes simplex virus infection from a physician to a neonate (32), and the author has seen a case of pharyngeal gonorrhea in a resident physician acquired by mouth-to-mouth resuscitation of a contaminated newborn.

Outbreaks of infection caused by *Pseudomonas aeruginosa* and other nonfermenting bacteria have been traced to contaminated eye wash (33,34), resuscitation equipment (35–37), and hand carriage by personnel (38). Contaminated

scrub brushes were responsible for an outbreak of *Serratia marcescens* infection (39). Contaminated hand lotions (40,41), topical ointments (42), phenolic disinfectants (43), intravenous fluids (44–46), laundry (47), umbilical cord wash (48), hexachlorophene disinfectants (49,50), and total parenteral nutrition fluids (51) have caused outbreaks of infection in nurseries.

Although fomites and contaminated liquids carry a potential risk for spreading infections in nurseries, outbreaks are far more often traced to personnel and poor aseptic techniques. Transmission of pathogens on hands of nursery personnel is the most common cause of outbreaks of infections in neonates (38,52–57). Nasal carriage of staphylococci in personnel can be responsible for outbreaks of skin infections in newborns (58,59). Group A streptococcal infections can occur in nurseries (60–65) as well as outbreaks of diarrheal illness caused by toxigenic coliform bacilli (66), rotaviruses (67), *Shigella* (68), *Salmonella* (69), and enteropathogenic *Escherichia coli* (70–72). In most such outbreaks, fecal-oral spread via hands of personnel is the mode of transmission.

Echovirus 11 (73–76) and respiratory syncytial virus (77) are spread both by airborne droplets and by the hands of personnel touching contaminated objects, since the viruses survive well on hard surfaces in the nursery environment. Coxsackie virus (78–80) and toxigenic *Clostridium difficile* (81) infections are spread by the fecal-oral route, but the mode of transmission of rotavirus infection is not entirely clear; it may involve fecal-oral, respiratory, and vertical routes of spread (82–85).

In years past, the sick or preterm newborn was thought to be a fragile thing that should be disturbed as little as possible. With the concept of aggressive intensive care and with technological advances came the common use of invasive procedures and devices to manage sick neonates. All carry the risk of nosocomial infection. Intravascular catheters are commonly used to administer fluids and medications and to obtain samples of blood for laboratory tests.

Placement of umbilical vein catheters may introduce bacteria on the umbilical stump into the circulation or dislodge contaminated thrombi (86–89). Culture of bacteria from the catheter tip following removal has been uncommon in some series (90,91), and more than 50% in others (86,92,93). The frequency of infection does not appear to correlate with age at time of insertion, local skin care, or duration of catheterization (86,92,93).

Infectious complications are less common with umbilical artery catheters (92–99), very rare with radial artery catheters (100), and virtually never seen with scalp vein needles (101,102).

Indwelling peripheral or central venous catheters are commonly used in sick newborns. In one series (102), bacteremia occurred in 8% of patients. Central venous catheters used for administering parenteral nutrition are a serious infection risk from preparation of the fluid, contamination when connections in the line are violated, and entry wound infections. In several reported series involving more than 2500 infants receiving parenteral nutrition, bacteremia occurred in a broad range from none to 23%. In most series, however, the frequency was from 3–8% (103–115). Candidemia was a more serious problem, occurring in about 10% of cases overall. Nosocomial fungemia has also been associated with intravascular pressure monitoring devices (116).

Insertion of an umbilical vein catheter in order to perform exchange blood transfusion induces a transient bacteremia in 10% of cases, but this is cleared spontanenously by the infant, and prophylactic antibiotics have no beneficial effect (88,117).

Banked breast milk that becomes contaminated during collection or storage has caused *Salmonella* (118) and *Klebsiella* (119) infections in preterm infants.

The instances of nosocomial infection in newborn nurseries and intensive care units are numerous. The foregoing examples are merely representative of the problem.

POPULATION

The newborn nursery, as with other areas of the hospital, has permanent residents—the hospital staff—and two types of transients—the neonates and their visitors. The unique feature of the population in the nursery is that most babies enter it without an established microflora of the skin and mucous membranes. An aim of infection control is to allow the infant to establish a microflora consisting of nonpathogenic organisms, rather than the potentially pathogenic organisms that are common in the hospital environment.

Unless there has been intrauterine infection, the infant's first exposure to microorganisms is the maternal vaginal flora. In a study of the endocervical flora during labor (120), 75% of women had a mixture of aerobic and anaerobic bacteria and 25% had only aerobes. The major aerobes were *Staphylococcus epidermidis*, diphtheroids, and *Gardnerella vaginale*. Various *Bacteroides* species were found, but *B. fragilis* was rare (120,121). Potential pathogens in the vagina or cervix are group B streptococci, gonococci, chlamydia, *Listeria monocytogenes*, cytomegalovirus, and herpes simplex virus, among others.

The newborn's nares commonly become colonized with *S. epidermidis* and nonhemolytic streptococci. Those organisms and *Klebsiella-Enterobacter* species colonize the umbilical stump (122). *Escherichia coli* colonization increases during summer months, and increased humidity favors *E. coli* and *P. aeruginosa* (123).

An anaerobic fecal flora develops rapidly, and by a week of age, the frequency of colonization with *B. fragilis* and other anerobes in babies born vaginally and formula-fed approaches that of adults (124,125). Breastfeeding or being delivered by cesarean section decreases substantially the rate of *Bacteroides* colonization (124) but not that of *Clostridium difficile* (125).

Being in an intensive care nursery has a profound effect on the types of organisms colonizing the skin, nasopharynx, and colon (126,127). *Klebsiella-Enterobacter* species and *Citrobacter* are prominent. Antibiotic therapy, which is commonly given to infants in an ICU setting, suppresses anaerobic bacteria and increases the likelihood of colonization with Gram-negative aerobes, especially those resistant to commonly used antibiotics (126–129). Nasotracheal tubes lead to the colonization of the trachea and bronchii with organisms that normally colonize the nasopharynx (130) and nasojejunal feeding tubes result in colonization of the proximal small bowel with coliform bacilli (131).

Besides possibly acquiring microorganisms from nursery personnel and from other infants, newborns can be infected by other sources. These include potential pathogens from other areas of the hospital via medical and surgical consultants and community-type organisms from visitors.

DIAGNOSIS
Recognition of Nosocomial Infections

Nosocomial infections in the nursery are more often insidious than explosive. When a cluster of cases break out within a short time span, it is an easy matter to recognize the situation. This is the pattern with organisms that have a high disease-to-colonization ratio, such as several infectious diarrheal agents and group A streptococci.

More commonly, nosocomial infections are caused by diseases with low disease-to-colonization ratios, such as group B streptococci and *Staphylococcus aureus*. There may be only one or two cases of overt disease for every 100 infants who are colonized with the microorganism. To complicate the matter of recognition, infants who become colonized with a potential pathogen may not develop disease until many days after discharge from the nursery. This is more likely to occur in a term nursery, whence infants are customarily discharged on the 2nd or 3rd day of life, than in a preterm nursery, where the babies stay for weeks or months. For example, in one outbreak of group A streptococcal infection in a term nursery that eventually involved 69 cases, there had been 20 cases spread over a 3-month period before the problem was recognized (60). Only four infants had developed disease while in the nursery during the 3 months. Thus, the magnitude of the outbreak was initially overlooked.

Appropriate bacterial, fungal and viral cultures, rapid antigen detection methods, and acute and convalescent serum specimens for antibody studies are variously needed to establish the pathogen involved in nosocomial infections, depending on the circumstances.

SURVEILLANCE

The nursery staff must be alert to occurrences of possible nosocomial infection and report them to the person or persons responsible for infection control. Inpatient education of nursing and technical personnel about infection control practices repeated at regular intervals helps to maintain awareness.

Monitoring for nosocomial infection problems requires a collaborative effort of the microbiology laboratory staff, the infection control practitioner, and the nursery staff. Ideally, information about numbers and types of infection and antibiotic resistance patterns should funnel to one person, the infection control practitioner or his or her designee. Alert laboratory technologists may be the first to notice unusual pathogens, development of antibiotic resistance in common pathogens, or unusual clusters of cases.

A system should be established to monitor infections and antibiotic susceptibilities. The frequency with which that is done depends largely on the usual census of the nursery and the numbers of high-risk, preterm babies. A community hospital unit with only 1000–2000 babies annually and one that refers complicated cases to a tertiary center would require only infrequent surveillance. On the other hand, a hospital like the one in which the author works, which has more than 12,000 deliveries annually and a 70-bed special care nursery, requires monthly surveillance.

Monitoring of events occurring in the nursery is relatively easy. It requires only a commitment of time and effort. Monitoring for diseases acquired in the nursery but first manifest after discharge to home is a difficult matter, unless the infants are followed in one clinic. Most often, the infants are followed by many physicians, and communication is not good. Physicians should be requested to report illnesses of possible nosocomial origin to the infection control practitioner in the nursery.

Identifying Sources of Infection

In general, routine surveillance cultures from neonates, personnel, and environmental sources in the nursery are not useful, recommended, or cost-effective (132–134). Most nosocomial infections are spread from baby to baby by hands or clothing of personnel. Transmission of infection from baby to personnel or from personnel to baby is an unusual event, and environmental surfaces, solutions, ointments, etc. are not often the source of infection in a modern nursery.

If nosocomial infections continue after a cohorting system has been established and after handwashing has been reinforced, thought should be given to the possibility of an environmental or personnel source of the problem. One should be selective in performing cultures of personnel or fomites. The nature of the organism and the anatomic site of the infection often give clues to the possible sources of contamination. For example, if the nosocomial pathogen is an enteric Gram-negative bacillus typically transmitted by the fecal-oral route, the overwhelming likelihood is that hands of personnel are responsible for transmission, and environmental cultures are not likely to be worthwhile. However, if the site of infection is the lower respiratory tract of intubated babies, one should look carefully at procedures for suctioning and possible contamination of suctioning equipment. If the pathogen is *Pseudomonas* or another "water bug," one should suspect standing water or mist as the source.

Careful thought about procedures, close scrutiny of their implementation, and good detective work are usually more productive than indiscriminate culturing of the inanimate and animate environment.

Whenever new procedures are introduced in the nursery, the potential for nosocomial infection should be considered. This is particularly important in the case of invasive procedures. Details of the procedure should be discussed with the infection control practitioner. Depending on the nature of the procedure, it may be desirable to do prospective surveillance cultures to monitor for nosocomial infection.

MANAGEMENT

Recommended isolation practices based on the guidelines developed by the Centers for Disease Control (132) are presented in Table 22.1. Details about the various types of isolation are presented in Chapter 25.

Congenital Infections

The literal meaning of the word congenital, namely, present at birth, has given way to medical jargon. By tradition, the phrase "congenital infection" has come to mean syphilis, rubella, toxoplasmosis, herpes simplex, listeriosis, cytomegalovirus infection, hepatitis, and varicella. Illogically, a baby with intrauterine infection caused by group B streptococcus or Gram-negative bacilli is not considered to have a congenital infection, although it is truly congenitally infected. Equally illogically, most infections with herpes simplex, cytomegalovirus, and hepatitis are acquired at or shortly after birth, yet those diseases are classified as being congenital infections.

Toxoplasmosis. Nosocomial infection with *Toxoplasma gondii* does not occur, so no isolation precautions are necessary for a congenitally infected infant. *Toxoplasma* organisms can be present in the lungs, saliva, sputum, kidneys, and intestine, suggesting a potential risk for nursery personnel. Transmission from such sources, however, has never been proved (135).

Syphilis. Skin and mucous membrane lesions of an untreated infant with congenital syphilis are teeming with spirochetes, and such infants may have spirochetemia. Therefore, blood precautions are necessary, and gloves should be worn when handling the infant. *Treponema pallidum* in the environment is rapidly killed by drying, heat, and soap (136–139). Once treatment with penicillin is started, the organisms are eliminated rapidly (140), and isolation precautions can be discontinued after 24 hours.

Herpes Simplex Infection. On rare occasions, intrauterine infection of the fetus with herpes simplex virus occurs (141), but in most cases, the infection is acquired during vaginal delivery. The risk of infection is greater when the mother has primary infection than when she has reactivation disease, and prematurity is also a risk factor (142). Cesarean delivery before or within 4 hours of rupture of amniotic membranes substantially reduces but does not eliminate the risk of infection when the mother has genital lesions.

Nosocomial transmission of herpes simplex infection is rare, but an outbreak in a nursery has been reported (143) in which the identity of the isolates was confirmed by restriction endonuclease cleavage of viral DNA. Herpes simplex virus type 1 was transmitted to a newborn during endotracheal suctioning by a physician with herpes labialis (32). It has also been transmitted by fetal scalp electrodes (30), from a maternal breast lesion (144), and from oral lesions of nursery personnel (145).

Antenatal maternal cultures are poorly predictive of the infant's risk of exposure to herpes simplex virus at delivery (146). Therefore, it is prudent to use contact isolation precautions on babies born vaginally to a mother with a history of genital herpes whether lesions are present or not. Vaginal cultures should be taken at delivery to guide future management.

The optimum management of an infant at risk for neonatal herpes simplex infection has not been developed by controlled studies, but a consensus opinion has emerged (147). The baby with herpetic lesions and the baby at risk for developing herpes should be managed with contact isolation precautions in the nursery. Breastfeeding is contraindicated only if the mother has a herpetic lesion on the breast. The mother with genital lesions should be instructed about hand-

Table 22.1
Guidelines for Isolation of Neonates

Disease or Condition	Strict	Contact	Respiratory	Enteric	Drainage/ Secretion	Blood/ Body fluids	Routine
AIDS						♦	
Candidiasis							♦
Chlamydia					♦		
Conjunctivitis[a]					♦		
Cytomegalovirus						♦	
Diarrhea				♦			
Gonorrhea		♦					
Hepatitis in mother							
A				♦			
B						♦	
Non-A, non-B						♦	
Herpes simplex		♦					
Meningitis, aseptic				♦			
Meningitis, bacterial							♦
Multiply resistant bacteria (Disease or colonization)		♦					
Necrotizing enterocolitis				♦			
Pneumonia		♦					
Respiratory viruses		♦					
Rubella		♦					
Sepsis							♦
Skin infections, funisitis or omphalitis							
Minor					♦		
Major[b]		♦					
Syphilis							
Mucosal or skin lesions					♦	♦	
Other						♦	
Toxoplasmosis							♦
Tuberculosis							♦
Urinary tract infection							♦
Varicella in mother	♦						

[a]Contact isolation for gonococcal conjunctivitis.
[b]Recommended for any staphylococcal or group A streptococcal infection.

washing, and the mother with herpes labialis should be instructed not to kiss the baby. On the 2nd day of life, viral cultures of the eye and oral cavity are taken from the baby at risk. If the baby has been born vaginally to a mother with primary genital herpes or, in the case of reactivation disease, if the baby has another risk factor (prematurity, invasive instrumentation, or lacerations) anticipatory antiviral chemotherapy is given until the results of cultures are known.

If an infant has been treated for active disease, and must remain in the nursery subsequently for other medical reasons, isolation precautions should be maintained because recurrence of skin lesions is common.

Personnel with genital herpes can work in the nursery, provided that strict handwashing techniques are used. Personnel with herpes labialis should not have direct contact with infants until the lesions are crusted.

Listeriosis. There have been several reports of clusters of cases of neonatal listeriosis and of protracted outbreaks in nurseries (148–150). In general, investigations have failed to uncover the source of infection and, specifically, nosocomial sources have not been implicated. Congenitally infected neonates with listeriosis are managed the same as babies with other types of sepsis or meningitis (see below).

Hepatitis. Transmission of hepatitis A from mother to newborn is extraordinarily rare. Nevertheless, if the mother had onset of jaundice within a week of delivery, the baby should be considered possibly contaminated by hepatitis virus in her feces, and enteric precautions should be used with the infant. The infant is given human immune serum globulin.

With hepatitis B infection in the mother, the risk of infection of her newborn is very great, particularly if she carries the e antigen (151). Vertical transmission is effectively prevented by combined use of hepatitis B immune globulin and hepatitis vaccine (152) or even by vaccine alone (153).

The infant should be considered potentially infected. Gloves should be worn when cleansing the baby's skin after birth. Blood and body fluid precautions are used until the immune status of the infant has been verified at 1 year of age.

Varicella. Infants whose mothers have varicella typically develop disease between the 5th and 10th day of life, unless effective prophylaxis is used (154). Severe infection is most likely if the mother's illness began between 4 days before delivery and 48 hours after delivery. Passive immunization with varicella-zoster immune globulin (VZIG) should be given immediately after birth (155,156). Prophylaxis is not uniformly effective (157), so strict isolation technique should be used until the infant is 10 days old.

Rubella. Congenital rubella has become uncommon in areas where rubella vaccination is widely used. Chronicity of infection is characteristic of intrauterine infection. The virus can be recovered from pharyngeal secretions, urine, conjunctival fluid, and feces for many months and occasionally years (158,159). Contact isolation precautions are used in the infant with congenital rubella for at least 1 year.

Cytomegalovirus Infection. Cytomegalovirus (CMV) infection is the most common congenital infection, and many additional babies acquire the virus during delivery or postnatally (160–162). The neonate can also acquire infection from breast milk (163,164) or from blood transfusions (165). CMV can survive on paper diapers for as long as 48 hours (166), posing a potential hazard to nursery personnel who handle diapers. Transmission of CMV infection

among neonates in an intensive care unit has been documented using restriction endonuclease digestion analysis (167). This technology has also been used to show that apparent nosocomial infections in nurseries were actually caused by different strains (168,169).

In spite of the pervasiveness of CMV in a nursery setting, transmission between babies and personnel is rare (169–173). The virus is present in saliva and urine of infected infants, but routine handwashing appears to be a very effective preventive measure. Although the risk of acquisition of infection by female personnel from an infant is remote, it is prudent to exempt pregnant personnel from attending an infant with known CMV infection, for emotional reasons rather than scientific ones. This practice is totally illogical, however, since for every baby in a nursery with known CMV infection there are many others with unknown, asymptomatic infection (174).

The diverse opinions about isolation precautions for CMV infection were summarized by Plotkin (173). This author agrees with Plotkin's recommendations:

1. Do not routinely screen neonates for CMV infection;
2. Use "pregnant women precautions" for infants with known CMV infection;
3. Screen female personnel who have the potential for becoming pregnant for their CMV serologic status.

Sepsis and Meningitis

Infants with neonatal sepsis or meningitis are often critically ill and require constant observation and intensive care. Excessive isolation precautions could interfere with their care. The risk of horizontal transmission of sepsis or meningitis in a nursery is virtually nonexistent, so routine precautions are sufficient. A possible exception is the case of *Citrobacter diversus*, an organism with unusual tropism for the central nervous system and a proclivity to cause brain abscesses. Outbreaks related to horizontal transmission of *C. diversus* have occurred (175). Because the reservoir of that organism is the gastrointestinal tract, enteric precautions are recommended.

Aseptic meningitis in the neonate is commonly caused by enteroviruses, and outbreaks are not uncommon (75,76,176). The aseptic meningitis or encephalitis may be accompanied by cardiac and hepatic involvement. Enteric precautions are important in preventing transmission of enteroviruses.

Skin, Soft Tissue, and Mucous Membrane Infections

Staphylococcus aureus is the most common cause of nosocomial skin infections in a nursery. Prolonged outbreaks are not unusual (58,59), and control can be difficult.

Daily bathing of infants with hexachlorophene-containing soap decreases skin colonization rates (177,178), but was not reliable for controlling outbreaks (179). Rates of skin and mucous membrane colonization do not always correlate with rates of disease (180). In 1971, the Food and Drug Administration recommended that routine bathing be discontinued because of rare but serious toxicity of absorbed hexachlorophene (181). In the late 1950s and early 1960s, nurseries in the United States were plagued with outbreaks caused by phage group I invasive strains of *S. aureus*. Since that time, outbreaks have usually been with phage group II organisms, which are not invasive, and produce bullous impetiginous lesions (58,59,182). Outbreaks of scalded skin syndrome (Ritter's disease) have occurred in nurseries (183).

When multiple cases of staphylococcal disease occur within a limited timeframe in a nursery, and it is determined by antibiograms and bacteriophage testing that a single strain is involved, the following steps can be undertaken sequentially to control the outbreak:

1. Surveillance cultures (anterior nasal swabs and skin or umbilical cord swabs) of all infants in the nursery will define the extent of colonization. Strict adherence to handwashing and other aseptic techniques should be enforced. Colonized babies should be segregated. Epidemiologic surveillance for new cases of disease is carried out. Investigation for a specific environmental source of the outbreak should be undertaken, but will usually be unrevealing. In the majority of instances, these measures suffice for control of the outbreak.

2. If, after 1 or 2 weeks of these measures, new cases of disease continue to occur, a cohorting program should be implemented, if physical facilities permit. The value of performing nasal cultures of hospital personnel is debatable, but on occasion a nasal carrier among the staff will be responsible (58,59). The carrier

should be treated with bacitracin ointment or gentamicin nose drops in an attempt to eliminate carriage. In almost all cases, the cohort system and strict enforcement of aseptic technique terminate the outbreak.

3. Only in the most prolonged and persistent staphylococcal outbreak would one consider implementation of a bacterial interference regimen with *Staphylococcus aureus* 502A (184). The methods and results of bacterial interference programs have been reviewed by Shinefield et al. (185). Passing an umbilical catheter through a stump colonized with *S. aureus* 502A is potentially hazardous (186).

Group A streptococcal nosocomial infection most commonly involves the umbilical cord stump. The funisitis is mild with little inflammation and minimal secretion, which is characteristically sticky and has a musty odor (60). In one outbreak, there were 51 cases of funisitis or omphalitis, two cases of infected circumcision wound, and one case each of meningitis, peritonitis, and conjunctivitis (60). Local measures, such as applying triple dye or bacitracin ointment to the umbilical stump, may stop the outbreak, but sometimes it is necessary to give an injection of benzathine penicillin (50,000 units/kg) to all newborns until the epidemic has been stopped (60–65).

Nosocomial chlamydial infection has not been reported, probably because the disease usually has its onset after babies have been discharged to home. In preantibiotic days, gonococcal infection in a nursery was exceedingly difficult to control (47), but with present-day therapy, gonococcal ophthalmia is not a nosocomial problem. Nevertheless, the CDC recommends that full contact precautions be used instead of drainage/secretion precautions. Contact precautions are also recommended for group A streptococcal and staphylococcal skin or mucous membrane infections.

Respiratory Infections

Pertussis (187) and influenza A (188) are uncommon causes of nosocomial respiratory infections. Most outbreaks are caused by viruses, especially respiratory syncytial virus (77,189–191). RSV infection in infants with underlying cardiopulmonary disease is often lethal (189). Gowning and use of masks is ineffectual in preventing transmission of respiratory infection between infants and personnel because RSV survives on hard surfaces such as the crib or bassinet and is transmitted by hands of personnel (190,191).

Anterior nasal swab specimens can be used for rapid diagnosis of influenza A or RSV infections by immunofluorescence or ELISA methods (77,192–195). This is an exceedingly valuable tool for rapid identification of the cause of an outbreak.

Infants with respiratory symptoms should be housed in nurseries separate from asymptomatic babies. In the intensive care unit, separate isolation facilities should be available. In addition to airborne transmission of virus to other infants and personnel, transmission of infected secretions by hands or fomites can occur, so it is recommended that gowns be worn when handling babies. Handwashing is important. In a controlled trial (191), gowning and masking were not significantly better than handwashing alone in preventing nosocomial transmission of respiratory syncytial virus; nevertheless, these procedures are generally employed during an outbreak for whatever minimal benefit might accrue from their use. Masks should be changed frequently. Wearing eye-nose goggles was the most effective means of preventing nosocomial transmission of RSV in one study (196). Aerosolized ribavirin therapy shortens the period of shedding of RSV and could help in control (197–199).

In pertussis outbreaks, affected infants and personnel are treated with erythromycin to reduce their infectivity. (The dosage for newborns is 10 mg/kg 2 or 3 times daily (200).) In large and persistent outbreaks, widespread antibiotic prophylaxis and vaccination programs for personnel may be necessary (187).

Diarrhea and Necrotizing Enterocolitis

Outbreaks of infectious diarrhea in nurseries can be caused by enterotoxigenic (66) or enteropathogenic (71,72) strains of *Escherichia coli*, *Shigella* (68), *Salmonella* (69), or viruses (67,82,85,201).

The syndrome of necrotizing enterocolitis (NEC) is probably multifactorial in origin, but clusters of cases associated with intestinal pathogens suggest an important role for infection in pathogenesis. Outbreaks of NEC have been temporally associated with *Enterobacter cloacae* (202), rotavirus (203), and enteric coronavirus

(204,205); however, in most outbreaks of NEC, no enteric pathogen is found. The role of toxigenic *Clostridium difficile* in diarrhea or NEC is difficult to assess because many asymptomatic neonates are colonized with these strains (81,206–208). Presumably, the neonate's intestinal mucosa lacks receptors for this toxin.

In isolated cases of diarrhea, or when outbreaks occur, all infants with diarrhea should be housed separately from other infants. Strict enteric precautions for handling soiled diapers and washing of hands should be stressed. Rectal swab or stool cultures for bacterial pathogens should be performed on sick infants and other infants cared for by the same personnel. Rapid diagnostic tests for rotavirus antigen in stool or electron microscopic examination for coronavirus can be done. When enteropathogenic serotypes of *E. coli* are involved, specific fluorescent antibody study of rectal swab specimens rapidly identifies asymptomatic carriers who could serve as reservoirs for perpetuation of the outbreak (209). When a bacterial pathogen is responsible for the outbreak, appropriate antibiotic therapy is instituted. The exception is *Salmonella* infection in which antibiotic therapy is not effective or desirable in the routine case (210), but is reserved for those with bacteremic complications, acute colitis, or protracted diarrhea and failure to thrive. Oral colonization has been implicated as epidemiologically important in nosocomial spread of *Salmonella* in a nursery outbreak (211); in such cases, care must be taken with formula bottles and other objects contaminated with oral secretions.

Formerly, it was recommended that nurseries for low birthweight infants be closed to admissions and new units opened when a substantial outbreak of diarrhea disease occurred (212). With the measures just outlined, this disruptive, impractical extreme solution should not be necessary.

Fungal Infections

Candidal infection of the oral mucous membranes and diaper area is common in neonates who have received broad spectrum antibiotics, but nosocomial transmission is not obvious in such cases. Candida sepsis is a major problem in infants receiving total parenteral nutrition (103–115), and nosocomial fungemia has been associated with contaminated transducer domes (116).

Mixed pulmonary fungal infections occurred in babies in a special care unit secondary to construction activities (213). The fungi were *Aspergillus*, *Rhizopus*, and *Cryptococcus*.

Rhizopus contamination of elastic surgical bandages has caused wound infection (214). Seven nurses working in a newborn nursery developed *Microsporum canis* dermatophytosis of the left forearm. The infection was attributed to their practice of cradling the head of an infant who had *M. canis* infection of the occiput on their unclothed left forearm while feeding the baby (215). Such episodes are peculiarities and, in general, nosocomial fungal infections other than *Candida* sepsis are rare.

Multiply Resistant Bacteria

Antibiotic usage is not common in a nursery for term infants, but in intensive care units, more than half the infants receive antibiotic therapy on one or more occasions (126,127). Antibiotics alter the normal respiratory and gut flora so that resistant bacteria often replace the antibiotic-susceptible flora. Aminoglycosides are the most commonly used anti-Gram-negative antibiotics in nurseries. The common use of one particular aminoglycoside frequently leads to the emergence of coliform bacteria resistant to that aminoglycoside (216). When kanamycin was the most commonly employed antibiotic, reports of outbreaks caused by kanamycin-resistant strains appeared (52-55,217). Then followed outbreaks of coliform infections resistant to both kanamycin and gentamicin (51,218,219), and finally with strains resistant to kanamycin, gentamicin, and amikacin (220). *Klebsiella* and *Serratia* strains are especially likely to develop resistance. The resistance is due to transferable plasmids.

With the advent of new cephalosporin drugs, treatment of disease caused by aminoglycoside-resistant coliform bacteria has been facilitated. However, widespread use of cefotaxime in a nursery because of a problem with gentamicin-resistant *Klebsiella* led to the emergence of cefotaxime-resistant *Enterobacter cloacae* as a problem (221).

Methicillin-resistant *Staphylococcus aureus* strains, which are resistant to all the penicillins and cephalosporins, are common in many tertiary centers. *Staphylococcus epidermidis* is a common nosocomial pathogen associated with intravascular catheters, and most *S. epidermidis* strains are resistant to β-lactams. To date, vancomycin-resistant staphylococci have not appeared.

Monitoring antibiotic susceptibilities allows one to detect the emergence of a problem with multiply resistant organisms. A search for a source should be undertaken, but generally one will not be found since the infections are usually endogenous from altered flora. All infants in the nursing unit should have cultures of appropriate mucosal surfaces (rectum, throat, trachea) to determine the frequency of colonization with the resistant strain. Identification is facilitated by incorporating an antibiotic to which the organism is resistant into the culture medium. Colonized infants are placed in a cohort, and scrupulous aseptic technique is used in handling them. Ill babies are treated with an appropriate antibiotic, but it is futile to try to eliminate asymptomatic colonization with antibiotics. Periodic surveillance cultures are taken, and new cohorts of colonized and uncolonized babies are formed until the epidemic has been controlled. Because some colonized infants require medical care in a low-birthweight nursery or intensive care unit for a prolonged time, it often takes months to rid the unit of all colonized babies.

PREVENTION

Modification of Isolation Precautions for Newborns and Infants

The following recommendations are reprinted verbatim from the CDC Guidelines for Isolation Precautions in Hospitals (132).

Isolation precautions for newborns and infants may have to be modified from those recommended for adults because 1) usually only a small number of private rooms are available for newborns and infants, and 2) during outbreaks, it is frequently necessary to establish cohorts of newborns and infants. Moreover, a newborn may need to be placed on isolation precautions at delivery because its mother has an infection.

It has often been recommended that infected newborns or those suspected of being infected (regardless of the pathogen and clinical manifestations) should be put in a private room. This recommendation was based on the assumptions that a geographically isolated room was necessary to protect uninfected newborns and that infected newborns would receive closer scrutiny and better care in such a room. Neither of these assumptions is completely correct.

Separate isolation rooms are seldom indicated for newborns with many kinds of infection if the following conditions are met:

1. An adequate number of nursing and medical personnel are on duty and have sufficient time for appropriate handwashing;
2. Sufficient space is available for a 4- to 6-foot aisle or area between newborn stations;
3. An adequate number of sinks for handwashing are available in each nursery room or area; and
4. Continuing instruction is given to personnel about the mode of transmission of infections.

When these criteria are not met, a separate room with handwashing facilities may be indicated.

Another incorrect assumption regarding isolation precautions for newborns and infants is that forced-air incubators can be substituted for private rooms. These incubators may filter the incoming air, but not the air discharged into the nursery. Moreover, the surfaces of incubators housing newborns or infants can easily become contaminated with organisms infecting or colonizing the patient, so personnel working with the patient through portholes may have their hands and forearms colonized. Forced-air incubators, therefore, are satisfactory for limited "protective" isolation of newborns and infants, but should not be relied on as a major means of preventing transmission from infected patients to others.

Isolation precautions for an infected or colonized newborn or infant, or for a newborn of a mother suspected of having an infectious disease can be determined by the specific viral or bacterial pathogen, the clinical manifestations, the source and possible modes of transmission, and the number of colonized or infected newborns or infants. Other factors to be considered include the overall condition of the newborn or infant and the kind of care required, the available space and facilities, the nurse-to-patient ratio, and the size and type of nursery services for newborns and infants.

In addition to applying isolation precautions, cohorts may be established to keep to a minimum the transmission of organisms or infectious diseases among different groups of newborns and infants in large nurseries. A cohort usually consists of all well newborns from the same 24- or 48-hour birth period; these newborns are admitted to and kept in a single nursery room and, ideally, are taken care of by a single group of personnel who do not take care of any other cohort during the same shift. After the newborns in a cohort have been discharged, the room is thoroughly cleaned and prepared to accept the next cohort.

Cohorting is not practical as a routine for small nurseries or in neonatal intensive care units or graded care nurseries. It is useful in these nurseries, however, as a control measure during outbreaks or for managing a group of infants or newborns colonized or infected with an epidemiologically important pathogen. Under these circumstances, having separate rooms for each cohort is ideal, but not mandatory for many kinds of infections if cohorts can be kept separate within a single large room and if personnel are assigned to take care of only those in the cohort.

During outbreaks, newborns or infants with overt infection or colonization and personnel who are carriers, if indicated, should be identified rapidly and placed in cohorts; if rapid identification is not possible, exposed newborns or infants should be placed in a cohort separate from those with disease and from unexposed infants and newborns and new admission. The success of cohorting depends largely on the willingness and ability of nursing and ancillary personnel to adhere strictly to the cohort system and to meticulously follow patient-care practices.

Nursery Design

The preceding CDC statement addresses certain issues about nursery design. It is difficult to generalize about this subject because there is no uniformity in construction or arrangement of newborn nurseries. Some have multiple small rooms and others have one large open area. Some have isolation rooms for individual infants, and others do not. Nevertheless, certain generalizations apply to all nurseries.

Detailed recommendations for design of newborn units are available (222,223). The amount of floor space per bassinet for adequate separation of infants is from 20–25 square feet in a full-term infant nursery, approximately 50 square feet in an intermediate care nursery, and between 80–100 square feet in an intensive care unit. Sinks should be conveniently located throughout the nursery so that it is no more than a few steps from any bassinet to a sink. Foot or knee controls of faucets are preferable to hand controls. Faucet aerators should not be used, and sinks should not be set in countertops.

Floors, walls, counters, bassinets, and other furniture should be made of materials that are easily cleaned and will withstand disinfectant solutions. Disinfectant detergents are recommended for routine cleaning. When a baby is discharged, the bassinet should be disinfected with an iodophor or quartenary disinfectant.

Routine Procedures

Many restrictive procedures in the past have been shown to be ceremonial rites with little or no impact on nosocomial infection rates (224–227). Caps, masks, hairnets, and beard bags have been discarded as routines. Families are no longer barred from nurseries or intensive care units, and medical and surgical consultants are encouraged to enter the newborn unit. Excessive precautionary procedures were not only ineffectual, but discouraged personnel from giving optimal hands-on care to babies and decreased the likelihood of adherence to effective procedures.

Handwashing. The key to effective infection control in the nursery is strict adherence to handwashing before and after handling babies.

At the time of entering the nursery, personnel should remove rings, watches, and bracelets and scrub the hands and forearms to the elbows for a 3–5 minute period. An antiseptic agent, such as an iodophor, 4% chlorhexidine or 3% hexachlorophene, should be used for this scrub. Thereafter, hands should be washed for 15 seconds before and after handling an infant or potentially contaminated object. These washes are preferably done with an antiseptic soap, but plain soap suffices if the individual's skin is sensitive to the antiseptic. Fifteen seconds of washing has no impact on the individual's resident (i.e., "permanent") skin flora, but effectively removes transient flora acquired by handling a contaminated person or object (228). Hands should also be washed after touching one's own hair, face, or other parts of the body.

Attire, Gowns, Caps, Masks, and Gloves. Personnel working in the nursery should wear scrub suits. When they leave the nursery temporarily, they should don a long-sleeved gown over the scrub suit. Visitors, consultants, and laboratory and housekeeping personnel should wear a long-sleeved gown over their street clothes.

Caps, masks, and hairnets need not be used routinely. Personnel with long hair falling to the shoulders should tie it in back so that it does not fall in front of the shoulders, or they should wear a cap.

A long-sleeved gown should hang at the side of each bassinet. This is worn whenever the baby's body will come in contact with the body of personnel, such as during feeding. If disposable gowns are not used, the gown should be replaced every 8 hours.

Gowns, caps, masks, and gloves are used when specified for babies on isolation precautions and for performing invasive procedures.

The foregoing recommendations for limited use of gowns are the author's preferences. However, many studies have failed to establish a significant benefit in reducing colonization or disease rates attributable to gowning in term or preterm nurseries (229–233). A study in an intensive care unit showed no change in handwashing rates, infection, or intravascular catheter colonization rates when gowns were used (234). More than 700 neonatologists in the United States were recently surveyed about gowning preferences for their nurseries and intensive care units (235). The results were wildly divergent practices. Clearly, there is no uniform standard, and each nursery should set policy that appears to be most appropriate for the quality of personnel and the types of problems encountered.

Linens. Traditionally, bassinet linens in the admission observation area and intermediate and intensive care areas have been sterilized by autoclaving. This is recommended by the American Academy of Pediatrics (223). The need for this practice is debatable since linens after routine laundering are essentially germ-free (236). Linens and infant clothing are not important sources of infection. Routine laundering is sufficient, provided the hospital's laundry facilities are good. Soiled linens should be placed into plastic bags in receptacles, sealed, and removed from the nursery every 8 hours.

Neonatal Cord and Eye Care and Bathing. Many topical agents and systemic penicillin have been shown to be effective in preventing gonococcal ophthalmia (237). In most states, the type and method of prophylaxis are precisely defined by law. Credè prophylaxis with 1% silver nitrate has the disadvantages of causing chemical conjunctivitis frequently and of being ineffective for preventing chlamydial conjunctivitis. Tetracycline or erythromycin ophthalmic ointments have been proposed to prevent both gonococcal and chlamydial conjunctivitis, but there are conflicting reports about efficacy in preventing chlamydial conjunctivitis (238,239).

An intramuscular injection of penicillin G (50,000 units for term babies and 25,000 units for preterm babies) has been used for combined prophylaxis of gonococcal ophthalmia and group B streptococcal sepsis. It was effective in one study (240) but not in another (241).

A single intramuscular dose of 125 mg of ceftriaxone was effective in preventing (242) and treating (243) ophthalmia caused by penicillin-resistant gonococci.

Some parents refuse to have anything put in the eyes of their newborn because of theoretical concerns about interference with parental-infant bonding. In such cases, an injection of penicillin G or ceftriaxone should be used.

Assuming that state law allows options for prophylaxis, the author's preference is 1% tetracycline ophthalmic suspension for routine use or an intramuscular dose of 125 mg ceftriaxone in areas where penicillin and tetracycline-resistant gonococci are prevalent. Whichever preparation is used, unit dosage containers should be used to avoid possible contamination of multidose vials of tubes or ointment.

Immediately after birth, the umbilical cord is tied with sterile tape and cut with sterile instruments. Use of contaminated string or application of contaminated poultices to the severed cord is a cause of tetanus neonatorum. Subsequent care of the umbilical stump is a disputed matter. Application of "triple dye," silver sulfadiazine cream, or bacitracin ointment is advocated by some investigators, while others prefer keeping the cord dry with periodic swabbing with alcohol. Such disparate results of the various methods of removing umbilical stump flora have been reported (60,244–246), that it is not possible to identify the most effective method, other than concluding that dyes or antimicrobials more effectively suppress flora than do alcohol or castile soap.

Care of the newborn's skin has also been a debated matter. Current opinion holds that the so-called "dry technique" decreases trauma, avoids potential toxicity from absorption of chemicals, and interferes least with acquisition of normal flora. Shortly after birth, the skin is cleansed using sterile cotton sponges and either sterile water or mild castile soap. Thereafter, the diaper area is cleansed similarly when necessary. For reasons mentioned earlier, routine bathing with hexachlorophene is not recommended. However, during an outbreak of staphylococcal infection, its use as an adjunct to the control program can be considered vis-à-vis its neurotoxic potential.

Equipment.   Equipment used on many babies, such as stethoscopes, should be cleaned between use on each baby with alcohol or an iodophor solution. In an intensive care unit it is common practice to provide a stethoscope for each baby.

Nebulization equipment is easily contaminated. It should be autoclaved or gas sterilized every 8 hours. Water reservoirs are filled only with sterile distilled water and are autoclaved daily. Suction catheters and equipment must be sterilized by autoclaving or gas sterilization.

The parts of x-ray equipment that come into contact with an infant should be cleaned with alcohol or an iodophor solution.

If closed incubators are used, there must be scrupulous attention to cleaning and disinfection. Porthole cuffs should be replaced daily, and water reservoirs drained and refilled with sterile distilled water each day.

Visitors.   Parents should follow the same procedure for scrubbing used by personnel before entering the nursery. A long-sleeved gown should be worn over street clothing. They should be instructed not to touch other babies. Parents with respiratory infections or infected lesions on the hand or face should not be permitted in the nursery. Most nurseries permit children who are siblings of critically ill babies to enter the intensive care unit. They are barred from visiting if they have an infectious illness or have been recently exposed to a contagious disease.

Special Procedures

Collection and Storage of Breast Milk. Many mothers like to provide breast milk for their babies who are unable to nurse because of illness or prematurity. Before collecting the specimen, the mother scrubs her hands with an iodophor or other antiseptic. The nipple area does not need special cleansing. The milk is expressed manually or collected by a mechanical device and stored in a sterile bottle under refrigeration until it is used. Milk obtained this way is generally sterile or has small colony counts of nonpathogenic bacteria from normal skin flora (247,248).

The milk can be safely stored under refrigeration for up to 48 hours (247) and perhaps as long as 5 days (248). It is not necessary to perform quantitative bacterial cultures of the milk for surveillance.

Formerly, some institutions used banked breast milk collected from multiple donors, but this practice has largely been abandoned and it is not recommended because of outbreaks of infection with *Salmonella* (118), *Klebsiella* (119), and other organisms. If banked milk is used, it is mandatory to perform cultures for bacterial pathogens before it is given to infants.

Blood Banking Procedures.   In addition to routine testing for hepatitis B antigen and human immunodeficiency virus antibody, it is recommended that only blood without cytomegalovirus antibody be given to neonates. In some hospitals, this restriction is applied only to preterm neonates. An alternative is to use frozen, deglycerolized blood, since that process inactivates CMV (249).

Blood banking procedures are discussed in detail in Chapter 9.

Intravascular Catheters.   Bacteremia is a small but important complication of intravascular catheters. In four studies (96,98,131,151) of umbilical vein catheters, 7 (3.7%) of 187 infants developed bacteremia. The risk was smaller with umbilical artery catheters; 18 (1.2%) of 1,500 infants became bacteremic (90,91,94,96,98,100,250,251). This is comparable to the 11 (1.2%) of 893 rate of bacteremia found in studies of neonates who had only peripheral vein needles (99,101,102,252). The infections were principally with coliform bacilli and staphylococci; *Pseudomonas* and *Candida* infections were uncommon. Percutaneous catheterization of the radial artery is a low-risk procedure in terms of infection. In one series of 147 radial artery catheterizations, there was only one instance of catheter-related bacteremia, although 25% of cultures of catheter tips following removal were positive (100). Risk of bacteremia secondary to scalp vein needles is minimal; no case occurred in two series involving 361 babies (101,102).

To insert a radial artery or umbilical vessel catheter, the skin area should be scrubbed with an iodophor and draped with sterile surgical drapes. The operator should wear a cap, mask, and gloves. A gown is optional. The entrance wound should be covered with a sterile dressing that is changed daily. It is common practice to cleanse the entrance wound daily with an iodophor or other antiseptic or to use an antibiotic

ointment, but the value of these procedures has not been established.

Insertion of central venous catheters into the jugular or subclavian veins is done in the surgical suite with full surgical sterile technique. Daily dressing changes are done with glove, mask, and cap precautions.

When an infant with an intravascular catheter shows signs of infection, the blood specimen for culture is drawn through the catheter. If the entrance wound becomes infected, the wound itself and the tip of the removed catheter should be cultured in addition to obtaining blood cultures.

It is not unusual for catheter tip cultures to be positive in the absence of bacteremia. There are opportunities for contamination of the tip by skin bacteria or in handling the specimen.

Prophylactic systemic antibiotics are *not* recommended for infants with intravascular catheters.

Intravascular catheters and central nervous system shunts are discussed in detail in Chapter 8.

Fluids for Total Parenteral Nutrition.   In 13 reported series of 2727 infants receiving total parenteral nutrition (TPN) through central venous catheters, bacteremia occurred in 2.5% and candidemia in 3.4% (103–115). Pore size of the filter in the line may be a critical factor. Holmes et al. (253) reported that *Pseudomonas* penetrated 0.45 μm pore size filters within 12 hours and *Klebsiella* or *Serratia* within 48 and 72 hours. No bacteria penetrated the 0.22 μm filters under the test conditions.

If fluids are mixed for TPN administration, this should be done under a positive-pressure filtered hood. The connections in the tubing line should not be violated. Because TPN fluids are most commonly given via central venous catheters, the precautions discussed above should be followed.

Antibiotic Usage

β-Lactam and aminoglycoside combinations are the mainstay of therapy in newborn nurseries. Because of the widespread use of these antibiotics in low birthweight nurseries and intensive care units, there is selective drug pressure, encouraging the emergence of resistance to aminoglycosides. As discussed earlier, a monitoring system to detect emerging resistance of pathogens to the aminoglycoside being administered should be used. Generally, the resistance will be specific for one or two of the aminoglycosides, and another aminoglycoside can be selected for routine use. For example, if gentamicin resistance appears, tobramycin or amikacin can be substituted.

A broad spectrum cephalosporin, such as cefotaxime or ceftriaxone, should not be used routinely. These valuable drugs should be held in reserve to be used in the event of nosocomial disease caused by bacteria that are resistant to all aminoglycosides. However, when there is an ongoing nosocomial infection problem with an organism resistant to all aminoglycosides, a cephalosporin should *temporarily* become the drug of choice for empiric therapy of suspected sepsis. Once the problem has disappeared, one should revert to an aminoglycoside for routine use. With continued use of the cephalosporin, resistance to that drug is likely to develop (221).

Infants with intravascular catheters are prone to infection with *S. epidermidis*, which is usually resistant to methicillin and other β-lactams. In that situation, or when there is a nosocomial problem with methicillin-resistant *S. aureus*, vancomycin should replace the β-lactam as empiric initial therapy for suspected sepsis. Antibiotic usage is discussed in detail in Chapter 28.

Immunotherapy

An experimental approach to the prevention of nosocomial infections in low birthweight babies is administration of intravenous gammaglobulin shortly after birth (254,255). There are attractive theoretical considerations to this approach (27). Antibody production and T cell function in the newborn function too slowly to have a significant impact on bacterial disease. The only specific immunity available to the infant is maternally derived immunoglobulin, which is deficient in preterm babies. In preliminary studies (254,255), there has been a decrease in the incidence of infection in preterm babies given intravenous gammaglobulin. Another approach is to administer gammaglobulin to the mother of a preterm baby during labor; however, the gammaglobulin does not cross the placenta until 32 weeks of gestation (256).

Employee Health

General aspects of employee health are discussed in Chapter 26 and in the CDC Guidelines for Infection Control in Hospital Personnel (257).

Female personnel in the nursery who are of childbearing age should be tested serologically for susceptibility to rubella and, if necessary, given rubella vaccine with appropriate precautions. As discussed earlier, transmission of cytomegalovirus from infected babies to pregnant personnel is a minimal hazard. Although this appears to be a rare occurrence, prudence dictates that pregnant personnel should not handle infants known to be infected with cytomegalovirus, and they should pay meticulous attention to handwashing after diapering any infant.

Personnel with active tuberculosis (258), pertussis (187,188), influenza (189,259), and other communicable diseases should be excluded from the nursery. Personnel with bacterial or viral lesions on exposed areas of skin should not handle infants. For other respiratory, gastrointestinal, and cutaneous infections, rigid criteria for exclusion from the nursery are more difficult to establish. Clinical judgment and common sense are weighed against the needs of the nursery. Upper respiratory viral infections are most transmissible during the acute febrile period, but since symptoms often linger for a couple of weeks, employees are often permitted to return before complete resolution of symptoms. Personnel with acute diarrheal illnesses are preferably excluded or permitted to work if it is believed that scrupulous handwashing will effectively eliminate risk of transmission of the agent. Individuals with acute pharyngitis and fever should be excluded until group A streptococcal infection has been ruled out or treated. Management of herpes simplex infection is discussed in Chapter 11.

REFERENCES

1. Horan TC, White JW, Jarvis WR, Emori TG, Culver DH, Munn VP, Thornsberry C, Olson DR, Hughes JM: Nosocomial infection surveillance, 1984. *MMWR* 35 (No. 1SS):17SS–29SS.
2. Welliver RC, McLaughlin S: Unique epidemiology of nosocomial infection in a children's hospital. *Am J Dis Child* 138:131–135, 1984.
3. Hemming VG, Overall JC Jr, Britt MR: Nosocomial infections in a newborn intensive-care unit: Results of forty-one months of surveillance. *N Engl J Med* 294:1310–1316, 1976.
4. Jarvis WR: The epidemiology of nosocomial infections in pediatric patients. *Pediatr Infect Dis* 6: (in press)
5. Maguire GC, Nordin J, Myers MG, Koontz KP, Hierholzer W, Nassif E: Infections acquired by young infants. *Am J Dis Child* 135:693–698, 1981.
6. Anthony BF, Okada DM, Hobel CJ: Epidemiology of the group B streptococcus: Maternal and nosocomial sources for infant acquisitions. *J Pediatr* 95:431–436, 1979.
7. Paredes A, Wong P, Mason EO Jr, Taber LH, Barrett FF: Nosocomial transmission of group B streptococci in a newborn nursery. *Pediatrics* 59:679–682, 1977.
8. Boyer KM, Vogel LC, Gotoff SP, Gadzala CA, Stringer J, Maxted WR: Nosocomial transmission of bacteriophage type 7/11/12 group B streptococci in a special care nursery. *Am J Dis Child* 134:964–966, 1980.

9. Weems JJ Jr, Jarvis WR, Colman G: A cluster of late onset group B streptococcal infections in low birth weight premature infants: No evidence for horizontal transmission. *Pediatr Infect Dis* 5:715–717, 1986.

10. LaGamma EF, Drusin LM, Mackles AW, Machalek S, Auld PAM: Neonatal infections: An important determinant of late NICU mortality in infants less than 1,000 g at birth. *Am J Dis Child* 137:838–841, 1983.

11. Pierce JR, Merenstein GB, Stocker JT: Immediate postmortem cultures in an intensive care nursery. *Pediatr Infect Dis* 3:510–513, 1984.

12. Harpin VA, Eutter N: Barrier properties of the newborn infant's skin. *J Pediatr* 102:419–425, 1983.

13. Rosebury T: *Life on Man*. New York, Viking Press, 1969.

14. Miller ME: Chemotactic function in the human neonate: Humoral and cellular aspects. *Pediatric Res* 5:487–492, 1971.

15. Pahwa S. Pahwa R, Grines E, Smithwick EM: Cellular and humoral components of monocyte and neutrophil chemotaxis in cord blood. *Pediatr Res* 5:487–492, 1977.

16. Klein RB, Fischer TJ, Gard SE, Biberstein M, Rich KC, Stiehm ER: Decreased mononuclear and polymorphonuclear chemotaxis in human newborns, infants, and young children. *Pediatrics* 60:467–472, 1977.

17. Dassett JH, Williams RC Jr, Quie PG: Studies on interaction of bacteria, serum factors and polymorphonuclear leucocytes in mothers and newborns. *Pediatrics* 44:49–57, 1969.

18. Miller ME: Phagocytosis in the newborn infant: Humoral and cellular factors. *J Pediatr* 74:255–259, 1969.

19. Coen R, Grush O, Kauder E: Studies of bactericidal activity and metabolism of the leukocyte in full term neonates. *J Pediatr* 75:400–406, 1969.

20. Park BH, Holmes B, Good RA: Metabolic activities in leucocytes in newborn infants. *J Pediatr* 76:237–241, 1970.

21. Cocchi P, Marianelli L: Phagocytosis and intracellular killing of *Pseudomonas aeruginosa* in premature infants. *Helv Paediatr Acta* 22:110–118, 1967.

22. Holroyde CP, Oski FA, Gardner FH: The "pocked" erythrocyte: Red-cell surface alterations in reticuloendothelial immaturity of the neonate. *N Engl J Med* 281:516–520, 1969.

23. McCracken GH, Eichenwald HF: Leukocyte function and the development of opsonic and complement activity in the neonate. *Am J Dis Child* 121:120–126, 1971.

24. Farman ML, Stiehm ER: Impaired opsonic activity but normal phagocytosis in low birth weight infants. *N Engl J Med* 281:926–931, 1969.

25. Gerdes JS, Yoder MC, Douglas SD, Polin RA: Decreased plasma fibronectin in neonatal sepsis. *Pediatrics* 72:877–881, 1983.

26. Kohler PF, Farr RS: Elevation of cord over maternal IgG immunoglobulin—Evidence for an active placental IgG transport. *Nature* 210:1070–1071, 1966.

27. Wasserman RL: Intravenous gamma globulin prophylaxis for newborn infants. *Pediatr Infect Dis* 5:620–621, 1986.

28. Reveri M, Kirshnamurthy C: Gonococcal scalp abscess. *J Pediatr* 94:819–820, 1979.

29. Feder HM, MacLean WC, Moxon R: Scalp abscess secondary to fetal scalp electrode. *J Pediatr* 89:808–809, 1976.

30. Parvey LS, Chien LT: Neonatal herpes simplex virus infection introduced by fetal-monitor scalp electrodes. *Pediatrics* 65:1150–1153, 1980.

31. Cushing AH: Omphalitis: A review. *Pediatr Infect Dis* 4:282–285, 1985.

32. Van Dyke RB, Spector SA: Transmission of herpes simplex virus type 1 to a newborn infant during endotracheal suctioning for meconium aspiration. *Pediatr Infect Dis* 3:153–156, 1984.

33. Foley JF, Gravelle CR, Englehard WE, Chin TDY: Achromobacter septicemia—fatalities in prematures. *Am J Dis Child* 101:279–288, 1961.

34. Plotkin SA, McKitrick JC: Nosocomial meningitis of the newborn caused by a flavobacterium. *JAMA* 198:662–664, 1966.

35. Fierer J, Taylor PM, Gezon HM: *Pseudomonas aeruginosa* epidemic traced to delivery-room resuscitators. *N Engl J Med* 276:991–1067, 1967.

36. Drewett SE, Payne DJH, Tuke W, Verdon PE: Eradication of *Pseudomonas aeruginosa* infection from a special-care nursery. *Lancet* 1:946–948, 1972.

37. Bobo RA, Newton EJ, Jones LF, Farmer LH, Farmer JJ III: Nursery outbreak of *Pseudomonas aeruginosa*: epidemiological conclusion from five different typing methods. *Appl Microbiol* 25:414–420, 1973.

38. Morehead CD, Houck PW: Epidemiology of *Pseudomonas* infections in a pediatric intensive care unit. *Am J Dis Child* 124:564–570, 1972.

39. Anagostakis D, Fitsialos J. Koretsia C, Messaritakis J, Matsaniotis N: A nursery outbreak of *Serratia marcescens* infection. *Am J Dis Child* 135:413–414, 1981.

40. Morse LJ, Schonbeck LE: Hand lotions—a potential nosocomial hazard. *N Engl J Med* 278:376–378, 1968.

41. Morse LF, Williams HL, Grenn FP Jr, Eldridge EE, Rotta JR: Septicemia due to *Klebsiella pneumoniae* originating from a hand-cream dispenser. *N Engl J Med* 277:472–473, 1967.

42. Wargo EJ: Microbial contamination of topical ointments. *Am J Hosp Pharm* 30:332–335, 1973.

43. Simmons NA, Gardner DA: Bacterial contamination of a phenolic disinfectant. *Br Med J* 2:668–669, 1969.

44. Felts SK, Schaffner W, Melley MA, Koenig MG: Sepsis caused by contaminated intravenous fluids. Epidemiologic, clinical and laboratory investigation of an outbreak in one hospital. *Ann Intern Med* 77:881–890, 1972.

45. Guynn JB Jr, Poretz DM, Duma RJ: Growth of various bacteria in a variety of intravenous fluids. *Am J Hosp Pharm* 30:321–325, 1973.

46. Lapage SP, Johnson R, Hoomes B: Bacteria from intravenous fluids. *Lancet* 2:284–285, 1973.

47. Cooperman MB: Gonococcus arthritis in infancy. *Am J Dis Child* 33:932–948, 1927.

48. McCormack RC, Kunin CM: Control of a single source nursery epidemic due to *Serratia marcescens*. *Pediatrics* 37:750–755, 1966.

49. Simmons NA: Contamination of disinfectants. *Br Med J* 1:842, 1969.

50. Ayliffe GA, Barrowcliff DF, Lowbury EJ: Contamination of disinfectants. *Br Med J* 1:505, 1969.

51. Munson DP, Thompson TR, Johnson DE, Rhame FS, VanDrunen N, Ferrieri P: Coagulase-negative staphylococcal septicemia: Experience in a newborn intensive care unit. *J Pediatr* 101:602–606, 1982.

52. Adler JL, Shulman JA, Terry PM, Feldman DB, Skaliy P: Nosocomial colonization with kanamycin-resistant *Klebsiella pneumoniae*, types 2 and 11, in a premature nursery. *J Pediatr* 77:376–385, 1970.

53. Hable KA, Matsen JM, Wheeler DJ, Hunt CE, Quie PG: *Klebsiella* type 33 septicemia in an infant intensive care unit. *J Pediatr* 80:920–924, 1972.

54. Armstrong-Ressy CT: Epidemiologic notes and reports of nosocomial *Serratia marcescens* infections in neonates. *Puerto Rico MMWR*, May 18, 1974.

55. Cichon MJ, Craig CP, Sargent J, Brauner L: Nosocomial *Klebsiella* infections in an intensive care nursery. *South Med J* 70:33–35, 1977.

56. Parry MF, Hutchinson JH, Brown NA, Wu C-H, Estreller L: Gram-negative sepsis in neonates: A nursery outbreak due to hand carriage of *Citrobacter diversus*. *Pediatrics* 65:1105–1109, 1980.

57. Markowitz SM, Veazey JM Jr, Macrina FL, Mayhall CG, Lamb VA: Sequential outbreaks of infection due to *Klebsiella Pneumoniae* in a neonatal intensive care unit: Implication of a conjugative R plasmid. *J Infect Dis* 142:106–112, 1980.

58. Nakashima AK, Allen JR, Martone WJ, Plikaytis BD, Storer B, Cook LM, Wright SP: Epidemic bullous impetigo in a nursery due to a nasal carrier of *Staphylococcus aureus*: Role of epidemiology and control measures. *Infect Control* 5:326–331, 1984.

59. Belani A, Sherertz RJ, Sullivan ML, Russell BA, Reumen PD: Outbreak of staphylococcal infection in two hospital nur-

series traced to a single nasal carrier. *Infect Control* 7:487–490, 1986.

60. Nelson JD, Dillon HC Jr, Howard JB: A prolonged nursery epidemic associated with a newly recognized type of group A streptococcus. *J Pediatr* 89:792–796, 1976.
61. Gezon HM, Schaberg MJ, Klein JO: Concurrent epidemics of *Staphylococcus aureus* and group A streptococcus disease in a newborn nursery—control with penicillin G and hexachlorophene bathing. *Pediatrics* 51:383–390, 1973.
62. Geil CC, Castle WK, Mortimer EA Jr: Group A streptococcal infections in newborn nurseries. *Pediatrics* 46:849–854, 1970.
63. Tancer ML, McManus JE, Belotti G: Group A, type 33, β-hemolytic streptococcal outbreak on a maternity and newborn service. *Am J Obstet Gynecol* 103:1028–1033, 1969.
64. Dillon HC Jr: Group A type 12 streptococcal infection in a newborn nursery. *Am J Dis Child* 112:177–184, 1966.
65. Langewisch WH: An epidemic of group A, type 1 streptococcal infections in newborn infants. *Pediatrics* 18:438–447, 1956.
66. Guerrant RL, Dickens MD, Wenzel RP, Kapikian AZ: Toxigenic bacterial diarrhea: Nursery outbreak involving bacterial strains. *J Pediatr* 89:885–891, 1976.
67. Cameron DJS, Bishop RF, Veenstra AA, Barnes GL: Non-cultivable viruses and neonatal diarrhea: Fifteen-month survey in a newborn special care nursery. *J Clin Microbiol* 8:93–98, 1978.
68. Salzman TC, Scher CD, Moss R: Shigellae with transferable drug resistance: Outbreak in a nursery for premature infants. *J Pediatr* 71:21–26, 1967.
69. Schroeder SA, Aserkoff B, Brachman PS: Epidemic salmonellosis in hospitals and institutions: A five-year review. *N Engl J Med* 279:674–678, 1968.
70. Olarte J, Ramos-Alverez M: Epidemic diarrhea in premature infants. *Am J Dis Child* 109:436–438, 1965.
71. Kaslow RA, Taylor A Jr, Dweck HS, Bobo RA, Steele CD, Cassady G Jr: Enteropathogenic *Escherichia coli* infection in a newborn nursery. *Am J Dis Child* 128:797–801, 1974.
72. Boyer KM, Petersen NJ, Farzaneh I, Pattison CP, Hart MC, Maynard JE: An outbreak of gastroenteritis due to *E. coli* 0142 in a neonatal nursery. *J Pediatr* 86:919–927, 1975
73. Nagington J, Wreghitt TG, Gandy G, Roberton NRC, Berry PJ: Fatal echovirus 11 infections in outbreaks in special-care baby unit. *Lancet* 2:725–728, 1978.
74. Modlin JF, Polk BF, Horton P, Etkind P, Crane E, Spiliotes A: Perinatal echovirus infection: Risk of transmission during a community outbreak. *N Engl J Med* 305:368–371, 1981.
75. Kinney JS, McCray E, Kaplan JE, Low DE, Hammond GW, Harding I, Pinsky PF, Davi MJ, Kovnats SF, Riben P, Martone WJ, Schonberger LB, Anderson LJ: Risk factors associated with echovirus 11 infection in a hospital nursery. *Pediatr Infect Dis* 5:191–197, 1986.
76. Modlin JF: Perinatal echovirus infection: Insights from a literature review of 61 cases of serious infection and 16 outbreaks in nurseries. *Rev Infect Dis* 8:918–926, 1986.
77. Mintz L, Ballard RA, Sniderman SH, Roth RS, Drew WL: Nosocomial respiratory syncytial virus infections in an intensive care nursery: Rapid diagnosis by direct immunofluorescence. *Pediatrics* 64:149–153, 1979.
78. Swender PT, Shott RJ, Williams ML: A community and intensive care nursery outbreak of coxsackievirus B5 meningitis. *Am J Dis Child* 127:42–45, 1975.
79. Farmer K, Patten PT: An outbreak of coxsackie B5 infection in a special care unit for newborn infants. *NZ Med J* 68:86–89, 1968.
80. Farmer K, MacArthur BA, Clay MM: A follow-up study of 15 cases of neonatal meningoencephalitis due to Coxsackievirus B5. *J Pediatr* 87:568–571, 1975.
81. Zedd AJ, Sell TL, Schaberg DR, Fekety FR, Cooperstock MS: Nosocomial *Clostridium difficile* reservoir in a neonatal intensive care unit. *Pediatr Infect Dis* 3:429–432, 1984.
82. Murphy AM, Albrey MB, Crewe EB: Rotavirus infections of neonates: *Lancet* 2:1149–1150, 1977.
83. Zissis G, Lambert JP, Fonteyne J, deKegel D: Child-mother transmission of rotavirus? (Letter) *Lancet* 1:96, 1976.

84. Lewis HM, Parry JV, Davies HA, Parry RP, Mott A, Dourmashkin RR, Sanderson PJ, Tyrrell AJ, Valman HB: A year's experience of the rotavirus syndrome and its association with respiratory illness. *Arch Dis Child* 54:339–346, 1979.
85. Rodriguez WJ, Kim HW, Brandt CD, Fletcher AB, Parrott RH: Rotavirus: A cause of nosocomial infection in the nursery. *J Pediatr* 101:274–277, 1982.
86. Balagtas RC, Bell CE, Edwards LD, Levin S: Risk of local and systemic infections associated with umbilical vein catheterization: A prospective study in 86 newborn patients. *Pediatrics* 48:359–367, 1971.
87. Lipsitz PG, Cornet JM: Blood cultures from the umbilical vein in the newborn infant. *Pediatrics* 26:657–660, 1960.
88. Nelson JD, Richardson J, Shelton S: The significance of bacteremia with exchange transfusion. *J Pediatr* 66:291–299, 1965.
89. Houck PW, Nelson JD, Kay JL: Fatal septicemia due to *Staphylococcus aureus* 502A. *Am J Dis Child* 123:45–48, 1972.
90. Casalino MB, Lipsitz PJ: Contamination of umbilical catheters. (Letter to the Editor) *J Pediatr* 78:1077–1078, 1971.
91. Powers WF, Tooley WH: Contamination of umbilical vessel catheters. Encouraging information. (Letter to the Editor) *Pediatrics* 49:470–471, 1972.
92. Krauss AN, Albert RF, Kannan MM: Contamination of umbilical catheters in newborn infant. *J Pediatr* 77:965–969, 1970.
93. Van Vliet PKJ, Gupta JM: Prophylactic antibiotics in umbilical artery catheterization in the newborn. *Arch Dis Child* 48:296–300, 1973.
94. Bard H, Albert G, Teasdale F, Daray B, Martineau B: Prophylactic antibiotics in chronic umbilical artery catheterization in respiratory distress syndrome. *Arch Dis Child* 48:630–635, 1973.
95. Gupta JM, Robertson NRC, Wigglesworth JS: Umbilical artery catheterization in the newborn. *Arch Dis Child* 43:382–387, 1968.
96. Cochran WD, Davis HT, Smith CA: Advantages and complications of umbilical artery catheterization in the newborn. *Pediatrics* 42:769–777, 1968.
97. Egan EA, Eitzman DV: Umbilical vessel catheterization. *Am J Dis Child* 121:213–218, 1971.
98. Sarrut S, Alain J, Alison F: Les complications precoces de la perfusion par la veine ombilicale chez le premature. *Arch Franc Pediat* 26:651–657, 1969.
99. Vidyasagar D, Downes JJ, Boggs TR Jr: Respiratory distress syndrome of newborn infants, II. Technic of catheterization of umbilical artery and clinical results of treatment of 124 patients. *Clin Pediatr* 9:332–337, 1970.
100. Adams JM, Speer ME, Rudolph AJ: Bacterial colonization of radial artery catheters. *Pediatrics* 65:94–97, 1980
101. Crossley KM, Matsen JM: The scalp-vein needle: A prospective study of complications. *JAMA* 220:985–987, 1972.
102. Peter G, Lloyd-Still JD, Lovejoy FH Jr: Local infection and bacteremia from scalp vein needles and polyethylene catheters in children. *J Pediatr* 80:78–83, 1972.
103. Fuchs PC: Indwelling intravenous polyethylene catheters. *JAMA* 216:1447–1450, 1971.
104. Maki DG, Weise CE, Sarafin HW: A semiquantitative culture method for identifying intravenous-catheter-related infection. *N Engl J.* Med 296:1305–1309, 1977.
105. Dudrick SJ, Groff DB, Wilmore DW: Long-term venous catheterization in infants. *Surg Gynecol Obstet* 129:805–808, 1969.
106. Wilmore DW, Dudrick SJ: Safe long-term hyperalimentation. *Arch Surg* 98:256–258, 1969.
107. Filler RM, Eraklis AJ: Care of the critically ill child: Intravenous alimentation. *Pediatrics* 46:456–461, 1970.
108. Ashcraft KW, Leape LL: Candida sepsis complicating parenteral feeding. *JAMA* 212:454–456, 1970.
109. McGovern G: Intravenous hyperalimentation. *Milit Med* 135:1137–1145, 1970.
110. Curry CR, Quie PG: Fungal septicemia in patients receiving parenteral hyperalimentation. *N Engl J Med* 285:1221–1225, 1971.
111. Winters RW, Santulli TV, Heird WC, Schullinger JN, Driscoll

JM Jr: Hyperalimentation without sepsis. (Letter to the Editor) *N Engl J Med* 286:321–322, 1972.

112. Peden VH, Karpel JT: Total parenteral nutrition in premature infants. *J Pediatr* 81:137–144, 1972.

113. Driscoll JM Jr, Heird WC, Schullinger JN, Gongaware RD, Winters RW: Total intravenous alimentation in low-birth-weight infants: A preliminary report. *J Pediatr* 81:145–153, 1972.

114. Goldmann DA, Maki DG: Infection control in total parenteral nutrition. *JAMA* 223:1360–1364, 1973.

115. Dillon JD Jr, Schaffner W, Van Way CW III, Meng HC: Septicemia and total parenteral nutrition. *JAMA* 223:1341–1344, 1973.

116. Solomon SL, Alexander H, Eley JW, Anderson RL, Goodpasture HC, Smart S, Furman RM, Martone WJ: Nosocomial fungemia in neonates associated with intravascular pressure-monitoring devices. *Pediatr Infect Dis* 5:680–685, 1986.

117. Anagnostakis D, Kamba A, Petrochilou V, Arseni A, Matsaniotis N: Risk of infection associated with umbilical vein catheterization: A prospective study in 75 newborn infants. *J Pediatr* 86:759–765, 1975.

118. Ryder RW, Crosby-Ritchie A, McDonough B, Hall WJ: Human milk contaminated with *Salmonella kottbus*: A cause of nosocomial illness in infants. *JAMA* 238:1533–1534, 1977.

119. Donowitz LG, Marsik FJ, Fisher KA, Wenzel RP: Contaminated breast milk: A source of *Klebsiella* bacteremia in a newborn intensive care unit. *Rev Infect Dis* 3:716–720, 1981.

120. Thadepalli H, Chan WH, Maidman JE, Davidson EC Jr: Microflora of the cervix during normal labor and the puerperium. *J Infect Dis* 137:568–572, 1978.

121. Brook I, Barrett CT, Brinkman CR III, Martin WJ, Finegold SM: Aerobic and anaerobic bacterial flora of the maternal cervix and newborn gastric fluid and conjunctiva: A prospective study. *Pediatrics* 63:451–455, 1979.

122. Evans HE, Akpata SO, Baki A: Factors influencing the establishment of the neonatal bacterial flora. I. The role of host factors. *Arch Environ Health* 21:514–519, 1970.

123. Evans HE, Akpata SO, Baki A: Factors influencing the establishment of the neonatal bacterial flora. II. The role of environmental factors. *Arch Environ Health* 21:643–648, 1970.

124. Long SS, Swenson RM: Development of anaerobic fecal flora in healthy newborn infants. *J Pediatr* 91:298–301, 1977.

125. Siegel JD, Milvenan B: The effect of antibiotics on the development of the anaerobic gut flora of the neonate. Presented at the 20th Interscience Conference on Antimicrobial Agents and Chemotherapy. New Orleans, September 22–24, 1980.

126. Goldmann DA, Leclair J, Macone A: Bacterial colonization of neonates admitted to an intensive care environment. *J Pediatr* 93:288–293, 1978.

127. Farmer K: The influence of hospital environment and antibiotics on the bacterial flora of the upper respiratory tract of the newborn. *NZ Med J* 67:541–543, 1968.

128. Franco JA, Eitzman DV, Baer H: Antibiotic usage and microbial resistance in an intensive care nursery. *Am J Dis Child* 126:318–321, 1973.

129. Bennet R, Eriksson M, Nord C-E, Zetterstrom R: Fecal bacterial microflora of newborn infants during intensive care management and treatment with five antibiotic regimens. *Pediatr Infect Dis* 5:533–539, 1986.

130. Harris H, Wirtschafter D, Cassady G: Endotracheal intubation and its relationship to bacterial colonization and systemic infection of newborn infants. *Pediatrics* 58:816–823, 1976.

131. Challacombe D: Bacterial microflora in infants receiving nasojejunal tube feeding. (Letter to the Editor) *J Pediatr* 85:113, 1974.

132. Garner JS, Simmons BP: Guideline for isolation precautions in hospitals. *Infect Control* 4:245–325, 1983.

133. Allen JR: The newborn nursery. In Bennett JV, Brachman PS (eds): *Hospital Infections*, ed 2. Boston, Little, Brown & Co, 1986, pp 299–313.

134. Donowitz LG: Infection in the newborn. In Wenzel RP (ed): *Prevention and Control of Nosocomial Infections*. Baltimore, Williams & Wilkins, 1987, pp 481–493.

135. Remington JS, Desmonts G: Toxoplasmosis. In Remington JS, Klein JO (eds): *Infectious Diseases of the Fetus and Newborn Infant*, ed 2. Philadelphia, WB Saunders, 1983, p 167.

136. Boak RA, Carpenter CM, Warren SL: Studies on the physiological effects of fever temperatures. III. The thermal death time of *Treponema pallidum* in vitro with special reference to fever temperatures. *J Exp Med* 56:741–750, 1932.

137. Turner TB, Bauer JA, Kluth FC: The viability of the spirochetes of syphilis and yaws in desiccated blood serum. *Am J Med Sci* 202:416–423, 1941.

138. Keller R, Morton HE: The effect of a hand soap and a hexachlorophene soap on the cultivatable treponemata. *Am J Syph* 36:524–527, 1952.

139. Reasoner MA: The effect of soap on *T. pallidum*. *JAMA* 67:1799–1805, 1916.

140. Tucker HA, Robinson RCV: Disappearance time of *T. pallidum* from lesions of early syphilis following administration of crystalline penicillin. *Bull Johns Hopkins Hosp* 80:169–173, 1947.

141. Hutto C, Arvin A, Jacobs R, Steele R, Stagno S, Lyrene R, Willett L, Powell D, Andersen R, Werthammer J, Ratcliff G, Nahmias A, Christy C, Whitley R: Intrauterine herpes simplex virus infections. *J Pediatr* 110:97–101, 1987.

142. Nahmias AJ, Josey WE, Naib ZM, Freeman MG, Fernandez RS, Wheeler JH: Perinatal risk associated with maternal genital herpes simplex infection. *Am J Obstet Gynecol* 110:825–837, 1971.

143. Hammerberg O, Watts J, Chernesky M, Luchsinger I, Rawls W: An outbreak of herpes simplex virus type 1 in an intensive care nursery. *Pediatr Infect Dis* 2:290–294, 1983.

144. Sullivan-Bolyai JZ, Fife KH, Jacobs RF, Miller Z, Corey L: Disseminated neonatal herpes simplex virus type 1 from a maternal breast lesion. *Pediatrics* 71:455–457, 1983.

145. Van Dyke RB, Spector SA: Transmission of herpes simplex virus type 1 to a newborn infant during endotracheal suctioning for meconium aspiration. *Pediatr Infect Dis* 3:153–156, 1984.

146. Arvin AM, Hensleigh PA, Prober CG, Au DS, Yasukawa LL, Witter AE, Palumbo PE, Paryani SG, Yeager AS: Failure of antepartum maternal cultures to predict the infant's risk of exposure to herpes simplex virus at delivery. *N Engl J Med* 315:796–800, 1986.

147. Overall JC Jr, Whitley RJ, Yeager AS, McCracken GH Jr, Nelson JD: Prophylactic or anticipatory antiviral therapy for newborns exposed to herpes simplex infection. *Pediatr Infect Dis* 3:193–195, 1984.

148. Lennon D, Lewis B, Mantell C, Becroft D, Dove B, Farmer K, Tonkin S, Yeates N, Stamp R, Mickleson K: Epidemic perinatal listeriosis. *Pediatr Infect Dis* 3:30–34, 1984.

149. Evans JR, Allen AC, Stinson DA, Bortolussi R, Peddle LJ: Perinatal listeriosis: Report of an outbreak. *Pediatr Infect Dis* 4:237–241, 1985.

150. Canfield MA, Walterspiel JN, Edwards MS, Baker CJ, Wait RB, Urteaga JN: An epidemic of perinatal listeriosis serotype 1b in Hispanics in a Houston hospital. *Pediatr Infect Dis* 4:106, 1985.

151. Stevens CE, Neuroth RA, Beasley RP, Szmuness W: HBeAg and anti-HBe detection by radioimmunoassay: Correlation with vertical transmission of hepatitis B virus in Taiwan. *J Med Virol* 3:237–241, 1979.

152. Beasley RP, Hwang LY, Lee GC, Lan CC, Roan CH, Huang FY, Chen CL: Prevention of perinatally transmitted hepatitis B virus infections with hepatitis B immune globulin and hepatitis B vaccine. *Lancet* 2:1099–1102, 1983.

153. Xu Z-Y, Lu C-B, Francis DP, Purcell RH, Gun Z-L, Duan S-C, Chen R-J, Margolis HS, Juang C-H, Maynard JE, the United States-China Cooperative Study Group on Hepatitis B: Prevention of perinatal acquisition of hepatitis B virus carriage using vaccine: Preliminary report of a randomized, double-blind place-controlled and comparative trial. *Pediatrics* 76:713–718, 1985.

154. Myers JD: Congenital varicella in term infants: Risk considered. *J Infect Dis* 129:215–217, 1974.

155. Committee on Infectious Diseases: Expanded guidelines for

use of varicella-zoster immune globulin. *Pediatrics* 72:886–889, 1983.

156. Centers for Disease Control: Varicella-zoster immune globulin for the prevention of chickenpox. *MMWR* 33:84–100, 1984.

157. Bakshi SS, Miller TC, Kaplan M, Hammerschlag MR, Prince A, Gershon AA: Failure of varicella-zoster immunoglobulin in modification of severe congenital varicella. *Pediatr Infect Dis* 5:599–702, 1986.

158. Alford CA, Neva FA, Weller TH: Virologic and serologic studies on human products of conception after maternal rubella. *N Engl J Med* 271:1275–1281, 1964.

159. Alford CA Jr, Kanich LS: Congenital rubella: A review of the virologic and serologic phenomena occurring after maternal rubella in the first trimester. *South Med J* 59:745–748, 1966.

160. Stagno S, Whitley RJ: Herpesvirus infections of pregnancy. Part 1: Cytomegalovirus and Epstein-Barr virus infections. *N Engl J Med* 313:1270–1274, 1985.

161. Stagno S, Pass RF, Cloud G, Britt WJ, Henderson RE, Walton PD, Veren DA, Page F, Alford CA: Primary cytomegalovirus infection in pregnancy. *JAMA* 256:1904–1908, 1986.

162. Kumar ML, Nankervis GA, Cooper AR, Gold E: Postnatally acquired cytomegalovirus infections in infants of CMV-excreting mothers. *J Pediatr* 104:669–673, 1984.

163. Dworsky M, Yow M, Stagno S, Pass RF, Alford C: Cytomegalovirus infection of breast milk and transmission in infancy. *Pediatrics* 72:295–299, 1983.

164. Dworsky M, Stagno S, Pass RF, Cassady G, Alford C: Persistence of cytomegalovirus in human milk after storage. *J Pediatr* 101:440–443, 1982.

165. Adler SP, Chandrika T, Lawrence L, Baggett J: Cytomegalovirus infections in neonates acquired by blood transfusions. *Pediatr Infect Dis* 2:114–118, 1983.

166. Schupfer PC, Murph JR, Bale JF Jr: Survival of cytomegalovirus in paper diaper and saliva. *Pediatr Infect Dis* 5:677–679, 1986.

167. Spector SA: Transmission of cytomegalovirus among infants in hospital documented by restriction-endonuclease-digestion analysis. *Lancet* 1:378–381, 1983.

168. Yow AD, Lakeman AD, Stagno S, Reynolds RB, Plavidal FJ: Use of restriction enzymes to investigate the source of a primary cytomegalovirus infection in a pediatric nurse. *Pediatrics* 70:713–716, 1982.

169. Adler SP: Nosocomial transmission of cytomegalovirus. *Pediatr Infect Dis* 5:239–246, 1986.

170. Dworsky ME, Welch K, Cassady G, Stagno S: Occupational risk for primary cytomegalovirus infection among pediatric health-care workers. *N Engl J Med* 309:950–953, 1983.

171. Friedman HM, Lewis MR, Nemerofsky DM, Plotkin SA: Acquisition of cytomegalovirus infection among female employees at a pediatric hospital. *Pediatr Infect Dis* 3:233–235, 1984.

172. Balfour CL, Balfour HH Jr: Cytomegalovirus is not an occupational risk for nurses in renal transplant and neonatal units: Results of a prospective surveillance study. *JAMA* 256:1909–1914, 1986.

173. Plotkin SA: Cytomegalovirus in hospitals. *Pediatr Infect Dis* 5:177–178, 1986.

174. Interview with Sergio Stagno: Isolation precautions for patients with cytomegalovirus infection. *Pediatr Infect Dis* 1:145–147, 1982.

175. Lin F-Y, Devoe WF, Morrison C, Libonati J, Powers P, Gross RJ, Rowe B, Israel E, Morris JG: Outbreak of neonatal *Citrobacter diversus* meningitis in a suburban hospital. *Pediatr Infect Dis* 6:50–57, 1987.

176. Jenista JA, Powell KR, Menegus MA: Epidemiology of neonatal enterovirus infection. *J Pediatr* 104:685–690, 1984.

177. Hargiss C, Larson E: The epidemiology of *Staphylococcus aureus* in a newborn nursery from 1970 through 1976. *Pediatrics* 61:348–353, 1978.

178. Gezon HM, Schaberg MJ, Klein JO: Concurrent epidemic of *Staphylococcus aureus* and group A streptococcus disease in a newborn nursery—control with penicillin G and hexachlorophene bathing. *Pediatrics* 51:383–390, 1973.

179. Gehlbach SH, Gutman LT, Wilfert CM, Brumley GW, Katz SL: Recurrence of skin disease in a nursery: ineffectuality of hexachlorophene bathing. *Pediatrics* 55:422–424, 1975.

180. Gooch JJ, Britt EM: *Staphylococcus aureus* colonization and infection in newborn nursery patients. *Am J Dis Child* 132:893–896, 1978.

181. Tyrala EE, Hillman LS, Hillman RE, Dodson WE: Clinical pharmacology of hexachlorophene in newborn infants. *J Pediatr* 91:481–486, 1977.

182. Light IJ, Brackvogel V, Watton RL, Sutherland JM: An epidemic of bullous impetigo arising from a central admission-observation nursery. *Pediatrics* 49:15–21, 1972.

183. Faden HS, Burke JP, Glasgow LA, Everett JR III: Nursery outbreak of scalded-skin syndrome: Scarlatiniform rash due to phage group 1 *Staphylococcus aureus*. *Am J Dis Child* 130:265–268, 1976.

184. Eichenwald HF, Shinefield HR, Boris M. Ribble JC: "Bacterial interference" and staphylococcic colonization in infants and adults. *Ann NY Acad Sci* 128:365–380, 1965.

185. Shinefield HR, Ribble JC, Boris M: Bacterial interference between strains of *Staphylococcus aureus*. 1960 to 1970. *Am J Dis Child* 121:148–152, 1971.

186. Houck PW, Nelson JD, Kay JL: Fatal septicemia due to *Staphylococcus aureus* 502A: Report of a case and review of the infectious complications of bacterial interference programs. *Am J Dis Child* 123:45–48, 1972.

187. Linnemann CC Jr, Ramundo N, Perlstein PH, Minton SD, Englender GS, McCormick JB, Hayes PS: Use of pertussis vaccine in an epidemic involving hospital staff. *Lancet* 2:540–544, 1975.

188. Bauer CR, Elie K, Spence L, Stern L: Hong Kong influenza in a neonatal unit. *JAMA* 223:1233–1235, 1973.

189. MacDonald NE, Hall CB, Suffin SC, Alexson C, Harris PJ, Manning JA: Respiratory syncytial viral infection in infants with congenital heart disease. *N Engl J Med* 307:397–400, 1982.

190. Hall CB, Douglas RG Jr: Modes of transmission of respiratory syncytial virus. *J Pediatr* 99:100–103, 1981.

191. Murphy D, Todd JK, Chao RK, Orr I, McIntosh K: The use of gowns and masks to control respiratory illness in pediatric hospital personnel. *J Pediatr* 99:746–750, 1981.

192. Kaul A, Scott R, Gallagher M, Scott M, Clement J, Ogra PL: Respiratory syncytial virus infection: Rapid diagnosis in children by use of indirect immunofluorescence. *Am J Dis Child* 132:1088–1090, 1978.

193. Minnich L, Ray CG: Comparison of direct immunofluorescent staining of clinical specimens for respiratory virus antigens with conventional isolation techniques. *J Clin Microbiol* 12:391–394, 1980.

194. McIntosh K, Hendry RM, Fahnestock ML, Pierik LT: Enzyme-linked immunosorbent assay for detection of respiratory syncytial virus infection: Application to clinical samples. *J Clin Microbiol* 16:329–333, 1982.

195. Kim HW, Wyatt RG, Fernie BF, Brandt CD, Arrobio JO, Jeffreies BC, Parrott RH: Respiratory syncytial virus detection by immunofluorescence in nasal secretions with monoclonal antibodies against selected surface and internal proteins. *J Clin Microbiol* 18:1399–1404, 1983.

196. Gala CL, Hall CB, Schnabel KC, Pincus PH, Blossom P, Hildreth SW, Betts RF, Douglas RG Jr: The use of eye-nose goggles to control nosocomial respiratory syncytial virus infection. *JAMA* 256:2706–2708, 1986.

197. Taber LH, Knight V, Gilbert BE, McClung HW, Wilson SZ, Norton HJ, Thurson JM, Gordon WH, Atmar RL, Schlaudt WR: Ribavirin aerosol treatment of bronchiolitis associated with respiratory syncytial virus infection in infants. *Pediatrics* 72:613–618, 1983.

198. Hall CB, Walsh EE, Hruska JF, Betts RF, Hall WJ: Ribavirin treatment of experimental respiratory syncytial viral infection. *JAMA* 249:2666–2670, 1983.

199. Hall CB, McBride JT, Walsh EE, Bell DM, Gala CL, Hildreth S, Eyck LGT, Hall WJ: Aerosolized ribavirin treatment of infants with respiratory syncytial viral infection. *N Engl J Med* 308:1443–1447, 1983.

200. Patamasucon P, Kaojarern J, Kusmiesz H, Nelson JD: Pharmacokinetics of erythromycin ethylsuccinate and estolate in infants under 4 months of age. *Antimicrobiol Agents Chemother* 19:736–739, 1981.
201. Srinivasan G, Azarcon E, Muldoon MRL, Jenkins G, Polavarapu S, Kallick CA, Pildes RS: Rotavirus infection in a normal nursery: Epidemic and surveillance. *Infect Control* 5:478–481, 1984.
202. Powell J, Bureau MA, Parè C, Gaildry M-L, Cabana D, Patriquin H: Necrotizing enterocolitis. *Am J Dis Child* 134:1152–1154, 1980.
203. Rotbart HA, Levin MJ, Yolken RH, Manchester DK, Jantzen J: An outbreak of rotavirus-associated neonatal necrotizing enterocolitis. *J Pediatr* 103:454–459, 1983.
204. Rousset S, Moscovici O, Lebon P, Barbet JP, Helardot P, Macè B, Bargy F, Vinh LT, Chany C: Intestinal lesions containing coronavirus-like particles in neonatal necrotizing enterocolitis: An ultrastructural analysis. *Pediatrics* 73:218–224, 1984.
205. Resta S, Luby JP, Rosenfeld CR, Siegel JD: Isolation and propagation of a human enteric coronavirus. *Science* 229:978–981, 1985.
206. Sherertz RJ, Sarubbi FA: The prevalence of *Clostridium difficile* and toxin in a nursery population: A comparison between patients with necrotizing enterocolitis and an asymptomatic group. *J Pediatr* 100:435–439, 1982.
207. Donta ST, Myers MG: *Clostridium difficile* toxin in asymptomatic neonates. *J Pediatr* 100:431–434, 1982.
208. Han VKM, Sayed H, Chance GW, Brabyn DG, Shaheed WA: An outbreak of *Clostridium difficile* necrotizing enterocolitis: A case for oral vancomycin therapy? *Pediatrics* 71:935–941, 1983.
209. Nelson JD, Whitaker JA, Hempstead B, Harris M: Epidemiological application of the fluorescent antibody technique: Study of a diarrhea outbreak in a premature nursery. *JAMA* 176:26–30, 1961.
210. Nelson JD, Kusmiesz H, Jackson LH, Woodman E: Treatment of Salmonella gastroenteritis with ampicillin, amoxicillin, or placebo. *Pediatrics* 65:1125–1130, 1980.
211. Sanborn WR, Lesmana M, Koesno: Oral infection in pediatric salmonellosis. *Lancet* 2:478, 1976.
212. Wheeler WE: Spread and control of *Escherichia coli* diarrheal disease. *Ann NY Acad Sci* 66:112–117, 1956.
213. Kransinski K, Holzman RS, Hanna B, Greco MA, Graff M, Bhogal M: Nosocomial fungal infection during hospital renovation. *Infect Control* 6:278–282, 1985.
214. Dennis JE, Rhodes KH, Cooney DR, Roberts GD: Nosocomial *Rhizopus* infection (zygomycosis) in children. *J Pediatr* 96:824–828, 1980.
215. Mossovitch M, Mossovitch B, Alkan M: Nosocomial dermatophytosis caused by *Microsporum canis* in a newborn department. *Infect Control* 7:593–595, 1986.
216. Franco JA, Eitzman DV, Baer H: Antibiotic usage and microbial resistance in an intensive care nursery. *Am J Dis Child* 126:318–321, 1973.
217. Hill HR, Hunt CE, Matsen JM: Nosocomial colonization with Klebsiella, type 26, in a neonatal intensive care unit associated with an outbreak of sepsis, meningitis, and necrotizing enterocolitis. *J Pediatr* 85:415–419, 1974.
218. Arbeter AM, Aff C, Dill P, Widzer H, Plotkin SA: Experiences with a multiple-resistant *Klebsiella pneumoniae* in an infant intensive care unit. (Abstract) *Pediatr Res* 11:433, 1977.
219. Eidelman AI, Reynolds J: Gentamicin-resistant *Klebsiella* infections in a neonatal intensive care unit. *Am J Dis Child* 132:421–422, 1978.
220. Cook LN, Davis RS, Stover BH: Outbreak of amikacin-resistant enterobacteriaceae in an intensive care nursery. *Pediatrics* 65:264–268, 1980.
221. Bryan CS, John JF Jr, Pai MS, Austin TL: Gentamicin vs cefotaxime for therapy of neonatal sepsis. *Am J Dis Child* 139:1086–1089, 1985.
222. Planning and Design for Perinatal and Pediatric Facilities. Columbus, OH, Ross Laboratories, 1977.
223. American Academy of Pediatrics and American College of Obstetricians and Gynecologists. *Guidelines for Perinatal Care.* Evanston IL, American Academy of Pediatrics, 1983.
224. Evans HE, Akpata SO, Baki A: Bacteriologic and clinical evaluation of gowning in a premature nursery. *J Pediatr* 78:883–886, 1971.
225. Forfar JO, MacCabe AF: Masking and gowning in nurseries for the newborn infant: Effect on staphylococcal carriage and infection. *Br Med J* 1:76–79, 1958.
226. Silverman WA, Sinclair JC: Evaluation of precautions before entering a neonatal unit. *Pediatrics* 40:900–901, 1967.
227. Williams CPS, Oliver TK Jr: Nursery routines and staphylococcal colonization of the newborn. *Pediatrics* 44:640–646, 1969.
228. Sprunt K, Redman W, Leidy G: Antibacterial effectiveness of routine hand washing. *Pediatrics* 52:264–271, 1973.
229. Renaud MT: Effects of discontinuing cover gowns on a post partal ward upon cord colonization of the newborn. *J Obstet Gynecol Neonatal Nurs* 12:399–401, 1983.
230. Nauseef WM, Maki DG: A study of the value of simple protective isolation in patients with granulocytopenia. *N Engl J Med* 304:440–453, 1981.
231. Moylan JA, Kennedy BV: The importance of gown and drape barriers in the prevention of wound infection. *Surg Gynecol Obstet* 151:465–470, 1980.
232. Agbayani M, Rosenfeld W, Evans H: Evaluation of modified gowning procedures in a neonatal intensive care unit. *Am J Dis Child* 135:650–652, 1981.
233. Williams CP, Oliver TK Jr: Nursery routines and staphylococcal colonization of the newborn. *Pediatrics* 44:640–646, 1969.
234. Donowitz LG: Failure of the overgown to prevent nosocomial infection in a pediatric intensive care unit. *Pediatrics* 77:35–38, 1986.
235. Cloney DL, Donowitz LG: Overgown use for infection control in nurseries and neonatal intensive care units. *Am J Dis Child* 140:680–683, 1986.
236. Meyer CL, Eitzen HE, Schreiner RL, Gfell MA, Moye L, Kleiman MB: Should linen in newborn intensive care units be autoclaved? *Pediatrics* 67:362–364, 1981.
237. Rothenberg R: Ophthalmia neonatorum due to *Neisseria gonorrhoeae*: Prevention and treatment. *Sex Transm Dis* 6:187–191, 1979.
238. Hammerschlag MR, Chandler JW, Alexander ER, English M, Chiang WT, Koutsky L, Eschenbach DA, Smith JR: Erythromycin ointment for ocular prophylaxis of neonatal chlamydial infection. *JAMA* 244:2291–2293, 1980.
239. Rettig PJ, Patamasucon P, Siegel JD: (Letter to the Editor) Postnatal prophylaxis of chlamydial conjunctivitis. *JAMA* 246:2321, 1981.
240. Siegel JD, McCracken GH Jr, Threlkeld N, DePasse BM, Rosenfeld CR: Single-dose penicillin prophylaxis of neonatal group B streptococcal disease: Conclusion of a 41 month controlled trial. *Lancet* 1:1426–1430, 1982.
241. Pyati SP, Pildes RS, Jacobs NM, Ramamurthy RS, Yeh TF, Raval DS, Lilien LD, Amma P, Metzger WI: Penicillin in infants weighing two kilograms or less with early-onset group B streptococcal disease. *N Engl J Med* 308:1383–1389, 1983.
242. Laga M, Naamara W, Brunham RC, D'Costa LJ, Nsanze H, Piot P, Kunimoto D, Ndinya-Achola JO, Slaney L, Ronald AR, Plummer FA: Single-dose therapy of gonococcal ophthalmia neonatorum with ceftriaxone. *N Engl J Med* 315:1382–1385, 1986.
243. Haase DA, Nash RA, Nsanze H, D'Costa LJ, Fransen L, Piot P, Brunham RC: Single-dose ceftriaxone therapy of gonococcal ophthalmia neonatorum. *Sex Transm Dis* 13:53–55, 1986.
244. Speck WT, Driscoll JM, Polin RA, O'Neill J, Rosenkranz HS: Staphylococcal and streptococcal colonization of the newborn infant: Effect of antiseptic cord care. *Am J Dis Child* 131:1005–1008, 1977.
245. Pildes RS, Ramamurthy RS, Vidyasagar D: Effect of triple dye on staphylococcal colonization in the newborn infant. *J Pediatr* 82:987–990, 1973.

246. Barrett FF, Mason EO, Fleming D: The effect of three cord-care regimens on bacterial colonization of normal newborn infants. *J Pediatr* 94:796–800, 1979.
247. Larson E, Zuill R, Zier V, Berg B: Storage of human breast milk. *Infect Control* 5:127–130, 1984.
248. Sosa R, Barness L: Bacterial growth in refrigerated human milk. *Am J Dis Child* 141:111–112, 1987.
249. Taylor BJ, Jacobs RF, Baker RL, Moses EB, McSwain BE, Shulman G: Frozen deglycerolyzed blood prevents transfusion-acquired cytomegalovirus infections in neonates. *Pediatr Infect Dis* 5:188–191, 1986.
250. Neal WA, Reynolds JW, Jarvis CW, Williams HJ: Umbilical artery catheterization. Demonstration of arterial thrombosis by aertography. *Pediatrics* 50:6–13, 1972.
251. Krauss AN, Caliendo TJ, Kannan MM: Bacteremia in newborn infants. *NY State J Med* 72:1136–1137, 1972.
252. Banks DC, Yates DB, Cawdrey HM, Harries MG, Kidner PH: Infection from intravenous catheters. *Lancet* 1:443–445, 1970.
253. Holmes CJ, Kunksin RB, Ausman RK, Walter CM: Potential hazards associated with microbial contamination of in-line filters during intravenous therapy. *J Clin Microbiol* 12:725–731, 1980.
254. Sidiropoulos D, Boehme U, Von Muralt G, Morell A, Barandun S: Immunoglobulin supplementation in prevention or treatment of neonatal sepsis. *Pediatr Infect Dis* 5:S193–S194, 1986.
255. Haque KN, Zaidi MH, Haque SK, Bahakim H, El-Hazmi M, El-Swailam M: Intravenous immunoglobulin for prevention of sepsis in preterm and low birth weight infants. *Pediatr Infect Dis* 5:622–625, 1986.
256. Sidropoulos D, Herrmann U Jr, Morell A, von Muralt G, Barandun S: Transplacental passage of intravenous immunoglobulin in the last trimester of pregnancy. *J Pediatr* 109:505–508, 1986.
257. Williams WW: Guideline for infection control in hospital personnel. *Infect Control* 4:326–349, 1983.
258. Steiner P, Rao M, Victoria MS, Rudolph N, Buynoski G: Miliary tuberculosis in two infants after nursery exposure: Epidemiologic, clinical, and laboratory findings. *Am Rev Respir Dis* 113:267–271, 1976.
259. Meibalane R, Sedmak GV, Sasidharan P, Garg P, Grausz JP: Outbreak of influenza in a neonatal intensive care unit. *J Pediatr* 91:974–976, 1977.

23

The Immunocompromised Patient

Jane Skelton, M.D. and Philip A. Pizzo, M.D.

INTRODUCTION

Tremendous progress has been made in the treatment of childhood cancers. Some malignant diseases that were once uniformly fatal are now curable. These advances have been achieved primarily by using highly intensive multimodality treatment regimens, including bone marrow transplantation. Unfortunately, these treatments are frequently accompanied by significant toxicities, particularly myelosuppression.

Similarly, progress has been made with organ failure in the pediatric population, with kidney transplants being the most established of the organ transplantations. Heart and liver transplants are rapidly becoming increasingly common as lifesaving measures. The enthusiasm for allogeneic transplantation is largely due to the recent development of effective immunosuppressive agents which decrease the incidence of graft rejection. As in cancer therapy, the successful outcome of these endeavors is largely related to the management of the treatment-related toxicities and complications.

Infection remains the major cause of morbidity and mortality in immunocompromised patients, regardless of the reason for immunosuppression. The recognition of the increased susceptibility of these patients to common microbial organisms and opportunistic pathogens is crucial to their successful treatment and survival. Both the immunologic alterations consequent to the patient's underlying disease and its treatment, as well as the acquisition of pathogens in the hospital environment predispose these patients to severe infections. For such patients, the institution of appropriate preventive or prophylactic measures, and the rapid initiation of optimal antimicrobial therapy when indicated, maximizes the chance for a successful outcome.

FACTORS THAT MAKE THE IMMUNOCOMPROMISED HOST SUSCEPTIBLE TO INFECTION

Disease-Related Defects

Alterations in the immune defense system occur at many levels in patients with cancer and those undergoing transplantation. Disturbances in humoral and cell-mediated immunity, neutrophil dysfunction, and leukopenia (particularly granulocytopenia) secondary to bone marrow failure from malignant involvement or antineoplastic therapy may each influence a patient's susceptibility to infection.

Abnormal humoral immune profiles, with low immunoglobulin levels prior to the institution of chemotherapy, have been described in some patients with a hematologic malignancy; antibody response to antigenic stimulus may also be impaired (1–4).

Cell-mediated immunity may also be impaired in patients with lymphoid malignancy, especially Hodgkin's disease. These abnormalities may persist even after cessation of successful therapy (5).

In these compromised hosts, granulocytopenia is the single most important factor for infection. In addition, neutrophil dysfuction has been described in patients with hematologic malignancies and carcinomas prior to the administration of chemotherapy (6–8) as well as following the administration of various chemotherapeutic agents and craniospinal irradiation (9–12). This may contribute further to the high risk for infection.

Treatment-Related Defects

Both humoral and cell-mediated immunity may be further suppressed by cytotoxic agents (3,13). Corticosteroids, used in both cancer treatment and transplant recipients, compound the cell-mediated deficiency inherent to certain diseases (14).

In patients undergoing transplantation, cyclosporin A serves as a potent immunosuppressive agent and, together with corticosteroids, is a major cause of immunosuppression. Cyclosporin A has no significant adverse effect on neutrophil or monocyte function but inhibits the activation of resting T cells, causing a deficiency in helper T-cells (15–17). This leads to an increased risk of infection with *Pneumocystis carinii*, viruses, and fungi.

Granulocytopenia (generally defined as less than 500 polymorphonuclear cells/mm^3) is well-recognized as the predominant factor influencing host defense in the cancer patient. The relationship of the degree of granulocytopenia and its duration to the incidence of infection has been well-established (18). These patients must be vigilantly monitored for any signs and/or symptoms of infection, however subtle, since untreated infection in the patient with severe granulocytopenia may be rapidly fatal. Management of these problems is discussed later.

Colonization-Infection

When considering the possible or predominant pathogens encountered in the hospitalized, immunosuppressed patients, the source of the infecting agent is of paramount importance, both for planning any preventive measures and for initiating appropriate therapy. Both serious illness and antibiotic exposure alter the patient's microbial flora. This is relevant since more than four-fifths of the infections that occur in immunocompromised cancer patients arise from their endogenous flora (19). Of particular importance is the acquisition of Gram-negative bacilli in the oropharyngeal and gastrointestinal mucosa. The changes occur within the first 4 days following hospitalization; this transformation will occur without the addition of antibiotics, although antibiotics may accelerate the process (20–22). The inherent virulence of the colonizing flora, coupled with the degree of pertubation of local and systemic host defenses, influence whether a specific organism will become invasive and lead to infection. For example, the organism *E. coli*, although frequently acquired, is less often associated with infection than is *P. aeruginosa*, which results in infection of 40–68% of patients who become colonized and then become granulocytopenic (23).

Patients can be colonized with potential pathogens from a variety of sources within the hospital setting. Among the most important are the hands of hospital personnel, since they can transmit a variety of organisms to the patient, including *S. aureus*, *S. epidermidis*, *Corynebacterium JK*, and Gram-negative bacilli. Ventilator support systems have been associated with the transmission of *Serratia* sp. or *Pseudomonas*, while food (fresh fruits and vegetables in particular) and water can be sources of *Pseudomonas*, *Klebsiella*, *E. coli*, and *Legionella* (24,25).

Colonization with fungal organisms is also a common occurrence in hospitalized immunocompromised patients. *Candida albicans* can be part of the host flora and can be cultured from 80% of patients who have received broad spectrum antibiotics (26). Antibiotic therapy and immunosuppression are associated with a marked proliferation of this organism, with frequent clinically evident mucosal infections (27,28). The precise relationship of subclinical colonization, clinically evident superficial infection, and the relative risk of invasive or systemic candidal infections is not entirely understood at this time, but it is the subject of intense investigation in the hopes of establishing the value of efforts to reduce or eradicate nosocomial colonization.

C. tropicalis, although less frequently isolated from oropharyngeal or stool flora of the hospitalized patient than *C. albicans*, may be more invasive in the cancer patient. In a study of 25 patients who were colonized with *C. tropicalis*, 14 developed infection, as compared with three infections in 60 patients who were colonized with *C. albicans* (29). Of interest, the incidence of *C. tropicalis* infections varies widely among institutions, suggesting that it is hospital-related.

Aspergillus represents a significant problem for patients receiving cytotoxic agents or immunosuppressive therapy (e.g., steroids). Infections with *Aspergillus* are more common at some institutions than others, and reservoirs of organisms have been demonstrated in some treatment center. Colonization of the patient's upper airway with *Aspergillus* spores is associated with a risk for either local infection (e.g., sinusitis) or pulmonary infection when the patient becomes neutropenic (30).

NOSOCOMIAL SOURCES FOR INFECTION

Intravenous Catheters

A major risk factor for development of infection is an alteration of mucosal and integumentary physical defense barriers. Patients hospitalized for cancer treatment or organ transplantation often require prolonged venous access, either with repeated peripheral intravenous lines, or with indwelling central venous access devices. Peripheral intravenous lines have a recognized, but generally low rate of infection, particularly when they are monitored and replaced on a regular basis (31).

During the last several years, indwelling Silastic catheters have become more commonplace, and may be left in place for weeks to many months. In spite of their many attributes, such catheters are clearly associated with an increased risk for infection and require careful evaluation. (Table 23.1). They include infection at the site of exit of the catheter, along its subcutaneous tunnel, and bacteremias and fungemias. The infection rate varies between 10–60%, depending on the series (32,33). The more recently popularized subcutaneously implanted venous access devices (Port-a-Cath®, Medi-Port®, Infusaid®) appear, in preliminary studies, to have a significantly lower rate of infectious complications, reported to be between 2–15% (34,35). It is important to note, however, that these reports are primarily in patients without prolonged granulocytopenia, and data comparing the incidence and complications of infections in patients with Hickman-Broviac type catheters to subcutaneously implanted ones are under study (36).

The predominant pathogens isolated in catheter-related infections, are Gram-positive bacteria (37–40). *Staphylococcus epidermidis* has been increasingly recognized as a significant pathogen in the immunocompromised patient, and is frequently associated with an intravenous catheter source. The other common isolate is *Staphylococcus aureus*, which may cause both local catheter site infections as well as bacteremias. Gram-negative infections (e.g., *Pseudomonas, Acinetobacter*) are also associated with indwelling catheters, and polymicrobial bacteremias may originate from an infected line (41,42).

Of note, organisms previously viewed as contaminants or as unlikely pathogens may be associated with catheter-related infection. These include *Bacillus* spp. (which have been difficult to treat without removal of the catheter), *Corynebacterium JK* (a resistant Gram-positive), atypical mycobacteria, and nonaeruginosa *Pseudomonas* spp. (*P. maltophilia, P. cepacia,* and *P. picketti*).

Fungemias may also originate from an indwelling catheter. With both bacteremias and fungemias, it is important to establish if a blood-borne infection is directly related to the infected catheter (Table 23.2). Evidence to support the catheter as the primary source includes concurrent local catheter site infection with the same organism; a positive blood culture drawn through the catheter with negative concurrent peripheral cultures; and a positive blood culture drawn through the catheter with concurrent positive peripheral cultures, usually with the colony counts

Table 23.1.
Guidelines for Evaluating Catheter-Related Infections

Culture Site	Recommendations
Exit Site	Swab if tender, erythematous, or draining.
Tunnel	If tender, erythematous, or indurated, and exit site shows no signs of infection, aspirate or biopsy the cellulitis (away from catheter).
Blood	Always culture peripheral and catheter blood. For multilumen catheters, culture each lumen, and label appropriately.

Table 23.2.
Criteria that Suggest a Catheter-Related Bacteremia

Suggestive
- Positive blood culture with concurrent local catheter site infection with the same organism.
- Positive blood culture drawn through the catheter with negative concurrent peripheral culture in a newly febrile patient.

Definitive
- Positive blood culture drawn through the catheter with concurrent positive peripheral cultures, but less growth on the peripheral plates.

on the culture plates being higher in the central blood sample compared with the peripheral sample. Those patients with multilumen catheters should have cultures drawn from each lumen, as one particular catheter hub may serve as a persistent, potentially unrecognized nidus of infection. Treatment of catheter-related infection is discussed later.

Intraventricular Reservoirs

Patients with leukemia, and occasionally those with solid tumors, may have an Ommaya reservoir placed in the lateral ventricle of the brain for optimal delivery of chemotherapeutic agents to the cerebrospinal fluid (CSF). This foreign body is implanted subcutaneously, but the reservoir is entered by needle puncture through the skin. It is not surprising, therefore, that these devices may become colonized or infected. At the National Cancer Institute, we reviewed our experience of infections in leukemia patients with Ommaya reservoirs (43) and found that in spite of their frequent use, contamination or infection occurred in only 20% of patients.

Treatment of these infections must be directed at the known or predominant pathogens; coagulase-negative staphylococci (predominantly *Staphylococcus epidermidis*) account for 60–75% of isolates (44). Systemic treatment with vancomycin, with the addition of oral rifampin, may clear the infection in some patients. Intrathecal injection of antibiotics (including vancomycin) is advocated by some, but the appropriate dose, schedule, and the pharmacokinetics have not been determined (45,46).

Blood-Transmitted Infections

Both cancer patients and transplant recipients receive multiple transfusions of blood products, including red blood cells, platelets, granulocytes, as well as volume expanders (fresh frozen plasma, albumen). These transfusions are not without significant infectious risks (Table 23.3).

With current routine screening of blood products, hepatitis B, and more recently, human immunodeficiency virus (HIV), are now uncommon transfusion-related infections.

Non-A non-B hepatitis remains a significant problem and is the leading cause of post-transfusion hepatitis, accounting for 60–90% of cases (47). Unfortunately, the agent of non-A non-B hepatitis has not been isolated, and no screening test exists. The natural history of non-A non-B

hepatitis includes persistent elevation of liver enzymes in over one-third of patients, occasionally progressing to cirrhosis (47–49).

Cytomegalovirus (CMV) can be a serious pathogen in the immunosuppressed patient. CMV is transmitted by the transfusion of leukocytes from seropositive donors; whole blood, packed red blood cells, and platelets contain large numbers of viable leukocytes and can thus transmit organisms. When possible, transmission can be avoided by selecting seronegative donors for recipients who are seronegative (50,51). Seronegative individuals who are undergoing transplantation or profoundly immunosuppressed patients may suffer significant morbidity and mortality from transfusion-acquired CMV. It is estimated that 2.5–12% of blood donors can transmit CMV (52–54), and there is a significant correlation between the volume of blood received and the likelihood of acquiring an infection (55,56). The possibility of reinfection in an already CMV seropositive patient has also received some attention, but these infections may likely represent reactivation of the primary host infection (57,58).

Who should receive CMV seronegative blood products? Of the enormous number of cancer or immunocompromised patients receiving transfusions [accounting for 20% of all transfused blood products (59)], who will suffer increased morbidity and mortality if they receive seropositive blood? Not all patients require CMV-screened blood (52); however, there are a number of groups who should be considered possible candidates.

Renal transplant recipients have a high incidence of CMV infections, and infection may be associated with organ rejection (60,61). Although CMV infection is most commonly a reactivation of endogenous virus, a primary infection acquired from the donor organ is a problem for seronegative recipients. Although the role of blood transfusions in the transmission of these infections is not firmly established (62,63), it is generally considered prudent to transfuse seronegative renal transplant patients with seronegative blood.

Heart transplant recipients are also at significant risk for morbidity and mortality from CMV infections. Moreover, CMV infections in these patients appeared to increase the risk for bacterial and fungal superinfections (64). Thus, seronegative blood products would seem war-

Table 23.3.
Potential Infections Associated with Blood Product Transfusions

Organism	Comment
Hepatitis B	Minimal risk since routine screening of donated blood became standard.
HIV	Minimal risk since routine screening of donated blood became standard.
Non-A/non-B Hepatitis	No screening test available. Donor carrier incidence unknown. Currently an unavoidable risk.
Cytomegalovirus	Serologic screening for antibody available. Seronegative donors may acquire infection from seropositive donor. Certain groups (BMT, organ transplant patients) warrant seronegative products for seronegative recipients.
Bacteria, toxoplasma	Unusual contaminant during processing of blood.

ranted in seronegative recipients. Although less data are available for the less common liver transplant patients, similar conclusions seem appropriate at this time.

Allogeneic bone marrow transplant (BMT) recipients have been the most extensively studied group of immunosuppressed patients. In these patients, CMV infections are frequently life-threatening. The most conclusive study demonstrating the acquisition and risks of CMV infections was done in BMT patients receiving granulocyte transfusions, where seronegative patients receiving seropositive leukocytes had a significantly increased rate of CMV pneumonitis, compared with those receiving seronegative leukocytes (58). Therefore, allogeneic BMT patients should always be screened for CMV status, and only seronegative blood products should be given to seronegative recipients.

The issue of CMV infection in patients receiving autologous bone marrow transplantation, or other highly intensive treatments (e.g., induction phase of antileukemic therapy) that are associated with severe, prolonged immunosuppression is less well-documented. Until more data are available, one ideal is to use standards similar to those for patients undergoing allogeneic bone marrow transplantation.

Whether those patients who have malignancy that is treated with less intensive chemotherapeutic regimens would benefit from CMV screening is not well-studied. Autopsy studies reveal that the incidence of active CMV infection in cancer patients may be twice that of those dying of other causes (65,66), but specific studies addressing the role of primary CMV infections related to transfusions are lacking. Thus, there is no clear indication supporting screening

of all cancer patients receiving blood products at this time.

Airborne Infections: *Aspergillus*

Infection with aspergillus is a well-recognized and dreaded complication in hospitalized patients with prolonged myelosuppression. Aspergillus spores are ubiquitous and have been found in unfiltered air virtually everywhere they have been sought. They are also found on spices, commercial peppers, and other organic materials (67). A relationship between exposure to airborne spores, nasopharyngeal colonization, and the relative risk for developing an invasive *Aspergillus* infection has been suggested. Rhame et al. (67) reviewed the reported outbreaks of nosocomial aspergillosis; most are related to construction in the hospital, or to a poorly functioning air filter system. It must be noted, however, that construction is by no means invariably associated with *Aspergillus* infections. Nonetheless, *Aspergillus* seems to be increasing as a fungal pathogen (68), although there is considerable variability in its incidence at different institutions.

Waterborne Organisms: *Legionella*

Another organism associated with nosocomial outbreaks is *Legionella pneumophilia*, particularly among immunosuppressed patients. *L. pneumophilia* is found in water sources, including shower systems and nebulizers (69,70). However, the organism has also been isolated from potable water at institutions where infection with *Legionella* has not been a problem. Thus, routine culturing of potable water is not recommended unless an outbreak has occurred (25).

Other Nosocomial Infections

Severely immunocompromised patients are at risk of suffering significant infections from unusual pathogens, often from unexpected sources. For example, disinfectant or sterile solutions used in the hospital, albeit presumed to be clean or sterile, may become colonized with organisms. For example, *Pseudomonas cepacia* has been isolated in povidone solutions used to cleanse dressing sites, including Hickman-Broviac catheters, and the organism can lead to serious infection in these high-risk patients (71). Similarly, contamination of sterile water, respiratory equipment, and blood collection equipment with *Pseudomonas maltophilia* may lead to nosocomial colonization and subsequent disease (72). It is crucial in the successful management of immunosuppressed patients to view even the most unusual organisms as potential pathogens and pursue the significance of positive cultures, including determining the source of the organism.

Recently, armboards for children with peripheral intravenous lines have been associated with cutaneous and disseminated infection (73). Presumably, the covering of the armboards was the source for local colonization, reminiscent of the outbreak of Rhizopus, which occurred with contaminated elastoplast tape some years ago (74). It is recommended that such coverings and tapes be gas sterilized or radiated prior to their use in the immunosuppressed patient.

PREDOMINANT PATHOGENS AND PATTERNS OF INFECTION

The successful management of nosocomial infections demands an awareness of the predominant pathogens encountered in hospitalized patients. Many factors influence the "hospital flora," and hence determine the clinically significant organisms that are isolated at any one institution. In addition, the infecting microorganisms in any one patient also changes over time. Optimal therapy necessitates attention to both these factors.

Pathogen Profiles: Changing Patterns in Bacterial Isolates

Bacteria remain the most common cause of primary infection in the immunocompromised host. Over the past 30 years, there has been a change in the predominant pathogens isolated in nosocomial infections. In the 1950s, infections due to staphylococci predominated, but by the 1960s, there was a reduction in the incidence of Gram-positive, specifically *Staphylococcus aureus* infections. This was coupled with an increase in infections due to Gram-negative bacillary organisms, especially *E. coli*, *Klebsiella* sp. and *Pseudomonas aeruginosa* (75,76). For inexplicable reasons, there has been a decrease in infections due to Gram-negative bacteria, particularly *P. aeruginosa* during the first half of the 1980s. Indeed, in most centers, Gram-positive isolates again constitute the predominant pathogens (77–79). This changing pattern reflects, in part, the increased use of indwelling catheters and their accompanying predisposition for infections with the coagulase-negative staphylococci (80).

The use of broad spectrum antibiotics in immunocompromised hosts has also contributed to the changing trends in bacterial isolates. Because of the morbidity and mortality associated with untreated infections, most broad spectrum antibiotic combinations have emphasized coverage against Gram-negative isolates. However, many of these regimens are inadequate against Gram-positive bacteria, particularly *S. epidermidis*, an organism of increased importance in the immunocompromised patient (81–84). It is important to recognize that for the coagulase-negative staphylococci, even when in vitro sensitivity to antistaphylococcal penicillins or cephalosporins is demonstrated, clinical failures have been described (85). Vancomycin is the drug of choice for the coagulase-negative staphylococci.

Staphylococcus aureus remains a serious pathogen in the immunocompromised host, and knowledge of its sensitivities at any given hospital is important. Methicillin-resistant *S. aureus* is not present in all hospital centers. However, in those where it is isolated, appropriate modifications in the initial antibiotic regimen, specifically the addition of vancomycin, must be strongly entertained.

Although methicillin-resistant staphylococci (both coagulase-negative and coagulase-positive) are the most notorious "resistant variants" of a common bacterial isolate, the specific sensitivity patterns of these microorganisms must also be monitored at an individual center: *Serratia* sp., *Klebsiella*, *Enterobacter*, *Citrobacter*, *P. aeruginosa*, and *H. influenzae*. Awareness of the sensitivity patterns of these or other organisms help to define the appropriate regimens for empiric therapeutic intervention of compromised hosts.

Pneumocystis carinii: Hospital Outbreaks

Pneumocystis carinii has a global distribution, with inactive cysts detectable in asymptomatic patients and antibody to *P. carinii* found in nearly 100% of normal children. This would suggest that most episodes of *P. carinii* pneumonia in immunocompromised hosts are caused by reactivation infection (86). Although horizontal transmission has not been conclusively demonstrated, several accounts from different institutions of time-space clustering of infectious episodes suggest there may be a role of patient to patient transmission in some cases of *Pneumocystis* pneumonia (87,88). Although trimethoprim-sulfamethoxazole can prevent *P. carinii* pneumonia, its use prophylactically should depend on the incidence of infection at a given center. It should be appreciated that the type of immunosuppressive and chemotherapeutic regimens influence the prevalence of *P. carinii* infections, and accordingly, the recommendations regarding prophylaxis (89,90).

UNDERLYING DISEASE: INFECTIONS TO ANTICIPATE

Cancer Patients

As discussed earlier, cancer itself may alter a patient's immune system. Far more commonly, however, the granulocytopenia induced by antineoplastic therapy is responsible for the infections encountered in these patients. With the advent of intensive chemotherapy treatments for solid tumors, infectious complications have increased in these patients, and they have joined the ranks of patients with hematopoietic malignancies. The spectrum of infectious organisms is not static and will change as the duration of immunosuppression and granuloctyopenia is sustained.

The initial episode of fever in a granulocytopenic cancer patient is most likely to be due to bacterial organisms. Aerobic organisms (either Gram-positive or Gram-negative) predominate; anaerobic bacteria are rarely the sole cause of infection but may contribute to mixed infections in certain body sites (e.g., oropharyngeal cavity, perineal area).

Despite a careful history and physical examination, along with cultures of blood and other possible sites of infection, 40–70% of neutropenic patients who become febrile will not have a clinically or microbiologically defined site of infection (78,91–93). For convenience, these patients are categorized as having unexplained fever or fever of unknown origin (FUO).

As granulocytopenia persists, patients with persistent or recurrent fevers must be evaluated for the possibility of second or superinfections. Secondary bacterial infections may occur, usually with organisms not covered by the initial antibiotic therapy. These can be organisms that fall outside of the spectrum of the primary antibiotics or that are resistant to the initial antibiotic reigmen. Anaerobes, although uncommon as primary pathogens, can contribute to mixed infection or second infections. Mucositis (particularly necrotizing gingivitis), perirectal cellulitis, or an intra-abdominal infection are the predominant sites for mixed aerobic-anaerobic infection, and the addition of a specific antianaerobic agent (e.g., clindamycin or metronidazole) may be beneficial. *Clostridia tertium*, though an uncommon pathogen in the normal host, may be associated with a bacteremia, particularly in the granulocytopenic patient with abdominal pain (94). It is important to recognize that this species of *Clostridia* is not always sensitive to the more common antianaerobic regimens, although it is generally sensitive to vancomycin.

Fungal infections, once associated almost exclusively with hematologic malignancies and transplantation, must now also be considered in all cancer patients with prolonged neutropenia and fever. There has been an apparent increase in the incidence of fungal infections during the last 40 years. With aggressive antibacterial support, patients are capable of surviving sustained periods of neutropenia, exposing them to the increased risk for developing a fungal superinfection (95–97). Maksymiuk et al. summarized a 4-year experience at the M.D. Anderson Hospital and Tumor Institute, reviewing all patients with either positive fungal cultures of sterile body fluid, or autopsy cases with systemic fungal infection. The predominant pathogen was *C. albicans* (40%), followed by *C. tropicalis* (23%), and *Aspergillus* (8%) (98). It is important to recognize that the incidence of fungal pathogens (particularly *C. tropicalis* and *As-*

pergillus) varies from center to center. It is notable that positive culture results were available antemortem in only two-thirds, underscoring the difficulty in diagnosing fungal infections and in identifying the patients at high risk for them.

In addition to the increased risk of fungal infections in patients with neutropenia, Horn et al. noted that the incidence of fungemias has increased over the last 10 years in patients with solid tumors who were not generally neutropenic while undergoing treatment at the Memorial Sloan Kettering Institution (99). In these patients, the administration of broad spectrum antibiotics was considered the predominant risk factor associated with developing a fungemia.

Patients Undergoing Bone Marrow Transplantation

The infections encountered in patients undergoing allogeneic bone marrow transplantation (BMT) can be divided into three stages: the post-transplant pre-engraftment phase, the period of acute graft-versus-host disease (GVHD), and the period of chronic GVHD (100,101). The post-transplant pre-engraftment phase is characterized by neutropenia and the resulting infectious complications. These include Gram-negative as well as Gram-positive bacterial infections. As in the cancer patient, infections with coagulase-negative staphylococci have assumed increased importance, primarily because of the use of Hickman-Broviac catheters during this phase of management.

Also, like the neutropenic patient with cancer, the incidence of fungal infections increases with the duration of neutropenia and immunosuppression. *Aspergillus* has been a particularly notorious pathogen in these patients and has been a major cause of mortality in some treatment centers (102). The lungs are the most common site of infection, followed by the sinuses (102,103). Infection at either of these sites requires biopsy tissue to make a definitive diagnosis of aspergillosis. In patients who succumb to these infections, systemic *Aspergillus* infection is often found. Of note, infection with *Aspergillus* may occur either during the period of neutropenia or after bone marrow recovery, particularly in those patients receiving corticosteroids or broad spectrum antibiotics. Recently, a subset of patients undergoing T-cell-depleted BMT have been observed to be at particularly high risk for fungal infection (104).

During the postengraftment period, patients suffer a number of immunological abnormalities consequent to the effect of chemotherapy, total body irradiation, immunosuppressive therapy (e.g., steroids, cyclosporin A) and graft-vs-host disease. These combine to render the patient at risk for a variety of pathogens, especially viruses and *P. carinii*.

The most frequent viral infection within the first months following BMT is herpes simplex (105). It occurs as a reactivation in 80% of seropositive patients (100). The virus is most frequently isolated from the oropharyngeal area, and is associated with gingivostomatitis herpes simplex esophagitis may occur, as may pneumonia and hepatitis, but the latter infections are uncommon (106). Treatment of established infections with herpes simplex is achieved with intravenous acycloguanosine (750 mg/m^2/day in 3 divided doses). Because of the high incidence of oral stomatitis following transplantation, and the suggestion that stomatotoxicity is worse in association with herpes simplex, it is notable that several recent randomized studies have demonstrated a significant reduction in the incidence of oral herpetic infections in patients receiving prophylactic acyclovir, administered either intravenously or orally (107–109).

Infection with cytomegalovirus occurs at a median of 8–9 weeks after transplant (110), often in association with GVHD. The incidence has usually averaged about 50%, with higher rates among patients who were seropositive before transplant (111). The clinical spectrum of infection is highly variable, ranging from asymptomatic, to fever, hepatitis, leukopenia, and fulminant fatal pneumonia. Whereas idiopathic interstitial pneumonitis carries a mortality rate of approximately 60%, cytomegalovirus pneumonia has been reported to be fatal in up to 91% of patients (102). It is notable that the incidence of CMV pneumonitis can be reduced by using CMV-seronegative donor blood products for individuals whose pretransplant serology shows them to be CMV-seronegative.

Varicella-zoster virus infection occurs in nearly 50% of transplant recipients (112), usually 4–5 months post-transplantation. Although the usual presentation is dermatomal, the risk for dissemination is heightened in this patient population (100,113). Patients should, therefore, be promptly treated with acyclovir (1500 mg/m^2/day in 3 divided dosages for 7–10 days).

Adenovirus infection has been described to cause pneumonia and nephritis, but is more usually associated with asymptomatic viral shedding. Of particular concern have been outbreaks, in certain centers, of life-threatening diarrheal syndromes due to rotaviruses, enteroviruses, and coxsackie viruses (114).

In addition to CMV, *Pneumocystis carinii* has also been associated with interstitial pneumonia in patients who have undergone bone marrow transplantation. Whereas in the past, *P. carinii* accounted for up to 10% of the cases of interstitial pneumonitis, this has decreased to near zero with the routine use of prophylactic trimethoprim-sulfamethoxazole (115).

Interstitial pneumonitis (IP) is a common complication of allogeneic BMT. It occurs in 35–40% of patients (116,117). An infectious etiology is never established, despite multiple cultures and investigations, in up to 50% of these cases. Cytomegalovirus does account for approximately 40%, with idiopathic IP being the final diagnosis in the majority of the remaining cases (116,117). Risk factors that increase a patient's likelihood to develop IP identified are listed in Table 23.4.

Late infections are also well-recognized, primarily because of deficits in immune functions secondary to chronic graft-versus-host disease (118–120). These include varicella-zoster as well as infections by encapsulated bacteria, especially the pneumococcus (119–121).

Organ Transplant Patients

The ultimate success of any organ transplantation is determined by the function of the transplanted organ, the toxicities that occur during the perioperative period, and chronic immunosuppression required to maintain the graft. Indeed, infection is the main cause of morbidity in organ transplantation (122).

Unlike cancer patients or patients undergoing bone marrow transplantation, granulocytopenia does not usually play a role in the development of infections in these patients. They are compromised because of other alterations in their host defense matrix. Patients undergoing kidney, liver, or heart transplants usually have been ill prior to the procedure, often with numerous prolonged hospitalizations and contacts with hospital microflora.

Early after transplantation, skin and wound infections, related to the operative procedures, are the most common sites of infection (122). Subsequently, the immunosuppressive therapies (e.g., corticosteroids, cyclosporin A, or azathioprine) contribute to opportunistic infection.

Renal Transplantation

As with bone marrow transplant patients, there is a typical timetable that characterizes the nature and timing of infectious complications commonly encountered in the patient undergoing renal transplantation (123). As in other hospitalized postoperative patients, bacterial infections predominate in the 1st month after transplantation, including wound, pulmonary, urinary tract, and intravascular-catheter-related infections. The severity of these infections may, however, be more pronounced in the renal transplant recipient. The incidence of wound infection varies among institutions and is increased when technical problems occur (e.g., hematoma, urinary fistula), underscoring the importance of technical expertise (124–127). Superior technical quality is imperative, as 75% of deep perinephric infections ultimately necessitate removal of the transplanted kidney (127,128). The

Table 23.4.
Factors Associated with Increased Risk of Developing Interstitial Pneumonitis

Reference Number	Variable	Category with Increased Risk
117	Age	Older
116,117	Graft-versus-host disease	Severe
117	Interval from diagnosis to transplantation	> 6 months
117	Performance status prior to transplantation	< 100%
117	Dose-rate of total body irradiation	> 4.0 cGy/min
117	Donor	Allogeneic

role of perioperative antibiotic prophylaxis, however, remains controversial and unresolved (123,126,128,129).

Urinary tract infections, usually with Gram-negative bacilli and often with accompanying bacteremia, pyelonephritis, and allograft dysfunction are also a significant problem when they occur in the first 5 months following transplantation (123). However, the more routine use of prophylactic trimethoprim-sulfamethoxazole for *Pneumocystis carinii* appears to have decreased the incidence of urinary tract infections (126,130). This is of added importance, as up to 60% of bacteremias in these patients originate from the urinary tract (131,132).

Pneumonia is less common than urinary tract infections, but carries a higher mortality rate (126,133,134). Pneumonias occurring within the 1st month following transplantation are usually bacterial, whereas opportunistic pulmonary infections occur during the period of 2–4 months post-transplantation, when patients are still heavily immunosuppressed. Cytomegalovirus is the most common cause of pneumonia during this time, but other opportunistic infections, including *Aspergillus*, *Candida* and *Nocordia asteroides*, *Legionella*, and *Pneumocystis carinii* may all be encountered. The risks for these opportunistic pathogens are perpetuated in patients who require intense immunosuppressive therapy because of graft dysfunction.

Cytomegalovirus (CMV) infection occurs in approximately 75% of renal transplant recipients when it is defined as at least a 4-fold increase in CMV serum titers (measured by complement fixation or indirect fluorescent antibody levels to CMV) or a positive CMV culture from any body site (122,123,126,135). In a prospective study of 141 renal transplant patients, Peterson et al. (135) reported, however, that only 31% of patients actually developed a clinical illness. The median onset of infection was 7 weeks post-transplant, with only 10% developing infection later than 4 months post-transplant. CMV was the single most common cause of fever in the Minnesota study and was the cause of all documented fevers lasting greater than 7 days. Pneumonia developed in 25 of the 59 patients, with a mortality rate of 48%. Other complications included relative neutropenia (less than 1,000 neutrophils/mm^3) in 29%, gastrointestinal bleeding secondary to ulcerations in 20%, and 3 cases of pancreatitis.

Milder manifestations of CMV infection include musculoskeletal pain, leukopenia, and elevation of liver enzymes. The most common source of viral isolates is from the urine, but a thorough evaluation should include repeated buffy coat blood cultures.

As in bone marrow transplant recipients, the vast majority of the CMV infections occurring in renal transplant patients are due to latent virus (136). However, CMV can be transmitted to seronegative recipients from blood products as well as from the donor kidney. Of note, donor kidneys have less commonly transmitted other pathogens, including *S. aureus*, hepatitis B, and *Cryptococcus neoformans* (136–139).

Non-CMV viral infections, particularly the other herpesviruses, can also be a problem in renal transplant recipients. Infections with herpes simplex usually occur during the 1st month following transplantation. Varicella-zoster infections usually occur in the 2nd–6th month following transplants, are found in less than 10% of patients, and are usually self-limited (123,140).

Heart and Heart-Lung Transplantation

Both heart and heart-lung transplant patients suffer significant infectious complications. The immunosuppressive therapy is similar to that given to kidney transplant patients, and many of the infections that occur are similar. Two important differences are notable. First, the mortality rate associated with infection is higher in the cardiac transplant than in the renal transplant patients (122,141,142). Second, the primary site of infection is intrathoracic, predominantly the lungs, accounting for approximately 40% of all infections in heart transplant, and even more in heart-lung transplant (142,143). Bacterial isolates, both Gram-negative and Gram-positive, account for 35–50% of isolates in these patients (122,141). Viral infections, predominantly CMV, and protozoa are also seen in the patients, primarily in the first 6 months following transplantation (141). Fungal infections also occur, predominantly in patients receiving broad spectrum antibiotics (142,144).

Liver Transplant

With the advent of cyclosporin A, liver transplantation has gained some popularity in the pediatric age group because of both the increased survival and the decreased toxicity associated with its use as an immunonsuppressive agent.

Infectious complications are a significant problem for patients undergoing liver transplantation. Early in the postoperative period, hepatic ischemia may occur. In the setting of hepatic artery thrombosis, bacteremia often occurs (145). If there are large areas of necrosis, hepatic gangrene may occur within a few days of surgery, with accompanying sepsis (146). More commonly, the early infectious problems reflect the extensive intra-abdominal surgery, with Gram-negative aerobes being the most common bacterial isolates (122). Fungal infections, primarily with *Candida* have been reported in up to 44% of these patients and can be associated with a high mortality rate (122,147).

Viral infections, predominantly CMV, but also herpes simplex, varicella-zoster, and the Epstein-Barr virus can also complicate the clinical course in liver transplant patients (122). The interpretation of elevated liver enzymes, for example, can be a perplexing problem in these patients. Viral infections, if disseminated to the liver, can be the cause of elevated liver transaminases. Graft rejection, however, may cause a similar picture and may occur simultaneously, making the choice of treatment (i.e., either reducing or increasing the intensity of immunosuppression) a difficult dilemma.

ATTEMPTS TO PREVENT INFECTIONS IN IMMUNOCOMPROMISED PATIENTS
Prophylactic Antibiotics

Efforts to prevent infection in immunocompromised patients, particularly in those undergoing intensive chemotherapy regimens or bone marrow transplantation, have included a variety of attempts to decontaminate the host. Given that the majority of the infections in these hospitalized patients arise from their endogenous flora, much of which has been acquired in the hospital setting, the elimination or modification of this flora has theoretical rationale (148–151).

Gastrointestinal Decontamination

A variety of prophylactic antibiotic regimens have been studied in an effort to modify the bowel flora. Attempts to totally decontaminate or partially sterilize the gastrointestinal (GI) tract include various combinations of oral nonabsorbable antibiotics (e.g., gentamicin, vanco-

mycin, polymixin, colistin, nystatin). Unfortunately, most regimens are poorly tolerated, with poor compliance, and have failed to show a beneficial effect, particularly when used alone (148–155). Because this therapy suppresses rather than eliminates the endogenous flora, rapid repopulation of the GI tract (including aminoglycoside-resistant organisms) has been reported (156). This approach is not recommended.

Selective Decontamination

Partial decontamination with selective suppression of the GI aerobic flora and maintenance of the host's anaerobic flora can offer a resistance to colonization by new Gram-negative bacilli and has indeed appeared to reduce the incidence of infectious complications. This approach has a strong experimental basis, and promising results have been reported in two studies of acute nonlymphocytic leukemia patients receiving intensive treatment (157,158). However, patients require frequent microbiological monitoring to assure the adequacy of the selective decontamination regimen (e.g., polymixin, naladixic acid, trimethoprim-sulfamethoxazole, nafloxin) (159–161). Infections, however, still occur, predominantly with Gram-positive bacteria.

Oral Absorbable Antibiotics

The use of prophylactic oral absorbable antibiotics has been extensively studied. Trimethoprim-sulfamethoxazole (T-S) has been the most widely evaluated. Although T-S has been demonstrated to reduce the incidence of documented infections in some neutropenic leukemia patients, the incidence of fever, and hence the need for empiric antibiotics, has not been consistently decreased, nor has there been any increase in patient survival (162–167). The negative aspects of T-S prophylaxis, including reports of resistant organisms, GI intolerance, and myelosuppression, must also be considered (166–169). Although T-S is effective prophylaxis for patients at risk for *P. carinii* pneumonia, it has fallen from favor as an antibacterial prophylaxis regimen.

With the advent of the quinolones, however, oral, antibiotic prophylaxis of the immunosuppressed host is again under reevaluation. The quinolones exhibit broad antimicrobial activity against both Gram-positive and Gram-negative bacteria, especially enterobacteriaceae and *P.*

aeruginosa, and achieve good serum levels following oral administration (170). A small preliminary report from the Netherlands (171) reported no Gram-negative infections in 15 patients who received ciprofloxacin for a mean duration of 42 days during remission-induction treatment for leukemia. In spite of this, some resistant Gram-negative bacilli were isolated from routine oropharyngeal and fecal cultures, and seven patients became colonized in the bowel with *S. epidermidis*. This preliminary study reemphasizes the importance of larger comparative clinical trials before the quinolones can be recommended for prophylactic treatment.

Pathogen-Specific Prophylaxis

Certain pathogens occur more predictably in certain subsets of hospitalized immunocompromised patients. Efforts to prevent specific organisms from causing clinical infection have met with mixed success. The incidence of *Pneumocystis carinii* pneumonia has been dramatically reduced with the use of prophylactic trimethoprim-sulfamethoxazole in patients who are at high risk to develop the infection, and is indicated in patients undergoing allogeneic bone marrow transplantation. Many centers now give T-S prophylaxis on a more limited (e.g., twice a week) schedule to minimize its myelosuppressive effect.

Antiviral prophylaxis for herpes simplex with acyclovir, either orally or intravenously, has been shown to reduce the incidence of gingivostomatitis in patients receiving intensive chemotherapy or who are undergoing bone marrow transplant (172–175). To date, however, there is no effective prophylactic antiviral drug therapy to prevent cytomegalovirus infections. Although some studies have recommended a benefit of either hyperimmune anti-CMV antisera or high-dose intravenous immunoglobulins in decreasing the incidence of CMV interstitial pneumonia (176,177), these findings have been refuted by more recent controlled clinical trials (178,179). Presently, it appears that the only consistently successful way of controlling CMV pneumonitis is by using CMV-negative blood products for seronegative recipients. Clearly, this approach has limited effectiveness, since more than half of transplant recipients are seropositive prior to the transplantation.

Although fungal infections are generally postulated to arise from the patients's endogenous mucosal colonization, antifungal prophylaxis with oral agents that decrease the number of colonizing fungi (e.g., clotrimazole, meconazole, ketoconazole) have not been successful in reducing the incidence of invasive fungal disease (180–182). Oral antifungal agents (e.g., clotrimazole, ketoconazole) can be used to prevent or treat mucosal *Candida* infections (e.g., oral mucositis).

Principles of Hygiene

The medical staff may be a major vector in the transmission of microorganisms to hospitalized patients. The importance of the simple act of careful handwashing by all medical personnel before caring for a patient cannot be overemphasized and must be strictly enforced. Other theoretically standard hygiene practices must also be stringently adhered to and monitored to reduce the incidence of nosocomial infection. These include careful skin cleansing with iodophor solutions prior to skin puncture, antisepsis of equipment (e.g., vaporizer, respiratory support devices), and limited use of indwelling catheters, whenever possible.

The question of what foods an immunosuppressed hospitalized patient should receive has not been well studied. However, given these patients' propensity to become colonized with Gram-negative bacilli, efforts to reduce exposure to the more virulent organisms, such as *P. aeruginosa*, that are found on fresh, raw vegetables, may be helpful. Therefore, cooked food, when possible, is a reasonable recommendation, particularly for patients anticipated to have prolonged neutropenia.

Protected Isolation

Reverse isolation, restricting the granulocytopenic patient to a private hospital room, enforcing strict gown, mask, and glove precautions on all health personnel and visitors, is still standard practice at some hospital centers. This form of "protective isolation" is often advocated as a means to remind staff and visitors to wash their hands. If strict handwashing is enforced, the expense and inconvenience of such reverse isolation is not indicated (183,184).

Total protected environments (TPE) are an attempt to decontaminate the patient's endogenous flora while limiting the exposure to new nosocomial pathogens. This approach has theoretical rationale, and the use of laminar airflow rooms, strict isolation, and GI and cutaneous decontamination have been shown to reduce the incidence of infection in the profoundly neutropenic leukemia patient (155,185–188). With the advent of improved antimicrobial therapy and supportive care, the benefits of TPE are less apparent, and protected isolation is not routinely recommended for the cancer patient who becomes neutropenic.

There are, however, certain subsets who may benefit from TPE:

1. Those patients in whom neutropenia is anticipated to last greater than 25 days, as TPE may decrease the morbidity and mortality of infections;
2. In centers with a high incidence of *Aspergillus* infections, patients with prolonged neutropenia may have a lower infection rate with the use of laminar airflow rooms with high-efficiency particulate air (HEPA) filters;
3. Patients with aplastic anemia undergoing allogeneic BMT were shown in one study to have a decreased incidence of graft-versus-host disease (189).

There have been repeated reports of outbreaks of nosocomial *Aspergillus* infections during hospital construction (67,190–192). During construction, the use of airtight plastic barriers to isolate the area or the use of HEPA air filtration have both been shown to decrease the number of isolates (190,191). Following one outbreak of *A. flavis*, Opal et al. successfully decontaminated the affected site by treating the area with an aerosolized antifungal agent copper-8-quinoline product (192).

ATTEMPTS TO PREVENT THE SPREAD OF INFECTION BETWEEN IMMUNOCOMPROMISED PATIENTS

The issue of physical isolation to protect the immunocompromised patient from acquiring an infection has been discussed above. Once such a patient is suspected or known to be infected, a decision regarding isolation or hygienic precautions to prevent nosocomial transmission to another patient must be taken.

Patients who are in a TPE environment at the time an infection is suspected generally remain in that setting to receive their antimicrobial therapy. The more common situation is a newly or recurrently febrile immunocompromised patient who is cared for on a general hospital ward, often in a multibed room. There are no data at this time to support protected isolation of the febrile immunocompromised patient with a fever of unknown etiology. Similarly, if a microbiologic or clinical documentation of the source of infection is established, hospital isolation procedures as recommended by the Centers for Disease Control, and outlined in Chapter 25, should be applied to the infected immunocompromised patient.

Bacterial infections generally require drainage/secretion precautions if the source is exposed. Certain respiratory infections (e.g., *H. influenza*, meningococcus, *S. aureus*, group A *Streptococcus*) require respiratory or strict isolation until effective therapy has been established.

Fungal infections do not require isolation of any sort, although handwashing remains imperative. Viral infections in the immunocompromised host require the same isolation procedures as for other pediatric patients, with the exception of varicella-zoster infections. Patients with dermatomal herpes zoster should be strictly isolated as for disseminated disease until all lesions have crusted, because of the unpredictable occurrence of dissemination in these patients. Exposed, susceptible patients should be placed on strict isolation beginning 10 days after exposure and continuing until 21 days after last exposure.

Gastrointestinal infections dictate the usual enteric precautions, and similarly, there are no specific recommendations for isolation of the immunocompromised patient with a documented protozoal or parasitic infection.

ATTEMPTS TO BOOST IMMUNITY

Active Immunization

Attempts to improve the humoral defenses of the cancer patient are still in the early stages of development. Though some progress has been made, the primary limitation remains the impaired immune responsiveness of patients receiving chemotherapy. Pneumococcal vaccine, when administered to patients with a hematologic malignancy receiving chemotherapy, has limited efficacy, as it results in a poor antibody response, and levels fall over time. Patients with solid tumors, however, have a more normal response (193). In patients undergoing allogeneic BMT, the degree of impaired response to the pneumococcal vaccine was related to the presence of corticosteroid usage at the time of vaccination and to the time elapsed since transplantation; the absence of steroids and the longer the time since transplantation were both associated with a better response (194).

The *H. influenza* vaccine, like the pneumococcal vaccine, has limited efficacy in patients receiving combination chemotherapy. Although routine use of meningococcal polysaccharide vaccine is not recommended in the United States, it has been advocated that asplenic patients with solid tumors receive this vaccine, even though clinical efficacy has not been documented (195).

Viral vaccines of clinical relevance to immunocompromised patients include those for influenza and varicella. The influenza vaccine in children on maintenance chemotherapy for various malignancies has resulted in variable levels of antibody response, and clinical efficacy has not been demonstrated (196,197).

There is increasing interest in the use of the varicella virus vaccine. Essentially, all normal children develop antibody after an exposure to the vaccine, with protective efficacy in controlled studies nearing 100% (198,199). Furthermore, there is evidence that children with leukemia who are suseptible to varicella and who are in remission benefit from receiving the vaccine (200,201). However, the vaccine has been given only to children receiving maintenance chemotherapy, and when administered, chemotherapy has been discontinued for 2 weeks prior to vaccination. Protection is approximately 80% with nearly 100% protection against severe disease on natural exposure to varicella (200–202). Immunity may not be of long-term duration, and mild zoster infection has been reported in a small number of vaccinated immunocompromised children (196). It is not clear how the vaccine would fare in patients undergoing more intensive regimens, where the efficacy of the vaccine may not be as good and where the administration of a live vaccine may, in fact, be deleterious.

Passive Immunization

Passive immunization has recently received attention in cancer patients. Intravenous antisera

has been raised against the core glycolipid of *E. coli* (referred to as "J5") and is considered to have an antiendotoxin activity. A randomized trial showed that passive immunization with J5-antisera enhanced survival for adults with proven or putative Gram-negative sepsis (203). Similar efficacy was demonstrated for patients admitted to an intensive care facility and who were at risk for Gram-negative infection (204). A monoclonal antibody against J5 will soon be ready for clinical testing and may help obviate the problems associated with pooled antisera. Similarly, pooled immunoglobulins and hyperimmune gammaglobulin preparations are also undergoing clinical testing. At this time, however, these modulations should still be considered investigational (205).

Passive immunization with varicella-zoster immune globulin (VZIG) is, however, known to be effective in preventing or attenuating primary varicella in seronegative children. It is recommended that immunocompromised pediatric patients who have been exposed to varicella or herpes zoster and who are seronegative, or have a negative history of varicella infection, or have undergone a bone marrow transplantation should receive VZIG within 96 hours of exposure (206). Protection lasts approximately 3 weeks. Similarly, patients exposed to hepatitis B should receive hyperimmune antihepatitis B immunoglobulin (HBIG).

During the next several years, a number of immunoregulatory agents will be introduced into clinical testing, some of which may have a beneficial effect on the immunocompromised host. These include the interleukins, γ interferons, and especially the colony-stimulating factors (CSF). By activating various aspects of the immune system and by having the potential to shorten the duration of neutropenia, many serious infectious complications will hopefully be better controlled.

WHAT TO DO WHEN PREVENTION FAILS

Evaluation of the Febrile Immunocompromised Patient

Initial Assessment

Prompt evaluation of the immunocompromised patient who becomes febrile, and the institution of appropriate antimicrobial therapy are crucial to guarantee the best chance for successful treatment (207).

Fever in the immunocompromised patient requires immediate attention. Following a detailed history to discern any suggestive symptoms, or particular risk factors (e.g., previous illnesses, exposure to illness, medications) a thorough physical examination is essential. The signs of inflammation may be reduced or absent, and attention must be paid to even the smallest complaints or abnormal findings. A complete evaluation should not overlook a funduscopic exam, the oropharynx, including periodontal findings, perirectal inspection, examination of all skin surfaces, and assessment of all intravascular catheters and wounds.

Investigations in the initial assessment are listed in Table 23.5, and should include cultures of all sterile fluids. If a patient has an intravascular catheter, separate blood cultures should be drawn from each lumen at initial evaluation. Lumbar puncture is not generally indicated in the first assessment of a neurologically asymptomatic patient. However, any patient with an Ommaya reservoir or neurologic symptoms or signs should have a cerebrospinal fluid (CSF) examination. Any suspicious sites, such as cellulitis, should be aspirated or biopsied.

Specific Diagnostic Tests

In addition to routine bacterial and fungal cultures, certain specific diagnostic tests may be helpful in various subsets of patients. A sample of blood for an acute phase serum should be appropriately stored. In renal or other organ transplant patients, viral cultures of urine and buffy coat for CMV are indicated.

Table 23.5.
Initial Evaluation of Febrile Immunocompromised Patients

- Complete history and physical examination
- CBC, differential
- Routine chemistries, including liver function tests
- Acute phase serum (storage)
- Urinalysis, urine culture
- Oropharyngeal culture for bacteria and Candida
- Blood cultures: peripheral × 2
  all catheter lumens
  buffy coat for virus[a]
- Chest x-ray
- Lumbar puncture[a]
- Culture/aspiration/biopsy of suspicious lesions[a]
- Wound culture[a]

[a]As clinically indicated.

Blood culture technologies have become more sensitive and may be helpful in the diagnosis of bloodstream infections in immunocompromised hosts. For example, the lysis-centrifugation system (i.e., Dupont Isolator) permits the more rapid diagnosis of bacteremias (especially Gram-positive) and fungemia (208). The diagnosis of invasive mycoses, however, is often difficult, and the biopsy of suspicious sites including the skin, esophagus, and liver may be necessary to document invasive or systemic fungal infections. In patients with persistent fever, particularly when it follows granulocyte recovery, and when the patient has complaints of abdominal discomfort and an elevated alkaline phosphatase, hepatosplenic candidiasis should be considered, and an ultrasound and CT scan should be considered, looking for "bull's eye" lesions.

Unfortunately, the role of serologic studies to detect fungal infections remains unreliable, particularly in the immunocompromised host, except for the detection of cryptococcal antigen (209–211).

Investigating Pneumonia

A chest radiograph should be part of the initial evaluation in any febrile hospitalized patient. If the films show no evidence of infection, and the patient has no respiratory or thoracic symptoms, the film need not be repeated when the patient remains persistently febrile, despite antimicrobial therapy.

Two clinical scenarios deserve mention, however: First, consider the patient who has respiratory symptoms in the setting of fever, and a normal chest x-ray. Lack of neutrophils may explain the paucity of findings in the neutropenic patient, or the fever may reflect an early infection. As discussed earlier, neutropenic patients may have bacterial, fungal, viral, or protozoal infections. In the nonneutropenic immunosuppressed patient, this clinical presentation is suggestive of an early viral or *Pneumocystis carinii* pneumonia. An arterial blood gas sample should be obtained, as hypoxia with dyspnea is characteristic of *Pneumocystis carinii* pneumonia (PCP).

A second clinical problem is posed by the febrile immunocompromised patient with a fever and an abnormal chest x-ray. Most often, sputum will not be produced, and the question of what diagnostic procedures to perform will be raised. If the infiltrate is lobar or localized (i.e., noninterstitial), and the patient has not recently undergone a bone marrow transplantation, the pneumonia is most likely bacterial (especially Gram-negative aerobes), and broad-spectrum empiric antibiotics should be started promptly. A bronchoscopy or other invasive procedure is generally not necessary at this time, unless specific clinical or laboratory findings suggest that the initial broad-spectrum regimens might not be adequate. However, if the patient does not improve after 48–72 hours of empiric antibiotic therapy, a diagnostic procedure is indicated. Similarly, if the new infiltrate has developed in a neutropenic patient already receiving antimicrobial therapy who is not showing signs of hematologic recovery, a diagnostic procedure is necessary. It is also important to remember that noninfectious etiologies account for 17–41% of pulmonary infiltrates, generally due to pulmonary hemorrhage, malignant infiltration, or toxicity from chemotherapy or radiotherapy (212–216).

Currently available diagnostic techniques include bronchoalveolar lavage, transbronchial brush and biopsy, transthoracic needle aspiration (TTNA), and open-lung biopsy (OLB). Needless to say, no procedure is without risk, and it is important to assess whether the diagnostic yield and the potential changes in therapy justify the risk. Overall, the diagnostic yield of the open-lung biopsy is between 61–94% (212,217–220)—higher than any other procedure. In spite of this, McCabe et al. (216) reviewed the results of open-lung biopsy in 15 neutropenic leukemia patients with pulmonary infiltrates. The OLB yielded a diagnosis in only 40% of patients; 4 with fungal disease (2 were already on amphotericin B prior to OLB) and 2 with leukemic infiltrates. Autopsies on 3 cases with negative OLB results revealed pulmonary fungal infections. Other studies have also reported a low diagnostic yield in patients with hematologic malignancy, particularly in those who are neutropenic (212,213,219).

Empiric antimicrobial therapy may be a reasonable approach in the immunocompromised patient with interstitial pneumonitis (IP). At the National Cancer Institute, we compared the efficacy of early OLB versus early empiric therapy in a prospective randomized trial in cancer patients with IP (221). The results of OLB revealed a diagnosis in 64% of patients, but the findings did not suggest the need to add anti-

biotics that were not part of the empiric regimen. Importantly, there were no significant differences in the clinical outcome or morbidity in the nonneutropenic patients randomized to either arm.

Bronchoalveolar lavage (BAL) may provide a viable alternative to the OLB in the immunocompromised patient. Stover et al. (222) reviewed the results of BAL performed on 97 immunocompromised non-AIDS patients with pulmonary infiltrates. The overall diagnostic yield was 66% (diagnosis was reliably confirmed). Moreover, 83% of the infections were diagnosed, including *P. carinii* (18/22), CMV (10/12), fungal pneumonia (5/8), and mycobacterium (4/5). Using immunofluoresence staining with CMV-specific monoclonal antibodies may further improve the diagnostic yield (223).

MANAGEMENT OF THE FEBRILE IMMUNOCOMPROMISED CHILD

The therapeutic management of the febrile immunocompromised patient can be divided into three general strategies, determined by the temporal setting, the patient's clinical condition, and the degree of immunosuppression (particularly the presence of granulocytopenia). First, for the newly febrile patient who is receiving no antimicrobial therapy, decisions are influenced dramatically by the level of circulating granulocytes. Second, there is the patient who is febrile but who has an apparent focus of infection. Third, there is the patient who develops evidence of a new infectious process while already receiving antimicrobial therapy.

Initial Empiric Antibiotics

The Neutropenic Patient. Following a full evaluation, as outlined above, a decision must be made as to the need for immediate antibiotic therapy in the immunocompromised patient who has no apparent focus of infection. The presence of granulocytopenia necessitates the immediate institution of empiric antibiotic therapy. Since the routine adoption of this approach, there has been a significant reduction in the morbidity and mortality of infection in the febrile neutropenic patient (107,224). It is impossible to distinguish a life-threatening infection from a nonlethal course of fever. Thus, all patients with a new fever and neutropenia should receive broad-spectrum antibiotics. This should provide coverage for both the predominant Gram-negative bacilli, as well as the Gram-positive cocci, as discussed earlier. The importance of the rapid initiation of treatment cannot be overemphasized.

The choice of an empiric antibiotic regimen has been extensively studied. Multiple antibiotic regimens have been effectively utilized for the initial phase of management in these patients. Most successful regimens have included a combination of an aminoglycoside, an antipseudomonal penicillin, and/or cephalosporin. With the advent of the third-generation cephalosporins, extended spectrum penicillins, and most recently, the quinolones, there is interest in nonaminoglycoside regimens: double β-lactams, or even monotherapy (93,225–229). Certain of these newer agents achieve high bactericidal levels, and have good activity against Gram-positive bacteria, enterobacteriaceae, and *P. aeruginosa*. A recent study evaluating monotherapy with the third-generation cephalosporin, ceftazidime, as initial empiric therapy in the newly febrile neutropenic cancer patient has shown it to be as effective as combination therapy for this particular patient subset (93). These results remain to be confirmed, and such regimens should still be considered investigational. It is important to emphasize that not all the new β-lactam antibiotics offer adequate anti-*Pseudomonas aeruginosa* coverage. Also, modifications of treatment must be dictated by clinical judgment; treatment with the third generation cephalosporins may be more frequently complicated by superinfections with Gram-positive organisms (when compared with standard combination antibiotic regimens), and thus require the subsequent addition of a second agent (93,225–227).

The Nonneutropenic Patient. The newly febrile, immunocompromised patient who is not neutropenic and not anticipated to become imminently neutropenic, presents a different clinical problem. Minor infections that may be clinically inapparent at initial evaluation are less threatening to these patients. Thus, although they are immunocompromised, there is generally not the urgency for empiric broad-spectrum antibiotics in a patient with no apparent focus of infection who is clinically stable. The specific antibiotic therapy must be individualized, and the need for immediate treatment will be dictated by the clinical presentation.

Antibiotic Modifications for the Neutropenic Patient

Early Modifications. Certain changes in the immunocompromised patient's clinical status may mandate a modification of the initial antibiotic regimen. These include

1. The presence of a catheter-related infection or coagulase-negative bacteremia which requires the use of vancomycin;
2. Persistent mucositis (marginal gingivitis) or perirectal tenderness, despite adequate aerobic coverage; in this instance, the addition of anaerobic coverage may be beneficial. Particular clinical settings will dictate specific modifications (Table 23.6).

Prolonged Fever. Persistent or recurrent fever is a common problem in the immunocompromised patient receiving antibiotic therapy. Vigilant monitoring, frequent reevaluation, including thorough physical examination, repeated cultures, and x-rays, are required because of the risk of a second infection. Patients may show obvious signs of a second infectious process (e.g., new cellulitis), but persistent or recrudescent fever may be the only sign.

Knowledge of the pathogens responsible for these superinfections facilitates patient management. Bacterial isolates, including both obvious omissions (e.g., anaerobes, *Legionella*) and resistant organisms, may cause new fever and/or clinical symptoms. The development of an interstitial pneumonitis suggests a nonbacterial pneumonia, e.g., viral or *P. carinii* pneumonia. Alterations in antimicrobial therapy should be guided by these findings.

The development of clinical deterioration with hypotension and no-focus or defined infection is not uncommon. Empiric changes in antibiotic therapy to broaden and optimize antimicrobial coverage are required and will be influenced by the current antibiotic regimen. The duration of the patient's previous treatment, the underlying disease, the presence or absence of neutropenia, and the presence of current immunosuppressive drugs all influence the decision-making process. Treatment must be individualized.

The risk for fungal infection increases with the duration of neutropenia. The addition of empiric antifungal therapy, amphotericin B (0.5 mg/kg/day intravenously) for patients with persistent neutropenia and fever after 4–7 days of

Table 23.6.
Modification of Therapy in the Immunocompromised Patient Already Receiving Antibiotic Therapy

Clinical Event	Possible Modifications of Therapy
Breakthrough Bacteremia	
Gram-positive isolate	Add vancomycin until sensitivities available
Gram-negative isolate	Presume resistance to current regimen; switch to new regimen
Fungal isolate (i.e., Candida)	Add amphotericin B
Catheter-Associated Infection	
Local tunnel site/exit site	Add vancomycin (as well as Gram-negative coverage if not already being given). Consider removing line if no improvement after 48–72 hours.
Severe Oral Mucositis or Necrotizing Gingivitis	Add specific antianaerobic agent (e.g., clindamycin or metronidazole). Culture for herpes simplex and *Candida*, and treat if positive.
Esophagitis	
Initially	Trial of oral clotrimazole, ketoconazole or i.v. amphotericin B
If no improvement in 48–72 hours	Addition of i.v. acyclovir
Perianal Tenderness	If patient is already receiving broad-spectrum antibiotics, add a specific antianaerobic agent. If patient is not on antibiotics, begin broad-spectrum therapy; add anaerobic coverage if no improvement at 48 hours.
Pneumonitis	
Diffuse or interstitial	Trial of trimethoprim-sulfamethoxazole and erythromycin (plus broad-spectrum antibiotics if the patient is granulocytopenic)
New infiltrate in a granulocytopenic patient	
granulocyte count rising	Watch and wait
persistent granulocytopenia	If patient can sustain a diagnostic procedure, consider: bronchoscopy with lavage and/or biopsy open-lung biopsy If patient cannot tolerate a diagnostic procedure, consider adding erythromycin. Trimethoprim-Sulfamethoxazole amphotericin B.
Persistent Fever and Neutropenia	Continue antibiotics and cultures. If fever persists or recurs (after 1 week of antibiotics), and patient is still neutropenic, add systemic antifungal therapy empirically.

antibacterial therapy appears to decrease the rate of fungal infections (230,231). The timing of antifungal therapy may be influenced by the predominant fungal isolate at a single institution. Those where *Aspergillus* is a primary or prominent pathogen may benefit from earlier institution (and perhaps higher doses) of empiric antifungal treatment. The use of oral ketoconazole in the setting of prophylactic antifungal treatment may be a reasonable alternative to amphotericin B in some patients, as shown in a study at the NCI (232). These results remain to be confirmed, particularly with experimental studies which suggest the possibility of amphotericin resistance induced by pretreatment with ketoconazole (233).

Patients who respond clinically to an initial empiric antibiotic regimen with defervescence of fever, but who remain neutropenic, are also complex. Continuing antibacterial therapy may increase the risk for fungal and/or second bacterial infections, while discontinuing antibiotics after 7 or even 14 days in the setting of persistent neutropenia may lead to inadequately treated occult infection. At the NCI, we have addressed this issue in a series of randomized trials. When afebrile but persistently granulocytopenic patients had their antibiotics stopped after 1 week of therapy, they frequently recrudesced within 2–3 days. This suggested that continuing systemic antibiotics during granulocytopenia was preferable. In a second recently completed study, afebrile but granulocytopenic patients remained on antibiotics for a full 14-day treatment course (i.e., as if they were being treated for a defined infection). When randomized to stop or continue antibiotic therapy on day 14, however, patients showed a comparable risk for recrudescence (approximately one-third of the patients in both groups), suggesting that a defined course of therapy was reasonable for afebrile but persistently granulocytopenic patients. Therefore, we currently recommend that antibiotics be continued for 2 weeks if the patient is persistently afebrile and neutropenic. After that, the antibiotics should be discontinued and the patient followed expectantly.

Specific Infections

During the evaluation of a febrile immunocompromised patient, a focus of infection may be evident by symptoms, signs, or as revealed by the investigations (i.e., cultures, radiologic studies). The documentation of a focus of infection may occur at the onset of fever, or while a patient is already receiving some form of antimicrobial treatment. The potential pathogens cover the entire spectrum of "infectious complications," in any hospitalized patient, but an awareness of those problems found more particularly in the immunocompromised patient and their management will influence therapeutic interventions and optimize patient care.

Bacteremias/Fungemias. Following the isolation and identification of a specific organism from a blood culture sample, three questions arise: First, what is the source of the organism? Second, what is the appropriate antimicrobial therapy? Third, what is the optimal duration of therapy?

Frequently the source of a bacteremia is not evident, even after a complete evaluation, as listed in Table 23.5. This may be due to the lack of inflammation at an infectious nidus in the immunocompromised patient, or because many bacteremias arise from minor breakdowns in the gastrointestinal barrier without gross evidence of pathology. An extensive search is only warranted in cases of recurrent or persistent bacteremia. Patients with indwelling catheters must, of course, be followed to ascertain if this is the focus.

In the nonneutropenic patient, antimicrobial therapy can be dictated by the organism and its sensitivity pattern. In the neutropenic patient, broad-spectrum antibiotics are important initially. The duration of therapy in the immunocompromised patient for a documented bloodborne infection generally requires 2 weeks

of a standard treatment, but longer courses may be necessary in patients with persistent neutropenia or with a residual nidus of infection.

Catheter-Related Infections. Patients with indwelling venous access catheters are at an increased risk for infection. The infection rate varies between 10–60%, depending on the series reviewed (32). The predominant pathogens for both local exit site/tunnel site infections and bacteremias are Gram-positive organisms, particularly *S. epidermidis*, but Gram-negative and polymicrobial infections do occur. On the basis of our experience and a review of the literature, the following guidelines for catheter-related infections seem reasonable.

Exit site tenderness, redness, or cellulitis. Gram stain and culture should be obtained of any discharge. In the nonneutropenic patient, if the local inflammation is not progressing rapidly, a trial of oral antibiotics (e.g., dicloxacillin, cephalothin, erythromycin) may be adequate therapy. If *S. epidermidis* is isolated, susceptibility testing must be done to determine if parenteral vancomycin is necessary, as the oral agents may not provide adequate coverage.

If the patient is neutropenic, the patient should be hospitalized to receive parenteral antibiotics. If the patient is febrile, broad-spectrum agents should be employed. If a patient fails to respond to standard antibiotics, the possibility of an unusual pathogen, including fungi and atypical mycobacteria must be considered. Aspiration and/or biopsy may be warranted to isolate the causative organism.

Tunnel infections. These infections may or may not have associated exit site inflammation. In our experience, parenteral (rather than oral) antibiotics are necessary to treat the infection, and treatment failures (i.e., progression, or no improvement after 48–72 hours of intravenous antibiotics) are not uncommon, and require catheter removal.

Fever in the patient with a Hickman-Broviac catheter. The management of the febrile neutropenic patient is discussed earlier. If a nonneutropenic patient becomes febrile, one cannot be certain that the fever is not related to a catheter-associated bacteremia. If there is no obvious cause for the patient's fever, we currently admit these patients to hospital, and after performing cultures, including blood cultures through all lumens of the catheter and we begin them on empiric antibiotics through a peripheral site. Because of our experience showing that Gram-negative as well as Gram-positive isolates may be important in these patients, we begin with a combination of vancomycin and an aminoglycoside. If the cultures are negative at 48–72 hours, we stop the patients and follow expectantly. If the cultures are positive, patients receive a full course (i.e., 10–14 days) of specific antibiotic therapy, provided that follow-up cultures are negative. Although this approach is conservative, we feel it is warranted until more data are available.

Ommaya Reservoirs.   Any patient with an Ommaya reservoir who becomes febrile should have a CSF sample taken. In addition, a lumbar puncture should be performed if the Ommaya sample is positive on culture. *S. epidermidis* or *P. acnes*, may only colonize the reservoir, or these organisms may cause a true central nervous system infection. Patients who have recurrent isolation of one of these organisms in association with headache and ventricular pleocytosis should be treated for this infection. Intravenous, or even oral antibiotics may clear the infection; however, intraventricular antibiotics may be required (43–46). Treatment failures do occur, necessitating surgical removal of the reservoir, but most infections can be cleared with antibiotics alone.

Respiratory Infections—Sinusitis/Rhinocerebral Syndrome.   Sinusitis in the immunocompromised patient may be bacterial or fungal. Investigations should include sinus films at the least sign of sinus tenderness. Aggressive culture procedures are warranted only after an initial trial of antibiotics. A specimen should be cultured for *Aspergillus* spp. Coverage should include the common pathogens, as well as Gram-negative bacilli in the hospitalized immunosuppressed patient.

Fungal sinusitis is an especially serious complication, particularly when it occurs in the patient with prolonged neutropenia. The duration of neutropenia appears to be the major risk factor for invasive aspergillosis, although this also depends on whether the patient has been colonized with *Aspergillus* (30). The infection may begin as a minor local lesion in the nasal turbinate or septum, but can progress rapidly to a

sinusitis with facial swelling and subsequent bony erosion if left untreated (234). Unfortunately, the disease may progress in spite of treatment with amphotericin B (235). The rhinocerebral syndrome, with destruction of paranasal sinuses, orbit(s), and extension to the brain, may occur in this setting (236).

Aspergillus is the most common pathogen causing fungal sinusitis in patients with leukemia (234,237). Phycomyces, though a potential pathogen, is most commonly associated with diabetes, and *Candida* is also a less common, though reported pathogen in the immunocompromised patient (236,238,239). The definitive diagnosis of invasive fungal infection can be made only by biopsy with demonstration of tissue invasion by fungal forms. Efforts to identify patients at risk for invasive *Aspergillus* by surveillance nasal cultures have met with mixed success. Given the variable correlation of positive nasal swab cultures with the presence of invasive fungal disease, the cultures are of questionable value (240).

Treatment of fungal paranasal sinusitis/rhinocerebral syndrome in the immunocompromised patient must include intravenous amphotericin B. Surgical debridement, sometimes repetitive, is frequently necessary to control the infectious process (30,237,238). However, treatment is often disappointing, despite current maximal therapy. Moreover, it is not infrequent for patients with fungal sinusitis to have disseminated fungal disease, particularly involving the lung, liver, and central nervous system. Thus, the presence of the rhinocerebral syndrome in the immunosuppressed, particularly the neutropenic patient, should heighten one's awareness for the possibility of more generalized fungal disease.

Pulmonary Infiltrates.   Principles of managing a patient with a pulmonary infiltrate can be divided according to the clinical setting in which the infiltrate becomes apparent. Blood cultures and sputum cultures (if obtainable) may occasionally help to establish a diagnosis. Management of the newly febrile immunocompromised patient with a new pulmonary infiltrate should include broad-spectrum antibiotic coverage for both Gram-positive and Gram-negative organisms. Potential pathogens that are not as well-covered by most standard "broad spectrum" antibiotic regimens include *Legionella* sp. and *Mycoplasma pneumoniae*. *Legionella pneu-*

monia has been described in leukemia patients and in bone marrow transplant recipients (69,241). The early addition of specific therapy, erythromycin, is advised if there are recently reported cases of *Legionella* infection in the hospital/region, or if the clinical setting is suggestive (i.e., accompanying headache, gastrointestinal symptoms, and/or pleuritic chest pain).

Most patients who are newly febrile and previously untreated will respond to broad-spectrum antibiotic therapy. Management of the patient who is not responding to broad-spectrum antibacterial therapy, or the patient who develops a new infiltrate on such a regimen, necessitates modification of the current therapy. Given that a microbiologic diagnosis is frequently not available, the potentially treatable pathogens must be considered. If the patient is not responding to the initial antibiotic regimen after a 48–72-hour trial, less typical treatable pathogens should be considered. Depending on the patient's tolerance, a diagnostic procedure (BAL or open-lung biopsy) should be pursued. If the patient cannot tolerate a diagnostic procedure, and if all cultures are negative, the empiric addition of erythromycin and trimethoprim-sulfamethoxazole must be considered as the next step. Viral etiologies (particularly the herpesviruses and adenovirus) should also be considered. This is particularly true in the transplant recipients in the 2nd–6th months post-transplant. It must be remembered that patients who have been persistently neutropenic or severely immunosuppressed and on broad-spectrum antibiotics are also at high risk for invasive fungal infection, and amphotericin B should also be considered, particularly if the patient has received a week or more of broad-spectrum antibiotics and has a progressive or new pulmonary infiltrate.

Patients who develop a *new* infiltrate while already receiving broad-spectrum antibiotics present a particular problem. In these patients, the question arises whether the infiltrate is an early sign of granulocyte recovery with leukocyte infiltration into an already infected site, or whether the infiltrate is a "breakthrough" bacterial infection or fungal superinfection. Neutropenic patients with recovering granulocytes tend to do well without modification of therapy. Those who remain neutropenic, or whose granulocyte count does not change may benefit from the early institution of antifungal therapy (242).

Interstitial pneumonitis (IP) presents yet another dilemma in the immunocompromised patient. Although the potential pathogens include those causing the localized infiltrates, certain etiologies more commonly present in an interstitial pattern, including *P. carinii* pneumonia (PCP), viral infections, malignant infiltrates, and other noninfectious problems: toxic pneumonitis, radiation pneumonitis related to total body irradiation, and the nonspecific interstitial pneumonitis associated with allogeneic bone marrow transplantation. A trial of empiric therapy is reasonable for the nonneutropenic patient who presents with an interstitial infiltrate. However, should the patient improve after the initiation of empiric therapy, it is important that the antibiotics be continued for a "full course" of therapy (i.e., T-S: 2 weeks for PCP; erythromycin: 3 weeks for *Legionella*).

Obviously, treatment plans must be individualized and guided by an awareness of high-risk pathogens in particular patient populations (e.g., CMV pneumonitis in BMT recipients and organ transplant recipients; PCP in patients tapering off steroids; and encapsulated bacteria in splenectomized patients).

Gastrointestinal Tract.   Abdominal symptoms and signs in the immunocompromised patient deserve close attention. Infections of the gastrointestinal (GI) tract and alimentary organs can sometimes occur in these patients. Certain pathogens and clinical presentations can be peculiar and deserve mention.

Typhilitis.   Abdominal pain in association with fever is worrisome in immunosuppressed patients, particularly those with hematologic malignancy. Signs which are usually present in the normal host may be minimal or absent: concurrent corticosteroid therapy may also mask peritoneal signs or evidence of perforation, and neutropenia and immunosuppression may reduce the likelihood of any localized, identifiable abscess formation. The diagnosis of typhilitis, a necrotizing inflammatory lesion of the cecum, must be considered. This entity has been described in cancer patients who are neutropenic secondary to chemotherapy (243–246). Typhilitis, or necrotizing enteropathy, is usually manifested by fever, abdominal pain, particularly in the right lower quadrant, and may be associated with a palpable mass, diminished bowel sounds, and signs of an acute abdomen. Sepsis and GI hemorrhage may complicate this serious, potentially fatal disease. The diagnosis and the management of this entity remain somewhat controversial. Assessment should include physical examination, blood cultures, abdominal ultrasound or CT scan to identify a mass or abscess, and a search for any evidence of GI hemorrhage. Treatment includes bowel rest, broad-spectrum antibiotic coverage, and supportive measures for hemorrhage or sepsis, should they occur. Surgical exploration and resection of abnormal areas of bowel is advised by most authors, particularly if the patient has not improved rapidly on medical management (243,247–250).

Hepato/Splenic Candidiasis. Systemic fungal infection is an increasingly recognized problem in patients with profound immunosuppression, particularly those who suffer prolonged episodes of neutropenia. It is a difficult diagnosis to establish, as discussed earlier. If documented, treatment is with amphotericin B, and patients may require prolonged therapy, the average being a total dose of over 5 g of amphotericin B. The addition of 5-flucytosine may be helpful, although no controlled studies have been done. A preliminary report suggests that liposomal amphotericin B may benefit patients who had progression of invasive fungal disease while on amphotericin B (251).

Varicella (VZV) Infections. Primary infection with varicella virus (chickenpox) in a previously unexposed immunocompromised patient is potentially fatal. Without treatment, there is a significant risk of visceral dissemination and death (252,253). The most common sites of dissemination with VZV are lungs, liver, other gastrointestinal sites, and the central nervous system, usually occurring between 3–7 days after the onset of skin lesions. The most common life-threatening complication of disseminated varicella is pneumonia. Chest radiographs generally show diffuse pulmonary involvement with fluffy nodular infiltrates (252). Bacterial superinfections are a common occurrence in patients with severe disease. Such patients should be vigilantly monitored with appropriate cultures.

Treatment for established varicella infection in an immunocompromised patient should be instituted immediately. Acyclovir is the drug of choice and should be administered intravenously at a dose of 500 mg/m^2 every 8 hours, along with at least twice the fluid maintenance.

Vigilant supportive care is the other crucial aspect of successful treatment.

Herpes Zoster. Herpes zoster infections occur with increased frequency in immunosuppressed patients. Because of the risk of dissemination in patients with hematologic malignancies and the proven efficacy of antiviral agents in reducing the incidence of dissemination, the time of active viral shedding and the severity and duration of pain, treatment is recommended in these patients within 72 hours of the initial skin lesion(s). The recommendations for other immunosuppressed patient populations are less clearly established.

Herpes Simplex. Herpes simplex infections often complicate the clinical course of the immunosuppressed patient. Antiviral therapy has been shown to decrease the duration and severity of cutaneous lesions (254,255). The dose of intravenous acyclovir is 250 mg/m^2 every 8 hours. Oral therapy dosing is less well-defined, but adults treated with 200 mg, 5 times daily have shown good responses. Herpes simplex pneumonia may occur with or without a preceding or coincident mucocutaneous infection. Chest x-ray findings are nonspecific. If the diagnosis of HSV pneumonia or a disseminated HSV infection is established or strongly suspected, treatment with intravenous acyclovir should be initiated.

Miscellaneous. Other specific infections may occur in particular subsets of the patient population discussed. For example, urinary tract infections (UTI) in renal transplant patients carry more significance than an uncomplicated UTI in a nonneutropenic cancer patient. In the former group, a UTI occurring within the first few weeks post-transplant requires intravenous antibiotic therapy to ensure that the infection is contained and eradicated, as the sequelae of pyelonephritis in these patients may be devastating. Obviously, each patient requires individualized care and attention.

REFERENCES

1. Khalifa AS, Take H, Cejka J, Zuelzer WW: Immunoglobulins in acute leukemia in children. *J Pediatr* 85:788–791, 1974.
2. Hitzig WH, Pluss HJ, Joller P, Pilgrim U, Tacier-Eugster H, Jakob M: Studies on the immune status of children with acute lymphocytic leukemia. *Clin Exp Immunol* 26:403–413, 1976.
3. Hersh EN, Gutterman JU, Mavligit GM: Effect of haematological malignancies and their treatment on host defense factors. *Clin Haematol* 5:425–448, 1976.

4. Leikin S, Miller D, Sather H, Albo V, Esber E, Johnson A, Rogentine N, Hammond D: Immunologic evaluation in the prognosis of acute lymphoblastic leukemia: a report from Children's Cancer Study Group. *Blood* 81:501–508, 1981.

5. Fisher RI, DeVita VT, Bostick F: Persistent immunologic abnormalities in long term survivors of advanced Hodgkin's disease. *Ann Intern Med* 92:595–599, 1980.

6. McCormack RT, Nelson RD, Bloomfield CD, Quie PG, Brunning RD: Neutrophil function in lymphoreticular malignancy. *Cancer* 44:920–926, 1979.

7. Pickering LK, Anderson DC, Choi S, Feigen RD: Leukocyte function in children with malignancy. *Cancer* 35:1365–1371, 1975.

8. Snyderman R, Seigler HF, Meadows L: Abnormalities of monocyte chemotaxis in patients with melanoma: effects of immunotherapy and tumor removal. *J Natl Cancer Inst* 58:37–41, 1977.

9. Pickering LK, Ericsson CD, Kohl S: Effect of chemotherapeutic agents on metabolic and bactericidal activity of polymorphonuclear leukocytes. *Cancer* 42:1741–1746, 1978.

10. Baehner RL, Neiburger RG, Johnson DE, Murrman SM: Transient bactericidal defect of peripheral blood phagocytes from children with acute lymphoblastic leukemia receiving craniospinal irradiation. *N Engl J Med* 289:1209–1213, 1973.

11. Al-Hadithy H, Cawley JC, Addison IE, Gandossini M, Souhami RL, Goldstone AH: Neutrophil function in advanced Hodgkin's disease: effect of therapy. *Leukemia Res* 6:261–267, 1982.

12. Sosa R, Weiden PL, Storb R, Syrotuck J, Thomas ED: Granulocyte function in human allogeneic marrow graft recipients. *Exp Hematol* 8:1183–1189, 1980.

13. Cline MJ: Drugs and phagocytosis. *N Engl J Med* 291:1187–1188, 1974.

14. Dale DC, Petersdorf RG: Corticosteroids and infectious disease. *Med Clin North Am* 517:1277–1287, 1973.

15. Ryffel B, Tammi K, Grieder A, Hess AD: Effect of cyclosporin on human T cell activation. *Transplant Proc* 17:1268-1270, 1985.

16. Szamel M, Berger P, Resch K: Inhibition of T lymphocyte activation by cyclosporin A: interference with the early activation of plasma membrane phospholipid metabolism. *J Immunol* 136:264–269, 1986.

17. Lafferty KJ, Borel JF, Hodgkin P: Cyclosporine-A (CsA): Models for the mechanism of action. *Transplant Proc* 15:2242–2247, 1983.

18. Bodey GP, Buckley M, Sathe YS, Freirich EJ: Quantitative relationships between circulating leukocytes and infection in patients with acute leukemia. *Ann Intern Med* 46:328–340, 1966.

19. Schimpff SC, Young VM, Green WH, Vermeulen GD, Moody MR, Wiernik PH: Origin of infection in acute non-lymphocytic leukemia: significance of hospital acquisition of potential pathogens. *Ann Intern Med* 77:707–714, 1972.

20. Johanson WG, Pierce AK, Sanford JP: Changing pharyngeal flora of hospitalized patients. Emergence of gram-negative bacilli. *N Engl J Med* 281:1137–1140, 1969.

21. Fainstain V, Rodriguez V, Turck M, Hermann G, Rosenbaum B, Bodey GP: Patterns of oropharyngeal and fecal floral in patients with leukemia. *J Infect Dis* 144:10–18, 1981.

22. Beachey EH: Bacterial adherence adhesion-receptor interactions mediating the attachment of bacteria to mucosal surface. *J Infect Dis* 143:325–345, 1981.

23. Schimpff SC, Greene LH, Young VM, Wiernik PH: Significance of *Pseudomonas aeruginosa* in patients with leukemia or lymphoma. *J Infect Dis* (Suppl) 130:524–531, 1974.

24. Neu HC: Unusual nosocomial infection. *Disease-a-Month* 30(13):3–68, 1984.

25. Meyer RD: Legionnaire's disease: Aspects of nosocomial disease. *Am J Med* 76:657–663, 1984.

26. Kramer RK, Pizzo PA, Robichaud KJ, Witebskey F, Wesley R: Role of serial microbiological surveillance and clinical evaluation in the management of cancer patients with fever and granulocytopenia. *Am J Med* 72:561–568, 1982.

27. Dreizen S, McCredie KB, Keating MJ, Bodey GP: Oral infections associated with chemotherapy in adults with acute leukemia *Postgrad Med* 71:133–146, 1982.

28. Dreizen S, Bodey GP, Valdivieso M: Chemotherapy-associated oral infections in adults with solid tumors. *Oral Surg* 55:113–120, 1983.

29. Wingard Jr, Merz WG, Saral R: *Candida tropicalis:* a major pathogen in immunocompromised patients. *Ann Intern Med* 91:539–543, 1979.

30. Gerson SL, Talbot GH, Hurwitz S, Strom BL, Lusk EJ, Cassileth PA: Prolonged granulocytopenia: the major risk factor for invasive pulmonary aspergillosis in patients with acute leukemia. *Ann Intern Med* 100:345–351, 1984.

31. Band JD, Maki DG: Steel needles used for intravenous therapy. *Arch Intern Med* 140:31–34, 1980.

32. Hiemenz J, Skelton J, Pizzo PA: Perspective on the management of catheter-related infections in cancer patients. *Pediatr Infect Dis* 5:6–11, 1986.

33. Press OW, Ramsey PG, Larsen EB, Fefer A: Hickman catheter infections in patients with malignancies. *Medicine (Baltimore)* 63:189–200, 1984.

34. Gyves JW, Ensminger WD, Niederhuber JE, Dent T, Walker S, Gilbertson S, Cozzi E, Saran P: A totally implanted injection port system for blood sampling and chemotherapy administration. *JAMA* 251:2538–2541, 1984.

35. Khoury MD, Lloyd LR, Burrows J, Berg R, Yap J: A totally implanted venous access system for the delivery of chemotherapy. *Cancer* 56:1231–1234, 1985.

36. Skelton J, Leong S, Hathorn J, Rubin M, McKnight J, Thaler M, Pizzo PA: A prospective randomized trial comparing external venous access Hickman catheter to subcutaneously implanted catheter, Port-a-Cath® in cancer patients. (Abstract) Presented at the 26th Interscience Conference of Antimicrobial Agents and Chemotherapy, 1981, p 851.

37. Hiemenz JW, Robichaud KJ, Johnston MR, Pizzo PA: Bacteremias in patients with indwelling silastic catheters. (Abstract). *ASCO* 1:57, 1982.

38. Blacklock HA, Hill RS, Clarke AG: Use of modified subcutaneous right atrial catheter for venous access in leukemic patients. *Lancet* 1:993–994, 1980.

39. Houston G, Maher JW, Vance RB: Infectious complications associated with the Broviac catheter (CATH). (Abstract). *Proc Am Soc Clin Oncol* 2:C–336, 1983.

40. Pollack PF, Kadden M, Byrne WJ, Fonkalsrud EW, Ament ME: 100 patient years' experience with the Broviac silastic catheter for central venous nutrition. *J Parenter Enter Nutr* 5:32–36, 1981.

41. Shapiro ED, Wald ER, Nelson KA, Spiegelman KN: Broviac catheter-related bacteremia in oncology patients. *Am J Dis Child* 136:679–681, 1982.

42. Abrahm J, Mullen JL, Jacobson N, Polomano R: Continuous central venous access in patients with acute leukemia. *Cancer Treat Rep* 63:2099–2100, 1979.

43. Browne MJ, Dinndorf PA, Perek D, Commers J, Bleyer WA, Poplack DG, Pizzo PA: Infectious complications of intraventricular reservoirs in cancer patients. *Pediatr Infect Dis* 6:182–189, 1987.

44. Yogev R: Cerebrospinal fluid shunt infections: a personal view. *Pediatr Infect Dis* 4:113–118, 1985.

45. Frame PT, McLaurin RL: Treatment of CSF shunt infections with intrashunt plus oral antibiotic therapy. *J Neurosurg* 60:354–360, 1984.

46. Pau AK, Smego RA, Fisher MA: Intraventricular vancomycin: observations of tolerance and pharmacokinetics in two infants with ventricular shunt infections. *Pediatr Infect Dis* 5:93–96, 1986.

47. Berman M, Alter HJ, Ishak KG, Purcell RH, Jones EA: The chronic sequelae of non-A, non-B hepatitis. *Ann Intern Med* 91:1–6, 1979.

48. Koretz RL, Stone O, Gitnick GL: The long-term course of non A, non B post-transfusion hepatitis. *Gastroenterology* 79:893–898, 1980.

49. Alter MJ, Gerety RJ, Smallwood LA, Sampliner RE, Tabor

E. Deinhardt F, Frosner G, Matanoski GM: Sporadic non-A, non-B hepatitis: frequency and epidemiology in an urban U.S. population. *J Infect Dis* 145:886–893, 1982.

50. Adler SP, Chandrika T, Lawrence L, Baggett J: Cytomegalovirus infections in neonates acquired by blood transfusions. *Pediatr Infect Dis* 2:114–118, 1983.

51. Yeager AS, Grumet FC, Hafleigh EB, Arvin AM, Bradley JS, Prober CG: Prevention of transfusion-acquired cytomegalovirus infections in newborn infants. *J Pediatr* 98:281–287, 1981.

52. Alder SP: Transfusion-associated cytomegalovirus infections. *Rev Infect Dis* 5:977–993, 1983.

53. Bayer WL, Tegtmeier GE: The blood donor: detection and magnitude of cytomegalovirus carrier states and the prevalence of cytomegalovirus antibody. *Yale J Biol Med* 49:5–12, 1976.

54. Diosi P, Modlovan E, Tomescu N: Latent cytomegalovirus infections in blood donors. *Br Med J* 4:660–662, 1969.

55. Armstrong JA, Tarr GC, Youngblood LA, Dowling JN, Saslow AR, Lucas JP, Ho M: Cytomegalovirus in children undergoing open-heart surgery. *Yale J Biol Med* 49:83–91, 1976.

56. Prince AM, Szmuness W. Millian SJ, David DS: A serologic study of cytomegalovirus infections associated with blood transfusions. *N Eng J Med* 284:1125–1131, 1971.

57. Cheung K-S, Lang DJ: Transmission and activation of cytomegalovirus with blood transfusion: a mouse model. *J Infect Dis* 135:841–845, 1977.

58. Hersman J, Meyers JD, Thomas ED, Buckner CD, Clift R: The effect of granulocyte transfusions on the incidence of cytomegalovirus infection after allogeneic marrow transplantation. *Ann Intern Med* 96:149–152, 1982.

59. Friedman BA, Burns TL, Shork MA: A study of national trends in transfusion practice. A report to the National Heart, Lung, and Blood Institute. Ann Arbor, MI, University of Michigan, 1980.

60. Glenn J: Cytomegalovirus infections following renal transplantation. *Rev Infect Dis* 3:1151–1178, 1981.

61. Richardson WP, Colvin RB, Cheeseman SH, Tolkoff-Rubin NE, Herrin JT, Cosimi AB, Collins AB, Hirsch MS, McCluskey RT, Russell PS, Rubin RH: Glomerulopathy associated with cytomegalovirus viremia in renal allografts. *N Engl J Med* 305:57–63, 1981.

62. Ho M, Dowling JN, Armstrong JA, Suwansirikul S, Wu B, Youngblood LA, Saslow A: Factors contributing to the risk of cytomegalovirus infection in patients receiving renal transplants. *Yale J Biol Med* 49:17–26, 1976.

63. Naraqui S, Jackson GG, Janasson O, Yamashiroya HM: Prospective study of prevalence, incidence, and source of herpes virus infections in patients with renal allografts. *J Infect Dis* 136:531–540, 1977.

64. Preiksaitis JK, Grumet C, Merigan TC: Cytomegalovirus (CMV) infection in cardiac transplant recipients: the role of the donor heart. (Abstract). *Clin Res* 30:99A, 1982.

65. Smith TF, Holley KE, Keys TF, Macasaet FF: Cytomegalovirus studies of autopsy tissue. I. Virus isolation. *Am J Clin Pathol* 63:854–858, 1975.

66. Macasaet FF, Holley KE, Smith TF, Keys TF: Cytomegalovirus studies of autopsy tissue. II. Incidence of inclusion bodies and related pathologic data. *Am J Clin Pathol* 63:859–865, 1975.

67. Rhame FS, Streifel AJ, Kersey JH, McGlave PB: Extrinsic risk factors for pneumonia in the patient at high risk for infection. *Am J Med* 76:42–52, 1984.

68. Pennington JE: *Aspergillus* pneumonia in hematologic malignancy. *Arch Intern Med* 137:769–771, 1977.

69. Tobin JO, Beare J, Dunnill MS, Fisher-Hoch S, French M, Mitchell RG, Morris PJ, Muers MF: Legionnaire's disease in a transplant unit: isolation of the causative agent from shower baths. *Lancet* 2:118–121, 1980.

70. Arnow PM, Chou T, Weil D, Shapiro EN, Kretzschmar C: Nosocomial Legionnaire's disease caused by aerosolized tap water from respiratory devices. *J Infect Dis* 146:460–467, 1982.

71. Craven DE, Moody B, Connolly MG, Kollisch NR, Stottmeier KD, McCabe WR: Pseudobacteremia caused by povidone-iodine solution contaminated with *Pseudomonas cepacia. N Engl J Med* 305:621–623, 1981.

72. Zuravleff JJ, Yu VL: Infections caused by *Pseudomonas maltophilia* with emphasis on bacteremia: Case reports and review of the literature. *Rev Infect Dis* 4:1236–1246, 1982.

73. Barson WJ, Ruymann FB: Palmar aspergillosis in immunocompromised children. *Pediatr Infect Dis* 5:264–268, 1986.

74. Gartenberg C, Bottone EJ, Keusch GT, Weitzman I: Hospital acquired mucormycoses (*Rhizopus rhizopodiformis*) of skin and subcutaneous tissue. *N Engl J Med* 299:1115–1118, 1978.

75. Bodey GP, Bolivar R, Fainstein V: Infectious complications in leukemia patients. *Semin Hematol* 19:193–226, 1982.

76. EORTC International Antimicrobial Therapy Project Group: Three antibiotic regimens in the treatment of infection in febrile granulocytopenic patients with cancer. *J Infect Dis* 137:14–29, 1978.

77. Pizzo PA, Ladish S, Simon RM, Gill F, Levine AS: Increasing incidence of gram-positive sepsis in cancer patients. *Med Pediatr Oncol* 5:241–244, 1978.

78. Kilton LJ, Fossieck BE, Cohen MH, Parker RH: Bacteremia due to gram-positive cocci in patients with neoplastic disease. *Am J Med* 66:596–602, 1979.

79. McGowan Jr JE: Changing etiology of nosocomial bacteremia and fungemia and other hospital-acquired infections. *Rev Infect Dis* 7:S357–370, 1985.

80. Cairo MS, Spooner S, Sowden L, Bennetts GA, Towne B, Hoder F: Long-term use of indwelling multipurpose silastic catheters in pediatric cancer patients treated with aggressive chemotherapy. *J Clin Oncol* 4: 784–788, 1986.

81. Lu C, Bishop C, Braine H, Ownsend T, Saral R: *Staphylococcus epidermidis* sepsis in cancer patients. (Abstract). *Proc Am Soc Clin Oncol* 2:96, 1983.

82. Joshi J, Newman K, Tenny J, Ruxer RR, Markus S, Schimpff S: *Staphylococcus epidermidis* pneumonia in granulocytopenic patients with acute leukemia. (Abstract). *Proc Am Soc Clin Oncol* 2:90, 1983.

83. Atkinson BA, Lorian V: Antimicrobial agent susceptibility patterns of bacteria in hospitals from 1971 to 1982. *J Clin Microbiol* 20:791–796, 1984

84. Wade JC, Schimpff SC, Newman KA, Wiernik PH: *Staphylococcus epidermidis* an increasing cause of infection in patients with granulocytopenia. *Ann Intern Med* 97:503–508, 1982.

85. Acar JF, Courvalin P, Chabbert YA: Methicillin resistant staphylococcemia: bacteriologic failure of treatment with cephalosporins. *Antimicrob Ag Chemother* 10:280–285, 1970.

86. Meuwissen JH, Tauber I, Leeuwenberg AD, Beckars PJ, Sieben M: Parasitologic and serologic observations in infection with *Pneumocystis* in humans. *J Infect Dis* 136:43–49, 1977.

87. Ruebush TK, Weinstein RA, Baehner RL, Wolff D, Bartlett M, Gonzles-Crussi F, Sulzer AJ, Schulte MG: An outbreak of *Pneumocystis* pneumonia in children with acute lymphocytic leukemia. *Am J Dis Child* 132:143–148, 1978.

88. Singer C, Armstrong D, Rosen PP, Shottenfield D: *Pneumocystis carinii* pneumonia: a cluster of 11 cases. *Am J Med* 82:772–777, 1975.

89. Browne MJ, Hubbard SM, Longo DL, Fisher R, Wesley R, Inde DC, Young RC, Pizzo PA: Excess prevalence of *Pneumocystis carinii* pneumonia in patients treated for lymphoma with combination chemotherapy. *Ann Intern Med* 104:338–344, 1986.

90. Hughes WT: *Pneumocystis carinii* pneumonia. *N Engl J Med* 297:1381–1383, 1977.

91. Fainstein V, Bodey GP, Bolivar R, Elting L, McCredie KB, Keating MJ: Moxalactam plus ticarcillin or tobramycin for treatment of febrile episodes in neutropenic cancer patients. *Arch Intern Med* 144:1766–1770, 1984

92. De Jongh CA, Wade JC, Schimpff SC, Newman KA, Finley RS, Salvatore PC, Moody MR, Standiford HC, Fortner CL, Wiernik PH: Empiric antibiotic therapy for suspected infection in granulocytic cancer patients: A comparison between the combination of moxalactam plus amikacin and ticarcillin plus amikacin. *Am J Med* 73:89–96, 1982.

93. Pizzo PA, Hathorn JW, Hiemenz J, Browne M, Commers J,

Cotton D, Gress J, Longo D, McKnight J, Rubin M, Skelton J, Thaler M, Wesley R: A randomized trial comparing ceftazidime alone with combination antibiotic therapy in cancer patients with fever and neutropenia. *N Engl J Med* 315:552–558, 1986.

94. Thaler M, Gill V, Pizzo PA: The emergence of *Clostridium tertium* as a pathogen in neutropenic patients. *Am J Med* 81:596–600, 1986.

95. Bodey GP: Candidiasis in cancer patients. *Am J Med* 77:13–19, 1984.

96. Bodey GP: Fungal infections complicating acute leukemia. *J Chronic Dis* 19:667–687, 1966.

97. Pizzo PA, Robichaud KJ, Gill FA, Witebsky FG: Empiric antibiotics and antifungal therapy for cancer patients with prolonged fever and granulocytopenia. *Am J Med* 72:101–111, 1982.

98. Maksymiuk AW, Thongprasert S, Hopfer R, Luna M, Fainstein V, Bodey GP: Systemic candidiasis in cancer patients. *Am J Med* 77:20–27, 1984.

99. Horn R, Wang B, Kiehn TE, Armstrong D: Fungemia in a cancer hospital: changing frequency, earlier onset, and results of therapy. *Rev Infect Dis* 7:646–655, 1985.

100. Meyers JD, Atkinson K: Infection in bone marrow transplantation. *Clin Haematol* 12:791–811, 1983.

101. Winston DJ, Ho WG, Champlin RE, Gale RP: Infectious complications of bone marrow transplantation. *Exp Hematol* 12:205–215, 1984.

102. Peterson PK, McGlave P, Ramsay NKC, Rhame F, Goldman AI, Kersey J: A prospective study of infectious diseases following bone marrow transplantation: Emergence of *Aspergillus* and Cytomegalovirus as the major causes of mortality. *Infect Control* 4:81–89, 1983.

103. McGill TJ, Simpson G, Healy GB: Fulminant aspergillosis of the nose and paranasal sinuses: a new clinical entity. *Laryngoscope* 90:748–754, 1980.

104. Pirsch JD, Maki DG: Infectious complications in adults with bone marrow transplantation and T-cell depletion of donor marrow: Increased susceptibility to fungal infections. *Ann Intern Med* 104:619–631, 1986.

105. Meyers JD, Flournoy N, Thomas ED: Infection with herpes simplex virus and cell-mediated immunity after marrow transplant. *J Infect Dis* 142:338–346, 1982.

106. Ramsey PG, Fife KH, Hackman RC, Meyers JD, Corey L: Herpes simplex pneumonia: Clinical, virologic and pathologic features in 20 patients. *Ann Intern Med* 97:813–820, 1982.

107. Saral R, Burns WH, Laskin OL, Santos GW, Lietman PS: Acyclovir prophylaxis of herpes simplex virus infections: a randomized double-blind, controlled trial in bone marrow transplant recipients. *N Engl J Med* 305:63–67, 1983.

108. Saral R, Ambinder RF, Burns WH, Angelopulos CM, Griffin DE, Burke PJ, Lietman PS: Acyclovir prophylaxis against herpes simplex virus infection in patients with leukemia. A randomized, double-blind, placebo-controlled study. *Ann Intern Med* 99:773–776, 1983.

109. Gluckman E, Lotsberg J, Devergie A, Zhao XM, Melo R, Gomez-Morales M, Nebout T, Mazeron MC, Perol Y: Prophylaxis of herpes infections after bone marrow transplantation by oral acyclovir. *Lancet* ii:705:708, 1983.

110. Meyers JD, Flournoy N, Thomas ED: Cytomegalovirus infection and specific cell-mediated immunity after marrow transplantation. *J Infect Dis* 142:816–824, 1980.

111. Hersman J, Meyers JD, Thomas ED, Buckner CD, Clift R: The effect of granulocytye transfusions upon the incidence of cytomegalovirus infection after allogeneic marrow transplantation. *Ann Intern Med* 96:149–152, 1982.

112. Atkinson K, Meyers JD, Storb R, Prentice RL, Thomas ED: Varicella-zoster virus infection after marrow transplantation for aplastic anemia or leukemia. *Transplantation* 29:47–50, 1980.

113. Meyers JD, Flournoy N, Thomas ED: Cell-mediated immunity to varicella-zoster virus after allogeneic marrow transplant. *J Infect Dis* 141:479–487, 1980.

114. Yolken RH, Bishop CA, Townsend TR, Bolyard EA, Barlett J, Santos GW, Saral R: Infectious gastroenteritis in bone marrow transplant recipients. *N Engl J Med* 306:1009–1012, 1982.

115. Meyers JD, Pifer LL, Sale GE, Thomas ED: The value of *Pneumocystis carinii* antibody and antigen detection for diagnosis of *Pneumocystis carinii* pneumonia after marrow transplantation. *Ann Rev Respir Dis* 120:1283–1287, 1979.

116. Meyers JD, Flournoy N, Thomas ED: Non-bacterial pneumonia after allogeneic marrow transplantation: A review of the years' experience. *Rev Infect Dis* 4:1119–1132, 1982.

117. Weiner RS, Bortin MM, Gale RP, Gluckman E, Kay HE, Kolb HJ, Hartz AJ, Rimm AA: Interstitial pneumonitis after bone marrow transplantation: Assessment of risk factors. *Ann Intern Med* 104:168–175, 1986.

118. Witherspoon RP, Matthews D, Storb R, Atkinson K, Cheever M, Deeg HJ, Doney K, Kalbfleisch J, Noel D, Prentice R: Recovery of in vivo cellular immunity after human marrow grafting: Influence of time postgrafting and acute graft-versus host disease. *Transplantation* 37:145–150, 1984.

119. Atkinson K, Storb R, Prentice RL, Weiden PL, Witherspoon RP, Sullivan K, Noel D, Nomas ED: Analysis of late infections in 89 long-term survivors of bone marrow transplantation. *Blood* 53:720–731, 1979.

120. Witherspoon RP, Lum LG, Storb R: Immunologic reconstitution after human marrow grafting. *Semin Hematol* 21:2–10, 1984.

121. Winston DJ, Schiffman G, Wang DC: Pneumococcal infections after human bone-marrow transplantation. *Ann Intern Med* 91:835–841, 1979.

122. Dummer JS, Hardy A, Poorsattar A, Ho M: Early infections in kidney, heart and liver transplant recipients on cyclosporine. *Transplantation* 36:259–267, 1983.

123. Rubin RH, Wolfson JS, Cosimi AB, Tolkoff-Rubin NE: Infection in the renal transplant recipient. *Am J Med* 70:405–411, 1971.

124. Burgos-Caldeion R, Pankey GA, Gigueroa JE: Infection in kidney transplantation. *Surgery* 70:334–340, 1971.

125. Schweizer RT, Kountz SL, Belzer FO: Wound complications in recipients of renal transplants. *Ann Surg* 177:58–62, 1973.

126. Peterson PK, Ferguson R, Fryd DS, Balfour HH, Rynasiewicz J, Simmons RL: Infectious diseases in hospitalized renal transplant recipients: A prospective study of a complex and evolving problem. *Medicine (Baltimore)* 61:360–372, 1982.

127. Kyriakides GK, Simmons RL, Najarian JS: Wound infections in renal transplant wounds: pathogenetic and prognostic factors. *Ann Surg* 186: 770–775, 1975.

128. Lee HM, Madge GE, Mendez-Picon G, Chatterjee SN: Surgical complications in renal transplant recipients. *Surg Clin North Am* 58:285–304, 1978.

129. Tilney NL, Strom TB, Vineyard GC, Merrill JP: Factors contributing to the declining mortality rate in renal transplantation. *N Engl J Med* 299:1321–1325, 1978.

130. Rubin RH: Infection in the renal transplant patients. In Rubin RH, Young LS (eds): *Clinical Approach to Infection in the Compromised Host.* New York, Plenum, 1981, p 533.

131. Myerowitz RL, Medeiros AA, O'Brien TF: Bacterial infections in renal homotransplant recipients: a study of fifty-three bacteremic episodes. *Am J Med* 53:308–314, 1972.

132. Nielson HE, Korsager B: Bacteremia after renal transplantation. *Scand J Inf Dis* 9:111–117, 1977.

133. Ramsey PG, Rubin RH, Tolkoff-Rubin NE, Cosimmi AB, Russell PS, Greene R: The renal transplant patient with fever and pulmonary infiltrates: etiology, clinical manifestations, and management. *Medicine (Baltimore)* 59:206–222, 1980.

134. William DM, Krick JA, Remington JS: Pulmonary infection in the compromised host. *Am Rev Respir Dis* 114:359–394, 593–627, 1976.

135. Peterson PK, Balfour Jr HH, Marker SC, Fryd DS, Howard RJ, Simmons RL: Cytomegalovirus disease in renal allograft recipients: a prospective study of the clinical features, risk factors and impact on renal transplantation. *Medicine (Baltimore)* 59:283–300, 1980.

136. Glenn J: Cytomegalovirus infections following renal transplantation. *Rev Infect Dis* 3:1151–1178, 1981.

137. Betts RF, Freeman RB, Douglas RG, Talley TE: Transmission

of cytomegalovirus infection with renal allografts. *Kidney Int* 8:387–394, 1975.

138. Wolf JL, Perkins HA, Schreeder MT, Vincenti F: The transplanted kidney as a source of hepatitis B infection. *Ann Intern Med* 91:412–413, 1979.

139. Ooi BS, Chen BTM, Lim CH, Khoo OT, Chan DT: Survival of a patient transplanted with a kidney infected with *Cryptococcus neoformans. Transplantation* 11:428–429, 1971.

140. Luby JP, Ramirez-Ronda C, Rinner C, Hull A: A longitudinal study of varicella-zoster virus infections in renal transplant recipients. *J Infect Dis* 135:659–663, 1977.

141. Dummer JS, Bahnson HT, Griffith BP, Hardesty RL, Thompson ME, Ho M: Infections in patients on cyclosporin and prednisone following cardiac transplantation. *Transplant Proc* 15:2779–2781, 1983.

142. Dummer JS, Montero CC, Griffith BP, Hardesty RL, Paradis IL, Ho M: Infections in heart-lung transplant recipients. *Transplantation* 41:725–729, 1986.

143. Brooks RG, Hofflin JM, Jamieson SW, Stinson EB, Remington JS. Infections in heart-lung transplant patients. (Abstract). Presented at the 24th Interscience Conference on Antimicrobial Agents and Chemotherapy, 1984.

144. Baumgartner WA, Reitz BA, Oyer PE, Stinson EB, Shumway NE. Cardiac homotransplantation. *Curr Probl Surg* 16:1–44, 1979.

145. Busuttil RW, Moderator. Liver transplantation today. *Ann Intern Med* 104: 377–389, 1986.

146. Starzl TE, Putnam CW: *Experience in Hepatic Transplantation*. Philadelphia, WB Saunders, 1969.

147. Walsh TJ, Hamilton SR: Disseminated aspergillosis complicating hepatic failure. *Arch Intern Med* 143:1189–1191, 1983.

148. Johanson WG, Pierce AK, Sanford JP. Changing pharyngeal flora of hospitalized patients: emergence of gram negative bacilli. *N Engl J Med* 281:1137–1140, 1969.

149. Schimpff SC, Young VM, Greene WH, Vermeulen GD, Moody MR, Wiernik PH: Origin of infection in acute non-lymphocytic leukemia: significance of hospital acquisition of potential pathogens. *Ann Intern Med* 77:707–714, 1972.

150. Fainstain V, Rodriguez V, Turck M, Hermann G, Rosenbaum B, Bodey GP: Patterns of oropharyngeal and fecal flora in patients with leukemia. *J Infect Dis* 144:10–18, 1981.

151. Knittle MA, Eitzman DV, Baer H: Role of hand contamination of personnel in the epidemiology of gram-negative nosocomial infections. *J Pediatr* 86:433–437, 1975.

152. Yates JW, Holland JF: A controlled study of isolation and endogenous microbial suppression in acute myelocytic leukemia patients. *Cancer* 32:1490–1498, 1973.

153. Levine AS, Siegel SE, Schreiber AD, Hauser J, Preisler H, Goldstein IM, Seidler F, Simon R, Perry S, Bennett JE, Henderson ES: Protected environments and prophylactic antibiotics. A prospective controlled study of their utility in the therapy of acute leukemia. *N Engl J Med* 288:477–483, 1973.

154. Bodey GP, Rodriguez V: Infections in cancer patients in a protected environment-prophylactic antibiotic program. *Am J Med* 59:497–504, 1975.

155. Lohner D, Debusscher L, Prevost JM, Klastersky J: Comparative randomized study of protected environment plus oral antibiotics versus oral antibiotics alone in neutropenic patients. *Cancer Treat Rep* 63:363–368, 1979.

156. Schimpff SC, Greene WH, Young VM, Fortner CL, Cusack N, Block JB, Wiernik PH: Infection prevention in acute non-lymphocytic leukemia. Laminar air flow room reverse isolation with oral, non-absorbable antibiotic prophylaxis. *Ann Intern Med* 82:351–358, 1975.

157. Sleijfer DT, Mulder NH, de Vries-Hospers HG, Fidler V, Nieweg HO, van der Waaij D, van Saene HK: Infection prevention in granulocytopenic patients by selective decontamination of the digestive tract. *Eur J Cancer* 16:859–869, 1980.

158. Guiot HFL, van der Meer JWM, van Furth R: Selective antimicrobial modulation of human microbial flora: infection prevention in patients with decreased defense mechanism by selective elimination of potentially pathogenic bacteria. *J Infect Dis* 143:644–654, 1981.

159. Clasner HAL, Vollard EJ, van Saene HKF: Long-term prophylaxis of infections by selective decontamination in leukopenia and in mechanical ventilation. *Rev Infect Dis* 9:295–328, 1987.

160. Wade J, Schimpff SC, Hargadon MT, Fortner CL, Young VM, Wiernik PH: A comparison of trimethoprim-sulfamethoxazole plus nystatin with gentamicin plus nystatin in the prevention of infections in acute leukemia. *N Engl J Med* 304:1057–1062, 1981.

161. Wade J, deJongh C, Newman K, Wiernik P, Schimpff S: A comparison of trimethoprim/sulfamethoxazole to nalidixic acid: selective decontamination as infection prophylaxis during granulocytopenia. Presented at the 21st Interscience Conference on Antimicrobial Agents and Chemotherapy, 1981, p. 76.

162. EORTC International Antimicrobial Therapy Project Group: Trimethoprim-sulfamethoxate in the prevention of infection in neutropenic patients. *J Infect Dis* 150:372–379, 1984.

163. Weiser B, Lange F, Fialk MA, Singer C, Szatrowski TH, Armstrong D: Prophylactic trimethoprim sulfamethoxazole during consolidation chemotherapy for acute leukemia: a controlled trial. *Ann Intern Med* 95:436–438, 1981.

164. Dekker AW, Rozenberg-Arska M, Sixma JJ, Verhoef J: Prevention of infection by trimethoprim-sulfamethoxazole plus amphotericin B in patients with acute nonlymphocytic leukemia. *Ann Intern Med* 95:555–559, 1981.

165. Kauffman CA, Liepman MK, Bergman AG, Mioduszewski J: Trimethoprim-sulfamethoxazole prophylaxis in neutropenic patients. Reduction of infections and effect on bacterial and fungal flora. *Am J Med* 74:599–607, 1983.

166. Gualtieri RJ, Donowitz GR, Kaiser CE, Hess CE, Sarde MA: Double-blind randomized study of prophylactic trimethoprim-sulfamethoxazole in granulocytopenic patients with hematologic malignancies. *Am J Med* 74:934–940, 1983.

167. Pizzo PA, Robichaud KJ, Edwards BK, Schumaker C, Kramer BS, Johnson A: Oral antibiotic prophylaxis in patients with cancer: a double-blind randomized placebo-controlled trial. *J Pediatr* 102:125–133, 1983.

168. Woods WG, Daigle AE, Hutchinson RJ, Robison LL: Myelosuppression associated with co-trimoxazole as a prophylactic antibiotic in the maintenance phase of childhood acute lymphocytic leukemia. *J Pediatr* 105:639–644, 1984.

169. Bow EJ, Louie TJ, Riben PD, McNaughton RD, Harding GK, Ronald AR: Randomized controlled trial comparing trimethoprim/sulfamethoxazole and trimethoprim for infection prophylaxis in hospitalized granulocytopenic patients. *Am J Med* 76:223–233, 1984.

170. Crump B, Wise R, Dent J: Pharmacokinetics and tissue penetration of ciprofloxacin. *Antimicrob Agents Chemother* 24:784–786, 1983.

171. Rozenberg-Arska M, Dekker AW, Verhoef J: Ciprofloxacin for selective decontamination of the alimentary tract in patients with acute leukemia during remission induction treatment: the effect of fecal flora. *J Infect Dis* 152:104–107, 1985.

172. Gluckman E, Lotsberg J, Devergie A, Zhao XM, Melo R, Gomez-Morales M, Nebart T, Mazeron MC, Perol Y: Prophylaxis of herpes infections after bone marrow transplantation by oral acyclovir. *Lancet* 2:705–708, 1983.

173. Wade JC, Newton B, McLaren C, Flournoy N, Keeney RE, Meyers JD. Intravenous acyclovir to treat mucocutaneous herpes simplex virus infection after marrow transplantation: a double-blind trial. *Ann Intern Med* 96:265–269, 1982.

174. Saral R, Bruns WH, Laskin OL, Santos GW, Lietman PS. Acyclovir prophylaxis of herpes-simplex-virus infections: a randomized, double-blind, controlled trial in bone-marrow-transplant recipients. *N Engl J Med* 305:63–67, 1981.

175. Saral R, Ambinder RF, Burns WH, Angelopulos CM, Griffin DE, Burke PJ, Leitman PS: Acyclovir prophylaxis against herpes simplex virus infection in patients with leukemia. *Ann Intern Med* 99:773–776, 1983.

176. Winston DJ, Ho WG, Lin CH, Budinger MD, Champlin RE, Gale RP: Intravenous immunoglobulin for modification of cytomegalovirus infections associated with bone marrow transplantation. *Am J Med* 76(3A)128–133, 1984.

177. Winston DJ, Pollard RB, Ho WG, Gallagher JG, Rasmussen

LE, Huang SN, Lin CH, Gossett TG, Merigan TC, Gale RP: Cytomegalovirus immune plasma in bone marrow transplant recipients. *Ann Intern Med* 97:11–18, 1982.

178. Meyers JD, Leszcynski J, Zaia JA, Fournoy N, Newton B, Syndman DR, Wright GG, Levin MJ, Thomas ED: Prevention of cytomegalovirus immune globulin after marrow transplantation. *Ann Intern Med* 98:442–446, 1983.

179. Bowden RA, Sayers M, Flournoy N, Newton B, Banaji M, Thomas ED, Meyers JD: Cytomegalovirus immune globulin and seronegative blood products to prevent primary cytomegalovirus infection after marrow transplantation. *N Engl J Med* 314:1006–1010, 1986.

180. Acuna G, Winston D, Young L: Ketoconazole prophylaxis of fungal infection in the granulocytopenic patient: a double-blind, randomized controlled trial. Presented at the 21st Interscience Conference on Antimicrobial Agents and Chemotherapy, 1981, p. 851.

181. Degregorio M, Lee W, Ries C: Candida infections in patients with acute leukemia: ineffectiveness of nystatin prophylaxis and relationship between oropharyngeal and systemic candidiasis. *Cancer* 50:2780–2784, 1983.

182. Williams C, Whitehouse JMA, Lister TA, Wrigley PFM: Oral anticandidal prophylaxis in patients undergoing chemotherapy for acute leukemia. *Med Pediatr Oncol* 3:275–280, 1977.

183. Albert RK, Condie F: Handwashing patterns in medical intensive care units. *N Engl J Med* 304:1465–1466, 1981.

184. Nauseff WM, Maki DG: A study of value of simple protective isolation in patients with granulocytopenia. *N Engl J Med* 304:448–453, 1981.

185. Armstrong D: Protected environments are discomforting and expensive and do not offer meaningful protection. *Am J Med* 76:685–689, 1984.

186. Bodey GP: Current status of prophylaxis of infection with protected environments. *Am J Med* 76:678–684, 1984.

187. Pizzo PA, Levine AS: The utility of protected-environment regimens for the compromised host: a critical assessment. In Brown E (ed): *Progress in Hematology*. New York, Grune & Stratton, 1977, pp 311–322.

188. Pizzo PA: Do results justify the expense of protected environments. In Wiernick PH (ed): *Controversies in Oncology*. New York, John Wiley, 1981, pp 267–277.

189. Storb R, Prentice RL, Buckner CD, Clift RA, Applebaum F, Deeg J, Doney K, Sanders, JE, Singer J, Sullivan KM, Witherspoon RP, Thomas ED: Graft-versus-host disease and survival in patients with aplastic anemia treated by marrow grafts from HLA-identical siblings: beneficial effects of protective environment. *N Engl J Med* 76:564–572, 1983.

190. Arnow PM, Andersen RL, Mainous PD, Smith EJ: Pulmonary aspergillosis during hospital renovation. *Am Rev Respir Dis* 118:49–53, 1978.

191. Sarubbi FA Jr, Kopf HB, Wilson MB, McGinnis MR, Ratula WA: Increased recovery of *Aspergillus flavus* from respiratory specimens during hospital construction. *Am Rev Resp Dis* 125:33–38, 1982.

192. Opal SM, Asp AA, Cannady PB, Morse PL, Burton LJ, Hammer PG: Efficacy of infection control measures during a nosocomial outbreak of disseminated aspergillosis associated with hospital construction. *J Infect Dis* 153:634–637, 1986.

193. Shildt RA, Boyd JF, McCracken JD, Schiffman G, Giolma JP: Antibody response to pneumococcal vaccine in patients with solid tumors and lymphomas. *Med Pediatr Oncol* 11:305–309, 1983.

194. Winston DJ, Ho WG, Schiffman G, Champlin RE, Feig SA, Gale RP: Pneumococcal vaccination of recipients of bone marrow transplants. *Arch Intern Med* 143:1735–1737, 1983.

195. Recommendations of the Immunization Practices Advisory Committee (ACIP): Meningococcal vaccine. *MMWR* 34:255–259, 1985.

196. Smithson W, Siem RA, Ritts RE Jr, Gilchrist GS, Burgert ED Jr, Ilstrop DM, Smith TF: Response to influenza virus vaccine in children receiving chemotherapy for malignancy. *J Pediatr* 93:632–633, 1978.

197. Sumaya CV, Williams TE: Persistence of antibody after the administration of influenza vaccine to children with cancer. *Pediatr* 69:226–229, 1982.

198. Hilleman MR: Newer directions in vaccine development and utilization. *J Infect Dis* 151:407–419, 1985.

199. Weibel RE, Neff BJ, Kuter BJ, Guess HA, Rothenberger CA, Fitzgerald AJ, Connor KA, McLean AA, Hilleman ME, Buynak EB: Live attenuated varicella virus vaccine: efficacy trial in healthy children. *N Eng J Med* 310:1409–1415, 1984.

200. Gershorn A, Steinberg S, Gelb L, Galasso G, Borkowsky W, LaRussa P, Farrara A: Live attenuated varicella vaccine. Efficacy for children with leukemia in remission. *JAMA* 252:355–362, 1984.

201. Brunell PA, Geiser C, Shehab Z, Waugh JE: Administration of live varicella vaccine to children with leukemia. *Lancet* 2:1069–1072, 1985.

202. Gershorn AA: The success of varicella vaccine. *Pediatr Infect Dis* 3:500–502,1984.

203. Ziegler EJ, McCutchan JA, Fierer JA, Glauser MP, Sadoff JC, Douglas H, Braude AI: Treatment of gram-negative bacteremia and shock with human antiserum to mutant *Escherichia coli. N Eng J Med* 307:1225–1230, 1982.

204. Baumgartner JD, Glauser MP, McCutchan JA: Prevention of gram-negative shock and death in surgical patients by antibody to endotoxin core glycolipid. *Lancet* 1:59–63, 1985.

205. Pollack M, Huang AI, Prescott RK, Young LS, Hunter KW, Cruess DF, Tsai CM: Enhanced survival in *Pseudomonas aeruginosa* septicemia associated with high levels of circulating antibody to *Escherichia coli* endotoxin core. *J Clin Invest* 72:1874–1881, 1983.

206. Centers for Disease Control, Department of Health and Human Services; Atlanta, Georgia. Varicella-zoster immune globulin for the prevention of chickenpox. *Ann Intern Med* 100:859–865, 1984.

207. Schimpff SC, Aisner J: Empiric antibiotic therapy. *Cancer Treat Rep* 62:673–680, 1978.

208. Henry NK, McLimans CA, Wright AJ: Microbiological and clinical evaluation of the isolator lysis-centrifugation blood culture tube. *J Clin Microbiol* 17:864–869, 1983.

209. Bailey JW, Sada E, Brass C, Bennett JE: Diagnosis of systemic candidiasis by latex agglutination for serum antigen. *J Clin Microbiol* 21:749–752, 1985.

210. Masan AB, Smith JMB: Germling protoplast antigens of *Candida albicans* in the serodiagnosis of invasive candidosis. *J Infect Dis* 153:146–150, 1986.

211. Kahn FW, Jones JM: Latex agglutination tests for detection of candida antigens in sera of patients with invasive candidiasis. *J Infect Dis* 153:579–585, 1986.

212. Singer C, Armstrong D, Rosen PP, Warzer PD, Yu R: Diffuse pulmonary infiltrates in immunosuppressed patients: prospective study of 80 cases. *Am J Med* 66:110–120, 1979.

213. Tenholder MF, Hooper RG: Pulmonary infiltrates in leukemia. *Chest* 78:468–473, 1980.

214. Canham EM, Kennedy TC, Merrick TA: Unexplained pulmonary infiltrates in the compromised patient: An invasive investigation in a consecutive series. *Cancer* 52:325–329, 1983.

215. Greenman RL, Goodall PT, King D: Lung biopsy in immunocompromised hosts. *Am J Med* 59:488–496, 1975.

216. McCabe RE, Brooks RG, Mark JBD, Remington JS: Open lung biopsy in patients with acute leukemia. *Am J Med* 78:609–616, 1985.

217. Hiatt JR, Gong H, Mulder DG, Ramming KP. The value of open lung biopsy in the immunosuppressed patient. *Surgery* 92:285–291, 1982.

218. Cheson BD, Samlowski WE, Tang TT, Spruance SL: Value of open-lung biopsy in 87 immunocompromised patients with pulmonary infiltrates. *Cancer* 55:453–459, 1985.

219. Jaffe JP, Maki DG: Lung biopsy in immunocompromised patients: one institution's experience and an approach to management of pulmonary disease in the compromised host. *Cancer* 48:1144–1153, 1981.

220. Burt ME, Flye MW, Webber BL, Wesley RA: Prospective evaluation of aspiration needle, cutting needle, transbronchial, and open lung biopsy in patients with pulmonary infiltration. *Ann Thorac Surg* 32:146–153, 1981.

221. Potter D, Pass HI, Brower S, Macher A, Browne M, Thaler M, Cotton D, Hathorn J, Wesley R, Longo D: Prospective randomized study of open lung biopsy versus empirical antibiotic therapy for acute pneumonitis in non-neutropenic cancer patients. *Ann Thorac Surg* 40:422–428, 1985.

222. Stover MB, Zaman AI, Hajdu SI: Bronchoalveolar lavage in the diagnosis of diffuse pulmonary infiltrates in the immunosuppressed host. *Ann Intern Med* 101:1–7, 1984.

223. Emanuel D, Peppard J, Stover D, Gola J, Armstrong D, Hammerling U: Rapid immunodiagnosis of cytomegalovirus pneumonia by bronchoalveolar lavage using human and murine monoclonal antibodies. *Ann Intern Med* 104:476–481, 1986.

224. Love LJ, Schimpff SC, Schiffer CA, Siernik PH: Improved prognosis for granulocytopenic patients with gram-negative bacteremia. *Am J Med* 68:643–648, 1980.

225. De Pauw B, Williams K, de Neeff J, Bothof T, De Witte T, Holdrinet R, Hanaan C: A randomized prospective study of ceftazidime versus ceftazidime plus flucioxicillin in the empiric treatment of febrile episodes in severely neutropenic patients. *Antimicrob Ag Chemother* 28:824–828, 1985.

226. Ramphal R, Kramer BS, Rand H, Weiner RS, Schands Jr JW: Early results of a comparative trial of ceftazidime versus cephalothin, carbenicillin, and gentamicin in the treatment of febrile granulocytic patients. *J Antimicrob Chemother* 12 (Suppl A): 81–88, 1983.

227. Kramer BS, Ramphal R, Rand KH: Randomized comparison between two ceftazidime containing regimens and cephalothin-gentamicin-carbenicllin in febrile granulocytopenic cancer patients. *Antimicrob Agents Chemother* 30:64–68, 1986.

228. Klastersky J, Glauser MP, Schimpff SC, Zinner SH, Gaya H, EORTC Antimicrobial Therapy Project Group: Prospective randomized comparison of three antibiotic regimens for empirical therapy of suspected bacteremic infection in febrile granulocytopenic patients. *Antimicrob Agents Chemother* 29:263–270, 1986.

229. Gaya H: Combination therapy and monotherapy in the treatment of severe infection in the immunocompromised host. *Am J Med* 80 (Suppl 6B):149–155, 1986.

230. Thaler M, Pizzo PA: Empiric antifungal therapy in neutropenic cancer patients. (Abstract) *Proc Am Soc Clin Oncol* 222, 1986.

231. EORTC Antimicrobial Cooperative Group: Empiric therapy with fungizone in febrile neutropenic patients. (Abstract) *Proc Am Soc Clin Oncol* 223, 1986.

232. Hathorn J, Thaler M, Skelton J, McKnight J, Browne M, Rubin M, Marshall D, Gress J, Pizzo P: Empiric amphotericin B versus ketoconazole in febrile granulocytopenic cancer patients. (Abstract) *Proc Am Soc Clin Oncol* 136,1985.

233. Schaffner A, Frick PG: The effect of ketoconazole on amphotericin B in a model of disseminated aspergillosis. *J Infect Dis* 151:902–910, 1985.

234. McGill TJ, Simpson G, Healy GB: Fulminant aspergillosis of the nose and paranasal sinuses: a new clinical entity. *Laryngoscope* 90:748–754, 1980.

235. Swerdlow B, Deresinski S: Development of Aspergillus sinusitis in a patient receiving amphotericin B: treatment with granulocyte transfusions. *Am J Med* 76:162–166, 1984.

236. Centeno RS, Bentson JR, Mancuso AA: CT scanning in rhino-cerebral mucormycosis and Aspergillosis. *Radiology* 140:383–389, 1981.

237. Romett JL, Newan RK: Aspergillosis of the nose and paranasal sinuses. *Laryngoscope* 92:764–766, 1982.

238. Stevens MH: Primary fungal infections of the paranasal sinuses. *Am J Otolaryngol* 2:348–35, 1981.

239. Meyer RD, Rosen P, Armstrong D: Phycomycosis complicating leukemia and lymphoma. *Ann Intern Med* 77:871–872, 1972.

240. Aisner J, Murillo J, Schimpff SC, Steere AC: Invasive aspergillosis in acute leukemia: correlation with nose cultures and antibiotic use. *Ann Intern Med* 90:4–9, 1979.

241. Kugler JW, Armitage JO, Helms CM, Klassen LW, Goeken NE, Ahmann CB, Gingrich RD, Johnson W, Gilchrist MJ: Nosocomial Legionnaires' disease. Occurrence in recipients of bone marrow transplants. *Am J Med* 174:281–288, 1983.

242. Commers JR, Robichaud KJ, Pizzo PA: New pulmonary infiltrates in granulocytopenic cancer patients being treated with antibiotics. *Pediatr Infect Dis* 3:423–428, 1984.

243. Abramson SJ, Berdon WE, Baker DH: Childhood typhilitis: its increasing association with acute myelogenous leukemia. *Radiology* 146:61–64, 1983.

244. Jones GT, Abramson N: Gastrointestinal necrosis in acute leukemia: a complication of induction therapy. *Cancer Invest* 1:315–320, 1983.

245. Matolo NM, Garfinkle SE, Wolfman EF: Intestinal necrosis and perforation in patients receiving immunosuppressive drugs. *Am J Surg* 132:753–754, 1976.

246. Moir DH, Bale PM: Necropsy findings in childhood leukemia, emphasizing neutropenic enterocolitis and cerebral calcification. *Pathology* 8:247–257, 1976.

247. Exelby PR, Ghandchi A, Lansigan N, Schwartz I: Management of the acute abdomen in children with leukemia. *Cancer* 35:826–829, 1975.

248. Meyerovitz MF, Fellows KE: Typhilitis: a cause of gastrointestinal hemorrhage in children, *AJR*143:833–835, 1984.

249. Marki AP, Armitage JO, Feagler JR: Typhilitis in acute leukemia. Successful treatment by early surgical intervention. *Cancer* 43:695–697, 1979.

250. Shaked A, Shinar E, Freund H: Neutropenic typhilitis: a plea for conservatism. *Dis Colon Rectum* 26:351–352, 1983.

251. Lopez-Berenstein G, Fainstein V, Hopfer R, Mehta K, Sullivan MP, Keating M, Rosenblum MG, Mehta R, Luna M, Hersh EM: Liposomal amphotericin B for the treatment of systemic fungal infections in patients with cancer: a preliminary study. *J Infect Dis* 151:704–710, 1985.

252. Feldman S, Hughes WT, Daniel CB: Varicella in children with cancer: seventy-seven cases. *Pediatrics* 56:388–397, 1975.

253. Simone JV, Holland E, Johnson W: Fatalities during remission in childhood leukemia. *Blood* 39:759–770, 1972.

254. Wade JC, Newton B, Flournoy N, Meyers JD: Oral acyclovir for the prevention of herpes simplex reactivation after bone marrow transplantation. *Ann Intern Med* 100:823–828, 1984.

255. Mitchell CD, Bean B, Gentry SR, Groth KE, Boen JR, Balfour HH Jr: Acyclovir therapy for mucocutaneous herpes simplex infections in immunocompromised patients. *Lancet* 2:1389–1392, 1981.

24

The Critical Care Patient

Leigh G. Donowitz, M. D.

BACKGROUND

The pediatric critical care patient is unique in the hospital setting. Unlike other hospitalized patients who are divided by age or diagnosis, these units generally care for patients from the neonatal period through adolescence who have any diagnosis or process requiring monitoring and/or life-support therapies. The typical pediatric intensive care unit may take care of infants with respiratory syncytial virus pneumonia, or disseminated herpes simplex disease at the same time that a new leukemia patient is receiving plasmapheresis, a multiple trauma patient is being monitored and supported, and a postoperative cardiac patient is being weaned from ventilatory support. The nosocomial infectious disease risks to these patients are very high due to the severity and possible immunocompromising nature of their illnesses, their need for invasive monitoring and support equipment, and their close proximity to other patients with transmissible bacterial, viral, and protozoan pathogens.

The 1978 National Nosocomial Infection Study reports a 3.37% overall nosocomial infection rate with a 1.2% rate on pediatric services (1). Gastrointestinal and respiratory tract infections were the most commonly infected sites in children. In a study at the Children's Hospital of Buffalo, the overall rate of nosocomial infections was 4.1% and the pediatric intensive care unit (PICU) specific rate was 11% (2). In a study at the University of Virginia Hospital, ward and intensive care unit nosocomial infection rates were compared. During this 1-year prospective study, 4.7% of medical and surgical patients on the wards developed a hospital-acquired infection, compared with 13.7% of patients admitted to the PICU. Of patients admitted to the PICU 1.1% developed a bloodstream infection, 2.9%

developed pneumonia, 2% developed a urinary tract infection and 1.4% developed a postoperative wound infection. All site specific rates for critical care patients were significantly greater than ward site-specific rates (Table 24.1) (3).

ANTIBIOTIC-RELATED COLONIZATION AND INFECTION

Patients admitted to critical care settings are known to become rapidly colonized on the skin, in the nasopharynx, and in the gastrointestinal tract with nosocomial bacterial flora, which is very different from organisms routinely colonizing normal hosts (4–8). Critical care patients and, specifically, those with longer hospital stays have a significant risk of becoming infected with these hospital-acquired organisms.

Skin colonization may change to more antibiotic-resistant strains of coagulase-negative staphylococci and increased numbers of *Staphylococcus aureus* with varying rates of methicillin-resistant strains (9–13). Nasopharyngeal colonization, particularly in the intubated, ventilated patient and the patient receiving antibiotics, rapidly switches from the usual mixed oropharyngeal flora to the more unusual Gram-negative rods, specifically *Klebsiella-Serratia-Enterobacter* spp., *Pseudomonas* spp. (14-18), and *Candida* spp. Gastrointestinal flora changes with increasing numbers of unusual organisms and, specifically, more resistant Gram-negative enteric bacilli and *Candida* spp. (5).

These changes reflect rapid colonization with the critical care microflora, which is transmitted to the patients by health care providers and monitoring and support equipment. Most patients in critical care units receive multiple antibiotics during their stay. This further destroys the pa-

Table 24.1.
Hospital-Acquired Infection Rates for Pediatric Ward vs. ICU Patients

Site of Infection	Ward Admissions (n = 2640)		ICU Admissions (n = 444)		P
	No. of Infections	Infection Rate[a]	No. of Infections	Infection Rate[a]	
Bloodstream	9	0.4	5	1.1	0.05[b]
Lung	22	0.9	13	2.9	<0.005[c]
Urinary tract	19	0.8	9	2.0	0.02[b]
Postoperative wound	11	0.5	6	1.4	0.03[b]
Other	63	2.6	28	6.3	<0.005[c]
Total	124	4.7	61	13.7	<0.005[c]

[a]Number of infections per 100 admissions.
[b]Fisher's exact test.
[c]Chi-Square.

tient's own normal flora and promotes colonization with unusual and resistant bacteria.

When infection is presumed or diagnosed in critical care patients, it is imperative that empiric therapy be initiated, which is effective against these more unusual and antibiotic-resistant hospital-acquired bacterial strains.

DEVICE AND PROCEDURE-RELATED INFECTION

Invasive Vascular Lines

Invasive vascular access lines, specifically intravenous, arterial, pulmonary artery, and central venous catheters, are widely used in the critical care setting and contribute significantly to the risk of bacteremia in these patients (19). With the widespread use of these monitoring and supportive vascular lines, there has been a marked increase in the incidence of coagulase-negative staphylococci and *Staphylococcus aureus* bloodstream infections in critical care patients. Presumably, these infections result from cannula colonization and infection with skin pathogens. Specific guidelines for insertion, care, and duration of cannulation at these different sites are addressed in Chapter 8. It should be noted that daily recordings of all indwelling vascular lines should be made with careful records maintained on their duration of use. Daily examination of the insertion site should be made to optimize early removal when necessary and to minimize the risk of systemic infection. Invasive vascular lines should be discontinued as soon as possible and if not needed, should not be "kept open" or "heparin locked" for later use.

Pressure-Monitoring Transducers

In-line pressure transducers, disposable and reusable, have been reported as sources of nosocomial infection (20-23). Scrupulous disinfection technique is required between patients and at set intervals in the patient requiring long-term use to prevent a reservoir of nosocomial pathogens on the transducer head, which is repeatedly handled by nurses and cardiovascular technicians and subsequently transmitted to the patient side of the transducing membrane.

Urinary Tract Catheters

Urinary catheters are another real source of nosocomial morbidity in critical care children, although less so than in adult patients where the reported risks are up to 50% by day 8 of urinary catheterization (24). Specific guidelines for catheter care and monitoring for infection are outlined in Chapter 3.

Intracranial Pressure Monitors

Infection associated with intracranial pressure (ICP) monitoring is unusual. Infection appears to be associated with the insertion of the catheter and is thus more common early in the monitoring period. The overall number of infections in one study of 65 children and 72 ICP monitors was 9 infections or a risk of 1.5 infections per 100 ICP monitor days (25).

Respiratory Therapy Equipment

Ventilators, inhalation equipment, and nebulizers have been a noted source of nosocomial pneumonia in sporadic and epidemic circumstances (26,27). The critical care patient requiring ventilatory assistance has a 15-20% risk of acquiring a nosocomial pneumonia (28-32) and, if intubated nasally, an increased but un-determined risk of acquiring nosocomial sinu-sitis (33-38). Specific guidelines for the diagnosis, prevention, and treatment of ventilator-associ-ated pneumonia are discussed in Chapter 2. Nosocomial sinusitis is a reported infectious complication of nasotracheal intubation, but the incidence of this complication is not known. Sinus roentgenograms should be performed to look for this infectious complication in patients with unexplained fever and prolonged nasotra-cheal intubation. Etiologic diagnosis should be attempted by needle aspiration of the usually involved maxillary sinus. Therapy involves re-moval of the nasotracheal tube, antibiotics, de-congestants, and possibly surgical drainage.

Another infectious risk in the ventilated pa-tient is corneal ulceration, usually with Gram-negative bacilli caused by secretions suctioned from the endotracheal or nasotracheal tube splat-tering and infecting an eye that is compromised by incomplete closure and decreased host clean-sing mechanisms in the patient with a depressed level of consciousness (39,40). Specific mea-sures to reduce the risk of corneal ulceration and infection secondary to respiratory suctioning are (a) suctioning should never be performed resting the hand on the patient's face; (b) in a patient with a depressed level of consciousness, careful eye care should be maintained with the use of artificial tears and careful lid closure; and (c) routine opthalmologic examinations should be performed so that progressive infection does not go undetected and untreated.

PREVENTION OF INFECTION

Space

The location and design of a pediatric intensive care unit is an important part of infection control success. Ideally, each patient is physically sep-arated from other patients, with sinks available between patients to remind others about and to facilitate handwashing between contact with pa-tients. Experts have suggested 300–400 square feet of patient-care space per patient and addi-tional space for storage, utility, and ancillary services. Since the ideal is rarely available, ad-equate floor space between patients and ade-quate storage areas for equipment, supplies, and medication separate from contaminated utility space is required to insure an orderly unit with uncluttered counters and patient-care areas that can be readily cleaned.

Isolation

Cohort isolation may be required during epi-demic periods when infected or colonized staff can care for infected or colonized patients. Spo-radic cases of specific infections should be iso-lated according to the routine guidelines provided in Chapter 25.

Certain specific isolation issues are important in the PICU setting because of the many dif-ferent kinds of patients cared for in the same location and by the same staffs. Neonates are often admitted to the PICU following corrective surgeries or when they are readmitted following discharge from a neonatal unit, particularly when an infectious etiology for their disease is under consideration. They remain immune-immature and require stringent protection from the herpes simplex virus, varicella-zoster virus, mycobac-teria tuberculosis, respiratory syncytial virus—to mention only some of the pathogens that cause devastating neonatal infection.

Pulmonary patients, cardiac patients, im-muno-compromised patients and, specifically, those with cyanotic disease or pulmonary artery hypertension should be very carefully admitted during the winter months to avoid any exposure to staff or other patients infected with the re-spiratory syncytial virus or any other viral pul-monary pathogens. Superimposed infection with these pathogens carries with it a mortality in excess of 40% in these patients (41). If more than one patient is admitted with this diagnosis proven by culture or fluorescent antibody screen, it is acceptable to cohort patients, preferably with cohorted staff (see Chapter 15).

Handwashing

Handwashing remains the most important method of interrupting the transmission of hospital path-ogens between patients and between staff and patients (41,42). A recent study in the PICU at the University of Virginia documented a 70% failure rate of hospital personnel to wash their hands after contact with patients or direct pa-tient-care equipment (43). Adequate and con-venient handwashing facilities should be available (32), and strict handwashing policies should be established and enforced for all personnel en-tering the units.

Hands are colonized with both a permanent and a transient flora (44). The permanent flora is generally not removed with routine hand-washing methods, but these organisms can be reduced in number and inactivated by some antibacterial soaps. By definition, transient flora is more easily removed by routine soap and water wash. In an attempt to reduce the resident flora and remove the transient flora, an iodophor or antiseptic soap should be used (45,46). Personnel with hand dermatitis usually have an increased number of bacteria with a potential for more pathogenic organisms on their hands. They should be treated, required to use gloves, and possibly be removed from clinical patient care until their dermatitis is improved.

Gown Use

Routine gown use is traditional, but of unproven advantage in interrupting transmission of microorganisms in the critical care setting. Nursery studies to date that address this issue have shown that there is delay in the colonization of the umbilical cord when gowns are used (47), but multiple other studies (48–54) show no difference in the incidence of staphylococcal colonization or in the incidence of infections in settings of gown use compared with no gown use. A recent study in a pediatric intensive care unit showed no change in handwashing rates, infection, or intravascular catheter colonization rates when gowns were employed (55). Gowns should be worn for specific isolation of infected patients but are not indicated for routine care.

Environmental Cultures

Routine environmental culturing for bacterial contamination is indicated, but only in the setting of investigation for a particular reservoir. Verification of sterile procedure in formula preparation and equipment maintenance may mandate specific routine surveillance culturing.

Traffic

Traffic through the PICU should be limited to essential staff and family members. Congested areas, such as the nurses' station, should be separated from patient care and storage space.

Housekeeping

Routine housekeeping of the PICU is difficult in times of high census, but it should remain a priority. Daily wet mopping of the floor and daily dusting of the shelves, light fixtures, ventilation ducts, etc. with a damp cloth should be performed. Every 1–2 months, the walls should be scrubbed with a phenolic or quaternary ammonium germicide. Any cleaning that has the potential of dispersing dust should not be done when patients with open wounds are in the room. The nursing station, medication area, phones, computers, and charts should be wiped with an antiseptic cleaning solution at least daily.

Visitation Policies

Visiting policies for infection control purposes should require that all visitors be well and not recently exposed to highly communicable infectious diseases (specifically chickenpox). It should be required that all family be verbally screened by a member of the health care team prior to their entry into the unit. Specific recommendations for visitation and screening of visitors are outlined in Chapter 27.

REFERENCES

1. Centers for Disease Control: National Nosocomial Infections Study Report, Annual Summary 1978. March 1981.
2. Welliver RC, McLaughlin S: Unique epidemiology of nosocomial infection in a children's hospital. *Am J Dis Child* 138:131–135, 1984
3. Donowitz LG: High risk of nosocomial infection in the pediatric critical care patient. *Crit Care Med* 14:26–28, 1986.
4. Eickhoff TC: Nosocomial infections due to Klebsiella pneumoniae: Mechanisms of intra-hospital spread. In *Proceedings of the International Conference on Nosocomial Infections*. Chicago, American Hospital Association, 1971, pp 117–122.
5. Selden R, Lee S, Wang WL, Bennett JV, Eickhoff TC: Nosocomial Klebsiella infections: intestinal colonization as a reservoir. *Ann Intern Med* 74:657–664, 1971.
6. Pollack M, Charache P, Nieman RE, Jett MP, Reimhardt JA, Hardy PH Jr: Factors influencing colonization and antibiotic-resistance patterns of gram-negative bacteria in hospital patients. *Lancet* ii:688–671, 1972.
7. Stamm WE: Nosocomial infections: etiologic changes, therapeutic challenges. *Hosp Pract* 16:75–88, 1981.
8. Goldmann DA, Leclair J, Macone A: Bacterial colonization of neonates admitted to an intensive care environment. *J Pediatr* 93:288–293, 1978.
9. Ponce de Leon S, Wenzel RP: Hospital-acquired bloodstream infections with *Staphylococcus epidermidis*. Review of 100 cases. *Am J Med* 77:639–644, 1984.
10. Kirchhoff LV, Sheagren JN: Epidemiology and clinical significance of blood cultures positive for coagulase-negative staphylococcus. *Infect Control* 6:479–486, 1985.
11. Wenzel RP: Methicillin resistant *S. aureus* and *S. epidermidis* strains: modern hospital pathogens. *Infect Control* 7:118–119, 1986.
12. Jarvis WR, Thornsberry C, Boyce J, Huges JM: Methicillin resistant *Staphylococcus aureus* at children's hospitals in the United States. *Pediatr Infect Dis* 4:651–655, 1985.
13. Thompson RL, Cabezudo I, Wenzel RP: Epidemiology of nosocomial infections caused by methicillin-resistant *Staphylococcus aureus*. *Ann Intern Med* 97:309–317, 1982.
14. Johanson WG, Pierce AK, Sanford JP: Changing pharyngeal bacterial flora of hospitalized patients. Emergence of gram-negative bacilli. *N Engl J Med* 281:1137–1140, 1969.

15. Sanderson PJ: The sources of pneumonia in ITU patients. *Infect Control* 7:104–106, 1986.
16. Sottile FD, Marrie TJ, Prough DS, Hobgood CD, Gower DJ, Webb LX, Costerton JW, Gristina AG: Nosocomial pulmonary infection: possible etiologic significance of bacterial adhesion to endotracheal tubes. *Crit Care Med* 14:265–270, 1986.
17. Baigelman W, Bellin S, Cupples LA, Berenberg MJ: Bacteriologic assessment of the lower respiratory tract in intubated patients. *Crit Care Med* 14:864–868, 1986.
18. Johanson WG Jr, Pierce AK, Sanford JP, Thomas GD: Nosocomial respiratory infections with gram negative bacilli. The significance of colonization of the respiratory tract. *Ann Intern Med* 77:701–706, 1972.
19. Sattler FR, Foderaro JB, Aber RC: *Staphylococcus epidermidis* bacteremia associated with vascular catheters: an important cause of febrile morbidity in hospitalized patients. *Infect Control* 5:279–283, 1984.
20. Donowitz LG, Marsik FJ, Hoyt JW, Wenzel RP: Serratia marcescens bacteremia from contaminated pressure transducers. *JAMA* 242:1749–1751, 1979.
21. Luskin RL, Weinstein RA, Nathan C, Chamberlin WH, Kabins SA: Extended use of disposable pressure transducers. A bacteriologic evaluation. *JAMA* 255:916–920, 1986.
22. Weinstein RA, Stamm WE, Kramer L, Corey L: Pressure monitoring devices. Overlooked source of nosocomial infection. *JAMA* 236:936–938, 1976.
23. Buxton AE, Anderson RL, Klimek J, Quintiliani R: Failure of disposable domes to prevent septicemia acquired from contaminated pressure transducers. *Chest* 74:508–513, 1978.
24. Garibaldi RA, Burke JP, Dickman ML, Smith CB: Factors predisposing to bacteriuria during indwelling urethral catheterization. *N Engl J Med* 291:215–219, 1974.
25. Kanter RK, Weiner LB, Patti AM, Robson LK: Infectious complications and duration of intracranial pressure monitoring. *Crit Care Med* 13:837–839, 1985.
26. Pierce AK, Sanford JP, Thomas GD, Leonard JS: Long-term evaluation of decontamination of inhalation-therapy equipment and the occurrence of necrotizing pneumonia. *N Engl J Med* 282:528–531, 1970.
27. Grieble HG, Colton FR, Bird TJ, Toigo A, Griffith LG: Fine-particle humidifiers. Source of *Pseudomonas aeruginosa* infections in a respiratory-disease unit. *N Engl J Med* 282: 531–535, 1970.
28. Brook I: Bacterial colonization, tracheobronchitis and pneumonia following tracheostomy and long-term intubation in pediatric patients. *Chest* 76:420–424, 1979.
29. Tobin MJ, Grenvik A: Nosocomial lung infection and its diagnosis. *Crit Care Med* 12:191–199, 1984.
30. Stevens RM, Teres D, Skillman JJ, Feingold DS: Pneumonia in an intensive care unit. A 30-month experience. *Arch Intern Med* 134:106–111, 1974.
31. Garibaldi RA, Britt MR, Coleman ML, Reading JC, Pace NL: Risk factors for postoperative pneumonia. *Am J Med* 70:677–680, 1981.
32. Hemming VG, Overall JC Jr, Britt MR: Nosocomial infections in a newborn intensive care unit. Results of forty-one months of surveillance. *N Engl J Med* 294:1310–1316, 1976.
33. Deutschman CS, Wilton P, Sinow J, Dibbell D Jr, Konstantinides FN, Cerra FB: Paranasal sinusitis associated with nasotracheal intubation: a frequently unrecognized and treatable source of sepsis. *Crit Care Med* 14:111–114, 1986.
34. Knodel AR, Beekman JF: Unexplained fevers in patients with nasotracheal intubation. *JAMA* 248:868–870, 1982.
35. Caplan ES, Hoyt NJ: Nosocomial sinusitis. *JAMA* 247: 639–641, 1982.
36. Gallagher TJ, Civetta JM: Acute maxillary sinusitis complicating nasotracheal intubation: a case report. *Anesth Analg* 55:885–886, 1976.
37. Arens JF, LeJeune FE Jr, Webre DR: Maxillary sinusitis, a complication of nasotracheal intubation. *Anesthesiology* 40: 415–416, 1974.
38. Pope TL Jr, Stelling CB, Leitner YB: Maxillary sinusitis after nasotracheal intubation. *South Med J* 74:610–612, 1981.
39. Hilton E, Adams AA, Uliss A, Lesser ML, Samuels S, Lowy FD: Nosocomial bacterial eye infections in intensive care units. *Lancet* 1:1318–1320, 1983.
40. Ommeslag D, Colardyn F, DeLaey J-J: Eye infections caused by respiratory pathogens in mechanically ventilated patients. *Crit Care Med* 15:80–81, 1987.
41. Steere AC, Mallison GF: Handwashing practices for the prevention of nosocomial infections. *Ann Intern Med* 83:683–690, 1975.
42. Mortimer EA Jr, Lipsitz PJ, Wolinsky E, Gonzaga AJ, Rammelkamp CH Jr: Transmission of staphylococci between newborns. Importance of the hands to personnel. *Am J Dis Child* 104: 289–295, 1962.
43. Donowitz LG: Handwashing patterns in a pediatric intensive care unit. *Am J Dis Child* 141:683–685, 1987.
44. Price PB: The bacteriology of normal skin; a new quantitative test applied to a study of the bacterial flora and the disinfectant action of mechanical cleansing. *J Infect Dis* 63:301–318, 1938.
45. Brawley RL, Cabezudo I, Guenthner SH, Hendley JO, Wenzel RP: Evaluation of handwash agents using brief contact time. Program and Abstracts of the 24th Interscience Conference on Antimicrobial Agents and Chemotherapy, 1984, p 184.
46. Maki D, McCormick R, Alvarado C, Hassemer C: Clinical evaluation of the degerming efficacy of seven agents for handwashing in hospitals. Program and Abstracts of the 24th Interscience Conference on Antimicrobial Agents and Chemotherapy, 1984, p 184.
47. Renaud MT: Effects of discontinuing cover gowns on a postpartal ward upon cord colonization of the newborn. *J Obstet Gynecol Neonatal Nurs* 12:399–401, 1983.
48. Forfar JO, MacCabe AF: Masking and gowning in nurseries for the newborn infant. Effect on staphylococcal carriage and infection. *Br Med J* 1:76–79, 1958.
49. Nauseef WM, Maki DG: A study of the value of simple protective isolation in patients with granulocytopenia. *N Engl J Med* 304:448–453, 1981.
50. Moylan JA, Kennedy BV: The importance of gown and drape barriers in the prevention of wound infection. *Surg Gynecol Obstet* 151:465–470, 1980.
51. Murphy D, Todd JK, Chao RK, Orr I, McIntosh K: The use of gowns and masks to control respiratory illness in pediatric hospital personnel. *J Pediatr* 99:746–750, 1981.
52. Agbayani M, Rosenfeld W, Evans H, Salazar D, Jhaveri R, Braun J: Evaluation of modified gowning procedures in a neonatal intensive care unit. *Am J Dis Child* 135:650–652, 1981.
53. Evans HE, Akpata SO, Baki A, Behrman RE: Bacteriologic and clinical evaluation of gowning in a premature nursery. *J Pediatr* 78:883–886, 1971.
54. Williams CP, Oliver TK Jr: Nursery routines and staphylococcal colonization of the newborn. *Pediatrics* 44: 640–646, 1969.
55. Donowitz, LG: Failure of the overgown to prevent nosocomial infection in a pediatric intensive care unit. *Pediatrics* 77:35–38, 1986.

4
PERSONNEL AND POLICIES

25

Isolation Guidelines

Sandra M. Landry, R.N., M.S., C.I.C.

INTRODUCTION

"It may seem a strange principle to enunciate as the very first requirement in a hospital that it should do the sick no harm."

Florence Nightingale

The concept of isolation for the control of disease in man has existed since man inhabited the earth. Some early societies avoided the sick, as they were thought to be possessed by dangerous or evil spirits; while others thought that diseases were punishments for sins. A great deal of emphasis was also placed upon the environmental causes of disease, such as wind, rain, and floods, as well as celestial bodies (1-2).

Over the years, as the knowledge of epidemiology of diseases has increased, theories of isolation have progressed. Patients are no longer segregated in contagious disease hospitals and wards. Today, patients needing isolation are housed in the general hospital on the ward either in a specially designed single isolation room or in a regular, single, or multiple-patient room. The disease is isolated based on the transmissibility of the infectious agent and the susceptibility of the host.

FACTORS INFLUENCING SPREAD OF INFECTION

The three essential factors influencing the spread of infection are the source or reservoir of the infectious agent, the mode of transmission of the agent, and the susceptibility of the host.

Source of Infection

The source or reservoir of the infectious agent in the hospital may be patients, health care personnel, or visitors, whether they have active disease, are incubating disease, or are asymptomatic carriers of disease. Inanimate objects in the hospital environment, such as soiled bed linens, bedpans, and contaminated equipment, are excellent sources of potentially pathogenic organisms.

Transmission

The mode of transmission of the infectious agent within the hospital environment can be by four routes: contact, air, vehicle, or vector.

Contact transmission may be direct person-to-person spread of infection; for example, *S. aureus* infections; indirect spread of infections via a contaminated inanimate object; for example, hepatitis B via a contaminated needle; or spread through infectious droplets that are coughed or sneezed within 3 feet of the susceptible host, such as streptococcal pharyngitis.

The transmission of airborne infectious agents occurs via droplet nuclei, which are particles that remain suspended in the air for long periods of time, or resuspended contaminated dust. The susceptible host subsequently inhales the infectious agent. Such diseases as varicella, measles, and *Mycobacterium tuberculosis* may be spread by the airborne route.

Contaminated food, water, and drugs serve as common vehicle for the transmission of an infectious agent to the susceptible host. Diseases that may be spread by a common vehicle include salmonellosis (food), shigellosis (water), or hepatitis B (blood).

Transmission of an infectious agent in the hospital by a vector is not common in the United States, but in South America, mosquito-transmitted malaria is prevalent.

Many infectious agents may be transmitted by more than one route, such as varicella, which may be spread by contact or airborne transmission.

Susceptible Host

Significant factors occurring in the host may lower the body's resistance to infectious agents. The very young or the very old; patients with chronic debilitating disease, such as certain types of cancer, leukemia, diabetes mellitus, renal disease; or patients treated with certain drugs, such as corticosteriods, immunosuppressive agents, or continuous use of antibiotics may be more susceptible to infection. Accidental or surgical trauma, radiation, and many diagnostic procedures, such as aspiration of fluid or catheterization, are associated with decreased resistance. Other host factors, such as nutritional status, alcoholism, and hypogammaglobulinemia, also influence susceptibility.

ISOLATION PRECAUTIONS FOR PEDIATRICS

The Centers for Disease Control (CDC) in conjunction with a consultative group of experts have developed two systems of isolation guidelines: category-specific and disease-specific. Category-specific isolation guidelines identify which secretions, excretions, discharges, body fluids, and tissues are infective or might be infective. The isolation precaution is selected based on the infective material. An alternative to category-specific isolation is disease-specific isolation, which allows individualization of isolation measures for the disease in question. This complex system is more difficult for hospital personnel to implement. Both systems of isolation are based on diagnosis of the patient. Until recently, little attention was given to the patient with an unknown infectious process. Following the report of three health care workers who seroconverted following nonparenteral exposure to human immunodeficiency virus–infected blood, the CDC recommends that health care workers consider *all* patients as potentially infectious. When the possibility for exposure to blood and other body fluid exists, vigorous adherence to infection control precautions to minimize the risk of exposure should be followed. The anticipated exposure may require gloves alone, or may require gown, mask, and eye coverings when performing procedures involving more extensive contact with blood or potentially infective body fluids. The use of universal blood and body fluid precautions could eliminate the need for the isolation category blood and body fluid precautions previously recommended by the CDC since *all* patients are now treated as potentially infectious (3). However, it seems prudent to continue to inform employees of patients with known blood-transmitted diseases via standard isolation recommendations, thus effecting maximal safeguards in the workplace. An alternative approach to universal precautions, body substance isolation, has been proposed by Lynch and colleagues. This system focuses on isolating body substances from the hands of personnel, which eliminates the need for the traditional practices of isolation (4).

Hospitals are encouraged by the CDC to tailor the *Guidelines For Isolation Precautions in Hospitals* to meet their own needs (5). The following recommendations (Tables 25.1 and 25.2) are category-specific and are simple and generally appropriate for each disease (5–8); they are in accordance with the most recent guidelines of the Centers for Disease Control and the American Academy of Pediatrics.

GENERAL CONSIDERATIONS FOR ISOLATION

Isolation precautions should be initiated by the medical or nursing staff, including the Infection Control Practitioner when a patient is suspected or diagnosed of having an infectious process. The necessary precautions must be followed until the infectious process has subsided or is ruled out. All hospital personnel are responsible for complying with isolation precautions. The appropriate precautions should be explained to the patient, family, and visitors.

Patients with infections should be assigned to a room according to the isolation specification. An infected patient should not be assigned to a room with a patient who is at increased risk for developing an infection. Room assignments for infants and children may have to be modified to accommodate special circumstances, particularly isolation categories that require a private room. A forced air incubator or sufficient space (4–6 feet) between infant stations may be used when a private room is not available, except when airborne transmission of disease is suspected; thus, a private room is mandated (6). Cohorting of patients with the same clinical syndrome may be necessary during an outbreak situation.

Table 25.1
Categories of Isolation

Type of Isolation/Precaution	Private Room	Gown	Gloves	Mask	Negative Pressure Ventilation
Strict	Yes	Yes	Yes	Yes	Yes
Contact	Yes	Indicated if soiling is likely	Indicated for touching infective material	Indicated for those who come close to patient	No
Respiratory	Yes	No	No	Indicated for those who come close to patient	No
Acid-Fast Bacilli (AFB)	Yes	No	No	Only when patient is coughing and does not reliably cover mouth	Yes
Enteric	Indicated if patient hygiene is poor. May share room with patient infected with same organism.	Indicated if soiling is likely	Indicated for touching infective material	No	No
Drainage/ Secretion	No	Indicated if soiling is likely	Indicated for touching infective material	No	No
(Universal) Blood/Body Fluid	Indicated if patient hygiene is poor. May share room with patient infected with same organism.	Indicated if soiling is likely	Indicated for touching infective material	No	No

The isolation unit should include the patient, the physical area of the patient or patient room, and all equipment and furniture (6).

Preferably, susceptible personnel should not be assigned to care for a patient with a communicable disease.

Isolation precautions should be documented on the patient chart, patient door and/or above patient bed, Kardex, nursing notes, nursing care plan, patient requisitions, and biological specimens of the isolated patient.

Needs of the patient should be anticipated whenever possible, and all equipment should be assigned to the room for the duration of isolation (i.e., tourniquet, sphygmomanometer and stethoscope). Whenever possible, disposable patient care equipment should be considered for use. Reusable articles that are used should be considered contaminated and should be properly decontaminated and reprocessed after use.

An infant or child on isolation should not share toys with other children (5).

Isolation rooms assigned to patients with contagious airborne infections should be kept at negative pressure in relation to the anteroom or hallway. Negative pressure can be obtained by supplying less air to the area than is removed by the ventilation system. An inexpensive exhaust fan (12-inch/1550 rpm) in the window of a private room can be used to create negative pressure for strict, respiratory or acid-fast bacilli isolation. (9).

Table 25.2.
Category—Specific Isolation Precautions for Hospitalized Children

Disease	Infective Material	Incubation Period	Isolation Category	Comments[a]
Abscess, etiology unknown				
Draining, major	Pus		Contact	Not adequately contained in dressing.
Draining, minor	Pus		Drainage/secretion	Contained in dressing.
Acquired Immuno-deficiency Syndrome (AIDS)	Blood, semen, and possibly other body secretions	Unknown	Blood/body Fluid	Avoid needlestick injury; the presence of opportunistic infections may require additional isolation precautions.
Actinomycosis all lesions			None	Clinical disease endogenous.
Adenoviral Infections		2–4 days		During epidemics, infected patients may be cohorted in the same room.
Respiratory	Respiratory secretions and feces		Contact	
Conjunctivitis	Purulent exudate		Drainage/secretion	
Gastroenteritis	Feces		Enteric	
Amebiasis		Variable. Few days to months to years. Commonly 2–4 weeks		
Dysentery	Feces		Enteric	
Liver abscess			None	
Anthrax		1–7 days, usually		Steam-sterilize or burn contaminated dressings or bedclothes to destroy spores.
Cutaneous	Pus			
Inhalation	Respiratory secretions	2–5 days	Drainage/secretion Drainage/secretion	
Arthropodborne				
Viral encephalitis			None	Transmitted by the bite of infective mosquito; no evidence of transmission person to person.
Viral fevers (Dengue fever, yellow fever, Colorado tick fever)	Blood		Blood/body Fluid	Not directly transmitted person to person.
Ascariasis Roundworm	Parasite		None	
Aspergillosis	Fungus		None	Not directly transmitted person to person.
Babesiosis	Blood	1–12 months	None	Person to person transmission unlikely, except by blood transfusion.
Balantidiasis	Protozoan		None	

[a]Isolate for duration of illness, unless specific directions given.

Table 25.2. cont.

Disease	Infective Material	Incubation Period	Isolation Category	Comments[a]
Blastomycosis (cutaneous or pulmonary)	Fungus		None	Not directly transmitted person-to-person.
Borrelia (relapsing fever)	Louse	5–11 days	Blood/body Fluid	Not directly transmitted person-to-person. Treat louse infestation if present.
Botulism, Infant			None	Possible sources of botulinal spores include foods and dust.
Bronchiolitis, etiology unknown	Respiratory secretions	Variable, depending on causative etiology	Contact	Respiratory syncytial virus, parainfluenza viruses, adenoviruses, and influenza viruses have been associated with this syndrome.
Campylobacter Enteritis	Feces	1–10 days	Enteric	
Candidiasis (thrush)			None	
Cat scratch fever			None	
Chickenpox (varicella)	Respiratory secretions and lesion secretions	8–21 days; Varicella-zoster Immune globulin (VZIG) may prolong incubation up to 28 days	Strict	Neonates born to mothers with active lesions should be placed in strict isolation at birth. Hospitalized exposed susceptible patients should be isolated 10–21 days following exposure. Exposed susceptible hospital personnel should not have patient contact from days 10–21 following exposure.
Chlamydial Infections:		5–12 days or longer		
Conjunctivitis	Purulent exudate		Drainage/secretion	
Genital	Genital discharge		Drainage/secretion	
Respiratory	Respiratory secretions		Drainage/secretion	
Cholera	Feces	A few hours to 5 days, usually 1-3 days	Enteric	
Clostridium perfringens Food poisoning		8–24 hours, usually 8–12 hours	None	

[a]Isolate for duration of illness, unless specific directions given.

Table 25.2. cont.

Disease	Infective Material	Incubation Period	Isolation Category	Comments[a]
Gas gangrene	Pus	6 hours– 6 weeks; usually 1–5 days.	Drainage/secretion	
Clostridium difficile Pseudo-membranous colitis	Feces	Unknown	Enteric	
Coccidioidomycosis (valley fever)			None	Not directly transmitted from person to person.
Colorado Tick Fever			None	
Common Cold			None	Most commonly caused by rhinovirus. Good handwashing is necessary to prevent nosocomial spread. Precautions may be indicated for most likely etiologic agent, such as RSV and parainfluenza virus.
Conjunctivitis (pink eye) Bacterial	Purulent exudate	24 to 72 hours	Drainage/secretion	
Chlamydia		5–12 days or longer	Drainage/secretion	Isolate for 48 hours of specific treatment
Gonococcal		1–5 days	Contact	Isolate for 24 hours of specific treatment.
Viral and etiology un-known		12 hours –3 days	Drainage/secretion	A private room may be indicated if patient hygiene is poor.
Coronavirus, Respiratory Infection	Respiratory secretions	1–10 days; usually 2–4 days.	Contact	
Coxsackievirus diseases	Feces and respiratory secretions	3–5 days	Enteric	Isolate for 7 days after onset.
Croup	Respiratory secretions	Few days –1 week	Contact	
Cryptococcosis			None	
Cryptosporidosis	Feces	Unknown	Enteric	
Cutaneous larvae migrans (creeping eruptions)			None	Infective larvae of cat or dog hookworms are cause of disease.

[a]Isolate for duration of illness, unless specific directions given.

Table 25.2. cont.

Disease	Infective Material	Incubation Period	Isolation Category	Comments[a]
Cytomegalovirus Infections	Urine and respiratory secretions possible		None	Handwashing after exposure to secretions should prevent spread of infection. Pregnant personnel who may be in contact with an infected patient may need counseling.
Dengue Fever			Blood/body Fluid	(See arthropodborne viral fevers)
Diarrhea, infective etiology suspected	Feces	Depends on cause	Enteric	
Campylobacter	Feces	1–10 days	Enteric	
C. difficile	Feces	Unknown	Enteric	
E. coli	Feces	12–72 hours	Enteric	
Diphtheria Cutaneous	Lesion secretions	2–5 days, occasionally longer	Contact	Isolate until 2 cultures form skin lesions are negative, taken at least 24 hours apart after cessation of antibiotics.
Pharyngeal	Repiratory secretions		Strict	Maintain isolation until 2 cultures from both nose and throat are negative, taken 24 hours apart after cessation of antibiotics.
Echovirus	Feces and respiratory secretions		Enteric	Isolate for 7 days after onset.
Eczema vaccinatum (vaccinia)	Lesion secretions		Contact	
Encephalitis; etiology unknown, but infectious agent suspected	Feces	Variable, depending on etiologic agent	Enteric	Precautions for enteroviruses are generally indicated until a definitive diagnosis can be made.
Enterobiasis (pinworms)	None			
Enterovirus (nonpolio) infections (coxsackieviruses, echoviruses and enteroviruses)	Feces and respiratory secretions	3–6 days	Enteric	Isolate for 7 days after onset.
Epiglottis, due to *Haemophilus influenzae*	Respiratory	Probably less than 10 days	Respiratory	Isolate for 24 hours of specific treatment.

[a]Isolate for duration of illness, unless specific directions given.

Table 25.2. cont.

Disease	Infective Material	Incubation Period	Isolation Category	Comments[a]
Epstein-Barr virus infection, including mononucleosis		None		
Erythema Infectiosum, (fifth disease)	Respiratory secretions	4–14 days; usually 12–14 days	Respiratory	Isolate for 7 days after onset.
Fever of unknown origin (FUO)				If patient has signs and symptoms compatible with a disease that requires isolation precautions.
Food Poisoning				
Botulism			None	
Clostridium perfringens			None	
Salmonellosis	Feces	6–72 hours, usually less than 24 hours	Enteric	
Staphylococcal			None	
Furunculosis Staphylococcal	Pus		Drainage/secretion	During a nursery outbreak, cohorting of ill and colonized infants and use of gowns and gloves are recommended
Gangrene, due to any bacteria	Pus	Variable, depends on etiologic agent	Drainage/secretion	
Gastroenteritis				
Campylobacter species	Feces	1–7 days or longer	Enteric	
Clostridium difficile	Feces	Unknown	Enteric	
Cryptosporidium species	Feces	Not precisely known probably 10 days	Enteric	
E. coli (pathogenic)	Feces	2–6 hours	Enteric	
Giardia lamblia	Feces	5–25 days or longer	Enteric	
Norwalk agent	Feces	24–48 hours	Enteric	
Rotavirus	Feces	Approximately 48 hours	Enteric	
Salmonella species	Feces	6–72 hours	Enteric	
Shigella species	Feces	1–7 days	Enteric	
Unknown etiology	Feces	Vary with specific agent	Enteric	
Vibrio parahaemolyticus	Feces	5–29 hours	Enteric	
Viral	Feces	Vary with specific agent	Enteric	
Yersinia Enterocolitica	Feces	1–3 weeks	Enteric	

[a]Isolate for duration of illness, unless specific directions given.

Table 25.2. cont.

Disease	Infective Material	Incubation Period	Isolation Category	Comments[a]
German Measles (rubella)	Respiratory Secretions	14–21 days, usually 16–18 days	Contact	Isolate for 7 days after onset of rash. Infants with congenital rubella require isolation for 1 year, unless culture-negative after 3 months of age.
Giardiasis	Feces		Enteric	
Gonococcal Infections	Purulent exudate	2–7 days	Contact	Isolate for 24 hours of specific treatment.
Granulocytopenia			None	Good handwashing is important before taking care of patient.
Granuloma Inguinale (donovaniasis)	Drainage (possibly)		None	
Haemophilus influenzae infections	Respiratory secretions	Probably less than 10 days	Respiratory	Isolate for 24 hours of specific therapy.
Hand, foot, and mouth disease	Feces	Usually 3–5 days	Enteric	Isolate for 7 days after onset.
Hemorrhagic Fevers (lassa fever)	Blood, body fluids, and respiratory secretions	6–16 days	Strict	Contact State Health Department for advice regarding management of a suspected case.
Hepatitis A (infectious)	Feces	15–50 days, usually 25–30 days	Enteric	A private room is required for a patient who is not toilet trained, has diarrhea, or poor personal hygiene.
Hepatitis B (serum)	Blood and body fluids	50–180 days	Blood/body Fluid	Infants born to HbsAg-positive mothers should be placed on blood and body fluid precautions.
Hepatitis Delta Virus	Blood and body fluids	Not firmly established in humans but approximately 2–10 weeks in experimental animals	Blood/body Fluid	Occurs only with existing or simultaneous active hepatitis B infection.
Hepatitis, Non-A/ Non-B				No known serologic tests are available.
Epidemic or A-like	Feces	15–64 days	Enteric	
Non-B Transfusion or B-like	Blood and possibly other body fluids	2 weeks to 6 months, usually 6–9 weeks	Blood/body Fluid	

[a]Isolate for duration of illness, unless specific directions given.

Table 25.2. cont.

Disease	Infective Material	Incubation Period	Isolation Category	Comments[a]
Herpangina	Feces	3–6 days	Enteric	Isolate for 7 days after onset.
Herpes Simplex Encephalitis		2–12 days	None	
Mucocutaneous disseminated or severe	Lesion secretions		Contact	
Mucocutaneous, recurrent	Lesion secretions		Drainage/Secretion	Exposed lesions should be covered for day-care and school-age children infected as newborn infants or sexually abused with recurrences of genital HSV. Exclusion from day-care or school is not indicated for oral lesions.
Neonatal with infection			Contact	
Exposed			Contact	Includes infants born vaginally or by cesarean if membranes have been ruptured more than 4–6 hours. Initial symptoms may occur up to 1 month after birth.
Herpes Zoster (shingles)	Lesion secretions and possibly respiratory secretions			Persons who are susceptible to varicella (chickenpox) should ideally stay out of room. Persons who are not susceptible do not need to wear a mask. Roommates should not be susceptible to varicella (chickenpox).
Normal Patient Localized Disseminated Immunocompromised Patient Localized or Disseminated			Drainage/secretion Strict Strict	
Histoplasmosis			None	
Human Immunodeficiency Virus, confirmed positive (HIV)	Blood, semen, and possible other body secretions	Unknown	Blood/body Fluid	Avoid needlestick injury.
Impetigo	Lesion secretions	Approximately 10 days	Contact or drainage/secretion depending on the extent of the infection	Isolate for 24 hours of specific therapy.
Infectious Mononucleosis	Respiratory secretions		None	

[a]Isolate for duration of illness, unless specific directions given.

Table 25.2. cont.

Disease	Infective Material	Incubation Period	Isolation Category	Comments[a]
Influenza	Respiratory secretions	1–3 days	Contact	Viral shedding usually ceases within 7 days, but may be longer in children. During epidemics, patients with influenza may be cohorted.
Kawasaki Syndrome			None	
Keratoconjunctivitis, infective	Purulent exudate	Probably 5–12 days	Drainage/secretion	
Lassa Fever	Blood, body fluids, and respiratory secretions	6–16 days	Strict	Contact State Health Department for advice regarding management of suspected case.
Legionellosis (Legionnaire's disease)			None	
Leishmaniasis			None	
Leprosy			None	
Leptospirosis	Blood and urine 2–26 days, usually 7–13 days	Blood/body Fluid		
Lice (Pediculosis)	Infested area	Approximately 8–10 days after eggs hatch	Contact	Isolate for 24 hours after specific therapy. Mask unnecessary.
Listeriosis			None	
Lyme Disease			None	
Lymphocytic Choriomeningitis			None	
Malaria	Blood	Varies from 6–16 days depending on the *Plasmodium* species involved	Blood/body Fluid	Usually vectorborne transmission.
Measles (rubeola)	Respiratory secretions	6–21 days, usually 8–12 days	Repiratory	Persons who are susceptible to measles should ideally stay out of the room. Persons who are not susceptible do not need to wear a mask. Isolate for a minimum of 4 days after rash onset.
Melioidosis			None	
Meningitis Aseptic (nonbacterial or viral)	Feces	Vary with specific Infectious agent	Enteric	Isolate for 7 days after onset.

[a]Isolate for duration of illness, unless specific directions given.

Table 25.2. cont.

Disease	Infective Material	Incubation Period	Isolation Category	Comments[a]
Fungal			None	
Haemophilus influenzae	Respiratory secretions	Probably 2–4 days	Respiratory	Isolate for 24 hours of specific therapy.
Listeria monocytogenes			None	
Neisseria meningitidis	Respiratory secretions	1–10 days; usually 2–4 days	Respiratory	Isolate for 24 hours of specific therapy. Prompt evaluation and follow-up of exposed persons is necessary.
Pneumococcal			None	
Tuberculosis			None	If pulmonary tuberculosis present, AFB precautions are necessary.
Other diagnosed bacterial			None	
Meningococcal Pneumonia	Respiratory secretions		Respiratory	Isolate for 24 hours of specific therapy. Prompt evaluations and follow-up of exposed persons is necessary.
Meningococcemia (meningococcal species)	Respiratory secretions		Respiratory	Isolate for 24 hours of specific therapy. Prompt evaluation and follow-up of exposed persons is necessary.
Molluscon Contagiosum			None	
Mononucleosis			None	
Multiply resistant organisms, infection or colonization				Include Gram-negative bacilli resistant to all tested aminoglycosides, *S. aureus* resistant to methicillin, *Pneumoncoccus* resistant to penicillin, and *H. influenzae* resistant to ampicillin and chloramphenicol. Private room preferred. In outbreaks, cohorting of infected and colonized may be indicated.
Gastrointestinal	Feces		Enteric	
Respiratory	Respiratory secretions and possibly feces		Contact	
Skin, wound, or burn	Pus and possible feces		Contact	
Urinary	Urine		Contact	
Mumps	Respiratory secretions	12–25 days, usually 16–18 days	Respiratory	Isolate for 9 days after onset. Persons who are not susceptible do not need to wear a mask.
Mycoplasma pneumonia			None	
Necrotizing enterocolitis	Feces (possibly)		Enteric	Cohorting of ill infants is recommended.

[a]Isolate for duration of illness, unless specific directions given.

Table 25.2. cont.

Disease	Infective Material	Incubation Period	Isolation Category	Comments[a]
Nocardiosis			None	
Norwalk agent gastroenteritis	Feces	1–2 days	Enteric	
Orf			None	
Parainfluenza virus infection (respiratory)	Respiratory secretions	2–6 days	Contact	During epidemics, infected patients may be cohorted in the same room.
Pediculosis (head, body, and pubic louse)	Infested area	Approximately 8–10 days after eggs hatch	Contact	Isolate for 24 hours of specific therapy. Mask not necessary.
Pertussis (whooping cough)	Respiratory secretions	7–21 days, usually 7–10 days	Respiratory	Isolate for 7 days of specific therapy. If not treated, isolate for 3 weeks after onset of paroxysms. Prompt evaluation and follow-up of exposed persons is necessary.
Pharyngitis, infective	Respiratory secretions	Varies with specific etiologic agent	None	
Pinworm infection (Enterobiasis)			None	
Plague				Isolate for 3 days of specific therapy.
Bubonic	Pus	2–6 days	Drainage/secretion	
Pneumonic	Respiratory secretions	2–4 days	Strict	
Pleurodynia	Feces	3–6 days	Enteric	Isolate for 7 days of specific therapy. Frequently caused by enteroviruses.
Pnemococcal Infections			None	Respiratory secretions may be infective until 24 hours after start of specific therapy. Strict handwashing indicated following contact with secretions.
Pneumonia				
Bacteria not listed elsewhere			None	Respiratory secretions may be infective.
Chlamydia	Respiratory secretions		Drainage/secretion	
Etiology unknown				Precautions indicated for most likely etiology.
Fungal			None	
Haemophilus influenzae	Respiratory secretions	Probably less than 10 days	Respiratory	Isolate for 24 hours of specific therapy.
Legionella			None	Respiratory secretions may be infective.

[a]Isolate for duration of illness, unless specific directions given.

Table 25.2. cont.

Disease	Infective Material	Incubation Period	Isolation Category	Comments[a]
Meningococcal	Respiratory secretions		Respiratory	Isolate for 24 hours of specific therapy. Prompt evaluation and follow-up of exposed persons is necessary.
Multiply resistant bacterial	Respiratory secretions and possibly feces		Contact	Includes Gram-negative bacilli resistant to all tested aminoglycosides, *S. aureus* resistant to methicillin, *Pneumococcus* resistant to penicillin, and *H. influenzae* resistant to ampicillin and chloramphenicol. In outbreaks, cohorting of infected and colonized patients may be indicated.
Mycoplasma			None	Respiratory secretions may be infective.
Pneumococcal			None	Respiratory secretions may be infective.
Pneumocystis carinii			None	
S. aureus	Respiratory secretions		Contact	Isolate for 48 hours of effective therapy.
Streptococcus, group A	Respiratory secretions		Contact	Isolate for 24 hours of effective therapy.
Viral	Respiratory secretions		Contact	
Poliomyelitis	Feces	3–35 days, usually 7–14 days	Enteric	Isolate until virus can no longer be recovered from the feces. Report suspected case promptly to local health department.
Psittacosis (ornithosis, parrot fever)	Respiratory secretions	7–14 days	Drainage/secretion	Person-to-person transmission is rare and only from severely ill individuals with productive cough.
Q Fever	Respiratory secretions	2–4 weeks	None	Person-to-person transmission is rare but may occur in cases of pneumonia.
Rabies	Respiratory secretions	9 days to 1 year or more, usually 2–8 weeks	Strict	Isolate despite the absence of proven risk of person-to-person transmission. Report suspected case promptly to local health department.

[a]Isolate for duration of illness, unless specific directions given.

Table 25.2. cont.

Disease	Infective Material	Incubation Period	Isolation Category	Comments[a]
Rat-bite Fever			None	
Relapsing Fever (Borrelia)	Louse	5–11 days	Blood/body Fluid	Not directly transmitted person to person. Treat louse infestation if present.
Resistant Bacteria				See multiply resistant bacteria.
Respiratory Syncytial Virus (RSV)	Respiratory secretions	5–10 days	Contact	During epidemics, infected patients may be cohorted in the same room.
Reye's Syndrome			None	
Rheumatic Fever			None	
Rhinovirus Infections (common cold)			None	Good handwashing is necessary to prevent nosocomial spread.
Rickettsial Disease (Q fever, Rocky Mountain spotted fever, rickettsialpox, typhus)			None	
Ringworm			None	
Ritter's disease (staphylococcal scalded skin syndrome)	Lesion drainage	Variable; commonly 1–14 days	Contact	
Rocky Mountain Spotted Fever			None	Blood may be infective.
Roseola infantum (exanthen subitum, sixth disease)			None	
Rotavirus Infection (viral gastroenteritis)	Feces	1–3 days	Enteric	Isolate for 7 days after onset or duration of illness, whichever is less.
Rubella (German measles)	Respiratory secretions	14–21 days, usually 16–18 days	Contact	Isolate for 7 days after onset of rash. Infants with congenital rubella require isolation for 1 year, unless culture-negative after 3 months of age.
Salmonellosis	Feces	6–72 hours for gastroenteritis; 3–60 days for enteric fevers	Enteric	

[a]Isolate for duration of illness, unless specific directions given.

Table 25.2. cont.

Disease	Infective Material	Incubation Period	Isolation Category	Comments[a]
Scabies	Infested areas	2–6 weeks in person without previous exposure; 1–4 days after repeat exposure	Contact	Isolate for 24 hours after effective therapy. Masks are not needed.
Scaled Skin Syndrome, staphylococcal (Ritter's disease)	Lesion drainage	Variable; commonly 1–4 days	Contact	
Schistosomiasis			None	
Shigellosis	Feces	1–7 days; usually 2–4 days	Enteric	
Smallpox	Respiratory secretions and lesion secretions		Strict	Contact State Health Department for advice about management of suspected case.
Staphylococcal Infections		Variable; usually 1–10 days for bullous impetigo and scalded skin syndrome		
Skin, wound, or burn infections				
Major	Pus		Contact	Major—not contained in a dressing.
Minor	Pus		Drainage/secretion	Minor—adequately contained in a dressing.
Enterocolitis	Feces		Enteric	
Pneumonia or draining lung	Respiratory secretions		Contact	Isolate for 48 hours of effective therapy.
Scalded skin syndrome	Lesion drainage		Contact	
Toxic shock syndrome			Drainage/secretion	No evidence of person-to-person transmission has been documented.
Streptococcal Infections, Group A		Usually 1–3 days		
Impetigo	Lesion secretions		Contact or drainage/secretion, depending on the extent of the infection	
Pharyngitis	Respiratory secretions		Drainage/secretions	Isolate for 24 hours of effective therapy.
Pneumonia	Repiratory secretions		Contact	Isolate for 24 hours of effective therapy.
Scarlet Fever	Respiratory secretions		Drainage/secretion	Isolate for 24 hours of effective therapy.
Streptococcal Infections, Group B			None	

[a]Isolate for duration of illness, unless specific directions given.

Table 25.2. cont.

Disease	Infective Material	Incubation Period	Isolation Category	Comments[a]
Strongyloidiasis			None	
Syphilis Congenital	Lesion secretions and blood	10–90 days	Drainage/secretion Blood/body Fluid	Isolate for 24 hours of effective therapy. Gloves must be worn when handling infant, as open lesions are highly infective.

Tapeworm
  Taeniasis
  Cysticerosis
  Other
			None	

Tetanus (lockjaw)			None	
Tinea (ringworm)			None	
TORCH syndrome				See separate listing for these diseases: toxoplasmosis, rubella, cytomegalovirus, herpes, and syphilis.
Toxic Shock Syndrome			Drainage/secretion	No evidence of person-to-person transmission has been documented.
Toxoplasmosis			None	
Trachoma, acute	Purulent exudate	Variable	Drainage/secretion	
Trench Mouth (Vincent's angina)			None	
Trichinosis			None	
Trichomoniasis			None	

Trichuriasis
  (whipworm
  infection)
			None	

Tuberculosis Extrapulmonary, draining lesion	Pus	2–10 weeks	Drainage/secretion	A private room is important for children.

Pulmonary
  (positive
  sputum or
  cavity)
	Respiratory secretions		AFB	Isolate 2–3 weeks after effective therapy initiated and sputum smears show reduction in number of TB organisms and cough decreasing.

Primary			None	Must be receiving chemotherapy.

Skin test positive
  with no evidence
  of active disease
			None	

Atypical (mycobacteria other than tuberculosis)			None	

[a]Isolate for duration of illness, unless specific directions given.

Table 25.2. cont.

Disease	Infective Material	Incubation Period	Isolation Category	Comments[a]
Tularemia	Lesion secretions	1–21 days, usually 3–5 days	Drainage/secretion	
Typhoid Fever	Feces	1–3 weeks, depending on the size of the infecting dose	Enteric	

Typhus
  Murine
  Epidemic
    (louseborne)
			None
			None	

Varicella (chickenpox)	Respiratory secretions and lesion secretions	8–21 days; varicella-zoster Immune globulin (VZIG) may prolong incubation up to 28 days	Strict	Neonates born to mothers with active lesions should be placed on strict isolation at birth. Hospitalized exposed susceptible patients should be isolated from days 10–21 following exposure. Exposed susceptible hospital personnel should not have patient contact from days 10–21 following exposure.
Vibrio para-haemolyticus diarrhea	Feces	Median 23 hours with a range of 5–92 hours	Enteric	
Vincent's angina (Trench mouth)			None	
Viral Diseases Meningitis	Feces	Vary with specific infectious agent	Enteric	
Respiratory			None	Precautions may be indicated for most likely etiologic agent, such as RSV and parainfluenza virus.
Whooping Cough (pertussis)	Respiratory secretions	7–21 days, usually 7–10 days	Respiratory	Isolate for 7 days of specific therapy. If not treated, isolate for 3 weeks after onset of paroxysms. Prompt evaluation and follow-up of exposed persons is necessary.
Wound Infections Major	Pus		Contact	Major—not contained in a dressing.
Minor	Pus		Drainage/secretion	Minor—adequately contained in a dressing.

[a]Isolate for duration of illness, unless specific directions given.

Table 25.2. cont.

Disease	Infective Material	Incubation Period	Isolation Category	Comments[a]
Yersinia enterocalitica gastroenteritis	Feces	1–3 weeks	Enteric	
Zygomycosis			None	

[a]Isolate for duration of illness, unless specific directions given.

Gowns, gloves, and masks should be worn as indicated by the type of isolation category. Gowns should be worn only once, and discarded. Disposable single use gloves are recommended; the wearing of gloves is not a substitute for handwashing. Masks should be worn only once, tied to cover the nose and mouth, and changed whenever moist.

Linen from an isolation room should be handled as little as possible. It should be placed in a laundry bag, then double-bagged and placed in appropriate area for pickup.

No special precautions are necessary for dishes unless they are visibly contaminated with infective material. The water temperature and dishwasher detergent used are sufficient to decontaminate dishes (3).

Routine and terminal cleaning of the isolation room is the same as used in other hospital patient rooms, except housekeeping personnel should follow isolation precautions during routine and terminal cleaning. Furniture and floor should be cleared with a disinfectant detergent (5).

If an isolated patient must be transported to another area, use gown, gloves, and mask, as indicated by the isolation category. The patient should wear a clean gown and dressings. A clean sheet should be placed over the stretcher or wheelchair and wrapped around the patient, leaving the face exposed of patient on strict, contact, respiratory, or AFB isolation. It is preferable to place a clean mask on the patient if indicated. The transporter should wear a mask when this cannot be done.

Handwashing before and after each patient contact is the single most important means of preventing the spread of infection. The use of an antimicrobial preparation should be considered for handwashing, especially after the care of a patient on isolation.

Personnel should use the same isolation precautions to protect themselves when handling a deceased patient as they would if the patient were still alive. Identify the body with the appropriate isolation category. Notify autopsy personnel, morgue, and funeral home of the patient's disease status so that appropriate precautions can be maintained. State or local regulations may require additional precautions for postmortem handling of bodies (10).

Isolation should be discontinued in accordance with the isolation recommendations.

The prevention of cross-infection within the hospital is the basic goal of an isolation program. Isolation procedures are based on methods to prevent the transmission of potential pathogens from infected patients to susceptible hosts. These procedures result in certain disadvantages to the hospital and to patients. Isolation procedures are expensive, both in time and money, and make increased demands on hospital personnel.

The inconvenience of special techniques required by isolation discourages hospital personnel from giving the best possible care. The solitude of isolation separates the infant or child from most visual and physical contacts, thus depriving the patient from normal social stimulation. These children may feel they are being punished or rejected, which may be psychologically injurious (11–12). A Swedish study has shown the children on isolation who can observe staff members have no negative effects (13).

The hospital is responsible for ensuring that appropriate isolation precautions are followed when indicated; therefore, it is essential that all hospital personnel understand the principles of isolation as well as the mode of transmission and communicability of disease for optimal placement and care of the patient. Well-informed caregivers will be better able to provide and care and emotional support to the patient.

ACKNOWLEDGMENTS

The author wishes to thank Suzanne Pointer for secretarial assistance and Mary Ann M. Searcy for reviewing this chapter.

REFERENCES

1. Aronson SR: *Communicable Disease Nursing*. Garden City, NJ, Medical Examination Publishing, 1981, pp 9–16.
2. Dubay EC, Grubb RD: *Infection Prevention and Control*. St Louis, CV Mosby, 1978, pp ix–xii.
3. Centers for Disease Control: Recommendations for prevention of HIV transmission in health-care settings. *MWWR* 36:3S–18s, 1987.
4. Lynch P, Jackson MM, Cummings MJ, Stamm WE: Rethinking the role of isolation precautions in the prevention of nosocomial infections. *Ann Intern Med* 107–246, 1987.
5. Garner JS, Simmons BP: Guidelines for isolation precautions in hospital. *Infection Control* 4 (Suppl):245–348, 1983.
6. Peters G (ed): *Report of Committee of Infectious Diseases: 1986 Red Book*, ed 20. Elk Grove Village, IL, American Academy of Pediatrics, 1986, pp 81–407.
7. Benenson AS (ed): *Control of Communicable Diseases in Man*, ed 14. Washington, The American Public Health Association, 1985, pp 1–445.
8. Mandell GL, Douglas RG, Bennett JE (eds); *Principles and Practice of Infectious Diseases*, ed 2. New York, John Wiley & Sons, 1985, pp 334–1602.
9. Landry S, Loving TJ, Wenzel RP: Use of simple exhaust fan to control airborne transmission of varicella zoster. *J Hospital Infect* 8:305–307, 1986.
10. Lowbury EJL, Ayliffe GAJ, Geddes AM, William JD: *Control of Hospital Infection*. New York, John Wiley & Sons, 1975, p 120.
11. Robertson BA: The child in hospital. *South Am Med J* 51:749–752, 1977.
12. Hollenbeck AR, Susman EJ, Nannis ED, Strope BE, Hersh SP, Leving AS, Pizzo PA. Children with serious illness: Behavioral correlates of separation and isolation. *Child Psychol and Human Dev 11*: pp 3–11, 1980.
13. Putsep E: Pediatric patients. In Putsep E (ed); *Modern Hospital*. London, Lloyd-Luke, 1981, pp 86–88.

26

Roles of the Infection Control Professional

Terry Yamauchi, M.D.

The roles of the individuals responsible for infection control within the hospital setting have changed considerably since Ignaz Semmelweis observed the increased incidence of mortality from puerperal sepsis after allowing medical students into the delivery area directly out of the autopsy suite (1,2). Indeed, these individuals now form a select group of health professionals with multiple areas of expertise (3,4). The purpose of this chapter will be to more clearly define the roles of these professionals.

THE INFECTION CONTROL PROFESSIONAL (ICP)

The ICP has traditionally been an individual with primary background training in nursing (5). This selection likely represents the overview that the nurse fulfills many roles within the hospital, especially those involving patient care. Today, the majority of ICPs continue to be nurses; however, more recently, microbiologists, epidemiologists, and physicians have become interested in infection control and have assumed the responsibilities for hospital infection control. Since hospital infection control involves all areas of the hospital environment, the ICP can have a broad spectrum of interests and expertise (6,7). Each hospital infection control program should have the person who is most interested in this position serve as the ICP. Therefore, while a nurse may best fill this role in one hospital, a microbiologist or physician may function equally well in another hospital. Interest and dedication are two important characteristics to consider and are of foremost concern. Additional training for the ICP is encouraged, and several good programs exist to provide up-to-date information. The two most widely known programs are provided by the Centers for Disease Control (CDC), and are entitled "Surveillance, Prevention and Control of Nosocomial Infections" and "Infection Control in Small Hospitals and Extended Care Facilities." Additional information can be obtained by writing to the CDC, Hospital Infections Branch, Atlanta, Georgia.

The responsibilities of the ICP must be clearly defined and understood by all hospital personnel. Whenever possible, these responsibilities should be outlined as specific hospital policy and approved by the hospital administrator, medical staff, and/or board of directors. The ICP should be allowed to make decisions regarding obtaining proper specimens for culturing, ordering (or discontinuing) isolation, and identifying nosocomial infections. Hospital infection control education, surveillance, outbreak management, and employee health are other areas of responsibility for the ICP (8–10).

The ICP at Arkansas Children's Hospital in Little Rock, Arkansas is a member of the Infectious Disease Division and reports to the Medical Director and to the Chief of Infectious Diseases. Although in many hospitals ICPs also serve in a number of other roles (quality assurance, medical records committee, etc.), our ICP works full-time in infection control. Education of new employees, medical students, house officers, visitors, and hospital personnel; infection surveillance (patient and environmental); outbreak investigation; and daily communication with the employee health nurse are the duties carried out by our ICP.

THE INFECTION CONTROL COMMITTEE

The Infection Control Committee should be one of the strongest and well-recognized committees in the hospital. To obtain this status, the composition of this committee must be carefully considered and those chosen urged to participate. Membership should be limited to those individuals who are interested and effective in the hospital. Members should also represent major groups within the hospital and be acknowledged as experts from those groups. Ideally, the chairperson should be an individual with interests in infection control, hospital epidemiology, infectious diseases, and should be able to communicate freely with other clinicians within the hospital. Unfortunately, most often, the chairperson selected for this position is a physician with little if any training in infectious diseases or infection control (6). When this occurs, the ICP must become the "leader behind the scenes." Other committee members should include representatives from administration, nursing, housekeeping, quality assurance, laboratory, medical staff, special care units, surgery, and central services. Each member should have clearly defined guidelines of their responsibilities to the committee. The Infection Control Committee at Arkansas Children's Hospital uses the agenda shown in Table 26.1 for its monthly meetings.

You will note on the sample Infection Control agenda that we include the infectious diseases reported to the state health department and compare statistics from previous year and month figures. This alerts the committee to unusual outbreaks either in the community and/or the hospital. Points raised for discussion in the old or new business portions of the meeting are clearly defined in the meeting. If further discussion is

necessary for a future meeting, specific persons are assigned at that time for follow-up at the next meeting.

An important function of the Infection Control Committee is the regular review of hospital infection control policies. This review is required by the Joint Commission on Accreditation of Hospitals (JCAH) and must be done on a yearly basis. By reviewing a few policies each month, all hospital infection control policies can be covered over a 1-year period. We ask the supervisor from the department whose policy is reviewed to attend the committee meeting and to discuss the policy. We want to know specifically if the policy correctly reflects what is being done in that department. In addition to the department supervisor, two other committee members are asked to review the policy and to bring their questions, comments, and suggestions to the meeting. All committee members are also supposed to review the policies and comment as they see fit. Over the years, policy review gets easier because fewer changes are necessary.

Finally, the Infection Control Committee's minutes and reports have been sought in relation to various medical-legal actions. Whether the hospital Infection Control Committee minutes and reports can be released for legal reasons remains unclear. It has been suggested that this will probably remain a state-by-state decision (11,12).

SURVEILLANCE

Ignaz Semmelweis, the father of hospital epidemiology, is acknowledged as the first to use surveillance methods to evaluate an infection outbreak in the early 1800s. Since that time, hospital surveillance has become an integral part of hospital infection control activities. In fact, by 1976, more than 80% of United States hospitals had infection surveillance programs (12–16).

Definitions

Nosocomial infection is defined as follows:

1. Infections not known to be present or incubating at the time of admission;
2. If the incubation period is unknown, but infection develops any time after admission;
3. Onset of clinical infection at a different site;
4. New different microorganisms at site of previous nosocomial infection.

Table 26.1.
Infection Control Agenda

I. Review minutes from previous month

II. Nosocomial Infection Monthly Report
   A. Review of selected cases
   B. Comparison statistics from previous year and month
   C. Infectious diseases reported to the State Health Department

III. Old Business

IV. Review of Infection Control policies
   A. Reviewer #1—Department supervisor
   B. Reviewer #2—Infection Control Committee member
   C. Reviewer #3—Infection Control Committee member
   D. Review by rest of committee

V. New Business

Surveillance is defined as the ongoing evaluation of all aspects of the occurrence of an infection that are necessary for effective control and management.

Objectives of Surveillance

These are the most widely used objectives of surveillance:

1. To detect infection in the hospital;
2. To determine the rate of infection during and just after hospitalization;
3. To provide the patient, visitors, and hospital personnel with all possible protection from the development of nosocomial epidemics;
4. To establish policies of surveillance and control;
5. To educate the hospital staff;
6. To meet the requirements of the JCAH (17).

Types of Surveillance

There are many types of surveillance being used in this country. The ICP must determine what type of surveillance system is best suited for their particular hospital setting (17–23). The individual case study is one example of a surveillance system. In this approach, infection is reported to the ICP, who decides whether the infection is nosocomial and if further investigation is necessary. Table 26.2 is an example of a surveillance worksheet that can be used to record data collected in individual case studies. This type of surveillance works well in smaller health facilities, but requires a reporting system to notify the ICP.

Review of microbiological data, such as blood cultures, is also frequently used to survey the infections within a hospital. This system requires the ICP to review microbiology laboratory reports on a regular basis, and to then review those patients with positive cultures. In larger hospitals, this may be the only workable system, since it allows the ICP to quickly scan the entire hospital for infections. Unfortunately, many hospital infections (e.g., viral diseases) may not be evidenced by standard cultures and would therefore be missed if this were the only type of surveillance being carried out.

Another type of surveillance sometimes used in large facilities is the reviewing of discharge diagnoses. To this author, this is the least satisfactory because it requires discharging the patient from the hospital to determine if a nosocomial infection occurred during hospitalization. Naturally, people are reluctant to admit that an infection occurred, and underreporting results.

Environmental surveillance involves monitoring the entire hospital environment for the detection of potential reservoirs of infections. In the past, this meant the culturing of the inanimate environment, such as tabletops, floors, carpets, etc., or the culturing of selected personnel for specific microorganisms, such as *Staphyloccoccus aureus* or *Salmonella*. This type of surveillance culturing has been demonstrated to be of no value except in the rare epidemiologic study. There are however, some situations in which environmental culturing may be necessary and significant:

1. Monitoring Sterilization Procedures. Most hospitals have steam or gas autoclaves, which should be tested on a periodic basis via a sporicidal test. This test is required on a uniform schedule for all autoclaves and can be included with any materials or instruments being sterilized.
2. Spot Checking Instruments. Spot checking instruments that have been treated with chemical disinfection is a desirable procedure. This should include materials and/or instruments used in inhalation therapy and anesthetic equipment.
3. Epidemiological Culturing. In an investigation of nosocomial outbreak, culturing of various environmental materials might be necessary. For example, an outbreak of staphylococcal disease in the newborn nursery might require culturing of bassinets (inanimate) and personnel (animate) in order to find the cause of the outbreak.

Data Collection

Effective surveillance programs must collect correct data that best characterizes the hospital patients, clinical course, microorganisms, hospital procedures, and infection control intervention.

When characterizing the hospital patient, one should record such items as admitting diagnosis, symptoms, length of illness, and similar or known diseases in family contacts are especially important in pediatric facilities. Patient demographics, such as name, hospital record number,

Table 26.2.
Surveillance Worksheet

DATE: _____

Patient Name: _____

Hospital Number: _____

Birthdate: _____

Race: _____

Sex: _____

Next of Kin: _____

Hospital Service: _____

Admitting Diagnosis: _____

Hospital Infection: _____

   Site _____

   Microorganism _____

Antibiotic Sensitivity: _____

Hospital Course Summary: _____
_____
_____

Special Procedures: _____
_____
_____
_____

Risk Factors: _____
_____
_____
_____

Infection Control Intervention: _____
_____
_____
_____

Outcome: _____
_____
_____
_____

Infection Control Practitioner: _____

age, sex, race, and next of kin are also necessary as a means of identifying individual cases. At the same time, a system that maintains patient confidentiality must be utilized.

The clinical course should be reviewed for duration of hospitalization (especially duration from time of admission to onset of symptoms of infection or diagnosis of infection), host factors (recognized either at admission or during hospital stay); host factors resulting from specific hospital procedures (e.g., catheterization, surgery) should also be noted, as well as specific treatment plans. Other important factors of the clinical course in infection control would include location in hospital, personnel, including physicians, technicians, and other hospital staff involved in day-to-day management. Special attention should be given to the microbiology results, looking at specific microorganisms (quantities of microorganisms), specific antibiotic sensitivity patterns, specimen collection, and site of specimen collection from the patient.

When a patient is discharged from the hospital, it is important to document his/her current condition and diagnosis. Some method of noting hospital-acquired infections should be in effect. Patients with ongoing hospital infections at discharge should also be identified because if they are readmitted within a short period of time, special documentation may be necessary (see definitions of nosocomial infections earlier in this chapter). Data collection after discharge is obviously difficult to obtain and interpret. Nevertheless, every attempt to follow the patient after discharge should be made. This may be limited to a telephone call requesting an update on the patient's progress or a change in condition, e.g., temperature elevation, redness at incision site in the surgical patient, or other systemic symptoms. Discharges from pediatric hospitals have the added variable of sending the patient back into an environment where sibling contact and exposure is poorly controlled, leading to infections shortly after discharge.

Once data have been collected, the interpretation becomes of major importance. The decision to further investigate or to introduce control measures will depend upon the administrative structure of your program. This means that interpretation may be carried out by the ICP, infection control committee, or others within the institution and acted upon as necessary.

Data collected throughout surveillance should then be used to inform and educate hospital personnel, including administrators as well as the medical staff. The administrators see the results of the hospital infection control program that assist in keeping the hospital free of unwanted infections. The data are also compared with that of previous months, years, etc. for educational purposes (e.g., rise in respiratory infections during certain months of the year). Data generated through surveillance and passed on to the medical staff may lead the staff to select alternative methods of managing patient care within the hospital and enable them to follow the success or failure of such changes.

Team Surveillance

Arkansas Children's Hospital uses a unique and effective type of surveillance called team surveillance (24). The team is composed of several individuals, including the ICP, physician (infectious disease specialist), microbiologist, house staff physicians, medical students, and special visitors. In addition to these persons, a nurse from within the hospital is also included. Acting with the nursing supervisor's approval, the volunteer nurse's role is to observe the infection control team's activities and to report back any information that might be usefully implemented.

Team surveillance rounds are held only twice a week and require that the ICP gathers and reviews the patient records prior to the rounding. The team goes from unit to unit within the hospital reviewing patients with infectious diseases. Patient care, treatment, isolation policy, and microbiology are reviewed for the selected patients. If isolation policy is not appropriate, changes are made as needed. We also continue to seek patients with as yet undiagnosed diseases, or new hospital-acquired infections. Culture reports on all patients are reviewed by the microbiologist prior to rounds, and cases needing clarification are discussed. Specimen collection and antibiotic sensitivities are also reviewed. The nursing supervisors from each unit also accompany the team on its rounds and are asked the following questions:

1. Is there anyone on this unit who needs isolation?
2. Is there anyone on this unit who is on isolation but who doesn't need to be isolated?
3. Are there any patients on this unit with fever, diarrhea, wound infections, Foley catheters, arterial lines, or other predisposing factors?
4. Are there any patients with infections or with pus from a wound site (including postoperative patients)?
5. Are there any patients you think need to be cultured?
6. What would you culture?
7. Have you had increased absenteeism lately?
8. Are any of your staff ill?

These questions involve the nurses in decision-making while showing concern for their role in the care of patients.

House staff and medical students are taught the principles of infection control through these rounds. Hopefully, they will carry this knowledge with them when they start medical practice. Besides serving as an educational device to teach infection control, these rounds can encourage hospital epidemiologists, infection control experts, and infectious disease professionals to share tasks more equally.

STAFF EDUCATION

In addition to surveillance, most ICPs are responsible for the education of hospital personnel in infection control matters. For many years, the primary emphasis of hospital infection control was to provide in-depth hospital surveillance. The ICP's time commitment was largely consumed by collecting and analyzing surveillance data. Shortly thereafter, staff education was recognized as a more effective measure in preventing the occurrence of hospital infections, and the ICP's role became one of an educator. The enthusiasm for providing quality hospital staff infection control education has been so overwhelming, that in some hospitals, the ICP now spends more time providing staff education than surveillance. Recognizing the various needs of individual hospitals, each ICP must decide what is required in infection control education and the amount of time necessary to provide that service.

Staff education is often crisis oriented, aimed at providing an educational program or experience after a problem is recognized, to prevent continuation or recurrence of the problem. For example, if hospital surveillance reveals an increase of staphylococcal infections in the neonatal intensive care unit, an educational effort for personnel regarding staphylococcal infections, handwashing procedures, or procedural techniques is then indicated before further infections occur.

More frequently, staff education is a continuous process, such as a regularly scheduled didactic lecture, self-teaching, reading, demonstrations, or other more innovative methods. The ICP must be prepared and willing to utilize any or all of these techniques.

Three successful methods to teach infection control to hospital staff at Arkansas Children's Hospital are Nosocomial Grand Rounds, "Infection Control in a Box," and "College Bowl."

Nosocomial Grand Rounds can best be explained as a regularly scheduled monthly conference during which a subject is covered in-depth by a number of persons representing different areas within the hospital. For example, the case of a hospitalized patient with *Salmonella* gastroenteritis might be featured at this conference. The nurse providing the daily nursing care presents the patient's history, physical findings, and nursing requirements. A representative from the microbiology laboratory then discusses proper specimen collection and processing, and any interesting features of the *Salmonella* microorganism. The ICP then explains disease transmission and hospital isolation policy and technique. The dietitian reviews the role of the food handler in *Salmonella* infections, as well as how to feed the patient with such an infection. A physician gives the medical overview of the patient, followed by a general discussion of *Salmonella* infections, including treatment. The conference is terminated by requesting questions from the floor to any of the speakers. The Nosocomial Grand Rounds Conference has been a popular method of providing staff education (25).

The catchy title, "Infection Control in a Box," is a second innovative approach for staff education. This teaching program can be carried throughout the hospital, used by anyone at any time, and easily updated as necessary. The materials in the box include an infectious disease quiz, crossword puzzle, word search, cartoon pictures depicting breaks in techniques leading to infection that the test-taker is asked to identify, and prizes. Hospital staff are asked to complete each of the teaching materials in the box, take a prize (a badge or button), and sign the log to document completion of the program. The advantages of this program include convenience to personnel, as they can use the program at their own pace; ease in transporting it to any area in the hospital; and the ability to alter the program material as needed.

A third method of teaching infection control has been modeled after the popular game show, "College Bowl." During this teaching session, the class is divided into two teams, and asked to sit together so that they can discuss questions and answers as a group. A scorekeeper is assigned for each team, and noisemakers are provided to each player. Questions regarding infection control are then asked, and the first person who knows the answer sounds their noisemaker. If the answer is correct, the team is allowed a chance at a bonus question, which is given to the entire team, to think over and discuss before answering. This program can be very general or quite specific, depending upon the immediate needs of the institution. By using team or group discussion, no single individual feels threatened, and information can be exchanged freely.

EMPLOYEE HEALTH

The Joint Commission on Accreditation of Hospitals Manual states:

1. The Infection Control Program shall include " . . . a practical system for reporting, evaluating and maintaining records of infections among patients and personnel . . . "
2. The Infection Control Program shall have " . . . input into the content and scope of the Employee Health Program" (17).

Employee health has special significance in pediatric hospitals because several childhood diseases are now recognized as infectious to the hospital employee (26–29). Former childhood illnesses, such as rubeola (measles), rubella (german measles), and pertussis (whooping cough) are being reported in older individuals whose vaccine-induced immunity has waned. Pediatric patients often lack good personal hygiene habits, and personnel caring for these patients may be exposed to multiple infectious agents on a regular basis. With this background, objectives of the employee health program in a pediatric hospital are to

1. Identify specific employees at risk for contracting infections within individual hospital areas;
2. Provide appropriate preventive medicine and health education for the hospital employee;
3. Monitor the hospital employees for outbreaks of infectious diseases and assist in preventing further infections;
4. Prevent transmission of infections to patients and visitors by employees;
5. Assist in detection of carrier states when implicated by surveillance studies.

Initial Employee Health Examination

A careful health history is necessary to determine employee susceptibility accurately. The history should examine previous infections, immunizations, and medications. Historical questioning should document the childhood diseases, such as measles, mumps, rubella, and chickenpox. Although less frequently, children continue to be hospitalized with these contagious illnesses, thus exposing personnel. Equally important is the immunization history to determine the employee's susceptibility to the vaccine-preventable diseases. As previously mentioned, immunity induced by some vaccines appears to lessen over a period of time; other vaccines do confer lifelong protection, and the protected employees should be recognized.

Employees on medications that may suppress the immune response are at increased risk for infections. Although corticosteroids are the medicines more frequently associated with decreasing the immune response, the usual dosage for acute treatment (i.e., allergic reactions) is not enough to compromise the normal host response. Even long-term corticosteroid therapy for such diseases as asthma or systemic lupus erythematosis do not suppress the normal host response enough to cause concern. Higher doses of corticosteriods or chemotherapeutic agents used in hematology-oncology and/or transplantation individuals are the only conditions that place the individual at increased risk of infection. If there is any question regarding the employee's immune status, a statement from the physician prescribing the medication is indicated.

The physical examination should assure that the employee is physically able to carry out the tasks assigned for the area of employment. Obvious physical disorders that may be conducive to disease transmission, such as dermatitis, must be cleared by a physician before being allowed to work in patient contact areas.

Preemployment culturing for enteric pathogens is still required in some states, and individual state health regulations should be reviewed. In general, culturing of the employee before employment is of little value and should not be necessary. However, the employee should be aware that personal culturing may be required if surveillance data so indicate during a hospital outbreak investigation.

Employee Immunizations

The following immunizations are highly recommended for pediatric hospital employees: influenza, diphtheria-tetanus, rubeola (measles), mumps, rubella (German measles), polio, pertussis, and hepatitis B.

Influenza viruses have been well-known causes of nosocomial infections (30–32). On pediatric services, hospital-acquired influenza has been responsible for hospital epidemics (33,34). The influenza vaccine is a killed virus vaccine. It is recommended that health care professionals be administered the vaccine yearly. When administered at the proper time and against the appropriate influenza strain, the vaccine will protect from clinical disease 70% of the time. I would personally urge all hospital staff to be vaccinated each year. Unfortunately, the influenza virus undergoes periodic changes (antigenic drift and/or shift), and if that occurs after the vaccine strains have been selected, the vaccine may not be protective. Historically, influenza strains most prevalent in the orient and South America one year, have caused disease in the United States the following year, and the vaccine strains are selected on that basis. The influenza vaccine induces protective antibody which has a relatively short life and requires yearly immunizations. Because the immune response to the vaccine requires about 2 weeks for antibody levels to become protective, in times of epidemics it may be necessary to administer prophylactically the antiviral agent amantadine (Symmetrel®) (35–37).

Diphtheria–tetanus toxoids have been widely used in the United States and have markedly decreased the incidence of these diseases. Although the risks from these two diseases appear minimal, mortality from disease remains high—45–55% from tetanus, and 10% from diphtheria (38). Because of the seriousness of these two diseases, and the fact that hospital workers are considered a high-risk group, diphtheria-tetanus toxoid vaccination should be administered every 10 years. It may be necessary to reimmunize employees who have suffered wounds thought to be dirty and if more than 5 years have lapsed since the vaccines were last administered.

Rubeola (measles), mumps, and rubella (German measles) vaccines are live, attenuated viruses. They are available in combination or singly. Each vaccine should be considered separately in regard to its efficacy and use by hospital personnel.

Rubeola is a highly contagious disease with potential for serious complications, including pneumonia, encephalitis, and otitis media (39,40). Although the incidence of measles has declined over the past decade, selective susceptible populations have been identified (41). Measles has also been recognized in medical facilities, including children's hospitals (42–44).

Hospital employees should be considered immune to measles if they can prove a history of measles; laboratory evidence of past disease or vaccine use; or immunization with live measles vaccine at 12 months or older (39). Persons not meeting these criteria should be reimmunized.

Mumps virus infections have declined by 97% since the introduction of the vaccine in 1967 (45,46). The mumps virus vaccine is usually given in combination with measles and rubella vaccines. While hospital employees are not at any greater risk of mumps virus infection than the general population, there are few contraindications to its use.

Rubella virus infections have not shown the drastic decline in incidence as have measles and mumps. Susceptible populations have changed from infants and children to adolescents and young adults (47). The majority of reported cases of rubella now occur in persons 15 years or older (48).

Hospital employees lacking a history of disease or immunization by laboratory testing (whenever possible) should receive the vaccine.

It is important to remember that although attenuated measles, mumps, and rubella virus vaccines have not demonstrated disease and/or transmission, the potential for infection in the compromised patient must be considered. Individuals receiving these vaccines can excrete the attenuated viruses for several weeks. Therefore, it seems prudent to limit exposure of newly vaccinated employees to the immunocompromised patient while vaccinees are shedding virus.

The controversy of whether to immunize or serologically test for preexisting antibody to specific diseases continues to be controversial. However, the vaccines are cheap, effective, and associated with few adverse reactions. In addition, no serious adverse reactions have been documented following reimmunization.

Poliomyelitis is another disease that has almost disappeared in the United States and accurately reflects the efficacy of the poliovirus vaccines (49–51). Currently, two types of poliovirus vaccines are available: inactivated poliovirus vaccine (IPV) and live attenuated oral poliovirus vaccines (OPV). Controversy exists as to which vaccine should be used in the United States (52). As a general rule, persons 18 years of age or older are at little risk to wild poliovirus infections and do not require vaccine. However, pediatric hospital personnel should be fully immunized. IPV is the vaccine of choice for unvaccinated health care workers and should be administered at 1- to 2-month intervals for 3 doses, with a 4th dose 6–12 months later (53).

The widespread use of pertussis vaccine in combination with diphtheria-tetanus toxoid vaccines has dramatically decreased the occurrence of pertussis (whooping cough). Although pertussis has declined, sporadic cases continue to be seen in pediatric facilities. Recent concerns about the adverse effects of the pertussis vaccine has led to a drop-off in the acceptance of this vaccine with a resulting increase in the number of infants and children now lacking protection. Speculation has also been raised as to increased susceptibility of adults previously immunized. Hospital outbreaks of pertussis with the transmission of disease from patients to hospital staff, other patients, and household contacts have been reported (54,55).

Reimmunization with the pertussis vaccine is not recommended because of the increased risk of adverse reactions (56). Currently, protection of the exposed hospital employee consists of administration of oral erythromycin for 14 days.

Hepatitis B virus is the major cause of acute and chronic hepatitis in this country. Because of frequent contact with hepatitis B virus carriers and patients, hospital personnel are considered a high-risk group for acquiring hepatitis B virus disease. Since the risk of acquiring hepatitis B virus disease may vary from hospital to hospital, ICPs may wish to evaluate their own hospital experience and screening programs for hepatitis B virus infection.

Hepatitis B virus vaccine is now available and is recommended for selected high-risk groups within the hospital, including the staff of institutions for the mentally retarded (57,58). Individuals not previously immunized who receive needle sticks from known hepatitis B patients (those known to be hepatitis B surface antigen-positive) should also receive the vaccine (59,60).

Recommendations for the Pregnant Employee

Transmission of infectious agents within the hospital setting causes special risks to the pregnant employee. Pregnancy itself may predispose an individual to infection. Such factors as anemia, increased weight, and fatigue may increase the risk of infections. Infections in the pregnant woman carries the added risk of causing congenital malformations in the developing fetus (61–69). Concerns about possible infections to herself and the fetus also result in increased anxiety. Therefore, employee health should make available special educational programming for the pregnant employee (70–73).

Foremost in the education of the pregnant employee is an understanding of how infectious agents are transmitted. Infectious agents of concern to the pregnant employee and the mode of transmission are listed in Table 26.3 (74,75).

After acquiring an understanding of how infectious agents can be transmitted, the employee needs to review infection control guidelines aimed at disease prevention within the hospital. These guidelines include preventive health care (immunizations, personal hygiene, regular physical examinations, etc.) and hospital isolation policies and techniques.

VISITATION POLICIES

The purpose of visitation policies is to establish rules that acknowledge the rights of parents, visitors, and patients while providing an environment that serves the best interests of those patients and at the same time promotes the highest standards of quality patient care.

Children's hospitals and pediatric wards are usually family-centered care facilities, and parents are entitled to see their child at any time, to call the unit at any time to know their child's condition, to hold and touch their child, to care for their child, and to know who is responsible for their child's medical and nursing care and how to contact them. Therefore, visitation policies should take into account these rights.

General Visitation Guidelines

1. The patient's parents (or legal guardians) are not, strictly speaking, "visitors," since they play an important role in the total care of the child. Therefore, every effort should be made to give parents access to their children at all times.
2. Members of the clergy may visit a child at any time, if requested by the child or family.
3. Regularly scheduled visiting hours must be observed by persons other than parents, legal guardians, and clergy.

Table 26.3.
Infectious Agents of Concern to the Pregnant Hospital Employee and Mode of Transmission

Agent	Mode of Transmission
Cytomegalovirus (CMV)	Thought to be a sexually transmitted disease; virus transmitted via infected blood and blood products; also in urine of symptomatic and asymptomatic newborns.
Chickenpox (varicella-zoster virus, VZV)	Respiratory route; close personal contact; virus shed in respiratory secretions and from skin lesions.
Coxsackievirus	Personal contact; possibly respiratory route; virus in stool and oropharyngeal secretions.
Echovirus	Same as coxsackievirus.
Human Immunodeficiency virus (HIV)	Sexual contact, parenteral routes; virus shed in multiple human secretions, including semen, tears, vaginal secretions, and breast milk, but only blood and blood products implicated to date.
Influenza virus	Respiratory route; personal contact; virus in oropharyngeal secretions.
Measles virus	Same as influenza virus.
Mumps	Oral route; personal contact; virus in saliva, respiratory secretions, and urine.
Poliovirus	Oral route; possibly respiratory; personal contact; virus in stool and respiratory secretions.
Rubella (German measles)	Respiratory route; personal contact; virus in respiratory secretions, urine, stool, skin lesions.
Syphilis (*Treponema pallidum*)	Sexual contact is usual mode of transmission; direct contact with infected lesions or infected materials.
Toxoplasmosis (*Toxoplasma gondii*)	Contact with cat feces; ingestion of poorly cooked or raw meat.
Tuberculosis (*Mycobacterium tuberculosis*)	Respiratory route; personal contact; microorganism shed in respiratory secretions.

4. Persons with contagious diseases or suspected infections should not be allowed to visit any patient.
5. No visitors under 12 years of age are allowed in patient care areas. Exceptions can be made for siblings under the age of 12 years (see "Sibling Visitation Guidelines").
6. No more than two people at a time (including parents) are allowed in the patient's room, except with special permission of designated hospital personnel (nursing supervisor, infection control professional, etc.).
7. Exceptions to the General Visitation Guidelines can be made with respect to a given patient by written order by the patient's physician, following consultation with the proposed visitors, the infection control professional, nursing supervisor, and selected others, as necessary.

Recognizing the unique characteristics of siblings, such as increased level of activity, exploring nature, unrecognized illness, etc., special sibling visitation conditions.

Sibling Visitation Guidelines

1. Sibling visitation must be approved by the patient's physician and the unit nursing supervisor prior to the visit. When a request for visitation by a sibling under age 12 is received, the Sibling Visitation Checklist (Table 26.4) must be completed and a copy sent to the ICP.
2. Siblings under 12 years of age or those older with recognized behavioral disorders (i.e., hyperactivity, disruptive behavior, unwilling to follow instructions, etc.), may visit during the regularly scheduled visiting hours for a maximum time period as determined by the previously mentioned individuals.
3. Siblings under the age of 12 years must be accompanied by an adult, preferably a parent.

Table 26.4.
Sibling Visitation Checklist

Patient's Name _____ Unit _____ Room No. _____

Name of Visiting Sibling _____ Phone No. _____

Date Checklist Completed _____ Age of Sibling _____ (if 12 or older, no need to complete this checklist.)

1. Has patient's physician written an order for sibling to visit?   Yes _____ No _____
2. Will visiting sibling be accompanied by an adult?   Yes _____ No _____
3. Has nurse manager (or nursing supervisor) given approval?   Yes _____ No _____
4. Has the visiting sibling been screened by the nurse manager or the charge nurse for exposure to or symptoms of contagious diseases (i.e., have the following questions all been answered, *No*?)   Yes _____ No _____

    A. Within last 4 weeks, has the visiting sibling had or been exposed to:

Chickenpox	Yes _____	No _____	_____
Measles	Yes _____	No _____	_____
Mumps	Yes _____	No _____	_____
German Measles	Yes _____	No _____	_____
Hepatitis	Yes _____	No _____	_____
Common Cold	Yes _____	No _____	_____
Any other contagious illness	Yes _____	No _____	_____

    B. Does the visiting sibling have now or has he/she within the last 4 weeks had:

Upper respiratory infection	Yes _____	No _____	_____
Strep infection such as strep throat or impetigo	Yes _____	No _____	_____
Diarrhea	Yes _____	No _____	_____
Vomiting	Yes _____	No _____	_____
Fever	Yes _____	No _____	_____
Rash	Yes _____	No _____	_____
Other infections	Yes _____	No _____	_____

    C. Has the visiting sibling received within the last 4 weeks a live virus immunization such as MMR or Polio?
    Yes _____ No _____

5. Has the nurse manager or charge nurse explained to the visiting sibling what he/she will see and hear while visiting the patient and to parents the effects of sibling visitation?   Yes _____ No _____

If questions 1–5 have all been answered *Yes*, visiting by the sibling may occur for a maximum of 30 minutes. Otherwise, the sibling must remain in the lobby with a responsible adult.

Visitation: APPROVED _____
             DENIED   _____

_____
Signature of person completing form

Original form remains with chart.   Comments of Infection Control Professional
Send copy to Infection Control   _____
   Professional   _____

---

4. The nursing staff (supervisor, manager, or charge nurse) is responsible for screening siblings to ensure that they are not demonstrating symptoms of illness or have a history of recent exposure to a contagious disease. This information is included on the Sibling Visitation Checklist (Table 26.4). It is important that the individual doing this screening have an understanding of disease transmission, incubation periods of virus infections, and rapid access to consultation with the infection control professional.

5. The nursing staff will explain to siblings what they will see and hear while visiting the patient.

6. Siblings who cannot comply with rules in specific patient care areas must remain with a responsible adult in the hospital lobby or other designated waiting areas.
7. Sibling visitation will be monitored by the hospital Infection Control Committee, specifically for number of visits, noncompliance, infections noted in the siblings, and nosocomial infections. Results of the monitoring will be included in the monthly Infection Control Committee minutes.

Special Care Areas

These areas are involved in the care of unique medical problems and include emergency room, intensive care burn, nurseries, and hematology–oncology units. Because of the often highly technical nature of medical care and the susceptibility of the patients in these units, visitation policies must be clearly defined and strictly enforced. Careful and thoughtful explanation of visitation to all visitors (including parents) is of foremost importance. Most visitors are willing to accept any rules if the time is taken to explain why the rule is necessary. In order to deliver optimal care, traffic through the area must be minimized. This allows the medical care personnel the time and space to meet the special needs of that particular patient.

Emergency Room

The emergency room, because of the urgency of many of the health problems seen, is one obvious area where easy, rapid access to the patient is essential. In most instances, visitation of the patient is unnecessary and should not be allowed. However, in some circumstances, it may be desirable to allow visitors (i.e., to calm a child). The same guidelines as described for the hospital General Visitation Guidelines would apply. Certainly, in the case of a documented or suspected infectious disease, appropriate isolation techniques should be initiated and followed by visitors as well as personnel. Careful attention should be paid to the individuals involved in the care, handling, and observation of any suspected infectious disease patient in case it is discovered that prophylactic therapy is indicated for close contacts.

Intensive Care Unit

The increased incidence of nosocomial infections in intensive care units is related to many factors, including: high-risk patients, compromised host defense systems, invasive materials, broad-spectrum antibiotic usage, and multi-antibiotic-resistant microorganisms. Other factors to consider are the requirements of sensitive monitoring systems, personnel to oversee the equipment, and multiple medical specialists and technicians involved in the daily care.

The immediate medical needs of these patients must take priority over visitation, and the ICP, physicians, and nurses involved with the patient must impress upon visitors the importance of this condition. In addition, minimizing the number of visitors helps to control traffic in this special care unit.

Burn Unit

The pediatric patient with burns is a high-risk patient. Normal barriers to infection, such as skin and mucous membranes, swallowing reflex, cough and normal bacterial flora, may be lacking or diminished. Exposed areas allow easy access to numerous microorganisms ordinarily unable to attack the normal host (76–78). The bacteria most commonly recovered from burn wound infections are shown in Table 26.5. *Staphylococcus aureus* is the most frequent pathogen in burn wound infections. The next most common causes of burn wound infections are the Gram-negative bacilli.

Hands of personnel and visitors remain the major vectors for transmission of pathogens to the burn wound. Hand carriage of Gram-negative bacilli has been reported from other special care units (79). Handwashing will remove this risk and must be strictly enforced. Visitors should be taught proper handwashing before they are

Table 26.5.
Burn Wound Pathogens, Centers for Disease Control, National Nosocomial Infections Study, 1980–1984

Pathogen	Percentage of Isolates
Staphylococcus aureus	24.5
Pseudomonas aeruginosa	19.3
Enterococci	11.8
E. coli	8.4
E. cloacae	7.8
Serratia marcescens	4.7
Coagulase-negative staphylococcus	3.5
Candidas albicans	2.8
Klebsiella pneumoniae	2.4
Proteus mirabilis	2.1

allowed to visit. Shulman, et al. reported an outbreak of *Pseudomonas aeruginosa* in their burn unit and demonstrated the bacteria on sink handles, faucets, towel racks, and soap (80,81). Visitors should also be carefully screened for any possible infectious diseases and advised as to proper gowning and appropriate contact with the patient. It is important to remember that burn patients may serve as a reservoir of microorganisms with potential to cross-infect other patients within the unit, and visitors can serve as vectors. Visitors should not be allowed to move from one patient to another without proper rewashing and regowning.

Nurseries

The neonate is at significant risk of infection. Even the normal newborn has an increased rate of infection during the first few weeks of life (82). Nosocomial infections occur in 5–25% of the infants in intensive care (83,84). The increased susceptibility to infection can be attributed to several risk factors, including: immature and/or deficiencies in the natural immune system, and increased permeability of skin. Environmental nursery factors, such as crowding, contact with multiple individuals, other infections within the nursery, multiple antibiotic-resistant microorganisms, and invasive procedures, may contribute to increased infections. Hospital strains of Gram-negative bacilli with varying antibiotic sensitivities have been attributed to aminoglycoside usage (85). We have not been able to confirm this observation in the neonatal intensive care unit at Arkansas Children's Hospital (T. Yamauchi, unpublished observation).

The parents, hospital personnel, and visitors can serve as vectors for colonization of the infant. These same individuals may also serve as vectors for infections. Most often, the method of transmission for outbreaks in nurseries has been the hands. Gram-positive and Gram-negative microorganisms have been documented in hand contamination outbreaks (86–91). Therefore, handwashing is the important aspect of the visitation policy for preventing infections in these patients.

Gowns, although widely used, have not demonstrated any effectiveness in modifying nosocomial infections in nurseries. However, we continue to use them and ask visitors to gown before handling infants at our hospital.

Hematology–Oncology Unit

These patients pose the greatest challenge to the ICP. In actuality, the hospital as a place where infected individuals are cared for, would seem to be a poor environment to treat persons unusually susceptible to infection. The hematology–oncology unit is one such place. In addition to being highly susceptible, infections once acquired may progress rapidly and result in death in these unfortunate patients. Visitors must be kept to an absolute minimum, and careful screening is essential. The screening procedure for visitors should include questioning in regard to recent immunization with live vaccines (oral polio, measles, mumps, and rubella). Although transmission of the attenuated viruses in these vaccines is rare, the immunocompromised patient is susceptible. Since many infectious diseases are contagious before any symptoms are present, screening personnel must be familiar with incubation periods for infectious diseases and be alert for the history of potential exposures, such as infections in the visitors' homes.

Enforcement

Visitors must be made aware of the need for visitation guidelines. Special visiting hours allow the patient rest periods and the hospital personnel time to carry out their responsibilities. Persons who cannot abide by the guidelines should not be allowed to visit. If needed, hospital security can be called upon to enforce visitation hours. Hospital security actions should be clearly defined and approved by the appropriate hospital governing body (executive committee, board of directors, etc.).

PETS IN THE HOSPITAL

Pet animals are currently found in many hospital and institutional settings. The use of pets in patient therapy is strongly advocated by several special care groups, including play therapists, child life personnel, psychologists, psychiatrists, and some nurses, physicians, and parents. Virtually all patient populations have been targeted as potential populations who could benefit from the use of pet therapy while in the health care facility. Children, the elderly, and extended care hospital patients are populations most frequently singled out for pet therapy programs. These individuals may benefit from improved mental health by enhancing wellness and contact with familiar living things from home and thus reduce feelings of isolation and loneliness. Pets also help to teach a sense of responsibility. Unfortunately, objective means of measuring these benefits have not yet been developed. Therefore, while there are several potentially positive therapeutic effects pets can have on hospitalized patients, hospitals utilizing pets must take precautions to insure the safety of all patients and remain in compliance with federal and state licensure regulations. In many states, it is illegal to bring animals other than seeing eye dogs and those used in research into the health facility.

If the use of pets in the hospital setting is considered, one must remember that pets may be vehicles for diseases. They may also initiate allergic reactions in some individuals; may cause accidents; unpleasant odors may result; and they may infringe on other patients' rights. Animals brought into a strange new environment may not act as they normally do in more familiar surroundings. Therefore, any program utilizing pet animals must assure that all patients, hospital staff, and visitors are protected from these possible complications.

There are many microorganisms, including bacteria, virus, fungi, and parasites, associated with animals commonly used as pets. The microorganisms, disease state, mode of transmission, and animals most commonly involved are listed in Table 26.6 (92–108).

Table 26.6.
Bacterial, Viral, Parasitic and Mycotoic Zoonoses

Agent	Disease	Transmission	Reservoir
Bacterial, Viral, Parasitic and Mycotoic Zoonoses			
Pasteurella multocida P. haemolytica P. pneumotropica	Pasteurellosis Pneumonia Septicemia Otitis Gastroenteritis Meningitis (rare)	Aerosol Direct contact Inoculation through bites and scratches	Dog (79.5% of tonsils of dogs) Cats (90% of gumlines of cats)
Yersinia pestis	Bacteremia Pneumonia Bubonic plague	Infected fleas Airborne	Rodents Rabbits
Francisella tularensis	Tularemia	Inhalation Inoculation for bite or scratch Direct contact	Rabbits Rodents
Salmonella spp.	Salmonellosis Gastroenteritis (70%) Septicemia (8–10%) Focal infection (8–10%)	Direct contact May also be fomite aerial and dustborne	Dogs Turtles (85% colonized) Rabbits Reptiles Chicks
Shigella spp.	Shigellosis (bacillary dysentery)	Transmission occurs from feces via fomites	Dogs Rodents
Brucella canis	Brucellosis	Direct contact	Dogs Cats
Yersinia pseudotuberculosis Yersinia entericolitica	Acute mesenteric lymphadenitis Enteritis Erythema nodosum Septicemia (rare)	Direct or indirect contact	Cat Dog Guinea-pig[a] Hamster Rabbit[a]
Spirillum minus Streptobacillus moniliformis	Rabbit bite fever	Rodent bite	Rat Mouse
Rickettsia rickettsi	Rocky Mountain spotted fever	Tick bite	Rodents Dogs Rabbits

[a]Most frequently affected.

Table 26.6, cont.

Agent	Disease	Transmission	Reservoir
Rickettsia prowazeki	Epidemic Typhus	Infected louse feces into broken skin	Rodents
Coxiella burnetti	Q fever	Inhalation of infectious aerosol, tick bite	Rodents Dogs Cats
Leptospira icterohae-morrhagiade	Leptospiroisi	Direct contact Immersion exposure	Dogs Almost all mammals and nonmammals

Group A β-hemolytic streptococcal infections	Pharyngitis
	Long-term risks
	  rheumatic heart disease
	  glomerulonephritis
	  scarlet fever
		Droplet	Dogs
			Cats

Chlamydia psittaci	Chlamydiosis	Airborne Contact	Cats
Viral Zoonoses Arenovirus (LCM)	Lymphocytic Chorio-meningitis	Host excretions and secretions	Rodents Swine
Virus	Rabies	Bites of infected animals	Dogs
Unknown	Cat Scratch Disease	Cat scratch	Cats
Parasitic Zoonoses Various species of mites	Acariasis	Contact with infested animal or environment	Cats Dogs
Various species of ticks	Tick Paralysis	Tick bite	Dogs
Stenocephalides spp. *Noropsyllus spp.* *Pulex spp.*	Flea bite dermatitis	Contact with infested animal or environment	Dogs Cats Rodents

Mycotic Zoonosis
  Curvularia geniculata
  Curvularia lunata
	Eumycotic Mycetoma	Contact	Dogs

Helminthosporium speciferum	Eumycotic Mycetoma	Contact	Cats
Emmonsia parva *Emmonsia crecens*	Adiaspiromycosis	Contact	Rodents
Microsporum canis *M. distortum* *Trichophyton erinacei* *T. mentagrophytes*	Dermatomycoses Ringworm	Direct contact	Kittens Cats Dogs Rodents
Histoplasma capsulatum	Histoplasmosis	Inhalation, contact	Dogs Cats
Sporothrix schenkii	Sporotrichosis	Break in skin	Dogs Cats
Blastomyces dermatitidis	Blastomycosis	Contact	Dogs Cats
Coccidiodes immitis	Coccidioidomycosis	Contact Airborne	Dogs Rodents
Aspergillus spp.	Aspergillosis	Contact	Dogs Cats Mammals

Two recent studies from Arkansas confirm the bacterial flora of several different animals commonly used as pet therapy and pet lending programs.

In the first study, animals from a local museum and used in a pet lending program were cultured both at the museum (pet's home environment) and upon arrival at the hospital. All animals were colonized with multiple bacterial agents, and some of these microorganisms were potentially significant in the hospital setting. However, the most intriguing finding in this study was the isolation of *Salmonella* spp. from numerous animals which were culture-negative for the same bacteria in their home environment, but became culture-positive following transportation across town. The investigators postulated that the stress of transportation, additional handling, and unfamiliar surroundings activated latent *Salmonella*. This phenomenon is well-known in the cattle and swine industry. An added point of interest was the lack of bacteria recovered from tarantulas (109).

The second study examined the bacterial flora of dogs and cats that were healthy, asymptomatic pets, rarely allowed out of the home. Again, multiple bacteria were recovered from all pets tested and included agents capable of causing disease in even healthy individuals. Of concern was the recovery of methicillin-resistant *Staphylococcus aureus* from pets with no history of exposure to hospital or medical personnel or other sources of this microorganism (T. Yamauchi, unpublished observation).

With this background information, hospitals considering the use of pets or other animals within the health care facility must carefully weigh the potential benefits of pet therapy with the potential risks of exposure of each and every patient, visitor, and staff member within the hospital.

If the hospital administration decides that pet therapy is an acceptable risk, strict guidelines must be formulated before the animals are ever brought into the health care facility. Persons involved in developing these guidelines should include hospital administrator, infection control professional, practicing veterinarian, infectious disease specialist, and individuals using the animals within the hospital. Until further information is available, it seems prudent to limit the area and patient exposure in which pets can be used in the hospital setting.

REFERENCES

1. Semmelweis IP: Classics in infectious diseases: childbed fever. *Rev Infect Dis* 3:808–811, 1981.
2. Miller PJ: Semmelweis. *Infect Control* 3:405–409, 1982.
3. Haley RW: The "hospital epidemiologist" in U.S. hospitals, 1976–1977. A description of the head of the infection surveillance and control program. *Infect Control* 1:21–32, 1980.
4. Wenzel K: The role of the infection control nurse. *Nurs Clin North Am* 5:89–98, 1970.
5. Pope R: Control and prevention in occupational health: the nurse's role. *Occup Health Nurs* 29:12–14, 1981.
6. Eickhoff TC: Hospital epidemiology: an emerging discipline. In Remington JS, Swartz MD (eds): *Current Clinical Topics in Infectious Diseases.* New York, McGraw-Hill, 1984, p 241.
7. Chavigny KH: Professional ethics for infection control: the changing role of the infection control practitioners. *Am J Infect Control* 13:183–188, 1985.
8. Hierholzer WJ: The practice of hospital epidemiology. *Yale J Biol Med* 55:223–230, 1982.
9. Booth AL, Weeks RM, Hutcherson RH, Jr., Schaffner W: A statewide characterization of hospital infection control practices and practitioners. *Infect Control* 1:227–232, 1981.
10. McArthur BJ, Pugliese G, Weinstein S, Shannon R, Lynch P, Jackson MM, Tsinzo M, Serky J, McGuire N: A national task analysis of infection control practitioners, 1982. Part one: methodology and demography. *Am J Infect Control* 12:88–95, 1984.
11. Nottebart HC, Jr.: Infection control committee records. *Infect Control* 1:47–49, 1980.
12. Nottebart HC, Jr.: Infection control committee minutes-revisited. *Infect Control* 5:295–297, 1984.
13. Haley RW, Shachtma RH: The emergence of infection surveillance and control programs in U.S. hospitals: an assessment, 1976. *Am J Epidemiol* 111:574–591, 1980.
14. Haley RW, Culver DH, White JW, Morgan TM, Emori TG, Munn VP, Hooten TM: The efficacy of infection surveillance and control programs in preventing nosocomial infections in U.S. hospitals. *Am J Epidemiol* 121:182–205, 1985.
15. Centers for Disease Control: Infection surveillance and control programs in U.S. hospitals: an assessment, 1976. *MMWR* 27:139–145, 1978.
16. Jarvis WR, White JW, Munn VP, Mosser JL, Emori TG, Culver DH, Thornsberry C, Hughes JM: Nosocomial infection surveillance, 1983. *MMWR* 33(suppl 255):9SS–22SS, 1984.
17. Joint Commission on Accreditation of Hospitals: *Accreditation Manual for Hospitals.* Chicago, Joint Commission on Accreditation of Hospitals, 1976.
18. Centers for Disease Control: Outline for Surveillance and Control of Nosocomial Infections. Atlanta, Centers for Disease Control, 1972.
19. Haley RW: Surveillance by objective: a new priority-directed approach to the control of nosocomial infections. *Am J Infect Control* 13:78–89, 1985.
20. Emori TG, Haley RW, Garner JS: Techniques and uses of nosocomial infection surveillance in U.S. hospitals, 1976–1977. *Am J Med* 70:933–940, 1981.
21. Wenzel RP: Surveillance and reporting of hospital acquired infections. In Wenzel RP (ed): *Handbook of Hospital Acquired Infection.* Boca Raton, FL, CRC Press, 1981, pp 35–72.
22. Wenzel RP, Osterman CA, Hunting KJ, Gwaltney JM, Jr.: Hospital-acquired infections. I. Surveillance in a university hospital *Am J Epidemiol* 103:251–260, 1976.
23. Fuchs PC, Gustafson ME: Inter-relationship of clinical microbiology and infection control. *Lab Med* 10:22–25, 1979.
24. Yamauchi T, Eisenach KD: Team surveillance: a working model in a small hospital. *Am J Infect Control* 7:32–33, 1979.
25. Furr S, Jackson M, Yamauchi T: Nosocomial grand rounds: an innovative approach to inservice education. *Am J Infect Control* 9:47A, 1981.
26. Valenti WM, Dorn MR, Andrews BP, Presley BA, Reifler CB: Infection control and employee health: epidemiology and

priorities for program development. *Am J Infect Control* 10:149–153, 1982.

27. Haley RW, Emori TG: The employee health service and infection control in U.S. hospitals, 1976–1977, I. Screening procedures. *JAMA* 246:844–847, 1981.

28. Haley RW, Emori TG: The employee health service and infection control in U.S. hospitals, 1976–1977. II. Managing employee illness. *JAMA* 246:962–966, 1981.

29. Klein JO: Management of infections in hospital employees. *Am J Med* 70:919–923, 1981.

30. Hall CB: Nosocomial viral respiratory infections: perennial weeds on pediatric wards. *Am J Med* 70:670–676, 1981.

31. Wenzel, RP, Deal EC, Hendley JO: Hospital-acquired viral respiratory illness on a pediatric ward. *Pediatrics* 60:367–371, 1977.

32. Douglas RGJ, Betts RF, Huska J, Hall CB: Epidemiology of nosocomial viral infections. In Weinstein L, Remington J (eds): *Seminars in Infectious Diseases*. New York, Grune & Stratton, 1979, pp 98–144.

33. Hall CB, Douglas RG, Jr.: Nosocomial influenza as a cause of intercurrent fever in infants. *Pediatrics* 55:673–677, 1975.

34. Gardner PS, Court SDM, Brocklebank JT, Downham MAPS, Weightman D: Virus cross-infection in pediatric wards. *Br Med J* 2:571–575, 1973.

35. Centers for Disease Control: Recommendations of the Immunization Practices Advisory Committee (ACIP): prevention and control of influenza. *MMWR* 34:261–268, 273–275, 1985.

36. Riddiough MA, Sisk JE, Bell JC: Influenza vaccination: cost-effectiveness and public policy. *JAMA* 249:3189–3195, 1983.

37. Bailowitz A, Kaslow RA: Use of amantadine in the United States, 1977–1982. *J Infect Dis* 151:372–373, 1985.

38. Centers for Disease Control: Recommendations of the Immunization Practices Advisory Committee (ACIP): diphtheria, tetanus, pertussis: guidelines for vaccine prophylaxis and other preventive measures. *MMWR* 34:405–414, 419–426, 1985.

39. Centers for Disease Control: Recommendation of the Immunization Practices Advisory Committee (ACIP): measles prevention. *MMWR* 31:217–224, 229–231, 1982.

40. Nolan TF, Jr., Goodman RA, Patriarca PA, Hinman AR: Hospitalizations for measles, 1970–78. *Am J Public Health* 72:1037–1039, 1982.

41. Krause PS, Cherry JD, Desada-Tous S, Champion JG, Strassburg M, Sullivan C, Spencer MJ, Bryson YJ, Welliver RC, Boyer KM: Epidemic measles in young adults: clinical, epidemiologic and serologic studies. *Ann Intern Med* 90:873–876, 1979.

42. Centers for Disease Control: Measles in medical settings—United States. *MMWR* 30:125–126, 1981.

43. Seavy D, Moloy M, Dasco C, Anderson D, Feigen R: Nosocomial measles in a children's hospital transmitted by adult health care personnel (abstract). *Am J Infect Control* 10:111–112, 1984.

44. Davis RM, Orenstein WA, Frank JA, Jr., Sacks JJ, Dales LG, Preblud SR, Bart KJ, Williams NM, Hinman AR: Transmission of measles in medical settings, 1980 through 1984. *JAMA* 255:1295–1298, 1986.

45. Centers for Disease Control: Mumps—United States, 1980–1983. *MMWR* 32:545–547, 1983.

46. Centers for Disease Control: Recommendations of the Immunization Practices Advisory Committee (ACIP): mumps vaccine. *MMWR* 31:617–620, 1982.

47. Chappell JA, Taylor MAH: Implications of rubella susceptibility in young adults. *Am J Public Health* 69:279–281, 1979.

48. Robinson RG, Dudenhoeffer FE, Holyroyd HJ, Baker LR, Bernstein DI, Cherry JD: Rubella immunity in older children, teenagers and young adults: a comparison of immunity in those immunized with those unimmunized. *J Pediatr* 101:188–191, 1982.

49. Schonberger LB, Kaplan J, Kim-Farly R, Moore M, Eddins DL, Hatch M: Control of paralytic poliomyelitis in the United States. *Rev Infect Dis* 6(suppl):S424–S426, 1984.

50. Nathanson N: Eradication of poliomyelitis in the United States. *Rev Infect Dis* 4:940–950, 1982.

51. Kim-Farley RJ, Bart KJ, Schonberger LB, Ovenstein WA, Nkowane BM, Hinman AR, Kew OM, Hatch MH, Kaplan JE: Poliomyelitis in the USA: virtual elimination of disease caused by wild virus. *Lancet* 2:1315–1317, 1984.

52. McBean AM, Thomas ML, Johnson RH, Gadless BR, MacDonald B, Verhood L, Cummins P, Hughes J, Kimnear J, Watts C, Kraft M, Albaecht P, Boone EJ, Moore M, Frank JA, Jr., Bernier R: A comparison of the serologic responses to oral and injectable trivalent polio vaccines. *Rev Infect Dis* 6(suppl):S552–S555, 1984.

53. Centers for Disease Control: Recommendations of the Immunization Practices Advisory Committee (ACIP): poliomyelitis prevention. *MMWR* 31:22–26, 31–34, 1982.

54. Kurt TL, Yeager DS, Guenette S, Dunlop S: Spread of pertussis by hospital staff. *JAMA* 221:264–267, 1972.

55. Valenti WM, Pincus PH, Messner MK: Nosocomial pertussis: possible spread by a hospital visitor. *Am J Dis Child* 134:520–521, 1980.

56. Linnemann CC, Jr., Ramundo N, Perlstein PH, Minton SD, Englender GS, McCormick JB, Hayes PS: Use of pertussis vaccine in an epidemic involving hospital staff. *Lancet* 2:540–543, 1975.

57. Centers for Disease Control: Recommendations of the Immunization Practices Advisory Committee. Inactivated hepatitis B vaccine. *MMWR* 31:317–322, 327–328, 1982.

58. Centers for Disease Control: Recommendations for protection against viral hepatitis. *MMWR* 34:313–324, 329–335, 1985.

59. Dienstaz JL, Werner BG, Polk BG, Snyderman DR, Craven DE, Platt R, Crumpacker CS, Ovellet-Hellstrom R, Grady GF: Hepatitis B vaccine in health care personnel: safety, immunogenicity, and indications of efficacy. *Ann Intern Med* 101:35–40, 1984.

60. American Hospital Association: Hepatitis B vaccine recommendations for hospital employees. October 1982. *Infect Control* 4:41–43, 1983.

61. Siegel M: Congenital malformations following chickenpox, measles, mumps, and hepatitis. Results of a cohort study. *JAMA* 226:1521–1524, 1973.

62. Siegel M, Fuerst HT, Peress NS: Comparative fetal mortality in maternal virus diseases. A prospective study of rubella, measles, mumps, chickenpox and hepatitis. *N Engl J Med* 274:768–771, 1966.

63. Brown, GC, Karumas RS: Relationship of congenital anomalies and maternal infection with selected enteroviruses. *Am J Epidemiol* 95:207–217, 1972.

64. Modlin JF, Polk BF, Horton P, Etkind P, Crane E, Spiliotes A: Perinatal echovirus infection: risk of transmission during a community outbreak. *N Engl J Med* 305:367–371, 1981.

65. Desmouths G, Conveur J: Congenital toxoplasmosis. A prospective study of 378 pregnancies. *N Engl J Med* 290:1110–1116, 1974.

66. Savage MO, Moosa A, Gordon RR: Maternal varicella infection as a cause of fetal malformations. *Lancet* 1:352–354, 1973.

67. Monif GRG, Egan EA, Held B, Eitzman DV: The correlation of maternal cytomegalovirus infection during varying states in gestation with neonatal involvement. *J Peditr* 80:17–20, 1972.

68. Stern H, Tucker SM: Prospective study of cytomegalovirus infection in pregnancy. *Br Med J* 2:268–270, 1973.

69. Grant S, Edmond E, Syme J: A prospective study of cytomegalovirus infection in pregnancy. I. Laboratory evidence of congenital infection following maternal primary and reactivated infection. *J Infect* 3:24–31, 1981.

70. Valenti WN, Hruska JF, Menegus MA, Freeburn MJ: Nosocomial viral infections. III. Guidelines for prevention and control of exanthematous viruses, gastroenteritis viruses, picornaviruses, and uncommonly seen viruses. *Infect Control* 2:38–49, 1981.

71. Nahmias AJ, Josey WE, Naib ZM: Significance of herpes

simplex virus infection during pregnancy. *Clin Obstet Gynecol* 15:929–938, 1972.

72. Nahmias AJ, Alford CA, Korones SB: Infection of the newborn with Herpesvirus hominis. *Adv Pediatr* 17:185–226, 1970.
73. Mann JM, Preblud SR, Hoffman RE, Brandling-Bennett AD, Hinman AR, Heymann KL: Assessing risks of rubella infection during pregnancy. A standardized approach. *JAMA* 245:1847–1852, 1981.
74. Votra EM, Rutala WA, Sarubbi FA: Recommendations for pregnant employee interaction with patients having communicable infections disease. *Am J Infect Control* 11:10–19, 1983.
75. Valenti WM: Infection control and the pregnant health care worker. *Am J Infect Control* 14:20–27, 1986.
76. McManus WF, Goodwin CW, Mason AD, Jr., Pruitt BA, Jr.: Burn wound infection. *J Trauma* 21:753–756, 1981.
77. Pruitt BA, Jr.: The diagnosis and treatment of infection in the burn patient. *Burns* 11:79–91, 1984.
78. Pruitt BA, Jr., Lindbery RB, McManus WF, Mason AD, Jr.: Current approach to prevention and treatment of *Pseudomonas aeruginosa* infections in burned patients. *Rev Infect Dis* 5(suppl): S889–S897, 1983.
79. Knittle MA, Eitzman DV, Baer HP: Role of hand contamination of personnel in the epidemiology of gram-negative nosocomial infections. *J Pediatr* 86:433–437, 1975.
80. Shulman JA, Terry PM, Hough EC: Colonization with gentamicin-resistant *Pseudomonas aeruginosa*, pyocine type 5, in a burn unit. *J Infect Dis* 124(suppl):518–523, 1971.
81. Fujita K, Lilly HA, Kidson A, Dyliffe GAJ: Gentamicin-resistant *Pseudomonas aeruginosa* infection from mattresses in a burns unit. *Br Med J* 283:219–220, 1981.
82. Plotkin SA, Stan SE: Symposium on perinatal infections. *Clin Perinatol* 8:617–637, 1981.
83. Hemming VQ, Overall JC, Britt MR: Nosocomial infections in a newborn intensive care unit: results of forty-one months of surveillance. *N Engl J Med* 294:1310–1316, 1976.
84. Goldmann DA, Leclair J, Macone A: Bacterial colonization of neonates admitted to an intensive care environment. *J Pediatr* 93:288–293, 1978.
85. Franco JA, Eitzman DV, Baer H: Antibiotic usage and microbial resistance in an intensive care nursery. *Am J Dis Child* 126:318–321, 1974.
86. Nahmias AJ, Eickhoff TC: Staphylococcal infections in hospitals: recent developments in epidemiologic and laboratory investigation. *N Eng J Med* 265:74–81, 120–128, 177–182, 1961.
87. Wolinsky E, Lipsitz PJ, Mortimer EA, Jr., Rammelkamp CH, Jr.: Acquisition of staphylococci by newborns. Direct versus indirect transmission. *Lancet* 2:620–622, 1960.
88. Adler JL, Shulman, JA, Terry PM, Feldman DB, Skaliz P: Nosocomial colonization with kanamycin-resistant *Klebsiella pneumoniae*, types 2 and 11, in a premature nursery. *J Pediatr* 77:376–385, 1970.
89. Kaslow RA, Taylor A, Jr., Dweck HS, Bobo RA, Steele CD, Cassady G, Jr.: Enteropathogenic *Escherichia coli* infection in a newborn nursery. *Am J Dis Child* 128:797–801, 1974.
90. Burke JP, Ingall D, Klein JO, GEzon HM, Finland M: *Proteus mirabilis* infections in a hospital nursery traced to a human carrier. *N Engl J Med* 284:115–121, 1971.
91. Watt J, Wegman, ME, Brown OW, Schliessman DJ, Maupin E, Hemphill EC: Salmonellosis in a premature nursery unaccompanied by diarrheal disease. *Pediatrics* 22:689–705, 1958.
92. Goscienski PJ: Zoonoses. *Ped Infect Dis* 2:69–81, 1983.
93. Schantz PM: Toxocariasis in dogs and humans. *Calif Vet* 7:17–18, 1981.
94. Hirsch MS, Moellering RC, Pope HG, Poskanzer DC: Lymphocytic-choriomeningitis-virus infection traced to a pet hamster. *N Engl J Med* 291:610–612, 1974.
95. Boyer KM, Cherry JD: Cat scratch disease. Feigin RD and Cherry JQ (eds): *Textbook of Pediatric Infectious Disease*. Philadelphia, WB Saunders, 1981, pp 1649–1654.
96. Gutman LT, Ottesen EA, Quan TJ, Noce PS, Katz SL: An intra-familial outbreak of Yersinia enterocolitica. *N Engl J Med* 288:1372–1377, 1973.
97. U.S. Department of Health Education and Welfare, Centers for Disease Control: Epidemiological aspects of some of the zoonoses. DHEW Publication No. (HSM) 73-8182, January, 1972.
98. Hubbert WT, McCulloch WF, Schnurrenberger PR (eds): *Disease Transmitted from Animals to Man*, ed 6. Springfield, IL, Charles C Thomas, 1975.
99. Marcy SM: Infections due to dog and cat bites. *Pediatr Infect Dis* 1:351–356, 1982.
100. Fox JG, Zanotti S: The hamster as a reservoir of *Camphylobacter fetus* subspecies *jejuni*. *J Infect Dis* 143:856, 1981.
101. Keymer JF: The unsuitability of nondomesticated animals as pets. *Vet Rec* 91:373–381, 1972.
102. Feigin RD, Lobes LA, Jr., Anderson D, Pickering LK: Human leptospirosis from immunized dogs. *Ann Intern Med* 79:777–785, 1973.
103. Bailie WE, Stowe EC, Schmitt AM: Aerobic bacterial flora of oral and nasal fluids of canines with reference to bacteria associated with bites. *J Clin Microbiol* 7:233–231, 1978.
104. Centers for Disease Control: Tularemia associated with domestic cats: Georgia, New Mexico. *MMWR* 31:39–41, 1982.
105. Reif JS, Marshak RR: Leptospirosis: A contemporary zoonosis. *Ann Intern Med* 79:893–894, 1973.
106. Baker EF, Jr., Anderson HW, Allard J: Epidemiological aspects of turtle-associated salmonellosis. *Arch Environ Health* 24:1–9, 1972.
107. Torphy DE, Bond WW: Campylobacter fetus infections in children. *Pediatrics* 64:898–902, 1979.
108. Frenkel JK, Dubey JP: Toxoplasmosis and its prevention in cats and man. *J Infect Dis* 126:664–673, 1972.
109. Yamauchi T, Baeyens MM, McCoy J, Carter D: The microflora of animals used in hospital pet therapy: is there patient risk? *Clin Res* 32:880A, 1984.

27

Microbiologic Aspects of Infection Control

Donald A. Goldmann, M.D.

INTRODUCTION

Infection control without high-quality microbiological support is unthinkable. More often than not, the first clue that there is a nosocomial infection problem comes from the clinical laboratory, and a visit to the laboratory is an integral part of the infection control practitioner's daily surveillance rounds. Epidemic investigation is impossible without prompt, accurate, reproducible microbiology data. Special infection control studies almost always depend on the good will and assistance of the laboratory director, and a successful relationship between laboratory and infection control staffs requires close cooperation, mutual understanding, and excellent communication. Infection control and microbiology are like partners at a dance: the failure of the partners to anticipate each other's next step and to be sensitive to their mutual abilities and limitations inevitably leads to bruised toes, damaged egos, and a stumbling performance.

Unfortunately, in the United States, infection control and microbiology laboratory personnel often enter the ballroom from opposite doors, and if they do manage to get together, they usually find that they don't know the same dances. The majority of American laboratory directors are clinical pathologists who have had little training and experience in infection control. Many are used to working in relative isolation; the laboratory receives specimens and sends out results with little regard for the concerns of more clinically oriented members of the hospital staff. In some hospitals, the relationship between microbiology and the clinician is, frankly, adversarial, and infectious disease physicians and hospital epidemiologists may be seen as rivals in a struggle for an important chunk of hospital turf. The situation seems to be improving as laboratory directors seek to build bridges to clinical departments, and there has been an encouraging trend to include infection control seminars in clinical pathology professional meetings. In a few cases, infectious disease specialists or hospital epidemiologists have acquired formal consulting positions in the laboratory, and in some institutions, they have even assumed the responsibilities of laboratory director. This may appear to be the ideal situation from the infection control point of view, but it is only fair to point out that many hospital epidemiologists are as ignorant about clinical microbiology as clinical pathologists are about infection control, and infectious disease specialists generally have received little training in either microbiology or infection control.

Perhaps American hospital epidemiologists and laboratory directors could learn important lessons from their British counterparts. In Great Britain, clinical microbiologists receive superb, intensive training in the more clinical aspects of their craft. On the one hand, the microbiologist is thoroughly schooled in the proper collection, transport, and processing of clinical specimens, and in the interpretation of culture results, so the information derived from cultures is likely to be maximally useful to both the infection control "sister" and the physicians caring for the patient. On the other hand, British clinical microbiologists recognize the epidemiological significance of the microorganisms isolated in their laboratory. They know the microorganism's ecological niche in the hospital, and how they are transmitted from patient to patient. A cluster of unusual isolates or important trends in antibiotic resistance are likely to be recognized quickly in the laboratory, so that a timely investigation can begin. In addition, clinical microbiologists take the meaning of their title literally and have the training, confidence, and trust to visit the wards as clinical consultants

ants to take an active role in the investigation of infection control problems.

If there is a weakness in the British system, it is the failure to provide the clinical microbiologist with training and experience in epidemiology and biostatistics. At the extreme, British microbiologists focus on organisms instead of patients, and this can lead to overzealous culturing of the environment, patients, and personnel, instead of careful infection surveillance and sound epidemiological investigation.

The relative lack of training that the American microbiologist and hospital epidemiologist receive in each other's specialty is even more evident at the level of the technologist and infection control practitioner. Medical technology training does not stress infection control or epidemiology (although some instruction concerning the pathophysiology and clinical manifestations of infectious diseases is provided). Most infection control practitioners are nurses who have had only rudimentary clinical microbiology training in nursing school.

Given the disparate backgrounds of clinical laboratory and infection control personnel, it is remarkable that excellent, productive working relationships have been established in so many hospitals. How do these programs bridge the chasm that separates them initially? Clearly, the approach must be individualized to the particular circumstances in each hospital, but some strategies are likely to be useful wherever they are applied. The most critical first step is to include a representative from the clinical laboratory on the infection control committee. In addition to satisfying the surveyor from the Joint Commission on Accreditation of Hospitals, he or she will be able to grapple firsthand with the practical problems of hospital epidemiology. The microbiologist will be in a position to advise the committee regarding the appropriate and parctical microbiological approach to a given infection control problem and will be able to plan for the corresponding allocation of laboratory resources needed to accomplish the committee's objectives. For their part, the other members of the committee and the infection control team will learn how to use the resources of the laboratory more effectively. It will become apparent, for example, that the microbiologist will be able to suggest epidemiologically useful laboratory techniques that may be unfa-

miliar to the infection control staff. The committee will soon realize that the resources of the laboratory are not inexhaustible, particularly in the current era of prospective payment and health care retrenchment when laboratory productivity and cost-effectiveness are being so closely scrutinized.

Since it is almost always inappropriate to charge patients for the cost of cultures ordered for infection control purposes, and since there is no mechanism under prospective payment for reimbursing the hospital for these cultures, regardless of how they are billed, the materials and personnel time devoted to infection control are a dead loss in the laboratory's budget. Therefore, special cultures should be ordered only if their potential value can be clearly defined. In general, requests for such cultures will be greeted more objectively by the laboratory director if the hospital designates a separate cost center for infection control microbiology. In allocating these funds, it is important to recognize the unpredictabilty of infection control problems. Although a few procedures, such as microbiological monitoring of sterilizers, have a foreseeable, relatively constant impact on the laboratory, there is no way to predict whether an outbreak of methicillin-resistant *Staphylococcus aureus* in intensive care will require widespread, long-term screening of patients and personnel. Therefore, the budget must have built-in flexibility.

The microbiology laboratory director sets laboratory policy, but it is the technologists who perform the tests requested by infection control and communicate with the infection control team on a day-to-day basis. A few large referral institutions have facilitated the interaction between technologists and infection control staff by setting up a separate, relatively independent infection control laboratory. However, it is difficult to staff, equip, and operate such small, freestanding laboratories. An appealing alternative is to designate an interested technologist to serve as the primary liaison to infection control and to attend infection control committee meetings. This approach can dramatically improve communication and efficiency.

It is obvious that the members of the infection control team can build good relationships with microbiology personnel if they visit the laboratory regularly to examine culture results, ask questions, and, most importantly, vent their problems and concerns. The computer terminal, while undeniably improving access to microbiology results, is a menace in this regard. The practitioner who can review computerized data in the comfort of his or her office or while working on the wards is likely to visit the laboratory less often. As an antidote to this dangerous trend, some laboratory directors have scheduled brief, routine daily rounds with infection control personnel to review pertinent results and set the agenda for the day's work. If the hospital has an infectious disease service, rounds can be enhanced and communication facilitated by asking the infectious disease consultant to attend on a regular basis. At the very least, periodic educational conferences should be scheduled to discuss important infection control problems and the relevant microbiology in depth.

REPORTING AND STORING DATA

No matter how well the microbiology laboratory performs its technical work, the infection control team will be at a great disadvantage if results are not made available in a timely, well-organized fashion. Some results are so critical that they should be phoned directly to the infection control practitioner as soon as they are ready. Although technologists should be encouraged to call infection control whenever they encounter a particularly alarming organism, it is best to decide on formal criteria for telephone reporting in advance and to modify them as necessary. For example, the infection control team may request that it be notified immediately when methicillin-resistant coagulase-negative staphylococci are isolated from any clinical specimen, *Salmonella* is recovered from the stool of a hospitalized patient, *S. aureus* is found in a surgical wound, or acid-fast bacilli are seen on a sputum smear. Additional requests will depend on the nature of the infections that are of particular concern to infection control at the time.

Routine reporting has been greatly facilitated by computerization of hospital laboratories. However, let the buyer beware, commercially available packaged systems are seldom designed with the epidemiologist in mind. In fact, most systems are geared to the relatively simple requirements of clinical chemistry and are not designed primarily to handle the more complex data base of the microbiology laboratory, let

alone to meet the demands of hospital epidemiology. Therefore, when the microbiology laboratory director begins negotiations with the hospital information department or with outside vendors for a computer system, the infection control team should be consulted early on in the process.

Careful attention should be paid to the data elements that will be stored by the computer. If potentially useful data are not entered initially, retrieval at a later date will be arduous, if not impossible, and the computer will have failed to perform its principal service. At the minimum, the following information should be recorded: patient name, hospital number, ward location, service, physician (this may be of little value in teaching hospitals where there are multiple responsible physicians who rotate frequently), type of specimen and culture site, date of specimen collection, organism(s) isolated (including "biotype" number, if available), and complete antibiotic susceptibility pattern (preferably including disc diffusion testing zone diameters or minimal inhibitory concentrations, if available). Since these data will be the foundation of all future epidemiological analyses, it is critical that repeated isolations of the same organism from the same site in a single patient be excluded so that the data base contains only "unique" isolates. This is necessary because patients with unusual pathogens or antibiotic-resistant organisms tend to be cultured repeatedly, thus skewing the data base toward these more notable isolates. As a result, the infection control team will receive reports that overemphasize the importance of certain microorganisms, and clinicians will conclude that the nosocomial strains in their hospital are, on the average, more resistant then they really are. Creating a computerized file of "unique" isolates is a complex, but certainly feasible programming task. The infection control team and microbiologists actually have the more difficult job of choosing reasonable criteria for defining an isolate as "unique." At the Children's Hospital in Boston, organisms are considered to be unique if they are not of the same species. If two organisms of the same species are isolated from a single site, they are classified arbitrarily as different if the minimal inhibitory concentrations of two or more antibiotics differ by 2 tube dilutions, or if the minimal inhibitory concentration of a single agent differs by ≥ 3 tube dilutions. Results of biotyping are not taken into account. These criteria are arbitrary, but have proved to be practical over a period of more than 3 years.

Computerized data should be readily retrievable for at least 15 months. This provides the infection control team with a long-term, seasonally adjusted baseline against which to evaluate current trends or outbreaks. Preferably, data from as long a period as possible should be kept on-line or in accessible data files, and infection control or microbiology staff should be familiar with the operation of software that can retrieve and manipulate the data base. Current technology permits great flexibility and individuality in the tabulation and analysis of microbiological data, and each infection control program should tailor its computer requests to its own needs. Many programs find it useful to generate tables summarizing the occurrence of specific site-pathogen, ward-pathogen, service-pathogen, and site-service combinations. Antibiotic susceptibility tables help the infection control team monitor the emergence of resistant nosocomial strains and guide the clinician in the choice of empiric antibiotic therapy. In outbreak investigations, it is important to be able to obtain a line listing of all isolates having specific epidemiologically relevant characteristics (e.g., specific species, antibiotic resistance pattern, isolation from a specific ward). Such line listings insure complete case-finding and serve as the basis for more refined analyses based on data obtained from patient records.

The Centers for Disease Control and a few hospitals have developed programs that can alert the infection control team when the incidence of a specific pathogen exceeds an arbitrary statistical threshold, based on prior experience with the organism in the institution. However, such programs are prone to issuing false alarms if the threshold is set too low, leading to needless labor by already overworked infection control teams. On the other hand, if the threshold is set too high, important events may be missed by epidemiologists lulled into complacency by the soft hum of the computer.

This emphasis on computerized analysis of microbiological data may be surprising to hospital epidemiologists and infection control practitioners who have followed diligently the bedside surveillance espoused by the Centers for Disease Control (1). After all, a positive culture might have been obtained from a patient with a nosocomial or community-acquired infection or from a patient who merely is colonized with the organism. The microbiology laboratory can increase the value of the culture report by separating out cultures obtained from patients who have been in the hospital for at least 48 hours, since strains recovered from these cultures are more likely to be hospital acquired. The number of positive cultures that reflect colonization rather than infection can be reduced by educating physicians and nurses in proper culturing techniques. Specimens that are clearly unsatisfactory, such as bag urine cultures and sputum specimens that contain epithelial cells on Gram strain, can be rejected at the planting bench (2), although uncontaminated clinical material is harder to obtain from young children than from adults.

But no matter how carefully specimens are collected and results reported, no one would argue that microbiological data can replace surveillance rounds by a clinically astute infection control staff, and epidemiological decisions should rarely be made on the basis of laboratory data alone. On the other hand, it is an error to disregard the results of contaminated cultures entirely. The transmission of potentially dangerous nosocomial pathogens on the wards of the hospital may be apparent in such culture material long before the first serious hospital-acquired infections occur. For example, the spread of a particularly antibiotic-resistant strain of *Pseudomonas aeruginosa* on the oncology ward of The Children's Hospital was detected when improperly obtained clean-catch urine specimens grew the organism. It is also important to note that more than 80% of nosocomial infections can be identified by reviewing laboratory reports (3).

It would be incorrect to assume that computerization of microbiology data is essential, and small hospitals may not find computers to be cost-effective. A well-organized manual data storage and retrieval system can be an extremely valuable resource. However, a box full of unorganized reports sitting in an off-site warehouse is an epidemiologist's nightmare.

While many laboratories have improved data storage and retrieval, few have paid equal attention to saving bacterial strains of potential importance to the infection control program. Often, isolates are discarded as soon as the laboratory report is finalized. This is a disservice to both clinicians and infection control staff. If possible, isolates should be saved on plates or slants for up to 7 days in case the physician decides that further workup or sensitivity testing is required. For example, the recovery of *Bacillus* from clinical specimens usually indicates contamination of the specimen, and full identification and susceptibility testing may be neither necessary nor practical initially. However, *Bacillus* does cause serious infections in critically ill immunosuppressed patients (4), and the physician should be given the opportunity to reflect on the culture result and request additional testing on the isolate. Likewise, the importance of a microbiological report might not be immediately obvious to the infection control team, but subsequent developments might suggest the need to save the isolate in order to perform more definitive typing procedures.

Outbreaks cannot be predicted in advance, and all too often, critical isolates are thrown away before appropriate tests can be performed. Certain pathogens should be frozen or lyophilized indefinitely because experience has shown that they are likely to be associated with outbreaks of infection. For example, it is prudent to save *S. aureus* isolates from surgical wound infections or nursery infections in case phage typing is required. Likewise, nosocomial strains of group A streptococci should be saved for possible M and T typing. At The Children's Hospital, all isolates from blood, cerebrospinal fluid, and other normally sterile body fluids are saved, as are multiply resistant Gram-negative rods and methicillin-resistant staphylococci.

Programs that routinely save nosocomial isolates such as these are occasionally rewarded when unexpected infection problems are clarified by subjecting strains to additional tests, some of which might not have been available when the collection was started. For example, the epidemiology of coagulase-negative staphylococcal infections following cardiac surgery was elucidated by retrospective phage typing and plasmid profiling (5,6). Regardless of the laboratory's policy for saving nosocomial pathogens, it should be periodically reviewed by the infection control team to be certain that it is still relevant. Storage space in laboratories is not unlimited, and purifying, storing, and cataloguing strains is labor intensive.

ROUTINE IDENTIFICATION PROCEDURES

It should go without saying that the microbiology laboratory must use standardized, reproducible procedures to identify organisms recovered from clinical specimens. Changes in methodology that might have an impact on culture results should be communicated promptly to the infection control staff. Improved detection of a pathogen due to the introduction of a new selective media could, for example, trigger an outbreak investigation by an infection control team unaware of the revised procedure. Similarly, changes in nomenclature must be well-advertised.

In general, microorganisms should be identified to the species level. Outbreak recognition depends on the ability to determine which strains are similar and represent a cluster of infections and which strains are different and unrelated (7). Strain differentiation can be difficult or impossible if only the genus is reported. For example, an epidemic of *Pseudomonas pickettii* urinary tract infections on the pediatric urology service might be overlooked by the infection control team if all pseudomonas isolates were reported as *Pseudomonas species*. However, speciation should not be performed just to display the laboratory's virtuosity, and speciation of all organisms is not cost-effective. Speciation of most anaerobic isolates does not benefit either the physician or the epidemiologist. Except for *Staphylococcus epidermidis* and *Staphylococcus saprophyticus*, it is probably not necessary to speciate isolates of coagulase-negative staphylococci in most circumstances. Speciation of viridans streptococci is usually not required. In other words, after a decade of obsession with speciation and even subspeciation, the pendulum has started to swing back the other way. It is doubtful that this bow to cost-containment will adversely affect the epidemiologist, but the infection control team should participate in the decision-making process.

Fortunately, speciation of most clinically relevant bacteria is now possible using a wide variety of reliable, relatively economical, and technically straightforward panels of biochemical tests. Some of the commercially available kits, such as the API-20E (Analytab Products, Inc., Plainview, NY), utilize lyophilized biochemical substrates that are metabolized by the growth of the bacterial inoculum. Preliminary results often are available within approximately 5 hours, but are more accurate if interpreted after overnight incubation. Other kits, such as the Micro-ID system (General Diagnostics, Morris Plains, NJ), detect preformed constitutive enzymes and other bacterial products and do not require bacterial growth, so results are usually available in about 4 hours. These manual procedures yield a "biotype" number based on the pattern of biochemical reactions. For example, the API-20E Gram-negative identification strip generates a 7-digit number based on the reactions of 20 biochemical tests. The identification of the organism can be ascertained by referring to the test manual, which is based on frequently updated, computerized results of a great number of strains encountered throughout the world.

Although these commercial panels provide excellent species identification, it is important to note that they were not specifically designed to subspeciate bacteria for epidemiological purposes. In fact, the term "biotype" probably should not be used in reference to these kits since none actually are biotyping systems. Moreover, some of the biochemical tests on the panels give variable results when tested by different technologists at different times (8,9). If biochemical testing of a particular strain reveals an unusual pattern of reactions that might provide a useful epidemiological marker, subsequent isolates should be collected and tested at the same time by a single technologist, using a carefully standardized inoculum (10). Even these measures will not guarantee stability of the biotype number, since most panels include reactions, such as H_2S production, which may be under the control of labile plasmids (11).

Despite their limitations, commercial identification panels may provide useful epidemiological information when used intelligently. When necessary, strains may be biotyped more precisely by performing additional biochemical tests not included in the panel. Alternatively, strains may be characterized by using a biotyping scheme developed expressly for the organism being studied. For example, a reliable and simple system for biotyping *Serratia marcescens* is avail-

able which uses 10 tests to differentiate among six pigmented and 13 nonpigmented biotypes within 5 days (12).

In the last few years, a number of semiautomated and automated systems that provide rapid identification of a broad range of bacteria have been marketed. Most of these devices provide accurate, reproducible information, and their speed and convenience have obvious allure. However, these attributes must be weighed against the considerable expense of the equipment, and microbiologists must try to predict whether automation will be cost-effective in an individual laboratory. It also is not clear that physicians need same-day bacterial identifications to provide quality patient care, except in very rare cases, and epidemiologists almost never need this information immediately. Moreover, epidemiologists who are accustomed to reviewing "biotype" numbers or the results of individual biochemical tests will find it much more difficult to retrieve this information from automated equipment that is geared to the bottom line of prompt, accurate species identification. Finally, the skill of the technologist who uses this equipment will tend to atrophy over time, and it will take a highly motivated individual to notice the emergence of a strain with an unusual biochemical profile.

ANTIBIOTIC SUSCEPTIBILITY TESTING

Like speciation, routine antibiotic susceptibility testing provides valuable epidemiological markers for tracing the spread of nosocomial bacterial strains in the hospital. This assumes that the antibiotic susceptibility pattern (often referred to as the "antibiogram") remains stable over time, but changes can occur resulting in a confusing epidemiological picture. For example, the antibiogram may change if a strain gains or loses plasmid genes. Some bacteria (e.g., *Enterobacter*) may suddenly become resistant to a wide variety of β-lactam agents when exposure to a β-lactam drug results in derepression of chromosomal genes responsible for constitutive β-lactamase production (13). *Pseudomonas aeruginosa* is notorious for developing resistance to β-lactam agents by reducing the permeability of the porin proteins in its outer membrane (14). Nevertheless, the antibiogram is one of the most useful, routinely available epidemiological markers for the infection control team.

The potential utility of antibiotic susceptibility patterns can be seriously compromised if the laboratory does not record the full results of the test and simply reports strains as "sensitive" or "resistant" to various agents. If Bauer-Kirby disc diffusion testing is used, the diameter of the zone of inhibition around each disc should be noted. If the procedure is standardized properly, these zone diameters can provide relatively stable, reproducible markers. Thus, a strain of *Klebsiella oxytoca* with a zone of 12 mm around the gentamicin disc may be different from a strain that consistently has a zone diameter of 6 mm, yet this distinction would be impossible if the laboratory reported both strains as "resistant" to gentamicin.

Disc diffusion testing has one major limitation of interest to the epidemiologist; since the diameter of the antibiotic disc is 6 mm, it is impossible to have a zone diameter less than 6 mm, regardless of the degree of resistance to the antibiotics on the test plate. Thus, two different strains of *Enterobacter cloacae*, one with a minimal inhibitory concentration of >128 µg/ml of gentamicin, the other with a minimal inhibitory concentration 32 µg/ml, may both have disc diffusion zone diameters of 6 mm. If the laboratory performed disc diffusion testing, the epidemiologist would be unaware that two different strains of *Enterobacter* were circulating in the hospital at the same time. Therefore, the current trend toward minimal inhibitory concentration testing in American laboratories might benefit the infection control team under certain, albeit unusual, circumstances. However, the value of minimal inhibitory concentration determinations has been seriously compromised by the simultaneous trend away from full-range testing towards "breakpoint" or limited-range commercial systems. To accommodate the profusion of new antibiotics that have been released in recent years, the manufacturers of these convenient susceptibility testing panels have reduced the number of concentrations of each antibiotic to the limited number required to characterize a strain as susceptible or resistant. Thus, antibiotic susceptibility testing has come full circle, and the epidemiologist has been left with neither the zone diameters of disc diffusion testing nor the precise minimal inhibitory concentrations of full-range broth dilution testing.

The proliferation of new antibiotics poses another problem for the infection control team.

The antibiotics tested by the laboratory tend to change rapidly as new drugs are added and older ones are displaced. If the epidemiologist is not vigilant, antibiotics that have proved to be useful epidemiological markers may be excluded inadvertently. Therefore, microbiologists should be encouraged to retain a core of key agents on the antibiotic susceptibility testing panel. In specific situations, it may be advantageous to test antimicrobials that are not routinely included in the panel. Plasmid-mediated silver resistance, for example, proved to be an extremely useful marker during a *Salmonella* epidemic in a Boston burn unit, presumably because the outbreak strain had developed resistance after prolonged exposure to silver nitrate on the surface of the burn wound (15). Occasionally, even drugs that are no longer used clinically may provide valuable information. In a nationwide outbreak of bacteremia caused by contaminated intravenous fluid, the epidemic strain of *Enterobacter agglomerans* was resistant to cephalothin, as expected, but surprisingly was susceptible to cephaloridine (16).

SPECIAL PROCEDURES FOR CHARACTERIZING BACTERIA

The procedures already described are sufficient to characterize most strains for epidemiological purposes. Speciation, occasionally supplemented by formal biotyping, and antibiotic susceptibility testing are all that are needed to solve most nosocomial infection problems. However, on occasion, it may be necessary to perform additional procedures, some of which may be beyond the capabilities of the clinical laboratory. The laboratory director and the infection control team should familiarize themselves with the cost, availability, interpretation, and limitations of these tests. A thoroughly researched review of available reference procedures has been published recently (17). However, this is a constantly evolving field as new epidemiological challenges are brought to the attention of the microbiology community. For example, *Pseudomonas cepacia* has emerged recently as an important pathogen in pulmonary exacerbations of cystic fibrosis (18). This development was of little concern to infection control programs in pediatric hospitals until it was discovered that *P. cepacia* was being isolated from cystic fibrosis patients in some institutes far more frequently than in others. This clustering of cases was apparent even after sensitive selective media were introduced at institutions across the country (19)—an epidemiologically useful case-finding technique that will be reviewed in greater detail later. Attempts to define the epidemiology and possible nosocomial transmission of *P. cepacia* among cystic fibrosis patients were frustrated by the lack of well-tested typing systems for subspeciating clinical isolates. Subsequently, biotyping, serotyping, and pycointyping systems have been developed (18,20-23) and are currently being tested on strains from cystic fibrosis patients.

One of the most useful and well-known procedures for subspeciating nosocomial pathogens is staphylococcal phage typing (24), which is widely available for testing *Staphylococcus aureus* and may also be useful for studying the epidemiology of *S. epidermidis* (5,25). In general, strains of *S. aureus* can be considered unique if they differ in more than two "strong" phage reactions. Since phage typing is tedious and expensive, it should only be performed to verify an epidemiological hypothesis concerning the transmission of staphylococcal disease. For example, it would be appropriate to submit strains isolated from an outbreak of nursery staphylococcal infections and from caregivers who have a strong epidemiological association with the infected babies. Phage typing of strains from personnel who clearly are not involved in the outbreak is wasteful and my yield misleading, potentially inflammatory data. Not all strains of *S. aureus* are typeable using currently available phages, limiting the usefulness of this technique. Moreover, when a particular phage type is prevalent in the community and hospital, it may be impossible to differentiate individuals who merely harbor the organism from those who are involved in an outbreak. Capsular serotyping (26) and plasmid typing (27) may be useful adjunctive techniques in studying the epidemiology of *S. aureus* infections.

Most laboratories differentiate among groups A, B, and D and viridans streptococci, but relegate other isolates to general categories, such as "betahemolytic streptococcus, not group A or D." Although this is sufficient for almost all clinical purposes, it will not permit the detection of clusters of infection caused by other serogroups. For example, a cluster of group C streptococcal infections following orthopaedic surgery at The Children's Hospital was recognized be-cause the laboratory routinely serogrouped streptococci recovered from surgical wound cultures (28). The resulting investigation revealed that an anal carrier of group C streptococci on the orthopaedic staff was responsible for these infections. Serogrouping of clinically important streptococci is now within reach of all clinical laboratories, since the required reagents are commercially available, and the procedures are technically straightforward. Streptococci can be further characterized by reference laboratories when necessary. For example, group A streptococci can be subdivided serologically by specific M and T antigens and by the ability of some strains to turn porcine serum opaque (serum opacity reaction) (29), and group B streptococci, which may be nosocomially acquired in some nurseries (30), can also be serotyped.

By far, the greatest number and variety of typing procedures have been developed to study the epidemiology of Gram-negative bacilli (7,17). For many organisms, a number of options are available, but most are performed primarily in reference laboratories. For example, *Klebsiella pneumoniae* may be subspeciated by biotyping (31), serotyping (32), phage typing (31), and bacteriocin typing (in this case, susceptibility to bacteriocins produced by a panel of standard bacterial strains) (33). *Serratia marcescens* can be characterized by biotyping (12), serotyping (34,35), bacteriocin typing (36), and phage typing (37). Techniques available for *Proteus mirabilis* include all of the above (17) plus the Dienes phenomenon (a line of demarcation where two unrelated swarming strains meet) (38). *Pseudomonas aeruginosa* poses an especially great challenge to the microbiologist, since strains tend to throw off multiple phenotypes on subculture. Thus, characterization of strains by phenotypic properties, such as colonial morphology, hemolysis, and pigment production is hazardous. Phage type (39) is not always a stable property of *Pseudomonas* strains. Susceptibility to *Pseudomonas* bacteriocins (known as pyocins) is also unreliable, although typing by pyocin production may be useful (40). Serotyping on the basis of *Pseudomonas* O-antigens (lipopolysaccharide) provides a stable epidemiological marker, although the availability of several different systems has created a confusing literature; the Fisher system of seven immunotypes has been used primarily by investigators studying *Pseudomonas* immunoprophylaxis (41), while the 17-serotype international system generally has been preferred by epidemiologists (42).

GENOTYPING PROCEDURES

Recent years have witnessed the explosive development of novel techniques that are useful not only in tracing the spread to unique nosocomial strains, but also in documenting the dissemination of antibiotic resistance genes and genes responsible for the expression of virulence properties (43-46). Progress has been most rapid in characterizing strains expressing plasmid-mediated antibiotic resistance. Rather than studying plasmids themselves, some investigators have elected to measure the products of plasmids, such as β-lactamases and aminoglycoside inactivating enzymes. For example, specific strains of aminoglycoside-resistant *Enterobacteriaceae* can be typed by their distinctive profiles of aminoglycoside-inactivating enzymes (47). These labor-intensive procedures are performed only in reference laboratories. Moreover, they are not as useful as originally anticipated, since gene expression and the resulting enzyme production can change dramatically as plasmids pass from strain to strain in the hospital setting.

Because of these problems, it is usually preferable to examine the genetic basis of antibiotic resistance directly. The simplest approach is to extract plasmids from bacteria and to measure their molecular weight by performing agarose gel electrophoresis. Although currently restricted to reference and research laboratories, there is nothing arcane or complex about this procedure. Since the technique is easily learned and does not require expensive equipment, it is reasonable to assume that it will be used by an increasing number of laboratories in the future, particularly as prepackaged commerical systems become available.

Examples of the utility of plasmid profiling by agarose gel electrophoresis abound in the recent literature (43-46). In some cases, application of this technique to refractory epidemiological problems has led to impressive breakthroughs. *Staphylococcus epidermidis* has resisted characterization by biochemical testing (5), and analysis of antibiotic susceptibility patterns has yielded misleading results. The limitations of biotyping and antibiogram analysis were dramatized by a cluster of patients who acquired *Staphylococcus epidermidis* prosthetic

valve endocarditis at the Seattle Veterans Administration Hospital over a 3-month period in 1982 (5). Twenty-three isolates of *S. epidermidis* were recovered from these patients, including isolates from the blood of all four patients, from the infected prosthetic valves retrieved from two patients, and from the pump blood obtained during two of the operations. These strains were then compared by biotyping and antibiotic susceptibility testing. Three strains differed from the other 20 in numerous respects and were assumed to be blood culture contaminants. The remaining 20 strains had a variety of biotypes and antibiograms. At least one strain from each of three patients was resistant to chloramphenicol, erythromycin, clindamycin, and gentamicin; a number of strains were susceptible to both clindamycin and erythromycin, while others were susceptible to either gentamicin or chloramphenicol. Despite these diverse antibiograms, all 20 strains had the same unusual phage type, and all shared a common core of three plasmids on agarose gel electrophoresis. Gels revealed the presence of distinct plasmid bands in strains that were resistant to specific antibiotics. Thus, strains that were resistant to clindamycin and erythromycin had a corresponding 1.7 megadalton plasmid band; strains resistant to chloramphenicol had a 2.5 megadalton plasmid; strains resistant to gentamicin had a 42 megadalton plasmid; and strains resistant to all of these antibiotics had all three plasmid bands. Remarkably, even strains from the same patient had different antibiograms and corresponding additions to or deletions from their plasmid profiles, but all had the unique plasmid core that betrayed their common origin. The four infections were attributed to a single surgeon who participated in all of the operations, although the microbiological and epidemiological evidence incriminating him was not conclusive.

Plasmid profiling has also been useful in elucidating the epidemiology of antibiotic-resistant Gram-negative bacilli. From 1976–1980, the Seattle Veterans Administration Hospital experienced a major outbreak of infection caused by strains of *Serratia marcescens* that were resistant to up to 11 antibiotics, including gentamicin and tobramycin (48). In addition, the same resistance pattern was observed in other isolates of *Enterobacteriaceae*, including strains recovered from urine cultures that also grew the multiply resistant *Serratia*. The epidemic antibiogram "invaded" a number of hospital wards and involved a growing list of pathogens, including *Citrobacter freundii*, *Proteus rettgeri*, *Providencia stuartii*, and *Enterobacter aerogenes*. In investigating this unusual and alarming outbreak, the Seattle investigators decided to focus on aminoglycoside resistance as a potentially promising epidemiological marker. All of the epidemic strains had similar zones of inhibition around gentamicin and tobramycin discs on Bauer-Kirby testing, and all produced a 2″ adenylating aminoglycoside inactivating enzyme, strongly suggesting that they contained a common plasmid. Indeed, a 45 megadalton plasmid mediating 2″ adenylase production was found, and this plasmid turned out to be the pLST 1000 plasmid that was subsequently found in nosocomial strains of *Enterobacteriaceae* in hospitals in several countries (49). The identity of these 45 megadalton plasmids was confirmed by digesting plasmid DNA with several restriction endonucleases and running the resulting DNA fragments on an agarose gel; all had the same genomic fingerprint, as revealed by the pattern of bands on the gel.

However, the Seattle story was not complete. The epidemic antibiogram began to appear in strains that did not contain the 45 megadalton plasmid, but instead had a much larger plasmid. Thus, spread of the resistance genes could no longer be monitored simply by performing agarose gel electrophoresis on suspect strains. Moreover, some strains no longer produced the 2″ adenylase, so outbreak strains could not be recognized by production of a specific gene product or by their resistance to aminoglycosides. As a result, resistance genes could spread undetected in the hospital until they were captured by a plasmid and organism in which they could be expressed. Faced with this challenging problem, the Seattle team constructed a specific radiolabelled DNA probe from a fragment of DNA isolated from pLST 1000 (50). This probe was able to recognize the DNA responsible for the production of the 2″ adenylase, regardless of the plasmid or bacterial strain in which it had taken up residence.

Probes capable of recognizing a variety of antibiotic resistance genes are being developed at a rapid pace (51) and should expand the hospital epidemiologist's armamentarium substantially in coming years. Some of these probes can even detect resistance genes on the bacterial chromosome of strains that do not harbor plasmids. For example, the Tn554 transposon-mediating spectinomycin and erythromycin resistance has been used as a chromosomal probe to demonstrate that *Staphylococcus aureus* toxic shock strains isolated from a neurosurgeon and the surgical wounds of two of his patients were identical (52). This approach was suggested by the observation that related isolates of *S. aureus* usually have specific transposons at the same chromosomal location, whereas unrelated strains have either transposons at different locations or no transposons at all. The strains in this small cluster of infections also shared the same antibiogram and phage type, so the information provided by the transposon probe turned out to be superfluous. However, this elegant approach may prove useful in studying the epidemiology of strains when more conventional techniques fail.

If bacteria do not have genes that are associated with distinctive antibiotic resistance patterns, molecular genetic techniques may still be useful to the epidemiologist. Restriction endonuclease digests of whole bacterial chromosomes (known as bacterial restriction endonuclease DNA analysis, or BRENDA) may produce characteristic patterns on gel electrophoresis (53). However, the banding patterns produced when large pieces of DNA are digested are extremely complex and may be difficult to interpret. Moreover, great care is required to be certain that the experimental methods and conditions are standardized. Faced with these problems, some investigators have attempted to design probes for specific regions of the chromosome. For example, Ogle and his colleagues have studied the epidemiology of *P. aeruginosa* by probing with a small PstI-NruI restriction fragment upstream from the exotoxin A structural gene (54). Even cloned random sequences of chromosomal DNA can be useful probes, as demonstrated in a recent epidemiological study of *Salmonella* (55).

In addition to helping the epidemiologist follow the transmission of specific strains in the hospital, gene probes may eventually be able to distinguish virulent strains that will tend to cause disease from those that are less likely to be a threat to hospitalized patients. While no nosocomial organisms have been studied in this manner, the virulence properties of a number of community-acquired pathogens can be detected by genomic probes. For example, Schoolnik's group at Stanford has described probes for the hemolysin virulence gene and the P pilus adhesin gene of uropathogenic *E. coli* (56). Probes are also being developed for the rapid diagnosis of bacterial pathogens which have been difficult to isolate and identify by traditional technologies. Rapid diagnosis using probes has already been applied successfully to several enteropathogens (57-59), and it is not difficult to imagine how such techniques might be useful in the investigation of hospital outbreaks.

INFECTION CONTROL ASPECTS OF DIAGNOSTIC VIROLOGY

Virtually every new textbook of medical microbiology contains an extensive discussion of infection control, but the important relationship between infection control and diagnostic microbiology is usually mentioned only in passing or ignored altogether. From the perspective of a pediatric hospital epidemiologist, this is a surprising omission, particularly considering the revolution in diagnostic techniques that has occurred in recent years. A decade ago, viruses could be identified only by growing them in tissue culture, a labor-intensive technique that was performed only in reference laboratories and that rarely yielded timely results. Now, rapid diagnosis is available for many nosocomial viral pathogens that affect children (60,61). Some tests can be performed directly on clinical specimens, permitting the laboratory to report same-day results. A number of tests are available as commercial kits, and the development of new rapid tests has become one of the most competitive sectors of the microbial diagnostics industry. Tests have become progressively easier to perform and interpret, and their use is already spreading beyond the reference laboratory and tertiary medical center. A broad range of diagnostic procedures is available routinely at The Children's Hospital, as summarized in Table 27.1. Although some of these tests employ reagents that are not generally available, all are technically quite straightforward and have commercial potential. Most are described in detail in a recent comprehensive review (60).

The potential value of rapid, accurate viral diagnosis to the infection control program is clear. Viral nosocomial infections have long been suspected to be a major cause of morbidity, increased length of hospitalization, and even mortality in the pediatric patient population (62,63), but elucidation of the extent and nature of the problem has awaited the availability of paractical diagnostic tests. The infection control practitioner need no longer classify obvious nosocomial infections as "probably viral" just because routine bacterial and fungal cultures do not reveal the etiologic agent, and the clinician's frustrated lament, "It must be the virus that's going around," is being heard less often. Fast, reliable identification procedures have greatly

Table 27.1
Availability of Rapid Viral Diagnostic Tests, The Children's Hospital, Boston.

Virus	Diagnostic Test	Specimen(s)
Adenovirus	IFA[a] for biopsies (IFA for respiratory specimens is investigational)	Biopsy, NP aspirate
Cytomegalovirus	Shell viral method (detection of early antigen)	NP aspirate, urine, buffy coat, others
Enterovirus	Not available	
Hepatitis B	RIA (detection of surface antigen)	Serum
Herpes simplex	IFA	Smear of lesion, biopsy
Herpes zoster	IFA	Smear of lesion
Influenza	IFA	NP aspirate
Measles	IFA	NP aspirate
Parainfluenza	IFA	NP aspirate
Respiratory syncytial virus (RSV)	IFA	NP aspirate
Rotavirus	ELISA	Stool
Rubella	Not available	

[a]IFA, indirect immunofluorescent antibody testing; RIA, radioimmunoassay; ELISA, enzyme-linked immunosorbent assay; NP, nasopharyngeal.

facilitated study of the epidemiology and modes of transmission of nosocomial viruses, and this in turn has permitted formulation of rational policies for interrupting the spread of viruses on the wards.

Particularly impressive strides have been made in recent years to clarify the epidemiology of respiratory syncytial virus (RSV) infections in pediatric hospitals, principally through the careful, imaginative work of Hall and her colleagues in Rochester (64–72). It is now known that RSV spreads rapidly through the pediatric wards each winter season, often reaching epidemic proportions. Nosocomial infection has particularly serious consequences for neonates, immunosuppressed children, and patients with congenital heart disease. The mode of transmission clearly is by direct contact with contaminated secretions and droplets, not via the air. Infected personnel, who generally develop symptoms of a cold, are important vectors in the spread of the virus. None of these significant epidemiological observations would have been possible without the full support of the virology laboratory. Now that specific therapy with ribavirin is available for patients with RSV infection, rapid diagnosis has assumed even greater significance (73).

Routine diagnostic techniques may not be adequate to define the spread of specific viral strains in the hospital. One herpesvirus isolate looks just like another by indirect immunofluorescent staining, and rotavirus strains detected by ELISA are indistinguishable. However, techniques are gradually becoming available that permit more definitive epidemiological studies of certain viruses. For example, at least two types of RSV can be differentiated serologically on the basis of their glycoprotein surface antigens, and both types can circulate in the community and hospital simultaneously (74). Of course, influenza viruses can be tracked with great precision as their hemagglutin and neuraminidase antigens change over time. The same genomic fingerprinting techniques that have proved so useful in studying bacteria have also been used to investigate the epidemiology of both RNA viruses, such as rotavirus (75), and DNA viruses, particularly the herpesviruses (76–82). For example, DNA fingerprinting of the cytomegalovirus genome by restriction endonuclease analysis has had direct application to clinical infection control problems. This technique has

been used to determine whether cytomegalovirus strains infecting pregnant health care workers were genetically distinct from the strains recovered from the patients under their care. In one especially striking case (80), a physician who had cared for an infant with congenital cytomegalovirus infection during the first trimester of pregnancy decided to have an abortion when she became ill and had a greater than 4-fold rise in her cytomegalovirus antibody titer. The restriction endonuclease fingerprints of the strains of cytomegalovirus recovered from mother and the abortus were identical, as expected, but the strain from the ill baby in the nursery had an entirely different band pattern. DNA fingerprinting has also been invaluable in studying the transmission of cytomegalovirus in day-care centers (83).

ENVIRONMENTAL CULTURES

Cultures of equipment, medical supplies, solutions, and the inanimate environment used to be a preoccupation of hospital infection control programs and a burden to diagnostic microbiology laboratories. Results of these cultures were dutifully reported to the infection control committee and cluttered the desks of infection control practitioners, but seldom provided useful information or led to specific interventions. Emphasis on environmental culturing has declined markedly in recent years, to the relief of both the epidemiologist and the microbiologist. Generally clinical laboratories are still involved in the microbiological monitoring of sterilizers, which are checked routinely for their ability to kill bacterial spores (*Bacillus stearothermophilus* for steam autoclaves and *Bacillus subtilis*, strain *globigii*, variety *niger* for ethylene oxide gas sterilizers). In addition, laboratories may perform quality control cultures on blood products (when patients have transfusion reactions), hemodialysis fluid, infant formula, banked breast milk, and other products or solutions prepared in the hospital. Routine culturing of commercially prepared products is not recommended.

The message that most environmental culturing is expensive and of doubtful utility has not reached the clinical staff of many hospitals, and it is not unusual for the infection control practitioner or microbiologist to be asked to "do a few cultures" to reassure concerned physicians and nurses that the environment is safe. For example, the first response of surgeons to an increase in the nosocomial wound infection rate might be to request cultures of the operating room air. Nurses worried about an increase in hyperalimentation line infections might ask for routine cultures of hyperalimentation fluid or catheter exit sites. A few cases of pneumonia in the intensive care unit might generate requests for cultures of just-sterilized respiratory therapy equipment. Of course, under certain circumstances, such requests might be legitimate. Perhaps there *is* a staphylococcal shedder in the operating room, a problem with contaminated hyperalimentation fluid, or an ineffective respiratory therapy equipment sterilization procedure, but culture surveillance should commence only if clearly indicated by available epidemiological data, and it should be carefully planned to yield meaningful results.

The indications for performing environmental culturing, along with descriptions of sensitive, standardized microbiological techniques have been summarized extensively in review articles and reference texts (17,84–87). Most solutions can be cultured satisfactorily by performing a quantitative culture of a small sample and passing the rest of the fluid through a $0.2 \mu m$ filter, which is then cultured on an agar plate. Environmental surfaces can be monitored by swabbing a standardized area (e.g., $4 \, cm^2$) using a precut template and a swab moistened with brain heart infusion or trypticase soy broth. To neutralize residual disinfectants on the surface being cultured, 0.07% soy lecithin and 0.50% Tween 80 may be added to the broth. Alternatively, Rodac contact plates may be used. Intravascular catheters should be cultured semiquantitatively by rolling the catheter tip on a nutrient agar plate following published recommendations (88) or examined directly by Gram stain (89).

Air sampling may be performed by placing uncovered agar plates (settle plates) in the environment, but it is preferable to culture large volumes of air quantitatively using an air sampler, such as the slit sampler manufactured by New Brunswick Scientific, Inc. (New Brunswick, New Jersey). The infection control team and laboratory director should be familiar with available techniques and have relevent references on hand. No matter how well-prepared that laboratory is for environmental cultures, advances in medical technology will provide new and unexpected challenges that will require consultation and collaboration between microbiology and infection control.

While the popularity of environmental culturing is generally on the wane, the increasing number of severely immunocompromised, neutropenic children on hospital wards has prompted renewed calls for monitoring the environment, particularly the air supply. The major concern is nosocomial infection due to *Aspergillus* and other invasive fungi. Clusters of *Aspergillus* infections have been attributed to contamination of hospital air with fungal spores, and there is ample evidence that spores originating from the environment outside of the hospital or generated within the hospital itself are a significant hazard to immunocompromised patients (Chapter 23). The best solution to this growing problem is to provide the patients with uncontaminated air cleansed by high efficiency (HEPA) filters. However, it is impossible to guarantee spore-free air in older institutions, so air sampling to determine the level of contamination has been advocated by some investigators in an attempt to determine if patients are being placed at excessive risk (90). While air sampling may be useful in investigating specific infection problems, it is doubtful that most hospitals will have the time or resources to mount the sustained effort required to obtain reliable, potentially useful data.

SURVEILLANCE CULTURES OF PERSONNEL AND PATIENTS

Except for states that require stool cultures of food handlers, there are no indications for routinely culturing hospital personnel. Only when epidemiological evidence suggests that an individual on the hospital staff is involved in the transmission of a pathogen, should personnel cultures be entertained. Culturing should be confined to those individuals who are linked epidemiologically to the problem, since indiscriminate culturing of the staff is expensive, yields misleading information, and fosters needless paranoia, which may impede further investigation. The site to be cultured depends on the pathogen. Although carriers of *S. aureus* may be heavily colonized on the skin and other body sites, cultures of the anterior nares have the highest yield, and cultures of the rectum or vagina are necessary only rarely (91). Group A streptococci are, of course, commonly found in the throat, but reported outbreaks generally have been attributed to anal or vaginal carriers (91). It is very unusual for Gram-negative infections to be traced to a carrier on the staff. A nursery outbreak of *Proteus mirabilis* infection, which was attributed to a nurse who had rectal and vaginal colonization with the organism, may be the exception that proves the rule (92). Even nosocomial bacterial gastroenteritis is more often caused by contaminated food or other environmental reservoirs than by carriers on the hospital staff.

When personnel *are* involved in the transmission of infections due to Gram-negative bacilli, it is ususally because their hands have become transiently colonized while caring for patients. Occasionally, Gram-negative bacilli may establish more long-term colonization on the hands, becoming part of the resident flora (93), although the clinical significance of this phenomenon is not known. Whether hand culturing is performed as part of an outbreak investigation or as an educational approach to persuading personnel to wash their hands, a simple, reliable method is needed. An inexpensive, convenient technique is to have personnel lightly touch their fingertips and palm to the surface of an appropriate selective agar medium. The probability of detecting hand colonization is greater if personnel vigorously wash their hands with 10 or 20 ml of Tween 80-supplemented nutrient broth containing either sodium thiosulfate broth to neutralize iodophor antiseptics or soy lecithin to neutralize chlorhexidine antiseptics. The hands can either be washed in a sterile plastic bag containing the broth, or the broth can be poured over the hands and collected in a sterile bowl.

Routine cultures to monitor the microbiological flora of pediatric patients in intensive care units and oncology and bone marrow transplantation wards are performed in many tertiary medical centers. Often, physicians request the laboratory to identify "all pathogens" isolated from cultures of a number of anatomical sites, and since cultures are obtained as often as several times weekly, the burden on the microbiology laboratory can be staggering. At The Children's Hospital, for example, it was estimated that one full-time technologist was required to process the routine surveillance cultures from approximately three bone marrow transplantation patients, so that as many as five technologists would be needed just to handle specimens from a planned 15-bed transplantation unit. The solution, of course, was not to hire more technologists, but rather to examine the evidence supporting the utility of screening cultures. In fact, the predictive value of a positive screening culture is poor, and the identification of a specific pathogen on a routine culture of throat or stool does not provide a reliable guide for empiric therapy.

Some studies suggest that isolation of *Aspergillus* from nose cultures (94,95), *Candida tropicalis* from urine cultures (96), and *Pseudomonas aeruginosa* from throat or stool cultures (95,97) may provide prognostic clues for the clinician, but few physicians are brave enough to tailor empiric therapy to the results of such screening cultures. Certainly, the results of surveillance cultures are of only marginal interest to the epidemiologist, although, as noted previously, the emergence and spread of a new pathogen can sometimes be detected in this fashion.

Routine periodic screening of throat and stool cultures for antibiotic-resistant bacteria is also practiced widely. Data supporting the usefulness of these cultures are hard to come by. However, if specific antibiotic resistance patterns are targeted by the infection control team for scrutiny, screening cultures can serve as an early warning system for the appearance of difficult-to-treat pathogens on the wards of the hospital. For example, isolation of a strain of gentamicin-resistant *Klebsiella* in a neonatal intensive care unit which had not had previous problems with aminoglycoside-resistant pathogens might prompt the infection control team to institute appropriate containment procedures. Recovery of methicillin-resistant staphylococci would also be cause for alarm. Since the value of these screening cultures has not been established by prospective studies, it is especially important that they be cheap and easy to perform. Fortunately, screening plates (e.g., MacConkey agar containing 10 µg/ml of gentamicin or Mueller-Hinton agar containing 6 µg/ml of oxacillin and 4% NaCl) are very inexpensive and can be processed rapidly.

Unlike routine surveillance cultures, the importance of screening cultures in outbreak investigation is indisputable. Since the primary goal of these cultures is case-finding, screening media that are extremely sensitive should be chosen, even if some specificity is sacrificed. Since clinical microbiologists are accustomed to using selective media in the laboratory, infection control personnel should consult the laboratory director for advice concerning the best screening technique. For example, the microbiologist may be able to advise the infection control practitioner that direct plating of specimens on methicillin-containing agar is satisfactory for routine surveillance, but that overnight growth in broth prior to plating on selective media will enhance detection of methicillin-resistant staphylococci (98).

PSEUDOEPIDEMICS

On occasion, the laboratory is the source of an apparent infection control problem, not its solution. A number of pseudoepidemics have been traced to contaminated devices, solutions, and medications used in patient care, but others have been caused by contamination of specimens during processing. These laboratory-based problems have been reviewed recently by Ristuccia and Cunha (84). Early recognition of pseudoinfections is critical, not only because patients may receive inappropriate therapy, but also because time-consuming, unnecessary epidemiological investigations are almost always precipitated. Pseudobacteremias have been reported particularly frequently because of cross-contamination of blood culture bottles in an automated detection device (99–101), although knowledge of this potential problem seems to have reduced the risk.

CONCLUSION

The microbiology laboratory is an indispensible resource for the infection control program. The complexity of present-day diagnostic microbiology and the rapid development of new procedures and technologies require ongoing collaboration between the laboratory and infection control programs. If a good working relationship has been established, investigation of nosocomial infection outbreaks and planning of special infection control projects are greatly facilitated. Constructive input from the laboratory director often leads to a more efficient, cost-effective infection control program, and feedback from the hospital epidemiologist can result in the curtailment of unnecessary, costly cultures and microbiology procedures.

REFERENCES

1. Haley RW, Garner JS: Infection surveillance and control programs. In Bennett JV, Bradman PS (eds): *Hospital Infections*, ed 2 Boston, Little, Brown & Company, 1986, pp 51–72.
2. Washington JA, II: Initial processing for cultures of specimens. In Washington JA (ed): *Laboratory Procedures in Clinical Microbiology*. New York, Springer-Verlag, 1981, pp 91–126.
3. Freeman J, McGowen JE, Jr: Methodologic issues in hospital epidemiology I. Rates, case-finding, and interpretation. *Rev Infect Dis* 3:658–667, 1981.
4. Tuazon CV, Murray HW, Levy C, Solny MN, Curtin JA, Sheagren JN: Serious infections from *Bacillus sp*. *JAMA* 214:1137–1140, 1979.
5. Mickelsen PA, Plorde JJ, Gordon KP, Hargiss C, McLure J, Schoenkrnecht FD, Condie F, Tenover FC, Tompkins LS: Instability of antibiotic resistance in a strain of *Staphylococcus epidermidis* isolated from an outbreak of prosthetic valve endocarditis. *J Infect Dis* 152:50–58, 1985.
6. Archer GL, Vishniavsky N, Stiver HG: Plasmid pattern analysis of *Staphylococcus epidermidis* isolates from patients with prosthetic valve endocarditis. *Infect Immunol* 35:627–632, 1982.
7. Goldmann DA, Macone AB: A microbiologic approach to the investigation of bacterial nosocomial infection outbreaks. *Infect Control* 1:391–400, 1980.
8. Butler DA, Lobregat CM, Gaven TL: Reproducibility of the Analytab (API 20-E) System. *J Clin Microbiol* 2:322–326, 1975.
9. de Silva MI, Rubin SJ: Multiple biotypes of *Klebsiella pneumoniae* in single clinical specimens. *J Clin Microbiol* 5:62–65, 1977.
10. Murray PR: Standardization of the Analytab Enteric (API 20-E) system in increase accuracy and reproducibility of the test for biotype characterization of bacteria. *J Clin Microbiol* 8:46–49, 1978.
11. Stoleru GH, Gerband GR, Bauanchaud DH, LeMinor L: Etude d'un plasmide transferable determinant la production d'H_2S et al resistance a la tetracycline chez "*Escherichia coli.*" *Ann Inst Pasteur* 123:743–754, 1972.
12. Grimont PAD, Grimont F: Biotyping of *Serratia marcescens* and its use in epidemiologic studies. *J Clin Microbiol* 8:73–83, 1978.
13. Sanders CC: Novel resistance selected by the new expanded-spectrum cephalosporins: a concern. *J Infect Dis* 147:585–589, 1983.
14. Quinn JP, Dudek EJ, DiVincenzo CA, Lucks DA, Lerner SA: Emergence of resistance to imipenem during therapy for *Pseudomonas aeruginosa* infections. *J Infect Dis* 154:284–294, 1986.
15. McHugh GL, Moellering RC, Hopkins CC, Swartz MN: *Salmonella typhimurium* resistant to silver nitrate, chloramphenicol, and ampicillin. *Lancet* 1:235–239, 1975.
16. Maki DG, Rhame FS, Mackel DG, Bennett JV: Nationwide epidemic of septicemia caused by contaminated intravenous products. I. Epidemiologic and clinical features. *Am J Med* 60:471–485, 1976.
17. McGowan JE, Jr: Role of the microbiology laboratory in prevention and control of nosocomial infections. In Lennette EH, Balows A, Hauser WJ, Jr., Shadomy EJ (eds): *Manual of Clinical Microbiology*, ed 4. Washington DC, American Society for Microbiology, 1985, pp 110–122.
18. Goldmann DA, Klinger JD: *Pseudomonas cepacia*: Biology, mechanisms of virulence, epidemiology. *J Pediatr* 108:806–812, 1986.
19. Gilligan PH, Gage PA, Bradshaw LM, Schidlow DV, DeCicco BT: Isolation medium for the recovery of *Pseudomonas cepacia* from the respiratory secretions of patients with cystic fibrosis. *J Clin Microbiol* 22:5–8, 1985.
20. Esanu JG, Schubert RHW: Zur taxonomie und nomenklatur von *Pseudomonas cepacia*. *Zentralbl Bakteriol Mikrobiol Hyg* (A) 224:478–483, 1983.
21. Richard C, Monteil H, Megraud F, Chatelain R, Laurent B: Characteres phenotypiques de 100 souches de *Pseudomonas*

cepacia: Proposition d' un schema de biovars. *Ann Biol Clin* 39:9–15, 1981.

22. Nakamura Y, Shigeta S, Yabuwchi E: Serological classification of *Pseudomonas cepacia*. Kamsenshogaku Zasshi 58:491–494, 1984.

23. Govan JRW, Harris G: Typing of *Pseudomonas cepacia* by bacteriocin susceptibility and production. *J Clin Microbiol* 22:490–494, 1985.

24. Blair JE, Williams REO: Phage typing of staphylococci. *Bull WHO* 24:771–784, 1961.

25. Parisi JT: Coagulase-negative staphylococci and the epidemiological typing of *Staphylococcus epidermidis*. *Microbiol Rev* 49:126–139, 1985.

26. Arbeit RD, Karakawa WW, Vann WF, Robbins JB: Predominance of two newly described capsular polysaccharide types among clinical isolates of *Staphylococcus aureus*. *Diagnostic Microbiol Infect Dis* 2:85–91, 1984.

27. Kozarsky PE, Rimland D, Terry PM, Wachsmuth K: Plasmid analysis of simultaneous nosocomial outbreaks of methicillin-resistant *Staphylococcus aureus*. *Infect Control* 7:577–581, 1986.

28. Goldmann DA, Breton SJ: Group C streptococcal surgical wound infections transmitted by an anal-rectal and nasal carrier. *Pediatrics* 61:235–237, 1978.

29. Richman DD, Breton SJ, Goldmann DA: Scarlet fever and group A streptococcal surgical wound infection traced to an anal carrier. *J. Pediatr* 90:387–390, 1977.

30. Parades A, Wong P, Manson EO, Tabor LH, Barrett FF: Nosocomial transmission of group B streptococci in a newborn nursery. *Pediatrics* 59:679–682, 1977.

31. Rennie RP, Nord CE, Sjoberg L, Duncan IBR: Comparison of bacteriophage typing, serotyping, and biotyping as aids in epidemiological surveillance of *Klebsiella* infections. *J Clin Microbiol* 8:638–642, 1978.

32. Murcia A, Rubin SJ: Reproducibility of an indirect immunofluorescent-antibody technique for capsular serotyping of *Klebsiella pneumoniae*. *J Clin Microbiol* 9:208–213, 1979.

33. Buffenmyer CL, Rycheck RR, Yee RB: Bacteriocin (Klebocin) sensitivity typing of *Klebsiella*. *J Clin Microbiol* 4:239–244, 1976.

34. Pitt TL: State of the art: Typing of *Serratia marcescens*. *J Hosp Infect* 3:9–13, 1982.

35. Ewing WH, Johnson JG, Davis BR: The occurrence of *Serratia marcescens* in nosocomial infections. Communicable Disease Center, U.S. Public Health Service, Atlanta. 1962.

36. Traub WH: Bacteriocin and phage typing of *Serratia*. In von Graevenitz A, Rubin SJ (eds): *The Genus Serratia*, Boca Raton, FL, CRC Press, 1980, pp 79–100.

37. Pitt TL, Erdman YJ, Bucher C: The epidemiological type identification of *Serratia marcescens* from outbreaks of infection in hospitals. *J Hyg Cambridge* 84:269–283, 1980.

38. Hickman FW, Farmer JJ, III: Differentiation of *Proteus mirabilis* by bacteriophage typing and the Dienes reaction. *J Clin Microbiol* 3:350–358, 1976.

39. Linberg RB, Latta RL: Phage typing of *Pseudomonas aeruginosa*: clinical and epidemiologic considerations. *J Infect Dis* 130(suppl):S33–S42, 1974.

40. Gillies RR, Govan JF: Typing of *Pseudomonas pyocyanea* by pyocin production. *J Pathol* 92:339–345, 1966.

41. Pennington JE: Immunotherapy of *Pseudomonas aeruginosa* infections. In Doggett RG (ed): *Pseudomonas aeruginosa Infections - Clinical Manifestation of Infection and Current Therapy*. New York, Academic Press, 1979, pp 192–218.

42. Farmer JJ, III, Weinstein RA, Zierdt CH, Brokopp CD: Hospital outbreaks caused by *Pseudomonas aeruginosa*: Importance of serogroup 011. *J Clin Microbiol* 16:266–270, 1982.

43. Wachsmuth K: Molecular epidemiology of bacteria infections: Examples of methodology and investigation of outbreaks. *Rev Infect Dis* 8:682–692, 1986.

44. John JF, Jr., Twitty JA: Plasmids as epidemiologic markers in nosocomial gram-negative bacilli: Experience at a university and review of the literature. *Rev Infect Dis* 8:693–704, 1986.

45. Schaberg DR, Zervos M: Plasmid analysis in the study of the epidemiology of nosocomial gram-positive cocci. *Rev Infect Dis* 8:705–712, 1986.

46. Shlaes DM, Currie-McCumber CA: Plasmid analysis in molecular epidemiology: A summary and future directions. *Rev Infect Dis* 8:738–746, 1986.

47. O'Brien TF, Ross DG, Guzman MA, Madeiros AA, Hedges RW, Botstein D: Dissemination of an antibiotic resistance plasmid in hospital patient flora. *Antimicrob Agents Chemother* 17:537–543, 1980.

48. Tompkins LS, Plorde JJ, Falkow S: Molecular analysis of R-factors from multiresistant nosocomial isolates. *J Infect Dis* 141:625–636, 1980.

49. O'Brien TF, Mayer KH, Kisui H, Syvanan M, Hopkins JD: Intercontinental spread of a new antibiotic resistance gene on an epidemic plasmid. *Science* 230:87–88, 1985.

50. Tenover FC, Gootz TD, Gordon KP, Tompkins LS, Young SA, Plorde JJ: Development of DNA probe for the structural gene of the 2″-O-adenyltransferase aminoglycoside-modifying enzyme. *J Infect Dis* 5:678–687, 1984.

51. Tenover FS: Studies of antimicrobial resistance genes using DNA probes. *Antimicrob Agents Chemother* 29:721–725, 1986.

52. Kreiswirth BN, Kravitz GR, Schlievert PM, Novick RP: Nosocomial transmission of a strain of *Staphylococcus aureus* causing toxic shock syndrome. *Ann Intern Med* 105:704–707, 1986.

53. Cook WL, Wachsmuth K, Johnson SR, Birkness KA, Samadi AR: Persistence of plasmids, cholera toxin genes, and prophage DNA in classical *Vibrio cholerae* 01. *Infect Immun* 45:222–226, 1984.

54. Ogle JW, Janda JM, Woods DE, Vasil ML: Characterization and use of a DNA probe as an epidemiological marker for *Pseudomonas aeruginosa*. *J Infect Dis* 155:119–126, 1987.

55. Tompkins LS, Troup N, Labigne-Roussel A, Cohen ML: Cloned, random chromosomal sequences as probes to indentify *Salmonella* species. *J Infect Dis* 154:156–162, 1986.

56. O'Hanley P, Low D, Romero I, Lark D, Vosti K, Falkow S, Schoolnik G: Gal:gal binding and hemolysin phenotypes and genotypes associated with uropathogenic *Escherichia coli*. *N Engl J Med* 313:414–420, 1985.

57. Yam WC, Lung ML, Ng MH: Evaluation and optimization of the DNA filter assay for direct detection of enterotoxigenic *Escherichia coli* in the presence of stool coliforms. *J Clin Microbiol* 24:149–151, 1986.

58. Tompkins LS, Mickelsen P, McClure J: Use of a DNA probe to detect *Campylobacter jejuni* in fecal specimens in *Campylobacter*. Proceedings of the Second International Workshop on *Campylobacter* Infections, Brussels, Belgium, September 6-9. 1983.

59. Tompkins LS, Troup N, Labigne-Roussel A, Cohen ML: Cloned, random chromosomal sequences as probes to identify *Salmonella* species. *J Infect Dis* 154:156–162, 1986.

60. McIntosh K, Pierik L: Immuno-fluorescence in viral diagnosis. In Coonrod JD, Kunz LJ, Ferraro MJ (eds): *The Direct Detection of Microorgamisms in Clinical Samples*. Orlando, Harcourt Brace Jovanovich, 1983, p 57.

61. Hsiung GD, Landry M: Rapid viral diagnosis. *Clin Microbiol Newsl* 23:173–177, 1986.

62. Valenti WM, Menegris MA, Hall CV, Pincus PH, Douglas RG, Jr: Nosocomial viral infections. I. Epidemiology and significance. *Infect Control* 1:33–37, 1980.

63. Welliver RC, McLaughlin S: Unique epidemiology of nosocomial infection in a children's hospital. *Am J Dis Child* 138:131–135, 1984.

64. Hall CB, Douglas RG, Geiman JM, Messner MK: Nosocomial respiratory syncytial virus infections. *N Engl J Med* 293:1343–1346, 1975.

65. Hall CB: Nosocomial viral respiratory infections: perennial weeds on pediatric wards. *Am J Med* 70:670–676, 1981.

66. MacDonald NE, Hall CB, Suffin S, Alexson C, Harris PJ, Manning JA: Respiratory syncytial viral infection in infants with congenital heart disease. *N Engl J Med* 307:397–400, 1982.

67. Hall CB, Kopelman AE, Douglas RG, Geiman JM, Meagher MP: Neonatal respiratory syncytial virus infection. *N Engl J Med* 300:393–396, 1979.

68. Hall CB, Powell KR, MacDonald NE, Gala CL, Menegus ME, Suffin SC, Cohen HJ: Respiratory syncytial viral infection in children with compromised immune function. *N Engl J Med* 315:77–81, 1986.

69. Hall CB, Douglas RG: Nosocomial respiratory syncytial virus infections—should gowns and masks be used? *Am J Dis Child* 135:512–515, 1981.

70. Hall CB, Douglas RG: Modes of transmission of respiratory syncytial virus. *J Pediatr* 99:100–103, 1981.

71. Hall CB, Douglas RG, Schnabel KC, Geiman JM: Infectivity of respiratory syncytial virus by various routes of inoculation. *Infect Immunol* 33:779–783, 1981.

72. Hall CB, Douglas RG, Geiman JM: Possible transmission by fomites of respiratory syncytial virus. *J Infect Dis* 141:98–102, 1980.

73. Hall CB, McBrid JT, Walsh EE, Bell DM, Gala CL, Hildreth S, Ten Eyck LG, Hall WJ: Aerosolized ribavirin treatment of infants with respiratory syncytial viral infection: A randomized double blind study. *N Engl J Med* 308:1443–1447, 1983.

74. Hendry RM, Talis AL, Godfrey E, Anderson LJ, Fernie BF, McIntosh K: Concurrent circulation of antigenically distinct strains of respiratory syncytial virus during community outbreaks. *J Infect Dis* 153:291–297, 1986.

75. Dolan KT, Twist EM, Horton-Slight P, Forrer C, Bell LM, Jr, Plotkin SA, Clark HF: Epidemiology of rotavirus electropherotypes determined by a simplified diagnostic technique with RNA analysis. *J Clin Microbiol* 21:753–758, 1985.

76. Sakaoka H, Saheki Y, Uzuki K, Nakakita T, Saito H, Sekine K, Fujinaga K: Two outbreaks of herpes simplex virus type 1 nosocomial infection among newborns. *J Clin Microbiol* 24:36–40, 1986.

77. Van Dyke RB, Spector SA. Transmission of herpes simplex virus type 1 to a newborn infant during endotracheal suctioning for meconium aspiration. *Pediatr Infect Dis* 3:153–156, 1984.

78. Linnemann CC, Jr, Light IJ, Buchman TG, Ballard JL, Roizman B: Transmission of herpes-simplex virus type 1 in a nursery for the newborn: Identification of viral isolates by DNA "fingerprinting." *Lancet* 1:964–966, 1978.

79. Halperin SA, Hendley JO, Nosal C, Roizman B: DNA fingerprinting in investigation of apparent nosocomial acquisition of neonatal herpes simplex. *J Pediatr* 97:91–93, 1980.

80. Wilfert CM, Huang E-S, Stagno S: Restriction endonuclease analysis of cytomegalovirus deoxyribonucleic acid as an epidemiologic tool. *Pediatrics* 70:717–721, 1982.

81. Spector SA: Transmission of cytomegalovirus among infants in a hospital documented by restriction-endonuclease-digestion analysis. *Lancet* 1:378–381, 1983.

82. Yow MD, Lakeman AD, Stagno S, Reynolds RB, Plavidal FJ: Use of restriction enzymes to investigate the source of a primary cytomegalovirus infection in a pediatric nurse. *Pediatrics* 70:713–716, 1982.

83. Adler SP: The molecular epidemiology of cytomegalovirus transmission among children attending a day care center. *J Infect Dis* 152:760–768, 1985.

84. Ristuccia PA, Cunha BA: Microbiological aspects of infection control. In Wenzel RP (ed): *Prevention and Control of Nosocomial Infections*. Baltimore, Williams & Wilkins, 1987, pp 205–207.

85. Weissfeld AS: Nosocomial infections and hospital epidemiology. In Sonnenwirth AC, Jarret L (eds): *Grudwohl's Clinical Laboratory Methods and Diagnosis*, ed 8. St Louis, CV Mosby, 1980, pp 1971-1977.

86. Weinstein RA, Mallison GF: The role of the microbiology laboratory in surveillance and control of nosocomial infections. *Am J Clin Pathol* 69:130–136, 1978.

87. Simmons BP. Centers for Disease Control guidelines for hospital environmental control - microbiologic surveillance of the environment and of personnel in the hospital. *Infect Control* 2:145–146, 1981.

88. Maki DG, Weise CE, Safafin HW: A semi-quantitative culture method for indentifying intravenous-catheter-related infection. *N Engl J Med* 296:1305–1309, 1977.

89. Cooper GL, Hopkins CC: Rapid diagnosis of intravascular catheter-associated infections by direct gram staining of catheter segments. *N Engl J Med* 312:1142–1147, 1985.

90. Rhame FS, Streifel A, Stevens P, Bozanich A, Bun FR, Hurd DS, McGlave SB, Kersey JH, Jr, Ramsay NKC: Endemic aspergillus airborne spore levels are a major risk factor for aspergillosis in bone marrow transplant (BMT) patients. Presented at the 25th Interscience Conference on Antimicrobial Agents and Chemotherapy, Minneapolis, MN 1985, Abstract No. 147.

91. Goldmann DA: Epidemiology of *Staphylococcus aureus* and Group-A streptococci. In Bennett JV, Brachman PS (eds): *Hospital Infections*, ed 2. Boston, Little, Brown & Co, 1986, pp 483–494.

92. Burke JP, Ingall D, Klein JO, Gezon HM, Finland M: *Proteus mirabilis* infections in a hospital nursery traced to a human carrier. *N Engl J Med* 284:115–121, 1971.

93. Knittle MA, Eitzman DV, Baer H: Role of hand contamination of personnel in the epidemiology of gram-negative nosocomial infections. *J Pediatr* 86:433–437, 1975.

94. Aisner J, Murillo J, Schimpff SC, Steere AC: Invasive aspergillosis in acute leukemia: Correlation with nose cultures and antibiotic use. *Ann Intern Med* 90:4–9, 1979.

95. Newman KA, Schimpff SC, Young VM, Wiernik PA: Lessons learned from surveillance cultures in patients with acute nonlymphocytic leukemia: Usefulness for epidemiologic, preventive, and therapeutic research. *Amer J Med* 70:423–431, 1981.

96. Sandford GR, Merz WG, Wingard JR, Cherache P, Saral R: The value of fungal surveillance culture as predictors of systemic fungal infections. *J Infect Dis* 142:503–509, 1980.

97. Schimpff SC, Greene WH, Young VM, Wiernik PH: *Pseudomonas septicemia*: incidence, epidemiology, prevention, and therapy in patients with advanced cancer. *Eur J Cancer* 9:449–455, 1973.

98. Kernodle DS, Barg NL, Kaiser AB: Evidence of widespread low level colonization with methicillin-resistant coagulase-negative staphylococci and emergence during antibiotic prophylaxis. Presented at the 26th Interscience Conference on Antimicrobial Agents and Chemotherapy, September 28 - October 1, 1986, New Orleans, Abstract No. 265.

99. Craven De, Lichtenberg DA, Browne KF, Coffey D, Treadwell TL, McCabe WR: Pseudobacteremia traced to cross-contamination by an automated blood culture analyzer. *Infect Control* 5:75–78, 1984.

100. Donowitz LG, Schwartzman JD: Pseudobacteremia and use of the radiometric blood culturing analyzer (letter). *Infect Control* 5:266, 1984.

101. Gurevich I, Tafuro P, Krystofiak S, Kalter R, Cunha BA: Three clusters of *Bacillus* pseudobacteremia related to a radiometric blood culture analyzer. *Infect Control* 5:71–74, 1984.

28

Antibiotic Restriction

Russell W. Steele, M.D. and Robert W. Bradsher, M.D.

BACKGROUND

Unlimited access to available therapeutic agents has traditionally been a very basic precept in the practice of medicine in the United States. Only recently have hospitals considered placing restrictions on the medications normally ordered by primary care physicians, and antibiotics have constituted the principal focus of such policies. These restrictions are placed on usage by physicians almost entirely because of the continued increasing costs of newer antibiotics.

In the past, efficacy as determined by controlled clinical trials was the single factor that determined selection of antibiotics. Penicillin replaced the sulfonamides for the treatent of pneumococcal infection in the 1940s, and ampicillin replaced penicillin in the 1960s as the drug of choice for otitis media and pneumonia in children because comparative trials clearly demonstrated improved cure rates. Comparative efficacy is rarely emphasized in currently published clinical trials of new antibiotics simply because analysis of results almost always demonstrates therapeutic equivalence rather than superiority of new compounds as compared with previous standard regimens. The major factor for selection of equally efficacious antibiotics has now shifted to relative toxicity, a more subtle issue. Ticarcillin is often selected over carbenicillin because of its reduced toxic effects on platelets. Piperacillin or mezlocillin might be chosen over these former two agents because it contains a monosodium salt thereby reducing the sodium load in the patient who may have poor cardiac function or hypokalemia. Relative toxicity between classes of antibiotics is summarized in Table 28.1.

If choices of antibiotics include two or more of equal efficacy and equal potential toxicity,

the choice is then usually made on the basis of comparative cost. Monitoring these cost issues has become the responsibility of pharmacy and therapeutics committees, or, in the case of antimicrobial agents, infectious disease specialists. This has led to formulary restriction as a simple but efficient method for the specialist to direct individual physician's prescribing habits (1).

Restriction may be defined in many ways, depending on reasons for its implementation and also on available subspecialty resources of the hospital. The most restrictive policy would be a closed pharmacy formulary in which certain antibiotics would not be stocked in the pharmacy. Other methods of restriction would be designed to limit the use of medicines that are stocked. In some cases, a formal written infectious disease consultation may be mandatory while other circumstances may warrant a telephone consult or perhaps only an explanation written on an audit form by the prescribing physician. Another subtle method of restriction would be simply not reporting the antibiotic on the results of the susceptibility testing.

Most important are the particular reasons for adopting restrictions that will, in large part, determine actions required of the primary care clinician. In addition to the relative cost issue already introduced, potential misuse of antibiotics is the

Table 28.1.
Relative Toxicity of Commonly Used Antibiotics

Highest	Chloramphenicol
	Aminoglycosides
	Sulfonamides
Lowest	Penicillins
	Cephalosporins
	Erythromycin

other major category that has resulted in restricting antimicrobial agents. Some studies which have critically evaluated therapy of pediatric infectious diseases have concluded that half of all antibiotic orders have been inaccurate in some way (2,3). Many experts feel that this observation alone dictates stringent monitoring and control of drug utilization.

Further discussion of this topic would best be accomplished by reviewing each of the five major areas that might justify antibiotic restriction (Table 28.2). For some antibiotics, a combination of these factors may apply and lead to their inclusion on a restricted list.

Even more importantly, new antibiotic education must emphasize an understanding of potential adverse reactions. The most significant clinical consequence of inappropriate antibiotic usage is unanticipated toxicity. In most cases, this could be prevented by a better awareness of reported untoward side effects. Sometimes, monitoring serum concentrations of antibiotics would allow adequate protection from toxicity. In one report (4,5), $\frac{1}{6}$ of all hospital patients developed medical complications caused by drugs whose adverse effects should have been predictable and preventable.

EDUCATION

Primary care physicians are now faced with a plethora of new antibiotics, each marketed by competitive pharmaceutical companies as having subtle advantages in clinical applications. This has been especially true since 1981 when the first third-generation cephalosporin was introduced. It is unrealistic for general physicians to critically evaluate the voluminous literature for each of these agents. It has therefore become the responsibility of infectious disease specialists to provide this service and summarize important clinical information for their colleagues. This may be accomplished through traditional continuing education programs either in the hospital itself or through regional and national symposia. However, voluntary participation is unlikely by itself to assure exposure to this information (6). The pharmaceutical companies attempt educational efforts, but these are often mixed with strong sales efforts. Antibiotic restriction allows the infectious disease specialist to monitor specific usage practices and to address deficiencies once they are identified during the interchange with primary care physicians that results from such restriction.

Table 28.2.
Rationale for Antibiotic Restriction

Education
Complexity of cases
Controlling bacterial resistance
Auditing drug utilization
Cost and contractual arrangements

In teaching hospitals, assurance of education is even more critical. In some centers, when newer antibiotics are added to the formulary, they are automatically restricted, regardless of relative toxicity or cost, until physicians in training have discussed their application with the infectious disease specialist. This may be accomplished once again either in hospital conferences or more effectively through one-on-one discussions of specific patients. During the time when the antibiotics are restricted, the educators will develop a general feeling for other physicians' understandings of proper use and when restrictions can be removed; this generally takes 3–6 months.

Education of private physicians is often more difficult. Attendance at conferences cannot be required, and the content of regional or national meetings may not always include a review of new antibiotics. Restriction of antibiotics offers the assurance of communication between the primary care physician and subspecialist. Once again, audits of antibiotic utilization are used to identify those antibiotics that are not being employed properly.

Hospitals are required by accreditation sources to monitor antibiotic utilization. This becomes a second method for evaluating adequacy of physician education. Once misuse of an antibiotic is identified (Table 28.3), the drug could be restricted while education efforts are again reinstituted.

Presently, there are computerized systems being developed for monitoring antibiotic usage. Briefly, physicians are usually required to spend approximately 2 minutes filling out a form indicating the reasons for an antibiotic selection. This information is then entered into a computer program by the ward clerk. Proper guidelines for antibiotic utilization, already contained within the computer program itself, allow rapid identification of inappropriate ordering practices. For instance, an antibiotic used for surgical prophy-

Table 28.3.
Inappropriate Use of Antibiotics Requiring Education of Physicians

Incorrect antibiotic (resistant organism)
Poor selection (another agent with lower MIC)
Improper dosage or dosing interval
Improper duration of therapy
Antibiotics not needed at all
Equally effective but less expensive agent

laxis that is ordered for greater than 48 hours' duration would be identified as one requiring justification. A selection of aminoglycosides or chloramphenicol would require that physicians indicate that they are monitoring antibiotic concentrations. For these two examples, all pertinent information would be contained on the very simple form the physician fills out at the time the antibiotics are ordered.

COMPLEXITY OF CURRENT INFECTIOUS DISEASES

The subspecialty of infectious disease has changed in many ways during the past two decades. Perhaps the most striking difference is the complexity of the clinical courses in patients who ultimately receive antimicrobial therapy. These are likely to be children who are immunosuppressed and who will remain hospitalized for long periods of time.

One of the most common clinical circumstances where the physician must make decisions for the immunocompromised host is fever in the neutropenic patient. For pediatricians, this individual is most commonly a child with leukemia who is neutropenic secondary to chemotherapy administered during treatment of the oncologic process. Selection of antibiotics must obviously provide coverage for the most likely pathogens, yet also be directed to cover the most difficult-to-treat organisms. In most settings, *Pseudomonas aeruginosa* is considered the most resistant organism to potentially cause infection early in the neutropenic phase. Most common pathogens will vary greatly among institutions and will change periodically within a given hospital. Careful monitoring of antibiograms is therefore required and is usually provided by an infectious disease specialist. It is this physician who might best make decisions for antibiotic selection. For example, in hospitals where *Staphylococcus epidermidis* and *Staphylococcus aureus* are common pathogens, often following placement of central venous lines, a combination of a first-generation cephalosporin with nafcillin or vancomycin should be selected, depending on the frequency of methicillin resistance in these strains.

Many combinations of antibiotics have been employed for empiric therapy in these patients, and there is presently little, if any, clinical evidence that one particular combination is more efficacious than another. This brings up the other issues of relative toxicity and cost in final selection of therapy.

Although a discussion of the compromised host usually focuses on the classic prototype of a neutropenic cancer patient on immunosuppressive chemotherapy, there are other pediatric patients much more commonly encountered who require management with many of the considerations used for that prototype. The largest such groups of patients are newborn infants. A number of immunologic defects have been documented during this age period which predispose these otherwise healthy individuals to life-threatening illness. It is not clear which defects might be more damaging and which may be related to specific disease processes. The absence of immunoglobulin M is considered one of the more important deficiencies and one that at least partially accounts for propensity to Gram-negative bacterial meningitis and bacteremia in this patient population.

Newborns are particularly vulnerable to treatment modalities that may further depress their immune function. Splenectomy is associated with a much higher long-term morbidity in the neonate as compared with older children and adults; steroid therapy is similarly fraught with more complications in this age group. The trauma of surgery and thermal burns will both suppress immune function in patients of all ages, but in neonates, it may have more potent influence on immune capabilities with resulting fatal infection.

Most of the basic principles that apply to the management of immunocompromised patients are, therefore, relevant to neonates. Maximum doses of bactericidal antibiotics should be given, with duration of therapy often being longer than for similar diseases in infants and children.

CONTROLLING BACTERIAL RESISTANCE

Bacteria which cause many of the clinical problems in infectious diseases today are different from bacteria less than half a century ago with respect to resistance patterns for antibiotics. Resistance now ranges from previously totally sensitive organisms such as *Staphylococcus aureus* and *Streptococcus pneumoniae* to organisms such as aerobic and anaerobic Gram-negative bacilli with highly resistant patterns. When Professor Guissepie Brotzu first isolated crude extracts from *Cephalosporium* species, activity was noted against the vast majority of clinical bacterial isolates. However, after three decades of intensive use with cephalosporins, only about half of the most common organisms causing hospital-acquired infections, *E. coli*, are killed by the first generation of cephalosporin antibiotics. Many consider the widespread use of this class of drug for surgical prophylaxis to be a reason for its inactivity against many organisms. It is because of this development of resistant strains that newer second- and third-generation cephalosporins, carbapenem and monobactam antibiotics, have been marketed and promoted as demonstrating activity against resistant bacteria. However, the most broad-spectrum antibiotics developed have not eliminated the potential of aerobic Gram-negative bacilli becoming resistant with continuing exposure to the drug, just as the parasites Paul Ehrlich used at the turn of the century became resistant to his "magic bullet" with repeated exposure.

Resistance to antibiotics by bacteria occurs typically by either inactivation of the drug, alteration of the biochemical or binding target of the antibiotic, or impermeability to penetration by the agent. The resistance may arise from genetic information contained in either the chromosomal material or in extrachromosomal pieces of DNA, called plasmids, or R factors. These plasmids may extend resistance to antibiotics in two separate ways. First, the genetic material typically encodes for resistance to more than a single antibiotic. Second, the plasmid may transfer resistance from one genus of bacteria to another through conjugation or transposition of DNA sequences from one plasmid to another.

A number of pressures on bacteria result in antibiotic resistance. These include inappropriate prescribing of oral antibiotics, use of an-tibiotics in animal-feed formulas, and self-administration of antibiotics by patients from leftovers of previous courses of therapy. An example of the scope of the problems that can result from all of these mechanisms was found in a report of an antibiotic-resistant *Salmonella* in contaminated beef, causing food poisoning (7).

Although community pressures have helped to account for the increasing isolation of ampicillin-resistance *Haemophilus influenzae*, penicillinase-producing *Neisseria gonorrhoeae*, and relatively-resistant pneumococci, the majority of resistance to antibiotics affecting clinical care has occurred in hospital settings. McGowan outlined several factors that associated the use of antibiotics in hospitals and the subsequent development of antibiotics in hospital bacteria (8). Resistance is more prevalent in bacteria causing nosocomial infection than in those causing community-acquired infection. In outbreaks of resistant nosocomial infections, one common risk factor is the prior use of antibiotics in infected patients. Moreover, the higher the dose of antibiotic given, the higher the rate of colonization and superinfection. Finally, McGowan noted that since antibiotics produce such marked changes in microbial flora, it is logical that this exerts pressure on resistance development. The focus of interest in this area has primarily been with aerobic Gram-negative bacilli and the use of either aminoglycosides or β-lactam antibiotics, and with methicillin-resistant staphylococci following cephalosporin use.

A number of studies have examined the effect on Gram-negative bacilli resistance patterns by restricting aminoglycoside use to one agent. The hypothesis for these studies has been that with the use of a drug other than gentamicin, e.g., amikacin, which has been associated with a lower incidence of resistance, the prevalence of gentamicin resistance in subsequent isolates will be reduced. This hypothesis has been confirmed in several studies as reviewed by McGowan (9), but a number of caveats were also listed. The studies were supported by a company marketing the antibiotics, which could present bias in the design. In addition, factors unrelated to the antibiotics that were not controlled may also be partially responsible for the observations. Although many of the studies showed a decrease in amikacin resistance, in a few hospitals the exclusive use of the drug was associated with a larger number of organisms resistant to the agent, just as occurs in individual patients who develop resistant bacteria while being treated (9,10). Therefore, restriction of the more broad-spectrum antibiotics may or may not be associated with changes in sensitivity to less broad-spectrum agents. It is the practice of many hospitals to reserve the use of more potent agents, like amikacin, to certain situations, since the efficacy of gentamicin and amikacin are equal if the organism is sensitive to both agents. If the organism is shown to be resistant or occurs in a hospital or area of the hospital where resistance is more common, then the more broad spectrum of the two agents is recommended.

With the development of new β-lactam antibiotics, such as the more broad-spectrum cephalosporins and carbapenems, new mechanisms of resistance have been demonstrated. The induction of β-lactamase enzymes that hydrolyze the antibiotic have been associated with some of the more difficult-to-treat Gram-negative bacilli, such as *Enterobacter*, *Serratia,* and *Pseudomonas*. This phenomenon, failure to cure infection caused by what appeared to be a sensitive organism that developed resistance during therapy, has been reviewed by Sanders (11). Whether restriction of certain antibiotics from use in hospitals will prevent bacteria from becoming resistant remains an open question.

To date, no resistance has been reported to vancomycin in methicillin-resistant *Staphylococcus aureus* isolates. The higher cost of vancomycin, the need for monitoring serum levels, and extensive use with β-lactam agents have discouraged the routine use of vancomycin in the usual infections caused by methicillin-sensitive strains. Whether restriction should be placed on empiric vancomycin use in the hospital will depend, as with other antibiotic restriction, on local factors such as sensitivity patterns reflected in antibiogram information and on cost factors unique to each hospital.

AUDITING DRUG (ANTIBIOTIC) UTILIZATION

The Joint Commission on Accreditation of Hospitals (JCAH) currently mandates that all hospitals institute some method for auditing drug utilization. The first group of drugs designated for auditing were antibiotics. One-half of community hospitals reviewed by JCAH were found deficient in this requirement. A major effort to correct this deficiency is currently in progress in many hospitals.

Hospital computer programs designed to provide physician education also generate readily accessible data for auditing antibiotic utilization. Two such programs currently in use are the Antibiotic Management System ™ (Medical Economics Company Inc., Oradell, NJ) and one developed at Albany Medical Center Hospital (Albany, NY). Both require the physician to fill out an antibiotic order sheet that includes clinical information, reasons for antibiotic use, i.e., prophylaxis, empiric, or therapeutic for documented infection, and methods for monitoring potential toxicity. The requirement for completing such a data form is a subtle method of antibiotic restriction but one that allows a month-to-month review of proper medical care.

Unfortunately, it is often difficult to motivate physician acceptance when it requires completion of "paperwork." In this case, however, accreditation loss for the hospital should be sufficient reason to institute strict policies and to assure compliance.

There are two alternatives for drug auditing, both with the disadvantage of being retrospective. One is the older method of random chart review by someone who would not have been involved directly with these patients' care. Minimum management criteria previously established by a consensus of staff physicians are used to evaluate these charts, and deficiencies are recorded. A committee then further evaluates variations from anticipated antimicrobial therapy to determine whether these deviations were appropriate. Responsible physicians may then be notified of documented deficiencies. The other method for auditing is accomplished by the pharmacy . Once again, predetermined management criteria are used to evaluate proper antibiotic utilization. The charts of all patients who received a particular antibiotic are reviewed for conformity with established guidelines. As with the other alternative, rapid correction of antibiotic errors cannot be provided with this retrospective audit.

A computer program requiring physician input at the time a patient is placed on antibiotics is the best method for immediate identification of antibiotic misuse. The programs mentioned above are designed to notify physicians, once they enter patient data, of any questionable antibiotic prescribing. A variation from established guidelines in the program is of course not always in error, so the physician may decie whether this is an appropriate exception.

COST AND CONTRACTUAL ARRANGEMENTS

Many studies have examined the impact of antibiotic restriction on cost containment, and conclusions have been quite variable; some have resulted in considerable savings (1–6), while others have demonstrated increased expenditures. The latter observations were unexpected, but quite readily explained. Many primary care physicians, faced with a requirement to obtain infectious disease consults to use a certain antibiotic, opted for another regimen that would not require notifying a specialist. Often, the alternative regimen would include two, or even three, antibiotics where one would have sufficed. Besides being more costly, this decision may also have included agents that were potentially more toxic. The usual circumstance has been selection of a penicillin plus an aminoglycoside rather than a restricted cephalosporin. Thus, the very purpose of restriction was defeated. This simply emphasizes the need for all physicians in a hospital to understand and concur with any policy designed to face the issue of cost containment and to support its implementation. Otherwise, such a program will never succeed. Likewise, the pharmacy and nursing services must be willing to examine their charges, make these known to physicians, and to reduce fees whenever possible. Only then can other cost factors be examined as discussed below. All factors constituting total antibiotic charges are summarized in Table 28.4.

Relative Cost

Where a number of antibiotics are considered equivalent both in efficacy and toxicity, one is

Table 28.4.
Antibiotic Cost Variables

Per gram cost
Dosage (mg/kg)
Frequency of administration
i.v. infusion set
pharmacy
nursing
duration for hospitalization
Monitoring

usually chosen on the basis of lower cost. This is especially true for oral antibiotics in children, since great pricing differences exist. For example, erythromycin is usually the drug of choice for skin and soft tissue infections as it offers coverage for the two common pathogens, Group A streptococcus and *Staphylococcus aureus*, at very low cost compared with cephalosporins and penicillinase-resistant penicillins.

However, the issue of drug cost is less relevant for parenteral antibiotics in the care of children, since the small size of treated individuals greatly reduces differences in expense as based on total dosages. Other cost considerations for antimicrobial therapy are of much greater import.

Per Gram (Acquisition Cost)

Cost per gram has become increasingly confusing in cost analysis, since recommended daily dosages can vary widely. Cost of an antibiotic for the entire treatment course is a more pertinent factor. Some newer cephalosporins are given at ¼–½ the daily dosage of others, making them less expensive, although the cost per gram may be greater.

Frequency of Administration

This variable determines many ancillary costs that constitute total patient antibiotic charges. The more frequently a drug is administered, the more intravenous infusion sets are used and the more involvement is required by pharmacy and nursing services. All of these must be reimbursed to the hospital.

Monitoring

Serum antibiotic concentrations of chloramphenicol, vancomycin, and aminoglycosides must be monitored. Unfortunately, this can add significant costs to the therapy. Aminoglycosides have a relatively narrow toxicity to therapeutic ratio as compared with penicillins or cephalosporins. To ensure efficacy in the treatment of serious Gram-negative bacillary infections, attempts are made to achieve peak serum levels of gentamicin, tobramycin, and netilmicin of 5–10 μg/ml while levels of 15-40 μg/ml are necessary for amikacin. To help reduce the nephrotoxicity and ototoxicity potential, trough levels of gentamicin, tobramycin, and netilmicin of less than 2 μg/ml and amikacin of less than 5 μg/ml are the goals of therapy. Since aminoglycosides are almost totally excreted by renal mechanisms, attempts to maintain appropriate levels have been directed by dosing nomograms, which are based on measurements of renal function (12,13).

Unfortunately, a number of studies have demonstrated individual variations between predicted and measured serum levels of aminoglycosides in patients with either normal or abnormal renal function. For example, patients with cystic fibrosis or extensive burns have a remarkably higher dosage requirement for gentamicin than the usual recommended maximum dose of 5 mg/kg/day. In one study of nine children with thermal injuries of 40–85% of body surface area, gentamicin dosages ranged from 7–30 mg/kg/day to achieve appropriate serum levels (14). Prediction of serum concentrations based on weight and renal function are also unpredictable in circumstances with altered absorption (cardiac disease, intramuscular route of administration), altered volume of distribution (edematous condition, obesity), and other variables, such as fever, hematocrit, and age. In one study, currently recommended nomograms for dosing were associated with levels that were appropriate only in a minority of the patients studied (15). Only 45 % of the patients had peak serum concentrations in the therapeutic range. A similar number of patients, 40%, had levels below the therapeutic range, while 15% had gentamicin levels in the toxic range (15).

The major reason for using aminoglycosides in clinical practice is in the treatment of Gram-negative bacillary bacteremia, which produces a mortality rate of 20–50%. Several studies have suggested an association between peak serum aminoglycoside levels early in therapy and a decrease in mortality from this infection (16). Since aminoglycoside levels cannot be predicted very accurately, even with the best dosing nomograms, serum levels should be measured early in the course, preferably with tests that can be completed rapidly. Bioassays, for example, are inadequate because they take too long. If the results are not available within a few hours because of requirements for sending the serum to a reference laboratory, or due to requiring growth of bacteria in a bioassay procedure, the value of the test for determining proper dosages diminishes.

The same lack of predictability of levels that occurs with gentamicin also occurs with tobramycin and amikacin, despite a few claims to the contrary by some of the pharmaceutical firms. In one study, instead of the recommended dosage of 15 mg/kg/day, a mean dosage of 29 mg/kg/day of amikacin was required for acceptable peak and trough concentrations, with a range from 12.9–50.8 mg/kg/day (17). Not only are aminoglycoside serum levels unpredictable, but the measured levels may not be acted upon in a proper fashion. In one study, appropriate action was taken on the aminoglycoside levels that were obtained from patients in only a minority of episodes; the majority of levels outside the desired range were simply ignored (18).

For the reasons of poor predictability of levels, need for adequate levels early in sepsis, the lack of understanding of how to utilize the levels that are obtained, and the narrow toxic-to-therapeutic ratio, the development of a computer-based pharmacokinetic model for aminoglycoside dosing run on a consult basis by clinical pharmacists, is a valuable program for a hospital to implement (13,14,17). If community hospitals are unable to provide this service, consideration of less toxic regimens than aminoglycosides might be considered as first-line type of therapy for Gram-negative sepsis.

Chloramphenicol administration requires monitoring for potential toxicity, including reversible marrow suppression, which begins at levels above 25 μg/ml and the gray baby or gray toddler syndromes at levels above 40 μg/ml. Levels of chloramphenicol below 3 μg/ml are considered subtherapeutic for the indications to use this drug. Chloramphenicol is probably better known for its adverse effects than any other antibiotic. This has caused most use of the agent to be for severe infections such as meningitis or rickettsial disease. This agent deserves further studies of its pharmacokinetic properties. A recent study indicated that the time-honored belief that intramuscular chloramphenicol is poorly absorbed may well be false. An appropriate peak level of drug was measured in each of the patients who received an intramuscular dose (19).

Flucytosine, an antifungal oral agent, is an important example where restriction is appropriately placed on drugs by requiring the monitoring of serum levels. This agent is primarily administered to patients in combination with amphotericin B for the treatment of cryptococcal meningitis. The usual dose of flucytosine in a patient with normal renal function is 150 mg/

kg/day in four equal doses, which usually results in blood levels of 50–100 µg/ml. The major toxicity is severe pancytopenia in conjunction with generalized bone marrow suppression. Toxicity correlates with worsening renal function and rising flucytosine levels. The drug is recommended to be given with amphotericin B, which consistently reduces renal function, and if blood levels cannot be followed closely, flucytosine should be restricted from use.

Vancomycin is the only reliable treatment for methicillin-resistant staphylococcal infections. The major reason for monitoring serum levels with this agent is to determine the appropriate dosing interval in patients with decreased renal function. The therapeutic-to-toxic ratio is broader than that for aminoglycosides, but vancomycin is cleared by renal mechanisms. If a patient is anephric, doses may be given once weekly with adequate serum levels maintained over the entire duration.

In hospitals unable to measure serum concentrations of antibiotics, restriction policies may be designed to encourage an alternative with low toxicity or a high safety index, thereby obviating the need to monitor levels. Cephalosporins, broad-spectrum penicillins, monobactams, or carbapenems, which might substitute for chloramphenicol or aminoglycosides, provide these alternatives.

Other Cost Factors

Most physicians assume that antibiotic charges to patients include only the acquisition price of the antibiotic plus an estimated market value for intravenous administration sets ($5 per set). These two calculations, however, are not the method most hospital pharmacies use to determine the price to the patient. A charge must be generated to support the pharmacy's operational costs. In some institutions, a factor (usually between 1.5–2.0) is multiplied by the acquisition price of the antibiotic, and the charge for consumable supplies (dispensing i.v. bag and tubing) is added. Some hospitals also use a higher factor for less expensive antibiotics. The cost for monitoring serum antibiotic concentrations must also be added, as discussed above.

Rather than the aforementioned formula, a majority of hospitals add a charge for each i.v. infusion to compensate for pharmacy operational costs. This ranges from $10–$50, with an average in U.S. hospitals of approximately

$25 per infusion. Using this method of charging, one can considerably reduce the comparative costs of antibiotics that can be given every 12 hours, and particularly every 24 hours.

SUMMARY OF CURRENT RECOMMENDATIONS

Teaching Hospitals. Antibiotic restriction should be instituted in all teaching hospitals, primarily as a method for assuring proper education of house officers who are responsible for writing most antibiotic orders. The infectious disease specialist should provide a teaching program for physicians in training, and drug restriction is presently the best method for identifying individual needs.

Community Hospitals. Routine antibiotic restriction is not an adequate method for controlling costs of antimicrobial therapy, and more frequently leads to increased expenditures, since the primary care physician may select two or three unrestricted antibiotics to avoid a single restricted agent. Periodic drug utilization review should identify misuse and direct proper educational methods for practicing physicians. A limited antibiotic restriction program may be employed when education itself fails to correct deficiencies.

REFERENCES

1. Moleski RJ, Andriole VT: Role of the infectious disease specialist in containing costs of antibiotics in the hospital. *Rev Infect Dis* 8:488–93, 1986.
2. Castle M, Wilfort CM, Cate TR, Osterhout S: Antibiotic use at Duke University Medical Center. *JAMA* 237:2819–22, 1977.
3. Naqir SH, Dunkle LM, Timmerman KF, Reichley RM, Stanley DL, O'Connor D: Antibiotic usage in a pediatric medical center. *JAMA* 292:1981–4, 1979.
4. Soumerai SB, Avorn J: Efficacy and cost-containment in hospital pharmacotherapy: state of the art and future directions. *Milbank Memorial Fund Quarterly/Health Society* 62:447–74, 1984.
5. Steel K, Gertman PM, Crescenzi C, Anderson J: Iatrogenic illness on a general medical service at a university hospital. *N Engl J Med* 304:638–42, 1981.
6. Lewis CE, Hassanein RS: Continuing medical education: an epidemiologic evaluation. *N Engl J Med* 282:254–9, 1970.
7. Holmberg SD, Osterholm MT, Senger KA, Cohen ML: Drug-resistant *Salmonella* from animals fed antimicrobials. *N Engl J Med* 311:617–622, 1984.
8. McGowan JE Jr: Antimicrobial resistance in hospital organisms and its relation to antibiotic use. *Rev infect Dis* 5:1033–1048, 1983.
9. McGowan JE Jr: Minimizing antimicrobial resistance in hospital bacteria: Can switching or cycling drugs help? *Infect Control* 7:573–576, 1986.
10. Murray BE, Moellering RC Jr: *In vivo* acquisition of two different types of aminoglycoside resistance by a single strain of *Klebsiella pneumoniae* causing severe infection. *Ann Intern Med* 96:176–180, 1982.

11. Sanders CC, Sanders WE Jr: Emergence of resistance during therapy with the newer beta-lactam antibiotics: Role of inducible beta-lactamases and implications for the future. *Rev Infect Dis* 5:639–648, 1983.

12. Chan RA, Benner ES, Hoeprich PD: Gentamicin therapy in renal failure: A nomogram for dosage. *Ann Intern Med* 76:773–778, 1972.

13. Hull JH, Sarubbi FA: Gentamicin serum concentrations: Pharmacokinetic predictions. *Ann Intern Med* 85:183–189, 1976.

14. Zaske DA, Sawchuk RJ, Gerding DN, Strate RG: Increased dosage requirements of gentamicin in burn patients. *J Trauma* 16:824–828, 1976.

15. Lesar TS, Rotschafer JC, Strand LM, Solem LD, Zaske DE: Gentamicin dosing errors with four commonly used nomograms. *JAMA* 248:1190–1193, 1982.

16. Moore RD, Smith CR, Lietman PS: The association of aminoglycoside plasma levels with mortality in patients with gram-negative bacteremia. *J Infect Dis* 149:443–448, 1984.

17. Finley RS, Fortner CL, DeJongh CA, Wade JC, Newman KA, Caplan E, Britten J, Wiernik PH, Schimpff SC: Comparison of standard versus pharmacokinetically adjusted amikacin dosing in granulocytopenic cancer patients. *Antimicrob Agent Chemother* 22:193–197, 1982

18. Anderson AC, Hodges GR, Barnes WG: Determinations of gentamicin levels; ordering patterns and use. *Arch Intern Med* 36:785–787, 1976.

19. Shann F, Linnemann V, MacKenzie A: Absorption of chloramphenicol after intramuscular administration in children. *N Engl J Med* 313:410–414, 1985.

Index